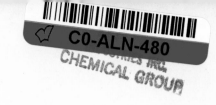

ANTIOXIDANTS

SYNTHESES AND APPLICATIONS

ANTIOXIDANTS
Syntheses and Applications

J.C. Johnson

NOYES DATA CORPORATION

Park Ridge, New Jersey   London, England

1975

FOREWORD

The detailed, descriptive information in this book is based on U.S. patents since 1972 relating to antioxidants. Where it was necessary to round out the complete technological picture, some earlier, but very relevant patents were included.

This book serves a double purpose in that it supplies detailed technical information and can be used as a guide to the U.S. patent literature in this field. By indicating all the information that is significant, and eliminating legal jargon and juristic phraseology, this book presents an advanced, technically oriented review of antioxidants and their synergists.

The U.S. patent literature is the largest and most comprehensive collection of technical information in the world. There is more practical, commercial, timely process information assembled here than is available from any other source. The technical information obtained from a patent is extremely reliable and comprehensive; sufficient information must be included to avoid rejection for "insufficient disclosure." These patents include practically all of those issued on the subject in the United States during the period under review; there has been no bias in the selection of patents for inclusion.

The patent literature covers a substantial amount of information not available in the journal literature. The patent literature is a prime source of basic commercially useful information. This information is overlooked by those who rely primarily on the periodical journal literature. It is realized that there is a lag between a patent application on a new process development and the granting of a patent, but it is felt that this may roughly parallel or even anticipate the lag in putting that development into commercial practice.

Many of these patents are being utilized commercially. Whether used or not, they offer opportunities for technological transfer. Also, a major purpose of this book is to describe the number of technical possibilities available, which may open up profitable areas of research and development. The information contained in this book will allow you to establish a sound background before launching into research in this field.

Advanced composition and production methods developed by Noyes Data are employed to bring our new durably bound books to you in a minimum of time. Special techniques are used to close the gap between "manuscript" and "completed book." Industrial technology is progressing so rapidly that time-honored, conventional typesetting, binding and shipping methods are no longer suitable. We have bypassed the delays in the conventional book publishing cycle and provide the user with an effective and convenient means of reviewing up-to-date information in depth.

The Table of Contents is organized in such a way as to serve as a subject index. Other indexes by company, inventor and patent number help in providing easy access to the information contained in this book.

15 Reasons Why the U.S. Patent Office Literature Is Important to You —

1. The U.S. patent literature is the largest and most comprehensive collection of technical information in the world. There is more practical commercial process information assembled here than is available from any other source.

2. The technical information obtained from the patent literature is extremely comprehensive; sufficient information must be included to avoid rejection for "insufficient disclosure."

3. The patent literature is a prime source of basic commercially utilizable information. This information is overlooked by those who rely primarily on the periodical journal literature.

4. An important feature of the patent literature is that it can serve to avoid duplication of research and development.

5. Patents, unlike periodical literature, are bound by definition to contain new information, data and ideas.

6. It can serve as a source of new ideas in a different but related field, and may be outside the patent protection offered the original invention.

7. Since claims are narrowly defined, much valuable information is included that may be outside the legal protection afforded by the claims.

8. Patents discuss the difficulties associated with previous research, development or production techniques, and offer a specific method of overcoming problems. This gives clues to current process information that has not been published in periodicals or books.

9. Can aid in process design by providing a selection of alternate techniques. A powerful research and engineering tool.

10. Obtain licenses — many U.S. chemical patents have not been developed commercially.

11. Patents provide an excellent starting point for the next investigator.

12. Frequently, innovations derived from research are first disclosed in the patent literature, prior to coverage in the periodical literature.

13. Patents offer a most valuable method of keeping abreast of latest technologies, serving an individual's own "current awareness" program.

14. Copies of U.S. patents are easily obtained from the U.S. Patent Office at 50¢ a copy.

15. It is a creative source of ideas for those with imagination.

CONTENTS AND SUBJECT INDEX

INTRODUCTION

Antioxidants can be defined as substances capable of slowing the rate of oxidation in an autoxidizable material. Commercially, antioxidants are used in plastics, elastomers, petroleum products, synthetic lubricants, food products, soaps and cosmetics. In plastics and elastomers they are particularly needed to overcome the exposure to heat and oxygen during processing and in use. The petroleum and synthetic lubricants are also required to withstand extremely high temperatures in today's automotive and jet engines without excessive breakdown.

Without the antioxidants our foods would become rancid, plastics become brittle and crack, tire sidewalls craze and eventually fail, and fuels and lubricants will corrode equipment and require shutdown for repair or replacement. Good antioxidants are therefore a valuable commercial commodity, particularly for the polymer (including elastomers) and petroleum industries.

In selecting patents to be covered in this review, the term antioxidant was applied in a strict sense of the term. Materials used to improve stabilization such as heat stabilizers for PVC, ultraviolet stabilizers for polyolefins, acid acceptors, dispersants and the like for lubricants were not included. However, antiozonants were considered a special form of antioxidants and were included in the review. Multicomponent stabilizing systems containing antioxidants or antiozonants were also included.

Most of the 247 patents covered in this review were issued since 1972. The old time standbys, the phenol and amine antioxidants, are still being synthesized. However, many of the new compounds produced as antioxidants combine a hindered phenol group with another group containing sulfides, triazine, phosphates, phosphites, etc. which give active materials hopefully having the advantage of two or more stabilizing moieties.

TEST METHODS

Various test methods have been used repeatedly throughout the book. To avoid unnecessary repetition, the procedures are given here for reference purposes.

Oven Aging Test

Unstabilized polymer powder is thoroughly blended with an antioxidant. The blended material is then milled on a two roller mill at 182°C for 10 minutes after which time the stabilized polymer is sheeted from the mill and allowed to cool.

1

The milled polymer sheet is then cut into small pieces and pressed for 7 minutes on a hydraulic press at 218°C and 2,000 psi pressure. The resultant sheet of 25 mil thickness is cut into small plaques and tested for resistance to accelerated aging in a forced draft oven at 150°C.

Fadeometer Test

The 25 mil plaques prepared as described in the Oven Aging Test are placed on a white card stock background and exposed in a Fadeometer. The specimens are tested for embrittlement at 20 hour intervals by bending them 180°. The result of this test is recorded as the number of hours the specimen stayed in the Fadeometer until a clean break is obtained.

Weatherometer Test

Solid polymer is milled in a two-roll heated mill and the additive is incorporated in the sample during the milling. The samples are pressed into sheets of about 17 mil thickness and cut into plaques of about 1⅜" x 1½". The plaques are inserted into plastic holders, affixed onto a rotating drum and exposed to carbon arc rays at about 52°C in a Weatherometer. The samples are examined periodically by infrared analysis to determine the carbonyl band at 1,715 cm^{-1} which is reported as the carbonyl number. The higher intensity of the carbonyl band indicates a higher carbonyl concentration (expressed as carbonyl number) and accordingly increased oxidation.

Falex Machine Test

This procedure is described in detail in *Lubricant Testing* by E.G. Ellis published by Scientific Publication Limited (Great Britain), 1953, pages 150–154. It is also described on pages 21-1 and 27-2 of the *Handbook of Lubrication Engineering,* O'Conner, editor, McGraw Hill 1968.

Briefly, the Falex machine consists of a rotating pin which runs between two V-shaped bearings which are spring loaded against the pin and provided with means for varying the load. The oil to be tested is poured into a metal trough in which the pin and bearings are partly submerged. The machine is operated for 5 minutes each at 250 and 500 pound loads and then 45 minutes at 750 pound load. The data collected include the temperature of the oil at each of the loads, as well as the wear which is determined by a ratchet wheel arrangement in which the teeth are advanced in order to maintain the desired load. Each tooth is equivalent to approximately 0.000022 inch.

In another series of tests the machine is operated for 5 minutes at each load from 250 lb to seizure at 250 lb increments. The maximum load, the time in minutes at this load to seizure are reported, as well as the temperature of the oil. In this case the higher temperature is preferred because it means that the oil is operating satisfactorily at a higher temperature.

PHENOLIC ANTIOXIDANTS

Phenolic compounds comprise one of the oldest and most frequently used category of antioxidants. Foremost among the phenols are the so called hindered phenols in which the aromatic ring contains alkyl groups, preferably branched groups such as tert-butyl. The hindered phenol moiety appears in many of the antioxidants produced in recent years, frequently combined with other active antioxidant groups.

HINDERED HYDROXYBENZYL ALCOHOL DERIVATIVES

Esters of 3-Hydroxybenzyl Alcohols

Antioxidants useful in many organic materials have been prepared by *J. Song and H. Richmond; U.S. Patent 3,795,700; March 5, 1974; assigned to American Cyanamid Co.* from phenol alcohols having three alkyl groups.

More particularly, these antioxidants are compounds of the formula:

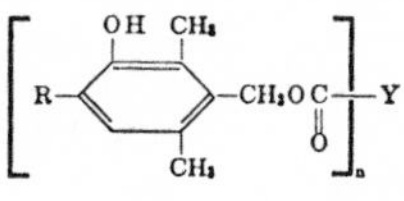

where R is branched chain alkyl group containing three to twelve carbons; Y is the residue of the carboxylic acid $Y(COOH)_n$, provided that when Y is alkyl and n is one, Y contains more than ten carbons; and n is one to four.

Illustrative of the branched chain alkyl groups represented by R ortho to the phenolic hydroxy group and para to the ester group are isopropyl, tert-butyl, sec-butyl, tert-amyl, sec-heptyl, sec-octyl, tert-octyl, tert-nonyl (1,1-dimethylheptyl), α,α-dimethylbenzyl, methylcyclopentyl, methylcyclohexyl, and the like.

Illustrative of the carboxylic acids $Y(COOH)_n$ of which the moiety Y forms part of these compounds are monocarboxylic acids such as stearic, myristic, palmitic, benzoic, naphthoic, salicylic, phenylglycolic, pyridinecarboxylic, mesitoic, oleic, and the like; dicarboxylic acids such as 3,3'-thiodipropionic, phthalic, hexahydrophthalic, terephthalic, adipic, p-phenylenediacetic, oxalic, malonic, succinic, pimelic, azelaic, sebacic, homophthalic, maleic, fumaric,

3

itaconic, and the like; and polycarboxylic acids such as trimesic, trimellitic, pyromellitic, aconitic, and the like.

These compounds may be prepared by known procedures such as the esterification of the 4-alkyl-2,6-dimethyl-3-hydroxybenzyl alcohol or halide with the carboxylic acid, acid salt, or acid halide. These compounds are especially useful for inhibiting oxidative degradation of organic materials normally subject to deterioration upon exposure to oxygen, such as polyolefins, ABS resins, polyamides, polyacetals, polystyrene, impact polystyrene, natural and synthetic rubbers including ethylene-propylene copolymers and carboxylated latices, fats, oils, greases, gasoline, etc.

Example 1: A mixture of 11.32 grams (0.05 mol) of 4-tert-butyl-3-hydroxy-2,6-dimethyl-benzyl chloride, 14.26 grams (0.05 mol) of stearic acid, and 58.6 grams (0.58 mol) of tri-ethylamine was allowed to react at a temperature of 88° to 96°C over a period of 14 hours. The reaction mixture was cooled and the salt collected. The filtrate was concentrated in vacuo to an oily residue, taken up in ether, and the unreacted stearic acid removed by treatment with 10% sodium bicarbonate solution.

The ether soluble fraction amounted to 14 grams. Purification by chromatography on alu-minum oxide using a benzene-hexane (1:1) mixture gave an oily product, 4-tert-butyl-3-hydroxy-2,6-dimethylbenzyl stearate. The infrared spectrum of a specimen showed the ex-pected major absorption bands. The assigned structure was also supported by NMR results.

This compound protected polypropylene films from embrittlement for 219 to 245 hours at 140°C whereas the corresponding prior art compound 3,5-di-tert-butyl-4-hydroxybenzyl stearate only protected such films for 55 to 94 hours. Unprotected polypropylene films lasted only 0 to 4 hours before embrittlement. Thus, this compound is about three times as effective as the corresponding prior art compound.

Example 2: A mixture of disodium terephthalate, 16.5 grams (0.08 mol) and 4-tert-butyl-3-hydroxy-2,6-dimethylbenzyl chloride, 35.7 grams (0.158 mol) in 200 ml of dimethyl-formamide was heated at reflux for 18 hours. The salt was then filtered off, and the filtrate poured into 400 ml of water. The resulting brown gum was dissolved in 50 ml of methanol and reprecipitated by addition of water. This procedure was repeated to give 18.9 grams (44%) of bis(4-tert-butyl-3-hydroxy-2,6-dimethylbenzyl) terephthalate, MP 227° to 230°C.

This compound protected polypropylene films from embrittlement for 880 to 890 hours at 140°C whereas the known compound most similar, bis(3,5-di-tert-butyl-4-hydroxybenzyl) terephthalate, only protected such films for 245 to 262 hours. Thus, this compound is about 3½ times as effective as the corresponding compound most similar to the prior art compounds.

Example 3: Bis(4-tert-butyl-3-hydroxy-2,6-dimethylbenzyl) terephthalate, was evaluated in an unstabilized ABS polymer at 0.5% in a formulation containing 1.0% zinc stearate as a lubricant, and 5% titanium dioxide pigment. The additive was incorporated into the above formulation by milling at 175°C and compression molded into 70 to 75 mil plaques. The plaques were oven aged at 150°C. The efficiency of the antioxidant was measured in terms of discoloration and hours to embrittlement at 150°C. Results are shown in the fol-lowing table.

| | | 150° C., oven aging | |
| | Brittle point (hrs.) | Δ(YI) | |
Sample		5 hours	12 hours
Control	5–12	19	42
Compound of Example 2	49–56	7	11

The data show that the compound of Example 2 affords protection against oxidative degradation (embrittlement) of from 5 to 10 times that of the control sample. Moreover, the increase in color on oven aging is considerably less in the stabilized sample. Additional examples in the original patent illustrate the use of these antioxidants in natural rubber and carboxylated latex (Pliolite 480).

Ethers of 2- or 4-Hydroxybenzyl Alcohols

A process for preparing antioxidant ethers has been developed by *B.R. Meltsner; U.S. Patent 3,692,691; September 19, 1972; assigned to Ethyl Corporation.* These dihydrocarbyl 2- or 4-hydroxybenzyl C_{4-20} alkyl ethers are prepared by reacting a dihydrocarbyl 2- or 4-hydroxybenzyl methyl ether with a higher primary alkanol in the presence of an acid catalyst under conditions such that methanol is distilled out. The dihydrocarbyl hydroxybenzyl methyl ether may be formed by reacting a dihydrocarbyl 2- or 4-hydroxybenzyl halide with a mixture of methanol and higher primary alkanols such that the methyl ether forms first and undergoes transetherification with the higher alkanol.

A preferred process for making the dihydrocarbyl 2- or 4-hydroxybenzyl C_{4-20} alkyl ethers, comprises reacting a dihydrocarbyl 2- or 4-hydroxybenzyl methyl ether with a C_{4-20} primary alkanol in the presence of an acid catalyst under conditions such that methanol is distilled out. Broadly, the dihydrocarbyl hydroxybenzyl methyl ethers used in the process are compounds having the formula:

(1)

where R_1 and R_2 are hydrocarbon groups, preferably C_{1-20} alkyl, C_{7-20} aralkyl and C_{6-20} aryl. In Formula (1) the methoxymethyl group is located ortho or para to the hydroxyl group.

Preferred compounds are 3,5-dialkyl-4-hydroxybenzyl methyl ethers with 3,5-di-tert-butyl-4-hydroxybenzyl methyl ether being most preferred. The higher alkanols which undergo the transetherification reaction can be any alkanol containing from 4 to 20 carbons. The preferred higher alkanols are mixtures consisting mainly of primary decanols and dodecanols because such alcohol mixtures lead to liquid products.

The transetherification is catalyzed by acids. The strong organic and inorganic acids are preferred, such as trifluoroacetic, trichloroacetic, sulfuric, sulfurous, phosphoric, hydrochloric, aromatic sulfonic acids such as p-toluenesulfonic acids, sulfonated ion exchange resins such as sulfonated polystyrene beads, and sulfonated aliphatics such as methanesulfonic acid.

Only a catalytic amount of acid is required. A useful range is from 0.05 to 5 weight percent. A preferred range is from 0.1 to 1 weight percent, based on the weight of the reaction mixture. The details of the transesterification reaction are shown in the following example.

Example: In a reaction vessel fitted with a stirrer, heating means and a distillation column was placed 25 parts of 3,5-di-tert-butyl-4-hydroxybenzyl methyl ether, 35 parts of a mixture of 43 weight percent n-decanol and 57 weight percent n-dodecanol, 40 parts of xylene, and 0.1 part of p-toluenesulfonic acid. The mixture was stirred and heated to about 157°C over a 1.5 hour period while distilling out 3.2 parts of methanol (65° to 70°C vapor temperature). The mixture was then cooled, washed with dilute aqueous sodium bicarbonate, and then with water. Xylene and excess C_{10-12} alcohol was distilled out under vacuum (0.3 mm Hg), up to a liquid temperature of 140°C. The product was 41 parts of 3,5-di-tert-butyl-4-hydroxybenzyl C_{10-12} alkyl ether, which was liquid at room temperature. The additives made by this process are excellent antioxidants in a wide range of organic materials. The product made using the preferred mixture of decyl and dodecyl alcohol is an especially useful product because it remains liquid at room temperature and is more readily handled in commercial applications.

Furthermore, it is much easier to disperse into organic substrates. For example, a stable lubricating oil is formed by adding 0.5 weight percent of this mixed ether to a neutral midcontinent mineral oil. Other additives normally used in lubricating oil formulations can be included such as zinc dialkyl dithiophosphates, calcium aryl sulfonates, polylauryl methacrylate VI improvers, and the like.

Likewise, the products can be added to a styrene-butadiene latex in an amount equal to 0.5 part per hundred of SBR. The latex is coagulated by addition to an aqueous sulfuric acid-sodium chloride solution. The SBR crumb which separates is very stable during storage over long periods of time and when formulated and vulcanized results in an excellent rubber.

ESTERS OF PHENOL SUBSTITUTED ACIDS

A series of ester antioxidants have been prepared by workers at the Ciba-Geigy laboratories based on carboxylic acids having a hindered phenol moiety, such as 3,5-di-tert-butyl-4-hydroxybenzoic acid or 3,5-di-tert-butyl-4-hydroxyphenylacetic acid.

Materials which are stabilized by these antioxidants include synthetic organic polymeric substances such as vinyl polymers and copolymers, poly-α-olefins, polyurethanes, polyamides, polyesters, polycarbonates, polyacetols, polystyrene, polyethyleneoxide, and copolymers such as those of high impact polystyrene containing copolymers of butadiene and styrene and those formed by the copolymerization of acrylonitrile, butadiene and/or styrene. Other materials include lubricating oil of the aliphatic ester type, vegetable derived oils, hydrocarbon material such as gasoline, waxes, resins and the like, fatty acids such as soaps and the like. In general these stabilizers are used from 0.005 to 10% by weight of the stabilized composition.

Esters of Hindered Hydroxybenzoic Acids

In one disclosure, *M. Dexter, J.D. Spivack and D.H. Steinberg; U.S. Patent 3,681,431; August 1, 1972; assigned to Ciba-Geigy Corporation* describe alkyl dialkylhydroxybenzoates of the formula:

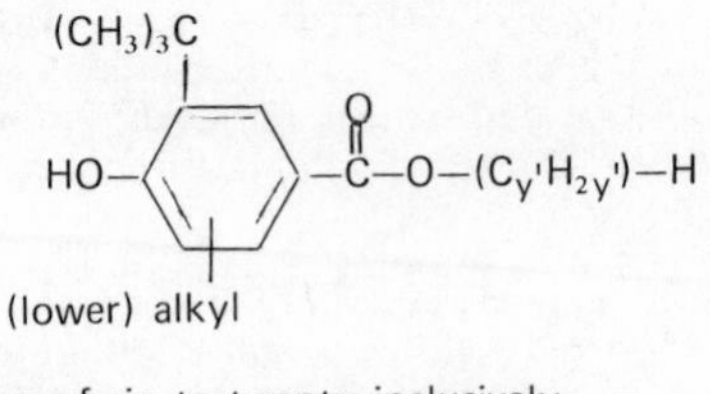

$$(CH_3)_3C$$

$$HO-\left\langle\bigcirc\right\rangle-\overset{\overset{O}{\|}}{C}-O-(C_{y'}H_{2y'})-H$$

(lower) alkyl

in which y' has a value of six to twenty inclusively.

These compounds may be prepared via usual esterification procedures from a suitable alcohol and the substituted benzoic acid or an acid halide, acid anhydride or mixed anhydride thereof. Similarly these esters may be prepared by conventional methods of transesterification or by treating a dialkylphenol with a halo-ester.

Example 1: 40 parts of 2,6-di-tert-butylphenol are dissolved in 150 parts by volume of methanol. To this solution are added 60 parts of sodium hydroxide as a 40% aqueous solution, followed by 1 part of cupric sulfate. The resulting mixture is then treated with 40 parts of carbon tetrachloride, which is added dropwise over a 15 to 20 minute interval.

This causes the reaction temperature to rise to 75° to 80°C. Stirring is continued for ten minutes after the addition of all reactants.

After cooling to room temperature, the reaction mixture is poured into 700 parts of water and the resulting solids are filtered to yield 68.5 parts of product. Further purification is achieved by recrystallization from aqueous acetic acid, benzene-hexane or, cyclohexane. Use of the last named solvent gives almost white crystals, MP 162° to 163°C of methyl 3,5-di-tert-butyl-4-hydroxybenzoate.

Methyl 3,5-di-tert-butyl-4-hydroxybenzoate (6.6 parts), 13.5 parts of n-octadecyl alcohol and 0.2 parts of sodium methylate are mixed at room temperature and then heated at 150°±5°C for 10 hours. During the final 2 hours of heating, an initial vacuum of 10-33 mm is applied, followed by a high vacuum of 0.5 to 1 mm for 0.2 hours. Removal of most of the impurities is accomplished by distillation of 125° to 185°C/0.25 mm. The residue (11.0 parts) is further purified by crystallization from acetone-cyclohexane to give a white crystalline product, melting at 65° to 67°C of n-octadecyl 3,5-di-tert-butyl-4-hydroxybenzoate.

Example 2: n-Hexanol (1.84 parts) and 1.82 parts of triethylamine are dissolved in 50 parts by volume of dry benzene. 3,5-Di-tert-butyl-4-hydroxybenzoyl chloride (4.72 parts) dissolved in 25 parts by volume of dry benzene is added dropwise with stirring at 25° to 30°C over a period of 10 minutes. The reactants are then heated under reflux for 3 hours after which time 1.6 parts of triethylamine hydrochloride are removed by filtration. The yellow filtrate is washed with saturated sodium chloride solution, twice with 2 N aqueous sodium carbonate solution and then again with saturated sodium chloride solution. After drying the solution over anhydrous sodium sulfate, the solvent is removed by evaporation. Six parts of a solid residue are thus obtained and purified by vacuum distillation. The n-hexyl 3,5-di-tert-butyl-4-hydroxybenzoate distills at 150° to 155°C/0.1 mm, MP 70° to 72°C. The yield of the pure product is 3 parts. Examples of the use of these stabilizers are given in U.S. Patent 3,285,855, page 14.

Esters of Hydroxyphenylalkanoic Acids

Similar antioxidant esters are also described by *M. Dexter, J.D. Spivack and D.H. Steinberg; U.S. Patent 3,330,859; July 11, 1967; assigned to Geigy Chemical Corporation.* Here the compounds have the formula:

(1)

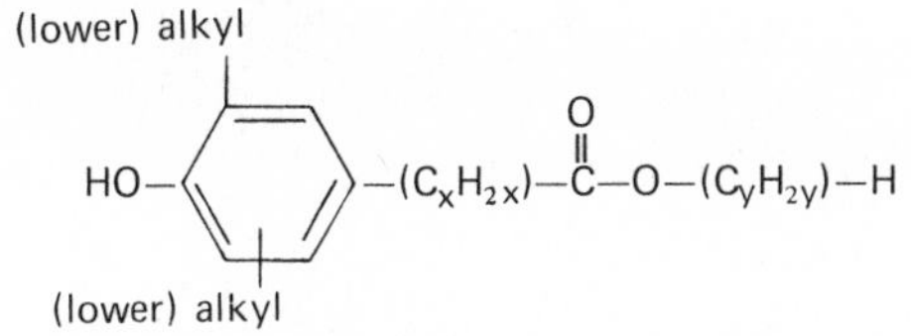

(lower) alkyl

$$HO-\langle\!\!\bigcirc\!\!\rangle-(C_xH_{2x})-\overset{\overset{O}{\|}}{C}-O-(C_yH_{2y})-H$$

(lower) alkyl

where x has a value of 0 to 6 inclusively and y has a value of 6 to 30 inclusively. The preferred species may be represented by the formula:

(2)

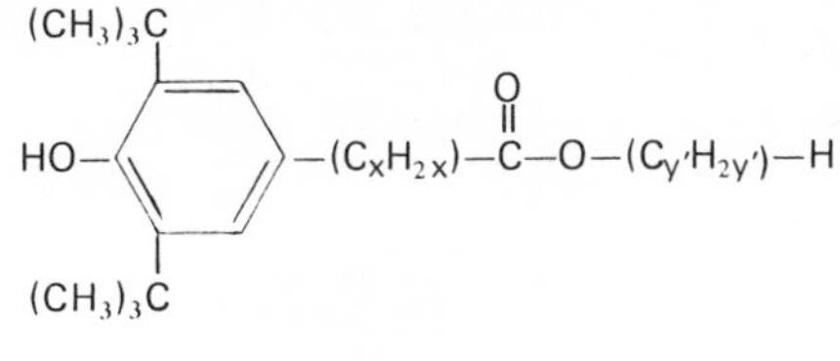

$(CH_3)_3C$

$$HO-\langle\!\!\bigcirc\!\!\rangle-(C_xH_{2x})-\overset{\overset{O}{\|}}{C}-O-(C_{y'}H_{2y'})-H$$

$(CH_3)_3C$

in which x is as above defined and y' has a value of from 6 to 20.

These compounds may be prepared via usual esterification procedures from a suitable alcohol and an acid, an acid halide, acid anhydride or mixed anhydride thereof or by transesterification. Alternatively when x = 2, the compounds may be prepared by treating a dialkylphenol in basic media with an olefinic ester of the formula:

$$CH_2{=}CH\overset{\overset{\displaystyle O}{\|}}{C}{-}O{-}(C_yH_{2y}){-}H$$

or by treating a dialkylphenol with a haloalkanoate ester of the formula:

$$Z{-}(C_xH_{2x}){-}\overset{\overset{\displaystyle O}{\|}}{C}{-}O{-}(C_yH_{2y}){-}H$$

in which A is halogen; e.g., Cl, Br, etc.

Example 1: Methyl 3,5-di-tert-butyl-4-hydroxyphenylacetate (7.2 parts), 7 parts of n-octadecyl alcohol and 0.1 part of sodium methylate are heated under nitrogen at 130°C for one and a half hours. The mixture is flushed with nitrogen and the methanol formed is collected in a Dry Ice-acetone cooled trap. After 1.2 parts of methanol are collected, the reaction mixture is heated at 150°C and 0.05 mm pressure for an additional 3 hours. The homogeneous reaction mixture is then dissolved in 40 parts by volume of hexane and cooled.

The crystalline precipitate, consisting of unreacted n-octadecyl alcohol, is filtered and the filtrate is concentrated under vacuum. The residue weighs 6.6 parts and is purified by high vacuum distillation. After a forerun, consisting of 2.3 parts of unreacted methyl 3,5-di-butyl-4-hydroxyphenylacetate, 4.3 parts of n-octadecyl 3,5-di-tert-butyl-4-hydroxyphenyl-acetate are collected at 230°C/0.075 mm. The n-octadecyl 3,5-di-tert-butyl-4-hydroxyphenyl-acetate thus obtained as an oily ester, solidifies on long standing and demonstrates a melting point of 33° to 35°C.

Example 2: 1-Octadecanol (3.63 parts) and 3.75 parts of β-(3,5-di-tert-butyl-4-hydroxy-phenyl)propionic acid are dissolved in 40 parts by volume of benzene. One half part of p-toluenesulfonic acid is added and the mixture refluxed with stirring for two and one-half hours. Approximately the theoretical amount of water (0.34 part) is collected during this time by azeotroping with benzene. At the end of the reflux period, the brownish solution is cooled, filtered and stripped of benzene in vacuo. The residue (7 parts), which crystallizes upon standing, is recrystallized from 3:2 methanol:ethyl acetate to yield 4 parts of the n-octadecyl β-(3,5-di-tert-butyl-4-hydroxyphenyl)propionate, which is a white, crystalline powder, MP 49° to 50°C. Examples of use of these stabilizers are given in U.S. Patent 3,285,855, page 14.

Esters of (Dialkyl-4-Hydroxyphenyl)Malonic Acids

Derivatives of malonic acid substituted with groups containing a hindered phenol are disclosed by *M. Dexter; U.S. Patent 3,721,704; March 20, 1973; assigned to Geigy Chemical Corporation.* A preferred compound is di-n-octadecyl 2,2-bis(3',5'-di-tert-butyl-4'-hydroxy-benzyl)malonate. The compounds are stabilizers suitable for numerous substrates of organic material subject to oxidative deterioration, in particular polypropylene. Synergistic combinations of these compounds and dialkyl thiodipropionates are also disclosed.

Broadly, these antioxidants have the following formula:

(1)

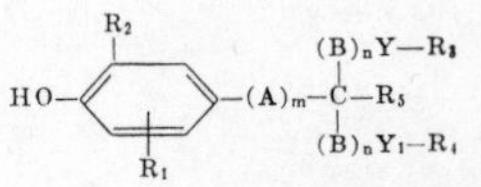

where R_1 is alkyl of one to 18 carbons; cycloalkyl of five to 12 carbons; alkyl of one to eight carbons is preferred, and most preferably is a tertiary butyl group ortho to the hydroxy group; R_2 is hydrogen or alkyl of 1 to 18 carbons; cycloalkyl of 5 to 12 carbons; an alkyl of one to eight carbons is preferred; and a tertiary butyl group is most preferable.

R_3 and R_4 are independently alkyl of 1 to 40 carbons, alkylthioalkyl, aryl including phenyl and substituted aryl, e.g., alkylaryl; when Y or Y_1 is carbonyl, R_3 or R_4 may also be amino, substituted amino, or thioalkyl respectively; and when Y or Y_1 is carboxyl, R_3 or R_4 may also be hydrogen or an alkali metal respectively; when $m = 0$ and $n = 1$, the combination of Y and R_3 and/or Y_1 and R_4 may then be cyano or cyanoloweralkyl; particularly preferred is alkyl of 1 to 24 carbon atoms and alkylthioalkyl.

R_5 is hydrogen, carbamyl, alkylcarboxyalkyl, cyano and alkyl of 1 to 22 carbons, or

the latter, hydrogen, and alkyl being preferred; m and n are 0 ot 1; Y and Y_1 are individually

$$-\overset{\overset{\textstyle O}{\|}}{C}-O-$$ or $$-\overset{\overset{\textstyle O}{\|}}{C}-$$

A is alkylene, straight and branched chain of one to twelve carbons, preferably one to six carbons, and most preferably methylene; and B is lower alkylene, i.e., one to six carbons, straight or branched chain.

Preferred stabilizers are diethyl 2,2-bis(3', 5'-di-tert-butyl-4'-hydroxybenzyl)malonate; dimethyl 2,2-bis(3',5'-di-tert-butyl-4'-hydroxybenzyl)malonate; di-n-octadecyl 2,2-bis(3',5'-di-tert-butyl-4'-hydroxybenzyl)malonate; ethyl 2,2-bis(3',5'-di-tert-butyl-4'-hydroxybenzyl)acetoacetate; 3,3-bis(3',5'-di-tert-butyl-4'-hydroxybenzyl)pentanedione; and di-n-octadecyl 2-(3',5'-di-tert-butyl-4'-hydroxybenzyl)malonate.

These compounds can be prepared by several known methods such as by condensation of a chloroalkylphenol with malonic acid esters, followed by ester interchange to form the final ester. This can be illustrated by the following example.

Example 1: 1.9 parts of sodium (0.08 mols) are dissolved in 100 parts by volume of ethanol at 25° to 50°C, cooled to room temperature and 5.8 parts of diethyl malonate added at room temperature, the colorless solution becoming yellow. 23.0 parts of 3,5-di-tert-butyl-4-hydroxybenzyl chloride (87%, 0.08 mols) are then added dropwise during 30 to 35 minutes at 10° to 12°C. The solution is then allowed to warm to 50°C over a period of 2 hours. The reaction is then diluted with 300 parts of water and extracted with two 100 parts by volume portions of ether and the separated ether extract dried over anhydrous sodium sulfate.

The ether is removed by distillation at 20 mm Hg pressure and the residue (24 parts) triturated twice with 50 parts by volume of petroleum ether yielding 14 parts of white crystals melting at 160° to 162°C. On recrystallization from a mixture of 100 parts by volume of hexane and about 5 parts of benzene, the diethyl 2,2-bis(3',5'-di-tert-butyl-4'-hydroxybenzyl)malonate (A) melts at 160° to 162°C.

5.5 parts of (A) (0.01 mols) and 5.40 parts of n-octadecanol (0.02 mols) are dissolved in 100 parts by volume of toluene. 0.100 parts of sodium methylate is dispersed in the above solution and 46.4 parts of the solvent slowly distilled over a period of one hour. The reaction mixture is then cooled to room temperature and neutralized with acetic acid, the color changing from reddish-brown to yellow. About 100 parts by volume of ether is added, the solution being washed with 5% aqueous hydrochloric acid. The solvent is stripped by distillation at 20 mm Hg pressure. The residue (10 parts) is recrystallized three times from isopropanol. Di-n-octadecyl 2,2-bis(3',5'-di-tert-butyl-4'-hydroxybenzyl)malonate is then obtained as white crystals melting at 98° to 100°C.

Example 2: Unstabilized polypropylene powder (Profax 6501) is blended with 0.5% by weight of di-n-octadecyl 2,2-bis(3'-5'-di-tert-butyl-4'-hydroxybenzyl)malonate and tested by oven aging test. The composition of 0.5% by weight of di-n-octadecyl 2,2-bis(3',5'-di-tert-butyl-4'-hydroxybenzyl)malonate and polypropylene is stabilized against oxidative deterioration for over 600 hours. The unstabilized polypropylene deteriorates after only three hours.

In the same manner, stable compositions of polypropylene are prepared having 0.5% by weight of the following compounds: diethyl 2,2-bis(3',5'-di-tert-butyl-4'-hydroxybenzyl)-malonate, stabilized for 155 hours; dimethyl 2,2-bis(3',5'-di-tert-butyl-4'-hydroxybenzyl)-malonate, stabilized for 65 hours, and ethyl 2,2-bis(3',5'-di-tert-butyl-4'-hydroxybenzyl)-acetoacetate, stabilized for 85 hours.

The same procedure was repeated, except that 0.1% of the stabilizer and 0.5% of dilauryl-β-thiodipropionate (DLTDP) was incorporated into the polypropylene. The resultant compositions were stabilized as indicated.

	Hours to Failure
Compositions of polypropylene, DLTDP, and:	
Diethyl 2,2-bis(3',5'-di-tert-butyl-4'-hydroxybenzyl)malonate	450
Dimethyl 2,2-bis(3',5'-di-tert-butyl-4'-hydroxybenzyl)malonate	385
Di-n-octadecyl 2,2-bis(3',5'-di-tert-butyl-4'-hydroxybenzyl)-malonate	1,050
Diethyl 2-butyl-2-(3',5'-di-tert-butyl-4'-hydroxybenzyl)-malonate	405
Ethyl 2,2-bis(3',5'-di-tert-butyl-4'-hydroxybenzyl)acetoacetate	390
3,3-bis(3',5'-di-tert-butyl-4'-hydroxybenzyl)-2,4-pentanedione	425
Di-n-octadecyl 4-(3',5'-di-tert-butyl-4'-hydroxyphenyl)-4-cyano-pimelate	710

Other examples show the effectiveness of these antioxidants in mineral oil, high impact polystyrene, ABS and cyclohexene.

Esters of Polyols

In this process, the antioxidants disclosed by *M. Dexter, J.D. Spivak and D.H. Steinberg; U.S. Patent 3,644,482; February 22, 1972; assigned to Ciba-Geigy Corporation* are compounds of the formula:

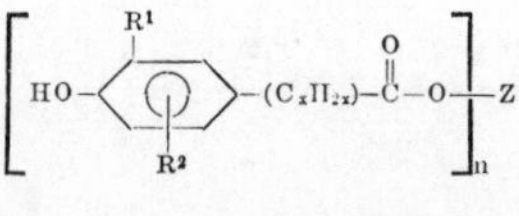

$$\left[HO-\underset{R^2}{\overset{R^1}{\underset{|}{\overset{|}{\bigcirc}}}}-(C_xH_{2x})-\overset{O}{\overset{\|}{C}}-O- \right]_n Z$$

where R^1 is methyl, ethyl or an α-branched alkyl group of 3 to 10 carbons; R^2 is hydrogen, methyl, ethyl or an α-branched alkyl group of from 3 to 10 carbons; x is 1 to 6; n is 2 to 6; and Z is an aliphatic hydrocarbon C_yH_{2y+2-n} in which y is 2 to 18 when n is 2 and is 3 to 6 when n is greater than 2, the value of y in all cases being equal to or greater than that of n.

It will be noted that these compounds have one alkyl group (R^1) ortho to the hydroxy group. A second like or different alkyl group (R^2) is optionally present either (a) in the other position ortho to the hydroxy group (the 3-position) or (b) meta to the hydroxy group and para to the first alkyl group (the 2-position).

These alkyl groups will be methyl, ethyl or when higher than ethyl, an α-branched alkyl group of 3 to 10 carbons. The α-branched alkyl group is one in which the carbons of the alkyl group bound to the phenyl group are also bound to at least two other carbons of the alkyl group. Thus the mono- or dialkylphenolic group includes for example the following,

3,5-di-tert-butyl-4-hydroxyphenyl
3,5-diisopropyl-4-hydroxyphenyl
2,5-dimethyl-4-hydroxyphenyl
2-methyl-4-hydroxy-5-tert-butylphenyl
3-methyl-4-hydroxy-5-tert-butylphenyl
3,5-diethyl-4-hydroxyphenyl

Preferred phenolic groups are those having at least one branched group such as isopropyl, tert-butyl or the like in a position ortho to the hydroxy group.

The mono- or dialkyl-4-hydrophenyl group is bound to an alkanoyl unit of 2 to 7 carbons. The hydrocarbon portion of this alkanoyl unit is represented by $-(C_xH_{2x})-$ and may be of a straight or, when x is greater than 1, branched chain. A preferred alkanoyl group is the 3-propionyl group.

Two or more (as determined by n) of these mono- or dialkylphenylalkanoyl groups are then bound through a like number of oxygen atoms to the hydrocarbon residue of a polyol. The polyol from which these esters are derived will thus consist of the straight or branched chain hydrocarbon residue of the formula C_yH_{2y+2-n} and a number of hydroxy groups equal to n.

When n is two, i.e., the polyol is a diol, this hydrocarbon residue will have 2 to 18 carbons. When n is greater than two; i.e., the polyol is a triol, tetrol, pentol or hexol, the hydrocarbon residual will have 3 to 6 carbons. In all cases the number of hydroxy groups and the resulting number of alkylphenylalkanoyloxy groups (as designated by n) will be equal to or less than the number of carbons (y) in the hydrocarbon residue; i.e., since each carbon of the hydrocarbon residue can bear only one hydroxy group, y is equal to or greater than n.

The esters can be prepared by standard esterification and the phenol acids can be obtained (where x is 1) through chloromethylation of an alkylphenol followed by treatment with sodium or potassium cyanide and hydrolysis of the resultant alkylhydroxyphenylacetonitrile. The acids (where x is two or greater) can be readily prepared by the methods of U.S. Patent 3,247,240 through the Friedel-Crafts reaction utilizing alkylphenol and alkyl ester of chloroformylalkanoic acid followed by reduction of the alkyl substituted 4-hydroxybenzoylalkanoate (or the saponified free acid) as for example through a Clemmensen reduction or through reaction of an alkyl metal phenolate with a halo substituted alkanoate.

Example 1: A mixture consisting of 16.7 parts 3-(3,5-di-tert-butyl-4-hydroxyphenyl)propionic acid, 1.90 parts propylene glycol, 2.5 parts p-toluenesulfonic acid monohydrate and 300 parts by volume of toluene is refluxed until a constant quantity of water has been collected in a Dean-Stark water trap.

After cooling, the mixture is diluted with 300 parts by volume of benzene and washed successively with the following: water, 0.5 N sodium hydroxide, water and saturated sodium chloride. After drying over sodium sulfate, the solvent is removed under reduced pressure to yield 1,2-propylene glycol bis[3-(3,5-di-tert-butyl-4-hydroxyphenyl)propionate] (13.1 parts). This material is further purified by chromatography over alumina. Elution with hexane produces a minor amount of yellow oil followed by the desired product which crystallizes spontaneously and demonstrates a MP of 70°C.

Example 2: Pentaerythritol (6.8 parts) and lithium hydride (0.0885 part) are added to a reaction vessel equipped with an agitator, Dean-Stark trap and nitrogen inlet. The mixture is heated until the contents are molten (220°C) and then cooled below 50°C. Methyl 3-(3,5-di-tert-butyl-4-hydroxyphenyl)propionate (64.5 parts) is then added and the reaction mixture heated at 185° to 190°C for 13 hours with stirring. During this time, nitrogen is continuously introduced to provide an inert atmosphere and remove the generated methanol. The reaction mixture is then cooled and 500 parts by volume of benzene are then added. The mixture is neutralized with glacial acetic acid and heated until a nearly complete solution is realized. After clarification and filtration, the reaction mixture is heated under reduced pressure to remove the solvent, cooled, then treated with 400 parts by volume of hexane and filtered. Chromatography over neutral alumina and elution with hexane produces an initial yellow impurity followed by pentaerythritol tetrakis [3-(3,5-di-tert-butyl-4-hydroxyphenyl)propionate], alternatively named tetrakis[methylene-3-(3,5-di-tert-butyl-4-hydroxyphenyl)propionyloxy] methane, is a clear amber glass which softens at 50° to 60°C. Examples of antioxidant activity of these compounds are also given in U.S. Patent 3,285,855, page 14.

Esters from Mixed Glycols

M. Dexter, J.D. Spivack and D.H. Steinberg; U.S. Patent 3,779,945; December 18, 1973; assigned to Ciba-Geigy Corporation have also prepared additional antioxidant materials of mixed esters. These mixtures contain 3-(3,5-dialkyl-4-hydroxyphenyl)propionic acid esters of at least two nonidentical alkanediols. The alkanediols will have 3 to 18 carbons, preferably 3 to 12, and may simply be structurally different, e.g., in carbon atom content. Alternatively the alkanediols may have the same number of carbons with the hydrocarbon chains differing in their branching so that as a result, each is a structural isomer of the other. Finally the alkanediols may have the same carbon content and the same branching but possess two centers of asymmetry and are diastereoisomers of each other. The groups X and Y are derived from and correspond structurally to the hydrocarbon residue of the alkanediols.

The ratio of the two components of this mixture can vary from 1:1 to 9:1. When X and Y differ solely by reason of diastereoisomerism, this ratio is preferably about 1:1; otherwise the range is preferably from about 1:1 to 3:1.

Esters of 3,5-dialkyl-4-hydroxyphenylalkanoic acids and alkanepolyols are described previously in U.S. Patent 3,644,482 are crystalline or vitreous solids which are highly effective stabilizers against thermooxidative aging, i.e., they are solid antioxidants. They generally have only limited solubility in those solvents employed technically in large amounts, such as aliphatic hydrocarbons.

These properties are highly advantageous in many applications but represent disadvantages in others. Thus it is difficult to use these compounds in technical processes in which the additives are pumped, proportioned and fed in fluid form, for example in solution polymerization processes.

The mixtures provided by this process are not only very suitable for the stabilization of organic material, they are liquids which can be pumped, proportioned and fed, or are very soluble in organic solvents, so that they can be employed in the form of highly concentrated solutions.

These mixtures are incorporated in the substrates in a concentration of 0.01 to 5% by weight calculated on the material to be stabilized, preferably 0.05 to 1.5% and especially 0.1 to 0.8%, by weight, calculated on the material to be stabilized.

The incorporation can be effected before or after polymerization, or before or after molding, for example, by mixing the mixtures according to the process and optionally other additives into the melt or solution of polymers by conventional methods. The dissolved or dispersed compounds may also be applied to the polymers, with optional subsequent evaporation of the solvent. It is a particular advantage that the mixtures, as such or as concentrated solutions, optionally at raised temperatures, can be pumped through pipes and fed in measured amount into the polymerization or finishing process. The following examples will illustrate the preparation and antioxidant use of these compounds.

Example 1: Sixty-four grams of a mixture of about 70% by weight of 2,4,4-trimethyl-1,6-hexanediol and about 30% by weight of 2,2,4-trimethyl-1,6-hexanediol together with 234 grams of methyl 3-(3,5-di-tert-butyl-4-hydroxyphenyl)propionate are placed in a three-necked flask fitted with a fractionating column and melted at 80°C with the introduction of nitrogen. To this melt is then added 0.8 grams of lithium amide. The mixture is heated with stirring, first at normal pressure, then under vacuum (about 12 mm) until the methanol ceases to be distilled. Two grams of glacial acetic acid are then added to the reaction mixture and the mixture is filtered. After filtering, a clear, light yellow viscous liquid is obtained which consists essentially of a mixture of about 70% by weight of 2,4,4-trimethyl-1,6-hexanediol bis[3-(3,5-di-tert-butyl-4-hydroxyphenyl)propionate] and about 30% by weight of 2,2,4-trimethyl-1,6-hexanediol bis[3,5-di-tert-butyl-4-hydroxyphenyl)-propionate] (Stabilizer No. 1).

Example 2: Stabilizing of Polypropylene — The test samples are prepared as follows. One hundred parts of polypropylene (melt index 3.2 grams) are kneaded in a Brabender plastograph for 10 minutes at 200°C with the stabilizer of Example 1. The resultant mass is then passed in a platen press at a plating temperature of 260°C to form sheets of 1 mm thickness from which strips 1 x 17 cm are cut.

The effectiveness of the additives is determined by heat aging the sheets in an air-circulation oven at 135°C and 149°C respectively. The beginning of visible decomposition of the test sample is taken as end point of the test, results are given in the table below.

Stabilizer	Time Until Decomposition in Days	
	135°C	149°C
Without stabilizer	1	<1
0.2% Stabilizer 1	158	39
0.1% Stabilizer 1+0.3% dilauryl-thiodipropionate	228	45

EPT was also stabilized by these compounds in another example in the complete patent.

Esters of Polyol Ethers

Stabilizing esters of dipentaerythritol or tripentaerythritol and 4-hydroxy-5-alkylphenyl-alkanoic acids having a second alkyl group in the 2 or 3 position of the phenyl ring are disclosed by *M. Dexter, J.D. Spivack and D.H. Steinberg; U.S. Patents 3,801,540; April 2, 1974; and 3,642,868; February 15, 1972; both assigned to Ciba-Geigy Corporation.* The compounds are obtained through transesterification techniques.

Broadly, these compounds have the formula:

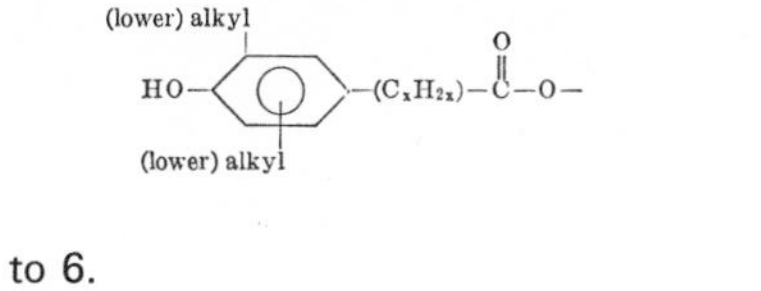

where s has a value of 0 or 1 and each R has the structure:

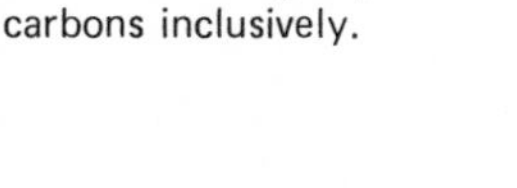

where x has a value of 1 to 6.

The (lower) alkyl in the above formula is a group containing a branched or straight chain hydrocarbon chain of 1 to 6 carbons inclusively.

Example 1: A reaction vessel is flushed with nitrogen and charged with 7.63 parts of dipentaerythritol and 50 parts by volume of dimethyl sulfoxide. This mixture is warmed to about 80°C and stirred until a complete solution is obtained. After cooling to 50°C, 0.177 part of lithium hydride is added and a nitrogen purge applied while stirring continuously. When frothing has subsided, 58.5 parts of methyl 3-(3,5-di-tert-butyl-4-hydroxyphenyl)propionate are added and the system evacuated to 20 mm. The mixture is heated at 85° to 90°C with stirring for 1¾ hours under the applied vacuum.

The main portion of the solvent is then removed over a 2 hour period of 90° to 100°C per 12 mm. Upon raising the temperature to 120° to 130°C and gradually reducing the vacuum to 0.3 to 0.5 mm over a 3 hour period, the remainder of the solvent is removed. After partially cooling to room temperature, but while still mobile, the reaction mixture is neutralized with 1.2 parts by volumn of glacial acetic acid. Excess starting ester is removed by vacuum distillation at 120° to 140°C/0.05 mm.

Further purification of the reaction product is accomplished by passing a benzene solution of the residue through a column of adsorbent (silica gel), washing with an additional quantity of the same solvent to remove colored impurities and finally eluting the product with a mixture of benzene and chloroform in the proportion of 1:1. After removal of the solvent, substantially pure dipentaerythritol hexakis [3-(3,5-di-tert-butyl-4-hydroxyphenyl)-propionate] is obtained having a MP of 70° to 80°C.

Example 2: A reaction vessel is flushed with nitrogen and charged with 22.34 parts of tripentaerythritol and 150 parts by volume of dimethyl sulfoxide. This mixture is heated to about 90°C with stirring and then allowed to cool to room temperature (about 25°C) and 0.212 part of lithium hydride is then added. After stirring for 30 minutes 154.8 parts of methyl 3-(3,5-di-tert-butyl-4-hydroxyphenyl)propionate are added. The system is then evacuated and heated at 80° to 82°C/15 to 20 mm for 4 hours, at 90°C/20 to 22 mm for 1¾ hours, at 73.5° to 75.5°C/13 to 23 mm for 2 hours and at 120°C/0.35 to 0.45 mm for 2 hours, collecting the solvent distillate.

The reaction mixture is then cooled, flushed with nitrogen and rendered neutral with glacial acetic acid. Excess starting ester is removed by vacuum distillation at 220°C/0.2 to 0.3 mm and the residue is then dissolved in hot benzene and chromatographed on silica gel to yield tripentaerythritol octakis [3-(3,5-di-tert-butyl-4-hydroxyphenyl)propionate], MP 65° to 85°C.

Stabilization with Alkylhydroxyphenyl Acid Esters

M. Dexter, J.D. Spivack and D.H. Steinberg; U.S. Patent 3,285,855; November 15, 1966; assigned to Geigy Chemical Corporation have further disclosed the stabilization of many polymeric and petroleum products with the esters described in several of the previous patents. They also include the use of compounds of the following formula not included in these disclosures.

where x' has a value of 0 to 6, inclusively, each of y' and z' has a value of 2 to 20, inclusively, R is hydrogen, hydroxy, alkanoyloxy or and B is a divalent sulfur atom, a divalent oxygen atom or the group >N—A in which A is alkyl or alkanoyl. Formula (1) includes compounds such as:

2-(n-octylthio)ethyl 3,5-di-tert-butyl-4-hydroxybenzoate

2-(n-octadecylthio)ethyl 3,5-di-tert-butyl-4-hydroxyphenyl-
acetate

2-(2-hydroxyethylthio)ethyl 3,5-di-tert-butyl-4-hydroxy-
benzoate

diethylene glycol bis[3-(3,5-di-tert-butyl-4-hydroxyphenyl)-
propionate]

n-butylimino N,N-bis[ethylene-3-(3,5-di-tert-butyl-4-hydroxy-
phenyl)propionate]

2-(2-stearoyloxyethylthio)ethyl 7-(3-methyl-5-tert-butyl-4-
hydroxyphenyl)heptanoate, and the like.

These compounds may be prepared via usual esterification procedure from a suitable alcohol and an acid.

Example 1: Unstabilized polypropylene powder (Hercules Profax 6501) is thoroughly blended with 0.5% by weight of 2-(n-octadecylthioethyl) 3,5-di-tert-butyl-4-hydroxyphenyl-acetate. The blended material is then milled on a two roller mill at 182°C for 5 minutes, after which time the stabilized polypropylene is sheeted from the mill and allowed to cool.

The milled polypropylene sheet is cut into small pieces and pressed for 7 minutes on a hydraulic press at 218°C and 2,000 pounds per square inch pressure. The resultant sheet at 25 mil thickness is then tested for resistance to accelerated aging in a forced draft oven at 149°C. The resultant composition of 0.5% by weight of 2-(n-octadecylthioethyl) 3,5-di-tert-butyl-4-hydroxyphenylacetate and polypropylene is stabilized against oxidative deterioration for 1,000 hours. The unstabilized polypropylene deteriorates after only 3 hours.

Example 2: Polypropylene compositions are prepared according to the procedure of Example 1 substituting for the 2-(n-octadecylthioethyl) 3,5-di-tert-butyl-4-hydroxyphenyl-acetate, equal amounts by weight of the following compounds prepared as described in U.S. Patents 3,330,859 and 3,681,431.

n-octadecyl 3,5-di-tert-butyl-4-hydroxyphenylacetate

n-octadecyl 3,5-di-tert-butyl-4-hydroxybenzoate (oven life,
15 hours)

n-dodecyl 3,5-di-tert-butyl-4-hydroxyphenylbenzoate (oven
life, 30 hours)

neo-dodecyl 3-(3,5-di-tert-butyl-4-hydroxyphenyl)propionate
(oven life, 30 hours)

Example 3: Polypropylene compositions are prepared according to the procedure of Example 1 substituting for the 2-(n-octadecylthioethyl) 3,5-di-tert-butyl-4-hydroxyphenyl-acetate equal amounts by weight of the following compounds prepared by the method of U.S Patent 3,644,482.

1,2-propylene glycol bis[3-(3,5-di-tert-butyl-4-hydroxyphenyl)-
propionate] (oven life, 780 hours)

ethylene glycol bis[3-(3,5-di-tert-butyl-4-hydroxyphenyl)-
propionate] (oven life, 820 hours)

neopentyl glycol bis[3-(3,5-di-tert-butyl-4-hydroxyphenyl)
propionate] (oven life, 510 hours)

Other examples in this patent and in U.S. Patents 3,681,431, 3,330,859 and 3,644,482 cover the stabilization of the following materials using these antioxidants: mineral oil, polystyrene, high impact polystyrene, linear polyethylene, nylon 6, polyvinyl chloride, ABS, polyurethane, gasoline, lard, synthetic ester lubricants, heptaldehyde, cyclohexene, and paraffin wax.

MISCELLANEOUS PHENOL COMPOUNDS

Halogenated Biphenols

H.-D. Becker and A.R. Gilbert; U.S. Patent 3,720,721; March 13, 1973; assigned to General Electric Company have prepared halobiphenols from precursor diphenoquinones by reacting the diphenoquinone with a hydrogen halide, such as hydrogen chloride. The biphenols can be used as antioxidants or as intermediates in the preparation of other diphenoquinones and polymeric compositions useful in polymeric coatings.

It was found that one can readily prepare halo-substituted hydrocarbon-substituted biphenols by effecting reaction between a hydrogen halide and a suspension of the corresponding tetra-hydrocarbon-substituted diphenoquinone in which the suspending medium is selected from water, alkanols of 1 to 4 carbons, and mixtures of water and these alkanols.

In addition to using relatively inexpensive solvents (alkanols and water), this reaction can take place within a relatively short period of time, generally in a matter of minutes to less than an hour, while at the same time preceeding at a relatively low temperature in the order of about 20° to 125°C. The yields of the biphenol obtained by this process are usually in excess of 75% of the theoretical yield, and for the most part exceed 90 to 95% of the theoretical value of the desired halogenated hydrocarbon-substituted biphenol.

Furthermore, the purity of the desired product is quite high after the initial reaction, thus significantly reducing the number and complexity of the processing steps required to isolate the pure product. What is equally important is that complicating quinhydrone formation is substantially repressed and the use of expensive acids, such as acetic acid, is avoided.

Included among the halobiphenols obtainable by this process are those of the general formula:

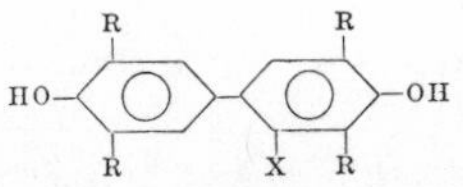

In the above formula, R may be the same or different monovalent hydrocarbon radicals of 1 to 6 carbons, and X is a halogen, for example, chlorine, bromine, fluorine.

These halobiphenols can be used as antioxidants for petroleum products, such as gasoline, and as stabilizers against polymerization of monomeric materials to maintain them in the essentially unpolymerized state until such time as they are ready for polymerization, for instance, with an organic peroxide.

In the following example, an inert atmosphere, in this instance, a nitrogen blanket, was maintained over the reaction mixture throughout the reaction; the temperature of the reaction was, in some instances, maintained by means of an ice bath. All parts are by weight unless otherwise stated.

Example: A slow stream of gaseous hydrogen chloride was introduced into a stirred suspension of finely ground 3,3',5,5'-tetramethyldiphenoquinone (120 g) in commercial grade absolute methanol (2,000 ml). The reaction mixture was kept under a nitrogen blanket and the temperature was held at 15° to 20°C. After five hours, the reaction mixture, which was clear, was diluted with 5 liters of water to cause deposition of an essentially colorless crystalline precipitate. The precipitate was removed by filtration, dissolved in methanol and reprecipitated by addition of water.

The colorless crystalline product, obtained in a yield of 98%, had a melting point of 208° to 210°C and was identified by spectroscopic means and by elemental analyses as being 3-chloro-2,2',6,6'-tetramethyl-p,p'-biphenol.

Other compounds prepared in examples of the patent include: 3-chloro-2,2',6,6'-tetraphenyl-p,p'-biphenol, 2-chloro-2',6,6'-tri-tert-butyl-4,4'-biphenol, 3-bromo-2,2',6,6'-tetramethyl-p,p'-biphenol, etc. No specific example was given to show the use of these compounds as anti-oxidants but they were stated to be useful as rubber antioxidants. Examples were shown using these biphenols in forming flame retardant polyester resins.

Improved Phenol-Cyclopentadiene Adducts

Phenolic antioxidants prepared by the reaction of cyclopentadiene with a phenol have been described in U.S. Patents 3,036,138 and 3,305,522. The emphasis in the former patent is on a one-step process wherein the latter discloses a two-step process involving an alkylation step subsequent to the phenolic/dicyclopentadiene reaction. When the reaction between the phenol and the dicyclopentadiene is carried out in the presence of a boron trifluoride catalyst, a highly colored reaction product results. Although the discoloration does not necessarily carry over into the polymer to which the antioxidant is added, it can sometimes tint the polymer and discolor the polymer on aging. It is desirable that the color of these phenolic antioxidants be improved and that their tendency to tint and/or discolor be reduced.

K.S. Cottman; U.S. Patent 3,746,654; July 17, 1973; assigned to The Goodyear Tire & Rubber Company has prepared these phenolic antioxidants with a reduced tendency to discolor polymer compositions by treating the product of the phenolic/dicyclopentadiene reaction with a phosphite compound.

The phenolic reaction products are prepared by reacting one mol of dicyclopentadiene with at least one mol of a phenolic compound conforming to the following structural formula:

where R and R^1 are selected from hydrogen and alkyl groups having 1 to 16 carbons. In the two-step reaction R is hydrogen and preferably R^1 is in a meta or para position. Preferred proportions of bound reactants in the resulting product are from 1.50 to 1.75 mols of phenolic compound per mol of the dicyclopentadiene. The reaction product of the dicyclopentadiene and phenolic compound can be subsequently alkylated with at least one-half mol of a tertiary olefinic material per mol of the dicyclopentadiene, the tertiary olefin having 4 to 16, preferably 4 to 12 carbons. When the one-step process is used, preferably R is a tertiary alkyl radical and is in a position ortho to the hydroxyl group. In both the one-step, and two-step processess, R^1 is preferably hydrogen, methyl or ethyl.

The treatment of the phenol/dicyclopentadiene reaction product normally comprises contacting the product with the phosphite while the product is in a solution. Increased agitation and/or higher temperatures reduce the time necessary to properly treat the reaction product.

The treatment generally is performed at 20° to 160°C. preferably from 60° to 140°C, under agitation. Preferably the phosphorus containing compounds and phosphites formed therefrom are added or formed under conditions conducive to their remaining in the reaction medium area for a period of time sufficient for them to improve color, e.g., at a temperature below their boiling point.

The following phosphorus containing compounds are used to treat the phenolic reaction products of this process. They consist of trisubstituted phosphites and compounds capable of reacting with a phenol to form a trisubstituted phosphite. The phosphorus containing compounds conform to the structural formula shown on the following page.

$$P{-}\begin{array}{l} \diagup R^7 \\ R^8 \\ \diagdown R^9 \end{array}$$

where R^7, R^8 and R^9 are selected from halogen radicals and radicals having the following structural formula, $-OR$, where R is selected from substituted and unsubstituted organic radicals. The substituents possessed by the organic radicals include nitro, hydroxy and halo, e.g., chloro radicals.

The substituted and unsubstituted organic radicals include radicals selected from alkyl radicals having 1 to 20 (preferably 1 to 6) carbons, aryl radicals having 6 to 20 (preferably 6 to 12) carbons, cycloalkyl radicals having 5 to 20 (preferably 5 to 12) carbons, aralkyl radicals having from 7 to 20 (preferably 7 to 12) carbons and alkaryl radicals having 7 to 20 (preferably 7 to 12) carbons. Preferably R^7, R^8 and R^9 are selected from chloro, and $-OR$ where R is methyl, ethyl, 1-chloroethyl, 2-chloroethyl, isopropyl, tertiary butyl, phenyl or p-tolyl. The following example will illustrate the preparation of color improved antioxidants.

Example: 648 grams of para-cresol and 18 grams of a 25% BF_3-para-cresol complex were heated to 90°C in a flask equipped with a stirrer, water condenser and thermometer. 264 g of dicyclopentadiene was then added at 88° to 99°C over a 35 minute period. After stirring 15 minutes, 19 grams of triethyl phosphite (1½ mol equivalent per mol BF_3) and 10 grams of Ca(OH)$_2$ were added. The reaction product was stirred at 90°C for 1¼ hours and then the excess para-cresol was removed by stripping the reaction product to a pot temperature of 195°C at 8 mm Hg. The resinous product was dissolved in 608 grams of toluene and filtered. The toluene was then removed from the filtrate by stripping to a pot temperature of 200°C at 8 mm Hg. The light amber resin weighed 608 grams.

The advantages of antioxidants produced by this process are shown in the following. Four batches (A, B, C and D) of antioxidant were prepared by reacting p-cresol and dicyclopentadiene, stripping off the excess p-cresol and butylating the reaction product.

Triethyl phosphite was added to two of the batches (C and D) prior to the stripping step. Gardner color determinations were made on 10% toluene solutions of the products of all four batches. Color data was also gathered on vulcanized (0.5 part of dicumyl peroxide) and unvulcanized portions of Plioflex 5000 (hot polymerized emulsion polybutadiene) containing two parts by weight per 100 parts by weight of polymer of the products of the batches. The results are listed in the following table.

Percent transmission, (10% toluene solutions)	A, 90.0	B, 92.2	C, 99.0	D, 100
R_d	70.8	74.3	77.8	76.9
a	−5.4	−6.0	−4.6	−3.9
b	29.4	24.9	16.6	12.8
ΔE	39	32	22	19
Visual	Amber	Amber	Straw	Straw
Polybutadiene: Unvulcanized:				
R_d	43.8	49.7	56.5	60.4
a	1.6	0.9	−0.9	−2.0
b	21.7	21.1	20.7	19
ΔE	44	40	36	33
Visual	(1)	(1)	(1)	(1)
Vulcanized:				
R_d	60.3	63.7	65.3	67.6
a	−2.2	−1.9	−2.0	−1.9
b	14.6	13.8	12.4	11.5

[1] Off-white.

The R_d value is high for white materials and low for black materials. Positive values of *a* indicate redness while negative values of *a* indicate greenness. Positive values of *b* indicate yellowness and negative values of *b* indicate blueness. The absolute values of *a* and *b* increase as the degree of discoloration increases. ΔE is a measure of color deviation from a given standard, in this case, magnesium oxide. Lower values of ΔE are desirable. As indicated by the above data, the phosphite treatment improved color characteristics. Staining and discoloring data was also gathered, but overall did not reveal significant differences.

Cycloalkylated Phenols

White, crystalline phenolic antioxidants are produced in the process disclosed by *E.A. Meier and H.H. Stockmann; U.S. Patent 3,683,033; August 8, 1972; assigned to National Starch and Chemical Corporation.* The compounds correspond to the formula:

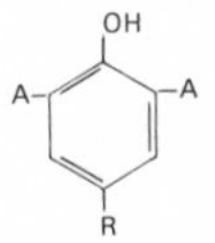

where A is a cyclododecyl radical, and R is methyl or a cyclododecyl radical. Thus, the compounds of this process include 2,4,6-tricyclododecylphenol and 2,6-dicyclododecyl-4-methylphenol.

These cyclododecyl substituted phenols are useful as antioxidants for substrates comprising hydrocarbons and substituted hydrocarbons such as natural and synthetic polymers, rubbers, oils, lubricants, and other compositions where it is desirable to inhibit thermal and oxidative degradation.

These compounds may function as primary antioxidants, i.e., they may be used as the sole antioxidant or, preferably, they may be combined with a secondary antioxidant which serves to enhance the stabilizing performance of the primary antioxidant. When used with a secondary antioxidant, the stabilizing effect achieved is synergistic and the performance substantially exceeds the sum total of the performances exhibited by the individual antioxidant components.

Secondary antioxidants suitable for use in combination with the compounds of this process include dilauryl thiodipropionate; dicetyl sulfide; didodecyl sulfide; bis(tetradecylmercapto)-p-xylylene; bis(octadecylmercapto)-p-xylylene; etc.

The method used to prepare the cyclododecyl substituted phenols may be described as follows. A phenolic reagent, selected from phenol, and 4-methylphenol, is first dissolved in cyclododecene whereupon an acidic catalyst, for example, sulfuric acid, phosphoric acid, aluminum chloride, boron trifluoroetherate, and the like, is added to initiate the reaction. About 2 or 3 mols of cyclododecene per mol of the phenolic reagent is used depending upon whether it is desired to prepare the disubstituted or trisubstituted cyclododecyl reaction product. Ordinarily, a slight excess of 5 to 7% of cyclododecene is used to insure its availability for a complete reaction with the phenolic reagent.

The initial reaction is exothermic and up to this point no external heat is applied to the mixture. However, when the initial exothermic reaction is completed, the mixture is heated to 110° to 160°C for 3 to 5 hours. The reaction need not be conducted in a solvent but such organic solvents as methylene chloride, benzene, chlorobenzenes, nitrobenzenes, alkylbenzenes, alkanes, chlorinated alkanes, and nitrated alkanes, etc. may be utilized in order to facilitate the reaction, if desired.

At the end of the reaction period, the resultant mass containing the crude product is worked up by washing and drying an organic solution of the product as illustrated in the following example.

Example 1: A reaction vessel fitted with a mechanical stirrer, thermometer, water-cooled condenser, and an injection port was charged with a solution of 18.8 parts of phenol dissolved in 140.0 parts of technical grade cyclododecene. At room temperature, 4 parts of boron trifluoride etherate was rapidly admixed with this solution while the latter was being subjected to mechanical agitation. After the initial exotherm had subsided, the reaction mass was heated to 120°C and maintained at this temperature for 4 hours. At the conclusion of this period, the reaction mass was cooled to room temperature and then dissolved in 200 parts of benzene. The benzene solution was washed, in turn, with small protions comprising a total of 100 parts of water, 100 parts of an aqueous 5% sodium bicarbonate solution and, finally, with additional water until the wash water was neutral to litmus.

The resultant benzene solution was then dried over anhydrous sodium sulfate and concentrated under reduced pressure so as to yield a viscous mass which was then crystallized from ethanol to yield a white crystalline solid. This solid was collected by filtration, dried, and recrystallized from ethanol to yield the purified 2,4,6-tris-cyclododecyl phenol having a melting point of 153.5° to 155.5°C.

Example 2: A stabilizer combination which comprised 0.3 parts of 2,4,6-tris-cyclododecyl phenol, prepared as described in Example 1, and 0.3 parts of dilaurylthiodipropionate was dissolved in 45 parts of methylene chloride. The resulting antioxidant solution was added to 100 parts of unstabilized polypropylene pellets and thoroughly blended for 15 minutes. The resulting mix was then milled for 5 minutes on a roller mill maintained at 370°F, to prepare a plastic, homogeneous mass.

Plastic sheets, 25 mils in thickness, were then prepared by pressing the plastic mass between two polished aluminum plates maintained at 350°F. Upon cooling, the plastic sheets were cut into 2 inch squares which were exposed to a degradative atmosphere for 48 hours by being suspended, by means of stainless steel clips, in a thermostatically controlled, forced-air oven which was set at 300°F.

The polypropylene sheets resulting from the above procedure were then compared with unstabilized polypropylene sheets, with polypropylene sheets containing 0.3 parts of dilauryl-thiodipropionate, as well as with polypropylene sheets containing 0.3 parts of 2,4,6-tris-cyclododecyl phenol. All of these sheets also had a thickness of 25 mils and had been prepared and tested in a manner similar to that used for the stabilized sheets described above. In each instance, four specimens of each plastic sheet were evaluated in order to check the reproducibility of the test procedure.

Those polypropylene sheets which contained a blend of 2,4,6-tris-cyclododecyl phenol and dilaurylthiodipropionate exhibited significantly less crazing than the sheets which contained only the 2,4,6-tris-cyclododecyl phenol. The latter samples were, however, far less degraded than the sheets which contained only the dilaurylthiodipropionate while they offered a rather substantial reduction in degradation when compared with the controls which did not contain any stabilizer.

Tetra-Phenol Compounds

Tetra-2,5-disubstituted phenolic derivatives of phthalaldehyde having the following formula are known as antioxidants:

(1)
$$\left[\text{HO} - \underset{Y}{\overset{X}{\bigcirc}} - CH-R-CH - \underset{Y}{\overset{X}{\bigcirc}} - OH \right]_2$$

where R is o-, m- or p-phenylene and X and Y are alkyl groups. *G.D. Brindell and J.P. Wuskell; U.S. Patent 3,796,685; March 12, 1974; assigned to The Quaker Oats Company* have found that the tetra-2,6-disubstituted phenolic derivatives are superior antioxidants. These are compounds having the formula shown on the following page where R_1, R_2, R_3, and R_4 are independently selected from alkyl and aralkyl; and R_5 is o-, m-, or p-phenylene. A process for stabilizing organic material is also disclosed which comprises incorporating the organic material with 0.01 to 10% by weight of a composition of Formula (2).

(2)

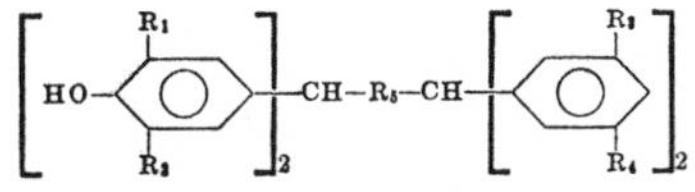

$$\left[\ HO-\langle\bigcirc\rangle\substack{R_1\\\\R_3}-CH-R_4-CH-\right]_2\left[\substack{R_1\\\\R_4}\langle\bigcirc\rangle\ \right]_2$$

Exemplary tetra-2,6-disubstituted phenolic derivatives of phthalaldehyde useful in this process include the following:

α,α,α',α'-tetrakis(4-hydroxy-3,5-dimethylphenyl)xylene
α,α,α',α'-tetrakis(4-hydroxy-3,5-diisopropylphenyl)xylene
α,α,α',α'-tetrakis(4-hydroxy-3,5-di-tert-butylphenyl)xylene
α,α,α',α'-tetrakis[4-hydroxy-3,5-di(p-bromobenzyl)phenyl] xylene
α,α,α',α'-tetrakis[4-hydroxy-3,5-di(p-methylbenzyl)phenyl] xylene

The condensation reaction between phenol and phthalaldehyde is preferably carried out in an inert solvent, for example an alcohol. Ethanol is the preferred solvent since it allows solubility of the reactants and, in many cases, crystallization of the product directly from solution. The reaction is most conveniently carried out at the reflux temperature of the solvent for 0.5 to 24 hours. The reaction is preferably carried out in the presence of a catalyst such as organic acids, inorganic acids, and Friedel-Crafts catalysts. Details of the condensation reaction are shown in Example 1.

Example 1: In a 500 ml 3-neck flask equipped with a stirrer, condenser, nitrogen inlet, and a thermometer, 50 ml of methanol and 20 ml of concentrated sulfuric acid were admixed and cooled to 15°C. Then 6.7 grams of terephthalaldehyde, 42 grams of 2,6-di-tert-butylphenol, and 50 ml of methanol were combined in a beaker and immediately added to the stirred mixture in the flask.

The reaction mixture was then held at 65°C under a nitrogen atmosphere for 5 hours. The reaction mixture was then cooled to room temperature (27°C) and allowed to stand overnight. The product was separated from the reaction mixture by filtration, was triturated with ethanol, washed with water until the water washes were neutral, and dried in an oven at 50°C. The product was identified as α,α,α',α'-tetrakis(4-hydroxy-3,5-di-tert-butylphenyl)-p-xylene, MP between 272° and 281°C.

Example 2: A number of candidate stabilizers were incorporated in 5 mil thick samples of polypropylene film, and the resulting materials evaluated by heat aging the films. In some of the tests where indicated dilaurylthiodipropionate was added as synergist.

In the heat aging test, polypropylene film samples 5 mil in thickness were maintained in an oven at 140°C. Each sample was tested for loss of structural integrity. The number of hours shown in the table are the total elapsed hours before the film cracked or embrittled when flexed. The film was embrittled when it crumbled to a powder. The resulting data are presented in the following table.

Test Number	Compound	Percent by Weight Tetraphenolic Derivative	Percent by Weight Synergist	Oven Hours Cracked	Oven Hours Embrittled
1	- - -	0	0	1	27
2	α,α,α',α'-tetrakis(4-hydroxy-3,5-dimethylphenyl)-p-xylene	0.1	0	31	31
3	α,α,α',α'-tetrakis(4-hydroxy-3,5-dimethylphenyl)-p-xylene plus dilaurylthiodipropionate	0.1	0.3	602	644
4	α,α,α',α'-tetrakis(4-hydroxy-3,6-dimethylphenyl)-p-xylene	0.1	0	30	30
5	α,α,α',α'-tetrakis(4-hydroxy-3,6-dimethylphenyl)-p-xylene plus dilaurylthiodipropionate	0.1	0.3	500	507

In Example 2, a comparison of Test 2 with Test 4 and more particularly of Test 3 with Test 5 shows the unexpected superiority of these tetra-2,6-disubstituted phenolic derivatives over the prior art 2,5-derivatives. The superiority of these compositions as stabilizers for polypropylene is most evident when used in conjunction with a synergist. The complete patent also includes an example of the stabilization of cis-polyisoprene with these tetra-phenols.

SYNERGISTIC PHENOL ANTIOXIDANTS FOR TRICHLOROETHYLENE

It is known to suppress oxidative deterioration of trichloroethylene by adding an inhibitor to the solvent, particularly a phenolic compound, for instance phenol itself, o-cresol, thymol, p-tert-butyl phenol, p-tert-amyl phenol or isoeugenol. When the stabilized solvent is used for the treatment of textile materials it is desirable to keep the concentration of phenolic additives as low as possible because residual odor can be imparted to the textile material by phenols adsorbed thereon from the solvent.

A. Campbell and P. Robinson; U.S. Patent 3,676,507; July 11, 1972; assigned to Imperial Chemical Industries Limited, England have found that a synergistic antioxidant effect can be obtained by adding to trichloroethylene a phenolic compound from each of two distinct classes of phenolic compounds. By working in this way an equivalent antioxidant effect can be obtained with a smaller total concentration of phenolic compounds than using one phenolic compound alone, or alternatively a higher degree of resistance to oxidation can be achieved with the same total concentration of phenolic compounds.

The synergistically co-operative inhibitors comprise a substituted phenol which carries at least one substituent in an ortho position with respect to a hydroxy group and phenol itself or a substituted phenol which carries no substituent in an ortho position with respect to a hydroxy group, the amount of each of the phenols being in the range 0.002 to 1.0% by weight of the trichloroethylene.

In general, it is preferred to employ approximately equal parts by weight of each of the two classes of phenolic compound. Proportions of each class of phenolic compound in the range 0.01 to 0.1%, calculated on the weight of the trichloroethylene, are most suitable.

Example: 180 ml of trichloroethylene with or without additions of phenols, as shown in the following table, and no other stabilizers were placed in a 500 ml conical flask together with 1.5 grams of iron powder. The flask was placed on an electric hot-plate with its vertical axis 4.5 inches from the center of an 80 watt Mazda mercury light bulb suspended vertically with its lower end 2 inches above the level of the top of the hot-plate.

A soxhlet extractor modified to act as a water-separator and give a continuous feedback of refluxing solvent to the flask was fitted to the main neck of the flask and 20 ml of the same trichloroethylene as in the flask were placed in the extractor and covered with 40 ml of distilled water, taking care to avoid any water entering the flask or the feedback arm. A dip-tube for the admission of oxygen to the liquid in the flask was fitted to a side neck.

A flow of oxygen (two bubbles/second) was passed through the solvent and the heat was switched on. When the solvent was refluxing at a steady rate the lamp was switched on and the test was continued for 18 hours. The lamp and heater were then switched off, the flask was allowed to cool and the oxygen flow was stopped. The results of the tests were evaluated by measuring the total chloride ion formed by decomposition of the solvent.

This was done by washing out the condenser with distilled water, adding the washings to the aqueous layer separated from the contents of the soxhlet extractor and titrating the total aqueous phase for chloride ion, then combining the solvent layer from the soxhlet extractor with the solvent in the flask and determining the total chloride ion in the solvent phase by titrating 50 ml of the solvent phase while stirring vigorously with 200 ml of distilled water. The results of the two titrations were combined, a blank figure for any chloride ion found in the distilled water used being subtracted. The results shown in the following table demonstrate the synergistic effect of employing two classes of phenolic compound together as inhibitors.

Inhibitors	Inhibitor Concentration % w/w	Chloride Ion Produced mg
None	- - - -	625
o-Cresol	0.02	12.1
p-Cresol	0.02	9.6
2,4-Dimethyl-6-tert-butyl phenol	0.02	24.9
p-Methoxy phenol	0.02	14.9
p-tert-Amyl phenol	0.02	23.3
o-Cresol+p-cresol	0.01+0.01	7.0
o-Cresol+p-methoxy phenol	0.01+0.01	3.9
o-Cresol+p-tert-amyl phenol	0.01+0.01	4.1
2,4-Dimethyl-6-tert-butyl phenol+p-cresol	0.01+0.01	5.7
2,4-Dimethyl-6-tert-butyl phenol+p-methoxy phenol	0.01+0.01	6.0
2,4-Dimethyl-6-tert-butyl phenol+p-tert-amyl phenol	0.01+0.01	7.7

SULFUR-CONTAINING PHENOLIC ANTIOXIDANTS

PHENOL SULFIDES

Hydroxymethyl Methylthiophenols

Substituted thiophenols are disclosed by *M.E. Cisney; U.S. Patent 3,699,172; October 17, 1972; assigned to Crown Zellerbach Corporation* which have use as antioxidants for organic materials, such as polymers, oils, rubber, fats and the like. In particular, polymerizable ethylenically unsaturated monomers are subject to degradation by oxygen. Polymers made from these monomers also are subject to degradation by oxygen so that antioxidant compounds are useful in this context. It is believed that these antioxidants absorb oxygen to react with sulfur atoms to result in formation of polymeric sulfoxides or sulfones. These phenols have the formula:

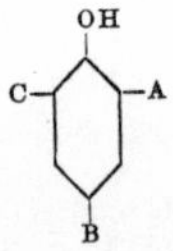

where A is a hydroxyalkyl having 1 to 3 carbons, B is alkylthio having 1 to 12 carbons and C is hydrogen or alkyl up to 12 carbons. These compounds are prepared by reacting alkylthiophenols with an aldehyde.

The preferred phenolic moiety used in forming these compounds is ortho-cresol. However, phenol itself may be used providing opportunities for greater molar amounts of aldehyde to react. That is, para-alkylthiophenol may be reacted with 2 mols of formaldehyde to form dimethylolalkylthiophenol. Other phenolic moieties that may be used are described in U.S. Patent 3,133,971 which covers the preparation of the starting phenol alkyl sulfide by decomposition of hydroxyaryl sulfonium chlorides.

The hydroxyalkyl group (A) in the above formula is derived from any reactive alkylaldehyde. That is, any alkylaldehyde may be used so long as the length of the alkyl chain does not affect the reactivity of the aldehyde. In practice, it is preferred to use formaldehyde, acetaldehyde, propionaldehyde or butyraldehyde in the reaction. Accordingly, alkylol group (A) in the formula is preferably up to 4 carbons in length. The following example gives the conditions for the preparation of these compounds.

Example: The reaction of formaldehyde with 4-methylthio-ortho-cresol takes place readily under alkaline catalysis and is essentially complete in 1 hour at a reaction temperature of 60° to 70°C. 1 mol (154 grams) of 4-methylthio-ortho-cresol was placed in 1 liter flask equipped with a nitrogen sweep and a condenser. 1 mol of sodium hydroxide was added as 400 grams of 10% aqueous NaOH. 1.5 mols formaldehyde was added as 125 ml of 36% formalin.

A nitrogen atmosphere was provided and the solution heated to about 50°C, whereupon the exothermic reaction raised the temperature further to 68° to 70°C. This occurred during the first 15 minutes. The temperature was allowed to fall to 60°C during the next hour. After a total heating time of 1 to 1¼ hours, the solution was cooled to room temperature, poured into about an equal volume of water and acidified with dilute hydrochloric acid to a pH of 9.5. The crude product was filtered, washed with water and dried to give 169 grams of light tan crystals, melting at 82° to 84°C. This represents 92% of the theoretical yield. Recrystallization of a sample from benzene-petroleum ether gave colorless crystals melting at 84.5° to 86°C. The compound is soluble in acetone, alcohols, benzene, chloroform and ether, and insoluble in carbon tetrachloride, petroleum ether and water.

Hydroxyphenyl Aminomethyl Hydroxybenzyl Sulfides

F.X. O'Shea; U.S. Patent 3,686,312; August 22, 1972; assigned to Uniroyal, Inc. has prepared a series of compounds which are useful as antioxidants for rubber, plastics, fats, petroleum products and other organic materials normally subject to oxidative deterioration. These compounds may be represented by the formula:

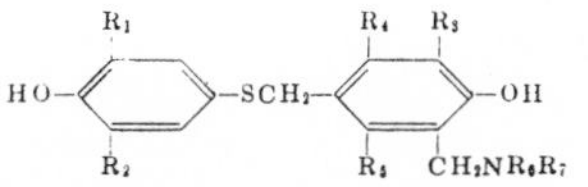

in which R_1, R_2 and R_3 may be alkyl groups of up to 12 carbons each, cycloalkyl groups of 6 to 8 carbons each or aralkyl groups of 7 to 9 carbons each, and R_2 may also be hydrogen, R_4 and R_5 may be hydrogen or methyl and R_6 and R_7 may be alkyl groups of up to 5 carbons each. In U.S. Patent 3,179,701, A.L. Rocklin described antioxidant compounds of the formula:

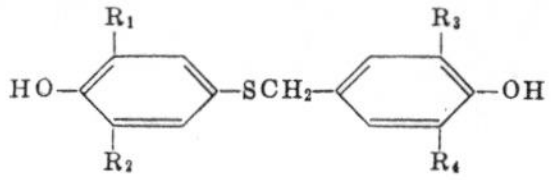

in which R_1, R_2, R_3 and R_4 are alkyl groups of up to 8 carbons each. The compounds of this process differ from the compounds described by Rocklin in that one of the groups on the benzyl portion of the molecule is a dimethylaminomethyl group rather than an alkyl group. This structural difference provides an unexpected and important advantage over the known compounds. This advantage is one of superior nondiscoloring properties while maintaining high activity.

These compounds are prepared by the reaction of a 3-hydrocarbyl-4-hydroxy-5-(dimethylaminoethyl)benzyl N,N-dimethyldithiocarbamate with a 4-mercaptophenol under alkaline conditions according to the following equation:

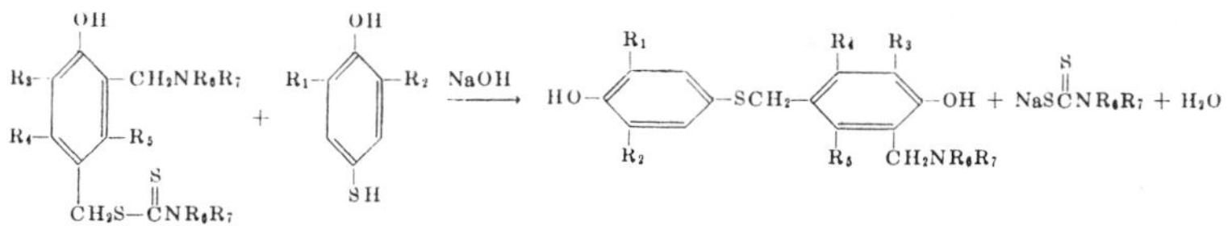

Preferred solvents for the reaction are methanol, ethanol and isopropanol. The preferred temperature is 50° to 100°C, the reaction ordinarily being carried out at or near the reflux temperature of the solution. The preferred time of the reaction is up to 4 hours. Longer times may be used but are not necessary, the reaction generally being complete in 30 minutes or less.

The reaction may also be carried out in a two-phase system such as benzene-water, xylene-water, etc. using good agitation. Although longer reaction times are generally used than in homogeneous solution, this heterogeneous system has the advantage of providing a simplified workup procedure. In such a two-phase system, the product is soluble in the organic phase which can be readily separated from the aqueous phase containing the alkali metal dialkyldithiocarbamate. The product is then obtained by removing the solvent from the organic phase. The following examples illustrate the preparation and testing of these compounds.

Example 1: To a solution of 9.8 grams (0.05 mol) of 2-methyl-4-mercapto-6-tert-butyl-phenol and 4.8 grams (0.06 mol) of 50% aqueous sodium hydroxide in 50 ml of ethanol was added 17 grams (0.05 mol) of 3-tert-butyl-4-hydroxy-5-(dimethylaminomethyl)benzyl N,N-dimethyldithiocarbamate. The solution was heated near reflux for about 15 minutes. It was then poured into water and the product which separated was extracted with ether. The ether extract was dried with anhydrous sodium sulfate and evaporated to an oily residue which was crystallized from hexane to yield 12.5 grams (60%) of 3-methyl-4-hydroxy-5-tert-butylphenyl 3-tert-butyl-4-hydroxy-5-(dimethylaminomethyl)benzyl sulfide, MP 82° to 84°C. Recrystallization from hexane raised the melting point to 83° to 85°C.

Example 2: A commercial cis-polyisoprene synthetic rubber containing 2,6-di-tert-butyl-p-cresol as a stabilizer was used as the base polymer. The polymer was dissolved in benzene to provide a 2% polymer solution. An aliquot portion of a benzene solution of the compound to be evaluated was added so as to provide 1% by weight of the additive based upon the weight of polymer in the solution. A thin film of rubber was then deposited on a sodium chloride disk by evaporating 10 drops of the solution on the 1" diameter disk.

The disks were then placed in a 130°C oven and removed after 30 minutes, 1 hour and ev every hour thereafter. At each interval, the infrared spectrum of the polymer film was obtained. Oxidation of the polymer film is evidenced by the appearance of a band at 5.85μ in the spectrum caused by the development of carbonyl groups in the polymer. The time of aging required for the appearance of this band in the spectrum is taken as the break time. The effectiveness of compounds as stabilizers can be evaluated by the length of time they protect the rubber against oxidation as determined by this carbonyl development test. The use of infrared spectrophotometry in following the oxidation of polymer films has been described by Bishop [*Anal. Chem.,* 33, 456 (1961)].

Added Stabilizer	Hours to Break
(1) None	½
(2) 3-Methyl-4-hydroxy-5-tert-butylbenzyl 3-methyl-4-hydroxy-5-tert-butylphenyl sulfide	4
(3) 3,5-Di-tert-butyl-4-hydroxybenzyl 3-methyl-4-hydroxy-5-tert-butylphenyl sulfide	4
(4) 3-tert-Butyl-4-hydroxy-5-(dimethylamino-ethyl)benzyl 3-methyl-4-hydroxy-5-tert-butylphenyl sulfide	9
(5) 3-Cyclohexyl-4-hydroxy-5-(dimethylamino-ethyl)benzyl 3-methyl-4-hydroxy-5-tert-butylphenyl sulfide	10

These results demonstrate the effectiveness of compounds of this process [(4) and (5)] as stabilizers and show their advantage over compounds of the prior art [(2) and (3)]. Additional tests also showed color stabilization by the compounds included in this process.

1,2-Bis[3-Alkyl-4-Hydroxy-5-(Dialkylaminomethyl)Phenylthio] Ethanes

A related series of antioxidants was also prepared by *F.X. O'Shea; U.S. Patent 3,686,313; August 22, 1972; assigned to Uniroyal, Inc.* These compounds contain two benzyl moieties having the dialkylaminomethyl group and may be represented by the formula:

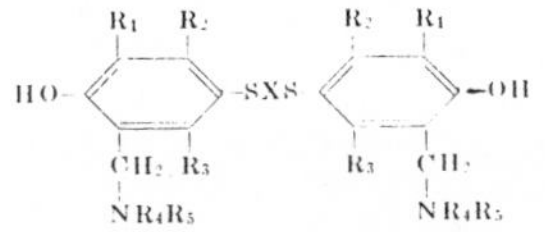

where R_1 may be an alkyl group of up to 12 carbons, a cycloalkyl group of from 6 to 8 carbons or an aralkyl group of from 7 to 9 carbons, R_2 and R_3 are hydrogen or methyl, R_4 and R_5 are alkyl groups of up to 5 carbons or R_4 and R_5 may be joined to form with the nitrogen atom, a radical selected from morpholinyl, pyrrolidinyl and piperidinyl, and X is diradical containing from 2 to 14 carbons and is selected from a wide variety of polymethylene, branched polyalkylene, aralkyl diradicals, etc. These compounds are prepared by the reaction of 1 molar equivalent of:

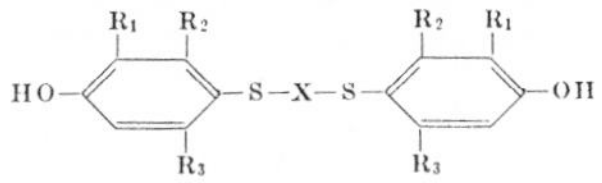

with 2 molar equivalents of formaldehyde and 2 molar equivalents of a dialkylamine of the formula, R_4R_5NH, where R_1, R_2, R_3, R_4, R_5 and x are as previously described. This Mannich type reaction is carried out under the usual conditions for this reaction. The amines which may be used to prepare the Mannich base (dialkylamine) include dimethylamine, methylethylamine, diethylamine, dipropylamine, dibutylamine, diamylamine, morpholine, pyrollidine and piperidine. The intermediate bis-phenol may be prepared by one of two general methods. The first involves the reaction of two molar equivalents of a mercaptophenol with two molar equivalents of an alkali metal hydroxide and one molar equivalent of an organic dihalide of the formula: Hal—X—Hal in which Hal represented a halogen atom and X is as previously described.

The second method involves the reaction of two molar equivalents of a mercaptophenol with one molar equivalent of a nonconjugated diolefin of from 5 to 30 carbons, under acid catalysis. This reaction may be carried out without a solvent or in a nonpolar organic solvent such as hexane, benzene, xylene, etc. at a temperature up to about 150°C. The acid catalyst which may be employed includes mineral acids such as sulfuric acid, Lewis acids such as $AlCl_3$ and BF_3, and heterogenous catalysts such as acid clays and acidic ion exchange resins.

Example 1: To a solution of 28 grams (0.2 mol) of 2-methyl-4-mercaptophenol and 16 grams (0.2 mol) of 50% aqueous sodium hydroxide in 150 ml of ethanol was added 10 grams (0.1 mol) of ethylene dichloride. The solution was heated gently for 10 minutes near reflux. The solution was then cooled and poured into water. The oil which separated was extracted with ether and the ether extract was dried with anhydrous sodium sulfate and evaporated down to an oil which crystallized. The product was triturated with a benzene-hexane mixture and filtered yielding 24.5 grams (80%) of 1,2-bis(3-methyl-4-hydroxyphenylthio)ethane, MP 93° to 96°C. The melting point was raised to 96° to 98°C by recrystallization from benzene.

To a solution of 30.6 grams (0.1 mol) of 1,2-bis(3-methyl-4-hydroxyphenylthio)ethane and 50 grams (0.22 mol) of 45% aqueous dimethylamine in ethanol was added 18 grams (0.22 mol) of 37% aqueous formaldehyde. The solution was then heated slowly to reflux and refluxed for 3 hours. The solution was then cooked and a crystalline precipitate formed.

It was filtered off, washed with aqueous ethanol and dried to give 37 grams (88% yield) of 1,2-bis[3-methyl-4-hydroxy-5-(dimethylaminomethyl)phenylthio]ethane, MP 93° to 95°C after recrystallization from hexane.

Example 2: A hexane solution of a commercial ethylene-propylene-dicyclopentadiene terpolymer containing no stabilizer was used as the base polymer. The solution was diluted with hexane to provide a 4% polymer solution. An aliquot portion of a benzene solution of the compound to be evaluated was added to provide 1% by weight of the additive based upon the weight of the polymer in the solution. A thin film of rubber was then deposited on a sodium chloride disk by evaporating five drops of the solution on the 1" diameter disk.

The disks were then placed in a 150°C oven and removed after 1 hour and every hour thereafter. At each interval, the infrared spectrum of the polymer film was obtained. Oxidation of the polymer film is evidenced by the appearance of a band at 5.85μ in the spectrum caused by the development of carbonyl groups in the polymer. The time of aging required by the appearance of this band in the spectrum is taken as the break time. The effectiveness of compounds as stabilizers can be evaluated by the length of time they protect the rubber against oxidation as determined by this carbonyl development test. The use of infrared spectrophotometry in following the oxidation of polymer films has been described by Bishop [*Anal. Chem.,* 33, 456 (1961)].

Added Stabilizer	Hours to Break
(1) None	2
(2) Bis(3-methyl-4-hydroxyphenylthio)-ethane	6
(3) Bis(3-tert-butyl-4-hydroxyphenylthio)-ethane	8
(4) Bis[3-methyl-4-hydroxy-5-(dimethylamino-ethyl)phenylthio]ethane	12
(5) Bis[3-tert-butyl-4-hydroxy-5-(dimethylamino-ethyl)phenylthio]ethane	12

The results demonstrate the value of the compounds of this process [(4) and (5)] as stabilizers compared to compounds representative of the prior art [(2) and (3)]. These compounds also gave improved nondiscoloring stabilization of the terpolymer elastomer.

HYDROXYPHENYLALKYL SULFIDES

Four disclosures have been made by J. Song on a series of antioxidants based on derivatives of hydroxyphenylmethyl sulfides. Similar compounds have also been prepared by Zaweski at Ethyl Corporation.

Hydroxybenzyl Sulfides

In the first disclosure by *J. Song; U.S. Patent 3,660,352; May 2, 1972; assigned to American Cyanamid Co.,* the antioxidants are based on the formula:

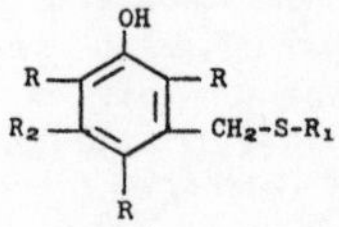

where each R is independently a lower alkyl group, R_1 is higher alkyl or higher alkylbenzyl, R_2 is hydrogen or the group $-CH_2SR_1$. These compounds are effective antioxidants for organic materials normally subject to oxidative deterioration, especially polyolefins.

It was found that phenol sulfides in which the sulfide group is oriented meta to a phenolic hydroxyl group and in which the positions ortho and para to the hydroxyl group are completely substituted exhibit a high degree of antioxidant activity for protection of oxidizable organic substrates and that the antioxidant protection is provided without any substantial discoloration of the substrate.

It is surprising that the compounds of the formula are as effective as they are since phenols having alkylthiomethyl groups in the ortho or para position generally discolor the substrate upon aging and afford a very low level of antioxidant protection as shown in the accompanying examples.

These compounds are prepared by the reaction of an appropriate higher alkyl (especially those of 8 to 18 carbons) or higher alkylbenzyl mercaptan with a meta-positioned chloromethyl group on a phenol which is completely substituted by lower alkyl groups in all ortho and para positions, in the presence of a basic material. The equivalent phenol esters (e.g., the acetate) may be used in place of the phenol. The chloromethyl group is introduced into the meta position of the substituted phenol (or phenol acetate) by reaction with HCl and formaldehyde or methylal in the presence of HCl and H_2SO_4, according to the procedure of R. Wegler and E. Regel, *Makromol. Chem.* 9, 1 (1952).

Suitable substituted phenols (or their equivalent acetates) include 2-tert-butyl-6-methyl-p-cresol, 2,4,6-trimethylphenol, 2-methyl-6-isopropyl-p-cresol, 2-sec-butyl-6-methyl-p-cresol, 2-cyclohexyl-6-methyl-p-cresol. Suitable higher alkyl or higher alkylbenzyl mercaptans include octyl mercaptan, decyl mercaptan, tetradecyl mercaptan, hexadecyl mercaptan, octadecyl mercaptan, and dodecylbenzyl mercaptan, and the like.

The reaction of the mercaptan with the chloromethyl compound is conducted in the presence of a base and usually in the presence of a solvent. Tertiary amines such as trimethylamine or triethylamine are useful bases. Others include sodium methylate or sodium ethylate. The solvent can be methanol, ethanol, tetrahydrofuran, ether, dimethylformamide and the like. The reaction temperature and time are not especially critical. The reaction can be accomplished in the temperature range of from room temperature to 100°C for from 4 to 24 hours, depending on the particular compound being synthesized. The following examples illustrate the preparation and use of these sulfides.

Example 1: A mixture of 11.5 grams (0.05 mol) of 6-tert-butyl-3-chloromethyl-2,4-dimethylphenol, 12.5 grams (0.066 mol) of tetradecylmercaptan, and 12.24 grams (0.12 mol) of trimethylamine in 76 ml of tetrahydrofuran was heated at 62° to 71°C for 11 hours. The mixture was cooled and added to 200 grams of ice. The oil which separated was purified by chromatography on alumina with hexane-chloroform (2:1) as the eluant. The structure of 6-tert-butyl-2,4-dimethyl-3-(tetradecylthiomethyl)phenol was confirmed by elemental analysis and by infrared and NMR spectroscopy.

Example 2: The following compounds were tested at 0.2% concentration for antioxidant activity in polypropylene using the oven aging test on page 1. The test compounds with identifying numbers referred to in the following table are as follows:

(1) 6-tert-butyl-2,4-dimethyl-3-(tetradecylthiomethyl)phenol
(2) 6-tert-butyl-2,4-dimethyl-3-(octadecylthiomethyl)phenol
(3) 3,5-bis(dodecylthiomethyl)-2,4,6-trimethylphenol
(4) 3,5-bis(tetradecylthiomethyl)-2,4,6-trimethylphenol
(5) 3,5-bis(octadecylthiomethyl)-2,4,6-trimethylphenol
(6) 6-tert-butyl-3-(p-dodecylbenzylthiomethyl)-2,4-dimethyl-phenol
(7) 2,6-di-tert-butyl-4-(p-nonylphenylthiomethyl)phenol
(control compound not included in this process)

Compound	Hours to Brittle Point at 140°C
None	0 - 4
1	260 - 270
2	620 - 640
3	1,180 - 1,200
4	1,118 - 1,128
5	1,234 - 1,244
6	620 - 630
7	10 - 15*

*Test sample was yellow at outset of brittle point test.

An example in the original patent also describes stabilization of ABS resins with these sulfides.

Hydrocarbon Bridged Thiomethylenephenols

The second series of antioxidants prepared by *J. Song; U.S. Patent 3,704,326; Nov. 28, 1972; assigned to American Cyanamid Company* are defined by the formula:

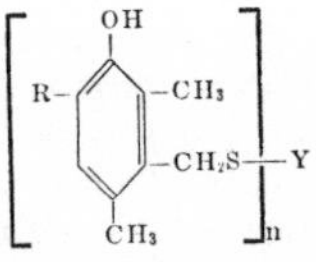

in which R is a branched-chain alkyl of 3 to 12 carbons, Y is a divalent or trivalent hydrocarbon radical of 2 to 18–20 carbons and n is 2 or 3. In all of these compounds the thiomethylene radical is also meta to the hydroxyl group as in U.S. Patent 3,660,352. The preferred compounds are those of the above formula in which n is 2 and Y is a straight-chain or branched-chain alkylene of 2 to 12 carbons or a mononuclear aromatic radical of the following formula:

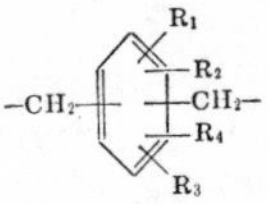

in which R_1, R_2, R_3 and R_4 are hydrogen or lower alkyl radicals, preferably of 1 to 3 carbons. These compounds are also prepared from the corresponding alkylphenols having a chloromethyl substituent meta to the hydroxyl group.

The 3-chloromethyl-2,4-dimethyl-6-secondary or tertiary alkylphenol, may be reacted with a hydrocarbon of 2 to 20 carbons containing two mercaptomethylene groups such as an alkyl dithiol of 2 to 12 carbons, a xylene dimercaptan such as α-α'-dimercapto-p-xylene, 1,4-dimercaptomethyldurene and the like or three mercaptomethylene groups as in mesitylene trimercaptan by a condensation reaction.

The reactions between these reagents are carried out in the presence of acid acceptors such as an alkali metal carbonate or alkoxide and preferably in a solvent or solvent mixture such as tertiary butanol, dimethylformamide or methyl isobutylketone. Reaction temperatures are not critical and may vary from room temperature to the boiling point of the mixture when reflux conditions are used. The desired reaction products may be purified by recrystallization and may be further purified by chromatography on aluminum oxide if desired.

These compounds are especially useful as antioxidants for polyolefins (e.g., homopolymers or copolymers of mono α-olefins of 2 to 6 carbons) in which they exhibit a high degree of activity and are nondiscoloring. The compounds can be similarly used in other organic material normally subject to oxidative deterioration, including ABS resins (acrylonitrile-butadiene-styrene copolymers), the polyamides, polyacetals (e.g., polyformaldehyde), polystyrene, impact polystyrene, natural rubber and the various synthetic rubbers including ethylene-propylene copolymer rubbers, and in oils, fats, greases, gasoline and the like. The following examples illustrate the preparation and antioxidant properties of these compounds.

Example 1: A mixture of 33.97 grams (0.15 mol) of 4-tert-butyl-3-hydroxy-2,6-dimethylbenzylchloride, 7.05 grams (0.075 mol) of 1,2-ethane dithiol and 60.72 grams (0.60 mol) of triethylamine in 225 ml of tetrahydrofuran was heated at 60° to 62°C for a period of 19 hours. The triethylamine hydrochloride was collected. The filtrate was concentrated to 150 ml and diluted with 250 ml of benzene. The benzene solution was washed with dilute hydrochloric acid, water and dried over anhydrous sodium sulfate. The salt was removed and the filtrate concentrated to give a mass (11.85 grams) of tan crystals, MP 125° to 128°C.

A recrystallization from benzene-hexane (1:1) mixture gave 8.6 grams of cream colored crystals, MP 131° to 133°C. An analytical specimen was obtained after chromatography of this material on aluminum oxide using benzene-chloroform (1:2) mixture as eluant. The colorless crystals of 3,3'-[ethylenebis(thiomethylene)]bis(6-tert-butyl-2,4-dimethylphenol) melted at 143° to 144°C.

Example 2: The following compounds prepared by this process were incorporated into unstabilized polypropylene in amounts of 0.2% of the weight of the polymer on:

    (1) 3,3'-[ethylenebis(thiomethylene)]bis(6-tert-butyl-2,4-dimethylphenol)
    (2) 3,3'-[tetramethylenebis(thiomethylene)]bis(6-tert-butyl-2,4-dimethylphenol)
    (3) 3,3'-[hexamethylenebis(thiomethylene)]bis(6-tert-butyl-2,4-dimethylphenol)
    (4) 3,3'-[ethylethylenebis(thiomethylene)]bis(6-tert-butyl-2,4-dimethylphenol)
    (5) 3,3'-[p-phenylenebis(methylenethiomethylene)]bis(6-tert-butyl-2,4-dimethylphenol)
    (6) 2,4-6-tris⟨[(4-tert-butyl-3-hydroxy-2,6-dimethylbenzyl)thio]methyl⟩mesitylene

by milling at 175° to 180°C. The polypropylene was then compression molded into films 15 to 20 mils in thickness. These were aged in a forced-draft oven at 140°C and the efficiency of the compound as an antioxidant was determined by noting the time in hours to embrittlement at this temperature. The results are shown in the following table.

Compound	Hours to Brittle Point
None	2 – 4
1	230 – 235
2	310 – 320
3	490 – 500
4	370 – 380
5	550 – 560
6	240 – 250

These results indicate that the effectiveness of these compounds as antioxidants increases when the molecular weight of the bridging hydrocarbon becomes a larger proportion of the total molecular weight of the compound. This is quite surprising, since the phenolic portions of the molecule are usually considered to be responsible for the antioxidant action.

Polycarboxylic Acid Bridged Thiomethylenephenols

The third series of antioxidants disclosed by *J. Song; U.S. Patent 3,810,929; May 14, 1974; assigned to American Cyanamid Company* have the following formula.

$$
\left[
\begin{array}{c}
\text{OH} \\
R\text{—}\underset{CH_3}{\overset{}{\bigcirc}}\text{—}CH_3 \\
\text{—}CH_3S\text{—}(CH_2CH_2O)_z\text{—}CO\text{—}
\end{array}
\right]_n \text{—Y}
$$

In the above formula R is a branched-chain alkyl of 3 to 12 carbons, z is zero or 1, n is a whole number from 2 to 4, and Y is the residue of the organic carboxylic acid $Y(COOH)_n$.

Representative branched-chain alkyls that may be present at the 6-position of the phenol are isopropyl, isobutyl, tert-butyl, dimethylpropyl, tert-octyl, 2,2-diethylhexyl, and di- and tripropylene and butylene radicals. Tert-butyl is the preferred substituent. The preferred compounds are those of the above formula in which n is 2 and Y is a straight-chain or branched-chain alkylene or thioalkylene of 2 to 12 carbons or a mononuclear arylene radical of the formula:

$$
\begin{array}{c}
R_1 \\
R_2 \\
\bigcirc \\
R_4 \\
R_3
\end{array}
$$

in which R_1, R_2, R_3 and R_4 are hydrogen or lower alkyls, preferably of 1 to 2 carbons. Representative polycarboxylic acids which contain these radicals, and which may be used in the form of their halides to prepare compounds of the first formula, are succinic acid, glutaric acid, pimelic acid, dimethylglutaric acid, adipic acid, oxalic acid, malonic acid, suberic acid, azelaic acid, diphenic acid, maleic acid, fumaric acid, itaconic acid, sebacic acid, o-phthalic acid, isophthalic acid, terephthalic acid and alkyl-substituted phthalic acids such as methylterephthalic acid, and 2,5-dimethylterephthalic acid, hexahydrophthalic acid, p-phenylenediacetic acid, and the like. The thioldicarboxylic acids of the formula:

$$
HOOC \cdot (CH_2)_n\text{—}S\text{—}(CH_2)_n \cdot COOH
$$

where n is a whole number from 1 to 4 such as thiolpropionic acid are particularly important in preparing antioxidants for polypropylene and other synthetic and natural rubbers.

The 3-chloromethyl-2,4-dimethyl-6-sec- or tert-alkylphenols used as starting material are reacted with 2-mercaptoethanol or they may be converted into the corresponding 3-mercaptomethyl-2,4-dimethyl-6-sec- or tert-alkylphenols by dissolving the chloromethyl compound in tetrahydrofuran, adding at least a molecular equivalent of an acid acceptor such as triethylamine, trimethylamine or anhydrous potassium carbonate and bubbling in hydrogen sulfide until the mercaptan formation is complete.

Reaction between the 3-chloromethyl-2,4-dimethyl-6-alkylphenol and 2-mercaptoethanol is preferably carried out in a mutual solvent such as methyl isobutyl ketone, acetone or the like using a base such as anhydrous potassium carbonate as acceptor for the hydrochloric acid evolved. The reaction is most advantageously carried out under reflux, after which the mixture is cooled, acidified with hydrochloric acid, and the organic layer is separated and washed with water. The solvent is then removed by vacuum distillation, leaving the 2,6-dimethyl-3-hydroxy-6-alkylbenzylthioethanol as an oily residue. From 2 to 4 mols of this material is used to esterify 1 mol of an organic dicarboxylic, tricarboxylic or tetracarboxylic acid, which is preferably reacted in the form of its chloride or other acid halide.

The compounds of this process are especially useful as antioxidants for polyolefins (e.g., homopolymers or copolymers of mono α-olefins of 2 to 6 carbons) in which they exhibit a high degree of activity and are nondiscoloring. The compounds can be similarly used in other organic material normally subject to oxidative deterioration, including ABS resins (acrylonitrile-butadiene-styrene copolymers), the polyamides, polyacetals (e.g., polyformaldehyde), polystyrene, impact polystyrene, natural rubber and the various synthetic rubbers including ethylene-propylene copolymer rubbers, and in oils, fats, greases, gasoline and the like.

Example 1: To a 2 liter 3-necked flask, equipped with a Dean-Stark trap, containing 900 ml of methyl isobutyl ketone was added 189 grams (0.83 mol) of 6-tert-butyl-3-chloromethyl-2,4-dimethylphenol, 65 grams (0.83 mol) of 2-mercaptoethanol, 115 grams (0.83 mol) of anhydrous potassium carbonate and 2 grams (0.012 mol) of potassium iodide. The stirred mixture was heated to reflux until the azeotropic distillation ceased. The mixture was cooled to 50°C and added to 750 ml of 0.61 N hydrochloric acid. The organic layer was separated and washed with four 200 ml portions of water. The solvent was removed by distillation in vacuo to give 217 grams (97%) of an oil residue.

A solution of 15.82 grams (0.20 mol) of terephthaloyl chloride in 30 ml of chloroform was slowly added to a stirred mixture of 33.4 grams (0.125 mol) of the 6-tert-butyl-3-[(2-hydroxyethylthio)methyl]-2,4-dimethylphenol, prepared as described above, and 15.82 grams (0.20 mol) of pyridine in 130 ml of chloroform. The reaction was heated at 35° to 40°C for a period of 17½ hours and cooled. The chloroform solution was washed with four 50 ml portions of water, dried over anhydrous sodium sulfate and concentrated in vacuo to give 44 grams of a tacky residue. Successive recrystallizations from methanol and chloroform, respectively, gave an analytical specimen of bis[2-(4-tert-butyl-3-hydroxy-2,6-dimethylbenzylthio)ethyl]terephthalate, colorless crystals, MP 142° to 145°C.

Example 2: The compounds below were incorporated into unstabilized polypropylene in amounts of 0.2% on the weight of the polymer by milling at 175° to 180°C. The polypropylene was then compression molded into films 15 to 20 mils in thickness. These were aged in a forced-draft oven at 140°C and the efficiency of the compound as an antioxidant was determined by noting the time in hours to embrittlement at this temperature. The results are shown in the following table.

Compound*	Hours of Brittle Point
1	540 – 550
2	390 – 410
3	130 – 140
4	970 – 990
5	2,020 – 2,040
6	1,767 – 1,775
7	1,563 – 1,603

*(1) bis[2-(4-tert-butyl-3-hydroxy-2,6-dimethylbenzylthio)ethyl]terephthalate
(2) bis[4-tert-butyl-3-hydroxy-2,6-dimethylbenzyl)thio]ethyl adipate
(3) tetrakis[2-(4-tert-butyl-3-hydroxy-2,6-dimethylbenzylthio)ethyl]pyromellitate
(4) bis(4-tert-butyl-3-hydroxy-2,6-dimethylbenzyl)-3,3'-thiobis(thioldipropionate)
(5) bis(4-tert-butyl-3-hydroxy-2,6-dimethylbenzyl)dithiolterephthalate
(6) bis[3-hydroxy-4-tert-butyl-2,6-dimethylbenzyl]dithiolisophthalate
(7) bis[3-hydroxy-4-(1,1,3,3-tetramethylbutyl)-2,6-dimethylbenzyl]dithiolterephthalate

1,3,4-Thiadiazole Bridged Thiomethylenephenols

Nonstaining antioxidants have been prepared by *J. Song; U.S. Patent 3,676,449; July 11, 1972; assigned to American Cyanamid Company* by reacting 2 mols of a 3-halomethyl-2,4-dimethyl-6-tert alkylphenol with 1 mol of 2,5-dimercapto-1,3,4-thiadiazole in the presence of an acceptor for the halogen acid evolved. The reaction is preferably carried out in an anhydrous solvent such as methyl ethyl ketone, methyl isobutyl ketone or tetrahydrofuran and at reflux temperatures. The reaction is continued until the product formation is substantially complete, after which the crystalline reaction product is washed with water and dried. It may be further purified by recrystallization from benzene and chloroform. These compounds have the formula:

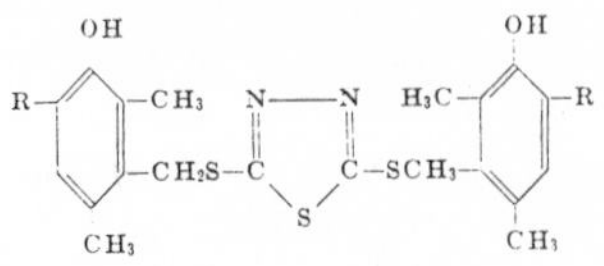

in which R is a tertiary alkyl or 4 to 12 carbons. These compounds are excellent antioxidants for oxygen-sensitive organic materials, particularly polyolefins of 2 to 6 carbons such as polypropylene plastics. The compounds can be similarly used in other organic material normally subject to oxidative deterioration, including ABS resins (acrylonitrile-butadiene-styrene copolymers), the polyamides, polyacetals (e.g., polyformaldehyde), polystyrene, impact polystyrene, natural rubber and the various synthetic rubbers including ethylene-propylene copolymer rubbers, and in oils, fats, greases, gasoline and the like.

Example 1: A mixture of 22.65 grams (0.10 mol) of 3-hydroxy-2,6-dimethyl-4-tert-butyl benzylchloride, 7.51 grams (0.05 mol) of 2,5-dimercapto-1,3,4-thiadiazole, 13.8 grams (0.10 mol) of anhydrous potassium carbonate, and 0.5 gram of potassium iodide in 250 ml of methyl isobutyl ketone was placed in a 500 ml 3-necked round bottom flask with an attached Dean-Stark water trap. The stirred mixture was heated to reflux for a period of 2½ hours.

The reaction was allowed to cool and the crystalline mass was collected, washed with water and dried in-vacuo to give 19.85 grams of crystals, MP 223° to 225°C. An additional quantity of 2 grams of product was isolated from the mother liquor. Recrystallizations from benzene and chloroform gave 1,3,4-thiodiazole-2,5-bis(3,3'-thiomethylene-2,4-dimethyl-6-tert-butylphenol), MP 230° to 232°C.

Example 2: The compound of Example 1 was incorporated into unstabilized polypropylene in an amount of 0.2% on the weight of the polymer by the process of the oven aging test, page 1. The polypropylene film containing the compound of Example 1 withstood heating for 725 to 750 hours before it became brittle while the control film reached its brittle point after only 2 to 4 hours.

Thiodimethylidynetetrakisphenols

Similar compounds, but having bis(hydroxyphenyl)methyl groups attached to the sulfur atom are disclosed by *E.F. Zaweski; U.S. Patent 3,694,357, September 26, 1972; U.S. Patent 3,522,315, July 28, 1970; and U.S. Patent 3,567,682, March 2, 1971; all assigned to Ethyl Corporation.* These thiodimethylidynetetrakisphenols are useful as antioxidants in various organic materials, particularly lubricants, polyolefins and elastomers. Broadly, these antioxidants have the following formula

(1)

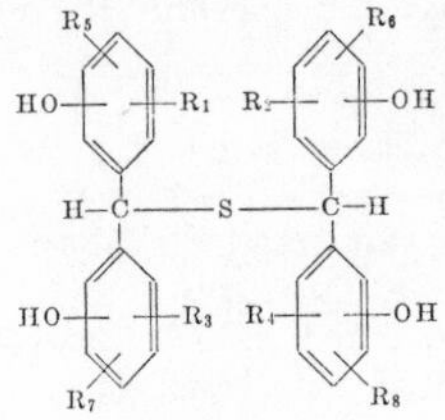

In the formula, R_1, R_2, R_3 and R_4 are C_{1-20} alkyl radicals, C_{6-20} aryl radicals, C_{1-20} aralkyl radicals, or C_{6-20} cycloalkyl radicals, and R_5, R_6, R_7 and R_8 are hydrogen or the same group as R_{1-4}. It is preferred that the thiodimethylidynetetrakisphenols have at least one substituent ortho to each phenolic hydroxyl radical and that each phenolic group be bonded to the methylene bridge at its para position.

It is highly preferred that the phenolic hydroxyl radicals be sterically hindered such as in the following compounds: 4,4',4'',4'''-(thiodimethylidyne)tetrakis(6-tert-butyl-o-cresol), 4,4',4'',4'''-(thiodimethylidyne)tetrakis(2,6-di-sec-butylphenol), 4,4',4'',4'''-(thiodimethylidyne)tetrakis[2,6-di-(α-methylbenzyl)phenol], with 4,4',4'',4'''-(thiodimethylidyne)tetrakis-(2,6-di-tert-butylphenol) being the most preferred. These compounds are made by reacting a hemiquinone selected from compounds having the formulas:

(2)

(3)

where R_1, R_3, R_5 and R_7 are the same as in Formula (1) with hydrogen sulfide at a temperature of from 0° to 250°C. The following example serves to illustrate the methods of making the thiodimethylidynetetrakisphenols. All parts are by weight unless otherwise specified.

Example 1: In a reaction vessel fitted with stirrer and means for introducing hydrogen sulfide was placed 16 parts of 2,6-di-tert-butyl-4-(3,5-di-tert-butyl-4-hydroxybenzylidene)-2,5-cyclohexadiene-1-one and 50 parts of toluene. There was then added 0.5 part of concentrated hydrochloric acid and, while stirring, hydrogen sulfide was bubbled through the solution at room temperature for 3 hours. The solvent was then evaporated off under vacuum, leaving a brown-orange solid. This was recrystallized from isopropanol, yielding 13 parts of 4,4',4'',4'''-thiodimethylidyne)tetrakis(2,6-di-tert-butylphenol) (MP 240° to 243°C), identified by elemental analysis and molecular weight determination.

In U.S. Patent 3,694,357, these antioxidants are used as stabilizers of natural and synthetic lubricants. The lubricant compositions can include the other ingredients normally added to formulated lubricants. For example, mineral oil and synthetic hydrocarbon oil lubricants generally include zinc dialkyldithiophosphates, calcium alkyl sulfonates, overbased calcium sulfonates containing colloidal calcium carbonate, calcium phenates, etc.

Example 2: In a blending vessel is placed 10,000 parts of a lubricant made by esterifying trimethylolpropane with a mixture of C and C_8 n-aliphatic carboxylic acids. Following this, there is added 100 parts of phenyl-α-naphthylamine, 100 parts of 4,4',4'',4'''-(thiodimethylidynetetrakis(2,6-di-tert-butylphenol), 10 parts of 1-salicylalaminoguanadine, 300 parts of tricresyl phosphate, and 0.05 part of dimethyl silicone. The mixture is warmed to 50°C and stirred for 15 minutes. It is then filtered to give a stable synthetic ester lubricant suitable for use in turbines and turbojet engines.

Tests were carried out to demonstrate the effectiveness of these antioxidants in protecting lubricating oils. These were Polyveriform Tests in which a neutral mineral oil containing a copper-lead bearing and lead bromide was heated to 300°F and subjected to air injection for a 48-hour period. Degradation of the oil was shown by increase in acid number and viscosity and also bearing weight loss. Results obtained in this test using an oil containing 1 weight percent 4,4',4'',4'''-(thiodimethylidyne)tetrakis(2,6-di-tert-butylphenol) compared to a nonadditive oil were as follows.

Additive	Bearing Wt Loss, mg	Acid Number Increase	% Viscosity Increase
None	135	17.9	Solid
4,4',4",4'''-(thiodimethylidyne)-tetrakis(2,6-di-tert-butylphenol)	8	8.7	168

In U.S. Patents 3,567,682 and 3,522,315 numerous additional examples were included which illustrated the use of these antioxidants in elastomers (natural rubber, SBR, NBR, ethylene-propylene terpolymer, cis-polybutadiene); polyolefins (polyethylene, polypropylene); ABS resins; foods (coconut oil, lard); and petroleum products (gasoline, diesel fuel, antiknock preparations). The following example will illustrate the use of these antioxidants in polypropylene.

Example 3: Test specimens are prepared by mixing the test stabilizers with polypropylene powder for 3 minutes in a Waring Blendor. The mixture is then molded into a 6" x 6" sheet with a thickness of 0.025" (25 mils). This is accomplished in a molding press at 400°F under 5,000 psi pressure. Each sheet is then cut into ½" to 1" test specimens in order to obtain the five replicate samples. These samples are then subjected to the Oven Aging Tests.

Additive	Conc, wt %	Sample Thickness, mil	Hours to Failure
None		25	2.5
4,4',4",4'''-(thiodimethylidyne)tetrakis-(2,6-di-tert-butylphenol)	⌈0.1 ⌊0.3	25 25	40 88

ESTERS OF SULFUR-CONTAINING HYDROXYPHENYLALKANOIC ACIDS

A broad series of sulfur-substituted phenolic acid ester antioxidants are disclosed by *I.A. Hechenbleikner, J.F. Hussar, A.F. Koeniger and R.E. Bresser; U.S. Patent 3,699,152; October 17, 1972; assigned to Carlisle Chemical Works, Inc.* These compounds have one of the following formulas:

(1) $HOR_1CH_2S(CH_2)_nCOOR_4$

(2) $HOR_1\overset{\displaystyle R_{14}}{\overset{|}{(CH)}}_yCH_2COOR_2$

(3) $HOR_1C_mH_{2m+1}[S(CH_2)_nCOOR_3]_2$

(4) $(HOR_1CH_2)_2C(COOR_2)_2$

(5) $HOR_1CH_2O(CH_2)_nCOOR_2$

(6) $HOR_1CH_2OCH_2CH_2OOCCH_2CH_2S(CH_2)_nCOOR_3$

(7) $HOR_1CH_2CH(COOR_2)_2$

(8) $HOR_1CH=C\begin{smallmatrix}\diagup COOR_2 \\ \diagdown COOR_2\end{smallmatrix}$

where HOR_1 is:

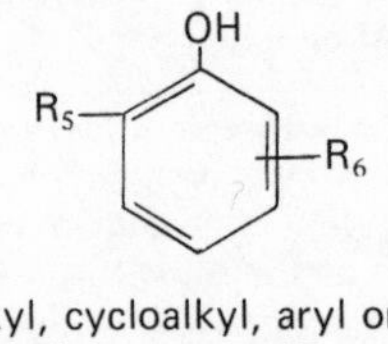

where R_5 and R_6 are hydrogen, alkyl, cycloalkyl, aryl or aralkyl, the total carbons in R_5 and R_6 is between 4 and 36, preferably not over 12, and R_6 is preferably in the ortho position.

R_2 is $-CH_2(C_nH_{2n})S(C_nH_{2n-1})COOR_3$ $CH_2S(CH_2)_nCOOR_3$
                              R_{15} $CH_2CHS(CH_2)_nCOOR_3$

or $\overset{\displaystyle C_nH_{2n-1}}{CH_2C}(CH_2OCH_2CH_2CH_2S(CH_2)_nCOOR_3)_2$

R_3 is hydrocarbyl preferably alkyl or alkenyl, e.g., of 1 to 18 carbons, R_{14} is hydrogen or $COOR_2$, R_{15} is hydrogen or lower alkyl, n is 1 or 2, m is 1, 2, 3 or 4, y is 0 or 1, and R_4 is either R_2 or R_3.

The compounds of Formula (1) are prepared by reacting HOR_1CH_2SH with $CH_2=CHCOOR_4$ or by reacting $HOR_1CH_2SCH_2CH_2COOCH_2CH=CH_2$ with $R_3OOC(CH_2)_nSH$. The compounds of Formula (2) can be prepared reacting:

$$HOR_1(CH_2)_nCOOCH_2\overset{\displaystyle C_nH_{2n+1}}{C}-(CH_2OCH_2CH=CH_2)_2$$

with $R_3OOC(CH_2)_nSH$. The compounds of Formula (3) can be prepared by reacting:

$$HOR_1\overset{\overset{\displaystyle R_2}{|}}{C}H\overset{\overset{\displaystyle R_3}{|}}{C}H\underset{\underset{\displaystyle O}{\|}}{C}R_{10}$$

where R_{10} is lower alkyl with $R_3OOC(CH_2)_nSH$ or by reacting HOR_1CHO with $R_3OOC(CH_2)_nSH$. The compounds of Formula (4) are prepared by reacting:

$$(HOR_1CH_2)_2C\overset{\displaystyle COOCH_2-CH=CH_2}{\underset{\displaystyle COOCH_2-CH=CH_2}{<}}$$

prepared by the procedure of Belgian Patent 710,873 or French Patent 1,536,020 with $R_3OOC(CH_2)_nSH$. The compounds of Formula (5) are prepared by reacting HOR_1CH_2Cl with allyl glycolate or allyl hydroxypropionate and then with a hydrocarbyl mercaptoacetate or mercaptopropionate. The compounds of Formula (6) can be prepared by reacting HOR_1CH_2Cl with hydroxyethyl acrylate and then with a hydrocarbyl mercaptoacetate or mercaptopropionate. The compounds of Formula (7) can be prepared by reacting HOR_1CH_2Cl or:

$$HOR_1CH_2N\overset{\displaystyle R_{11}}{\underset{\displaystyle R_{12}}{<}}$$

where R_{11} and R_{12} are alkyl with $HCH(COOR_2)_2$. The compounds of Formula (8) are prepared by reacting a compound HOR_1CHO with $HCH(COOR_2)_2$.

These compounds are primarily useful as anitoxidants and stabilizers for hydrocarbon resins and elastomers but are also useful with any resin requiring stabilization against atmospheric exposure. Thus, they can also be used with halogen-containing resins. As the halogen-containing resins there can be used resins made from vinylidene compounds such as vinyl chloride, vinylidene chloride, vinyl chloroacetate, chlorostyrenes, vinyl bromide and chlorobutadienes.

The compounds are employed usually in an amount of 0.1 to 10% by weight of the polymer they are intended to stabilize. The following examples show the preparation of only a limited number of the compounds covered by the disclosure.

Example 1: A mixture of 26.33 parts of N,N-dimethyl-3,5-di-tert-butyl-4-hydroxybenzyl-amine, 50.87 parts of methylene bis(butyl-3-thiopropoxycarbopropionate), 75 parts of toluene and 1 part of magnesium methylate was heated to reflux in an inert atmosphere for 14 hours. The batch was then worked up by washing with water and dilute hydrochloric acid and the organic layer solvent stripped to yield 2,6-di-tert-butyl-4-[ethylene bis(butyl-3-thiopropoxycarbopropionate)] in an amount of 61 parts (84%) as a viscous amber oil, n_D^{25} 1.5088.

Example 2: An amber liquid was prepared by refluxing 27.6 parts of 1-(3,5-di-tert-butyl-4-hydroxyphenyl)-3-butanone and 54.8 parts of lauryl mercaptopropionate in 150 parts of toluene using 1 part of p-toluenesulfonic acid (PTSA) as a catalyst until the theoretical amount of water was removed. The product was then worked up as in Example 1 to yield 77 parts (95% yield) of 1-(3,5-di-tert-butyl-4-hydroxyphenyl)-3,3-bis(dodecoxycarboethyl-thio)butane as a viscous amber oil, n_D^{25} 1.498.3.

Example 3: 12.4 parts of diallyl bis(3,5-di-tert-butyl-4-hydroxybenzyl)malonate and 6.5 parts of butyl mercaptopropionate were reacted in 100 parts of hexane at reflux using 0.0004 mol azoisobutyronitrile (AIBN) as the catalyst and the solvent removed by distillation. Bis(3,5-di-tert-butyl-4-hydroxybenzyl)bis(butoxycarboethylthiopropyl)malonate was obtained in a yield of 18.7 parts (99%) as an amber liquid.

Examples in the patent also covered the use of these antioxidants specifically in the following materials: polypropylene; natural rubber latex adhesive; carboxylated SBR latex; ethylene/vinyl acetate copolymer adhesive; and polyamide adhesives.

NITROGEN-CONTAINING PHENOLIC DERIVATIVES

DICARBOXYLIC ACID DIAMIDES OF PHENOL AMINES

Numerous diamides of hindered phenolamines have been prepared at the research laboratories of Ciba (or Ciba-Geigy). These are derivatives of dibasic acids and phenolic compounds having an amino nitrogen attached to the phenol nucleus.

Sulfur Bridged Carboxylic Acid Diamides

Antioxidants useful in polymers, particularly polyolefins have been prepared by *H.R. Biland and M. Duennenberger; U.S. Patent 3,676,494; July 11, 1972; assigned to Ciba Limited, Switzerland.* These are carboxylic acid amides of formula

(1)

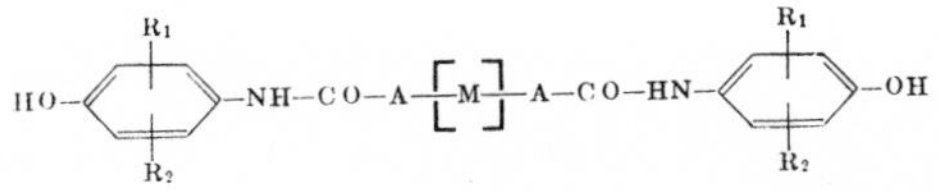

$$HO\!-\!\langle\rangle\!-\!NH\!-\!CO\!-\!A\!-\![M]\!-\!A\!-\!CO\!-\!HN\!-\!\langle\rangle\!-\!OH$$

where M is a divalent bridge of the series $-S\!-\!CH_2\!-\!CH_2\!-\!(O\!-\!CH_2\!-\!CH_2)_p\!-\!S\!-$ and $-S\!-$, $-S\!-\!A\!-\!S\!-$, A denotes an alkylene residue containing 1 to 18 carbons, p is one to three, R_1 is an alkyl group with 1 to 8 carbons and R_2 denotes hydrogen or an alkyl group with 1 to 8 carbons. The total of A member carbons may be 36, preferably no more than 26. Preferably R_1 and R_2 are branched and in the ortho position to the OH group.

These compounds can appropriately be obtained by reacting about two mols of a chlorinated carboxamide of formula

(2)

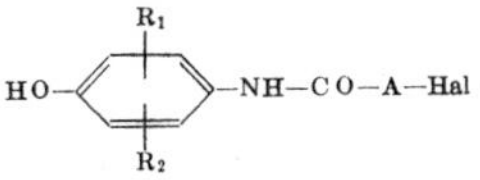

$$HO\!-\!\langle\rangle\!-\!NH\!-\!CO\!-\!A\!-\!Hal$$

with about one mol of a mercaptan of formula

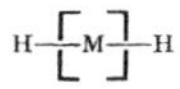

$$H\!-\![M]\!-\!H$$

in the form of its alkali salt, with R_1, R_2, A and M having the abovementioned significance and Hal representing a halogen atom.

The alkali salts of the dithiols can be manufactured in the presence of a solvent by using the alkali metal, or through the use of the stoichiometric amount of an alkali alcoholate. The compounds of formula (2) required as starting substances are obtained by the known reaction of acid halides, preferably acid chlorides of formula Hal—A—CO—Hal with the p-aminophenols.

Example 1: 1.6 grams of crystalline 61% strength sodium sulfide are dissolved in 100 ml of methanol. 7.425 grams of N(3,5-di-tert-butyl-4-hydroxyphenyl)-chloroacetamide, dissolved in 10 ml of methanol, are added. The reaction solution is heated for 30 minutes to reflux temperature and is then mixed with activated charcoal, filtered and concentrated to dryness. Yield of crude product: 6.0 grams (86.5%). The N,N'-bis(3',5'-di-tert-butyl-4'-hydroxyphenyl)-2-thiapropane-1,3-dicarboxamide, recrystallized from methylene chloride/cyclohexane, had a MP of 228° to 229°C.

Example 2: The mercaptide of 1,2-ethanediol is manufactured by introducing 580 mg of sodium into a solution of 1,2-ethanedithiol in 20 ml of absolute alcohol. 7.45 grams of N(3,5-di-tert-butyl-4-hydroxyphenyl)-chloroacetamide, dissolved in 70 ml of absolute ethanol, are added added to this solution. The reaction is then heated to reflux temperature for one hour and subsequently concentrated to dryness in vacuo, and the residue is taken up in methylene chloride and extracted by shaking with water. 4.0 grams of crude N,N'-bis(3',5'-di-tert-butyl-4'-hydroxyphenyl)-2,5-dithiahexane-1,6-dicarboxamide are obtained from the dried methylene chloride extracts. After recrystallizing from acetone/water, the product melted at 200° to 201°C.

Example 3: A mixture of 100 grams of unstabilized polypropylene (Profax 6501, Hercules Powder) and 0.2 gram of a compound according to the table given below is worked into a sheet on a calender at 170°C and subsequently pressed into a one mm thick sheet at 230°C and a pressure of 40 kg/cm². The sheets thus obtained are subjected to an accelerated oxygen aging at 140°C (air, normal pressure). The time which elapses until the first visually perceptible cracks arise is a measure of the antioxidative effect of the added compound.

Added Compound	Time Until Cracks Form, hours at 140°C
Without additive	5
A. Commercially available antioxidants:	
2,6-di-tert-butyl-4-methylphenol	25
Methylene-bis(3-methyl-4-hydroxy-5-tert-butylbenzene)	28
B. Compounds according to process:	
N,N'-bis(3',5'-di-tert-butyl-4'-hydroxyphenyl)-2-thiapropane-1,3-dicarboxamide	850
N,N'-bis(3'5'-di-tert-butyl-4'-hydroxyphenyl)-2,5-dithiahexane-1,6-dicarboxamide	620

The patent also contains examples of these compounds used to stabilize polyethylene and olive oil.

Some of the compounds disclosed in U.S. Patent 3,676,494 are also prepared by *M. Knell and M. Dexter; U.S. Patent 3,694,375; September 26, 1972; U.S. Patent 3,679,744; July 25, 1972; both assigned to Ciba-Geigy Corporation,* using different synthetic routes. The compounds in these disclosures are limited to the following formula

where R_1 is an alkyl group containing 1 to 8 carbons or a cycloalkyl group containing 5 to 12 carbons, R_2 is hydrogen, an alkyl group containing 1 to 8 carbons or a cycloalkyl containing 5 to 12 carbons and m and n are numbers 1 to 10.

Examples of alkyl groups are methyl, ethyl, propyl, isopropyl, butyl, amyl, hexyl, octyl, and the like. Included within designation of alkyl groups are tert-alkyl groups which have been found to be particularly effective and examples of such are tert-butyl, tert-amyl, tert-octyl, and the like. Illustrative cycloalkyl groups include cyclopentyl, cyclohexyl, cyclooctyl, cyclododecyl, and the like.

The thiodialkanoamidophenol compounds are prepared by the reaction between the selected alkylaminophenol and the thiodialkanoyl acid chloride. The reaction is carried out in a solution containing the reacting materials and useful solvents include, for example, acetone, pyridine, dimethylformamide, water, methylethylketone, methylisobutylketone, dioxane, and the like.

Stoichiometric amounts of the reactants are employed and a ratio of at least about 2 mols of the alkylaminophenol to about 1 mol of the acid chloride is used; generally an excess of the aminophenol, that is, an excess up to about 20%, has been found to be particularly useful.

In the reaction, hydrogen chloride is liberated forming the amine hydrochloride and consequently an alkaline material is used to neutralize the hydrogen chloride. Suitable alkaline materials which are used include, for example, sodium or potassium hydroxide, sodium or potassium acetate, sodium or potassium carbonate, sodium or potassium bicarbonate, and the like. Included among the acid chlorides which can be used are illustratively, acid chlorides of thiodiacetic acid, thiodipropionic acid, thiodibutyric acid, and the like.

Example 1: 11.05 grams (0.05 mol) 4-amino-2,6-di-tert-butylphenol are dissolved in acetone and 4.68 grams (0.025 mol) of thiodiacetyl chloride in acetone are added thereto portionwise, over a period of about 10 minutes, accompanied by agitation. It is noted that the reaction is only mildly exothermic. 10 ml of 5N sodium hydroxide is added portionwise, over a period of about 5 to 10 minutes, accompanied by agitation and here too, the reaction is mildly exothermic. The reaction mixture was allowed to stand for two hours, accompanied by occasional agitation. There was then added to the reaction mixture, 200 ml water and a dark oil separated, which solidified on cooling. The solid material was filtered, washed four times with 50 ml cold petroleum ether and then dried in vacuo over paraffin wax.

The product thus obtained was dissolved in 125 ml boiling 80% ethanol, filtered, treated with activated charcoal, filtered and then allowed to crystallize slowly. After cooling the crystals were filtered, washed with 80% ethanol and then air dried. The product was recrystallized from 80% ethanol and air dried. There was obtained a yield of 3.42 grams of the desired product, i.e., N,N'-bis(3',5'-di-tert-butyl-4'-hydroxyphenyl)-2-thiapropane-1,3-dicarboxamide which melted between 227.5° and 228.5°C.

Example 2: Following the procedure described in Example 1 supra, except for the use of 2,6-di-tert-butyl-4-aminophenol and thiodipropionyl chloride, there was obtained N,N'-bis(3',5'-di-tert-butyl-4-hydroxyphenyl)-3-thiapentane-1,5-dicarboxamide.

Example 3: Following the procedure described in Example 1 supra, except for the use of 2-methyl-6-tert-butyl-4-aminophenol and thiodibutyryl chloride, there was obtained N,N'-bis(3'-methyl-5'-tert-butyl-4'-hydroxyphenyl)-4-thiaheptane-1,7-dicarboxamide.

Example 4: The Tests were made following oven aging in a tubular oven, with an air flow of 400 feet per minute at a temperature of 150°C. See page 1. Unstabilized polypropylene powder (Hercules Profax 6501) was blended with 0.5% by weight of N,N'-bis(3',5'-di-tert-butyl-4'-hydroxyphenyl)-2-thiapropane-1,3-dicarboxamide. It was found that on exposure of unstabilized polypropylene the sample failed within three hours. However, the polypropylene containing the N,N'-bis(3',5'-di-tert-butyl-4'-hydroxyphenyl)-2-thiapropane-1,3-dicarboxamide had an oven life of 860 hours. Other examples in the patent illustrate the stabilization of Havea latex crepe and high impact polystyrene.

Bisoxalic Acid Diamides

Antioxidants have also been prepared by *M. Dunnenberger and H.R. Biland; U.S. Patent 3,734,884 and 3,706,798; May 22, 1973; assigned to Ciba-Geigy AG, Switzerland* by reacting an oxalic acid monoamide with an alkylenediamine. These bisoxalic acid diamides correspond to the formula

(1)

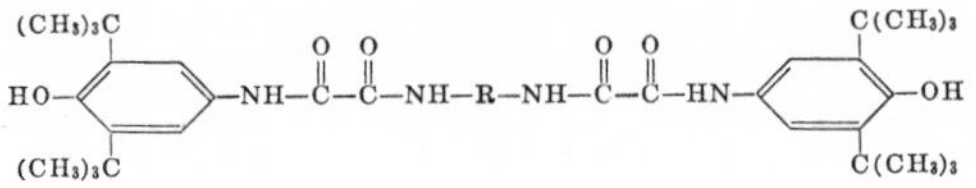

where R is an alkylene radical having 5 to 18 carbons. The alkylene radical R can be branched or, preferably, unbranched. Of particular practical interest, especially as antioxidants for poly-α-olefins, are bisoxalic acid diamides where R has 6 to 8 carbons.

Basically, a compound of the formula

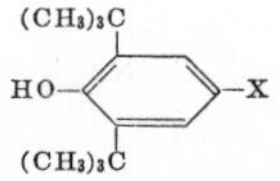

is reacted with a compound of the formula X'—R—X' where X and X' represent either —NH$_2$ or —NH—CO—CO—Y where Y is Cl, OH or an alkoxy having 1 to 12 carbons. R has the above given meaning. X and X' must be different in the two reactants.

These compounds constitute valuable antioxidants, i.e., they are suitable for the stabilization of organic materials to oxidative decomposition, by which is meant, in particular, thermally accelerated oxidations. To be specially emphasized is the excellent antioxidant effect of the above compounds in the case of polymerizate synthetic materials, particularly poly-α-olefins such as polypropylene. Sufficient for a good antioxidant effect is, in general, an amount of 0.01 to 5%, preferably 0.1 to 2% of the compounds, relative to the substrate to be protected.

Example 1: An amount of 6.4 grams of the compound of the formula

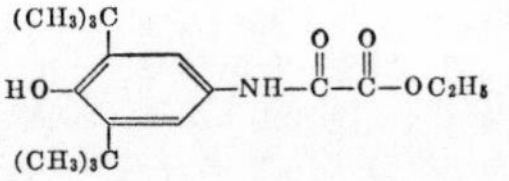

(produced by reaction of 1-amino-3,5-di-tert-butyl-4-hydroxybenzene with oxalic acid monoethyl ester olefride in benzene with pyridine as the HCl-acceptor; MP 139° to 140°C), is refluxed, with stirring, in 60 cc of ethanol with 1.2 grams of 1,6-diaminohexane for 3 hours. The reaction mixture is subsequently cooled to 10°C, whereby the product of the formula

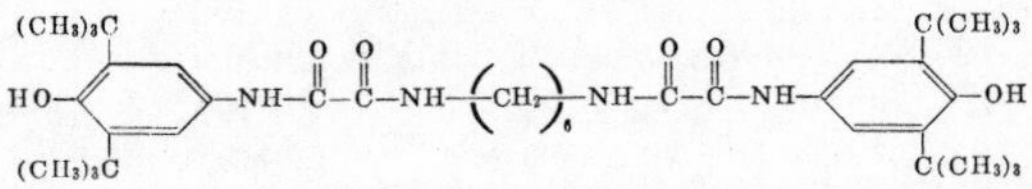

precipitates in the form of colorless crystals. Yield: approximately 7 grams. After recrystallization three times from ethanol, the analytical product melts at 230° to 231°C.

Example 2: A mixture of 100 parts of stabilizer-free polypropylene (Profax 6501, Hercules Powder) and 0.2 part of antioxidant is processed on a calendering machine at 170°C into a soft sheet, and subsequently pressed at 230°C, and under a pressure of 40 kg/cm^2, to form a plate of 1 mm thickness. The plates are subjected at 140°C (air, normal pressure) to an accelerated oxygen aging treatment. The time passing before the appearance of the first cracks detectable with the eye is a measure of the antioxidative effect of the added compound.

TABLE 1

Added Compound	Time Until Cracks Form, hours at 140°C
Without addition	5
Commercial antioxidants:	
2,6-di-tert-butyl-4-methylphenol	25
Methylene-bis(3-methyl-4-hydroxy-5-tert-butylbenzene)	28
Thio-bis(2-methyl-4-hydroxy-5-tert-butylbenzene)	100

TABLE 2

Antioxidant of Formula 1	Time Until Cracks Form, hours at 140°C
R = (CH$_2$)$_6$	2,250
R = (CH$_2$)$_7$	2,250
R = (CH$_2$)$_8$	2,000
R = (CH$_2$)$_{10}$	1,830

N,N'-Bis(3,5-Dialkyl-4-Hydroxyphenyl) Dicarboxamides

A series of bis-amides of adipic and sebacic acid have been prepared and tested as antioxidants by *M. Dexter and M. Knell; U.S. Patent 3,754,031; August 21, 1973; assigned to Ciba-Geigy Corporation.* These antioxidants are represented by the formula

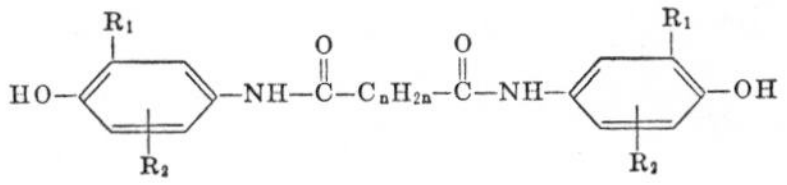

where R$_1$ and R$_2$ are independently lower alkyl groups having from 1 to 6 carbons, and n is 2 to 10.

Examples of alkyl groups are methyl, ethyl, propyl, isopropyl, butyl, sec-butyl, tert-butyl, amyl, tert-amyl, hexyl and the like. The branched alkyl groups have been found to be particularly effective and the preferred groups are tert-alkyl, such as tert-butyl, tert-amyl, and the like. The acyl moiety of the antioxidant compounds are derived from dicarboxylic acids containing 4 to 12 carbon atoms. Illustrative dicarboxylic acids include succinic acid, glutaric acid, adipic acid, pimelic acid, suberic acid, azelaic acid and sebacic acid.

The phenyl acylamide compounds are prepared by reacting an aminophenol and an acyl chloride. The reaction is carried out in a solution containing the reacting materials. The useful solvents include ketones, hydrocarbons and aldehydes. Examples of such solvents are acetone, pyridine, dimethylformamide, water, methyl ethyl ketone, methyl isobutyl ketone, dioxane, and the like.

Stoichiometric amounts of the reactants are used and a ratio of 1 mol of acyl chloride to 4 mols of aminophenyl can be used; a mol ratio of 1:2 has been found to be particularly useful. In the course of the reaction, hydrogen chloride is liberated forming the amine hydrochloride and consequently an alkaline material is used to neutralize the hydrogen chloride. Suitable alkaline materials which are used include, for example, sodium or potassium hydroxide, sodium or potassium acetate, sodium or potassium carbonate, sodium or potassium bicarbonate, and the like. Illustrative examples of acyl chlorides which can be used are acid chlorides of adipic acid, succinic acid, sebacic acid, and the like.

Example 1: 11.05 grams of 2,6-di-tert-butyl-4-aminophenol (prepared by the procedure described in U.S. Patent 3,156,690) is dissolved in 90 ml acetone and 4.57 grams adipoyl chloride in 10 ml acetone is added portionwise thereto. The reaction is mildly exothermic and some solid material separates. Dilute sodium hydroxide (50 ml of 1N) is added portionwise, accompanied by shaking. After the exothermic reaction is ended, 50 ml water is added to the reaction mixture followed by cooling and the mixture is then filtered.

The solid material is washed twice with 50 ml portions of cold petroleum ether to remove most of the red coloration and this is followed by drying. The weight of the product obtained is 8.87 grams; melting point 269° to 272°C. After recrystallization from ethanol, N,N'-bis(3,5-di-tert-butyl-4-hydroxyphenyl)adipamide is obtained in a yield of about 35%; a melting point of 274° to 276°C dec.

Example 2: Following the procedure described in Example 1, except for the use of 2-methyl-6-tert-butyl-4-aminophenol (prepared by the procedure described in U.S. Patent 3,156,690) and sebacoyl acid chloride, N,N'-bis(3-methyl-5-tert-butyl-4-hydroxyphenyl)-sebacamide is obtained.

Example 3: The tests conducted on the following material were made following oven aging in a forced draft oven, at a temperature of 300°F. Unstabilized polypropylene powder (Hercules Profax 6501) was thoroughly blended with 0.5% by weight of N,N'-bis(3,5-di-tert-butyl-4-hydroxyphenyl)adipamide. The blended material was then processed for the oven aging test, see page   , and tested at 300°F. Unstabilized polypropylene began to decompose within three hours. However, under the same conditions, the polypropylene containing the antioxidant showed signs of decomposition only after 205 hours.

Similar results are obtained when N,N'-bis(3-methyl-5-tert-butyl-4-hydroxyphenyl)sebacamide and N,N'-bis(3,5-dimethyl-4-hydroxyphenyl)adipamide are employed in place of the compound used in the above example. Examples are also given in the the patent illustrating the stabilization of Havea crepe and high impact polystyrene.

PHENOL AMIDES

Alkylthioalkanoylaminophenols

The active compounds of the process are obtained by *M. Dexter and M. Knell; U.S. Patent 3,687,892; August 29, 1972; assigned to Ciba-Geigy Corporation and U.S. Patent 3,590,083; June 29, 1971; assigned to Geigy Chemical Corporation* by the reaction of a selected alkylaminophenol with an alkylthioalkanoyl chloride. These antioxidant compounds are used to prevent oxidative deterioration of a wide variety of commercial products such as synthetic polymers, oils, plastics, and the like. These alkylthioalkanoylaminophenols are represented by the formula:

$$HO-\underset{R_2}{\overset{R_1}{\text{C}_6\text{H}_3}}-NH-\overset{\overset{O}{\parallel}}{C}-C_nH_{2n}-S-R_3$$

where R_1 is an alkyl group of one to eight carbons or a cycloalkyl group of five to twelve carbons, R_2 is hydrogen, an alkyl group of one to eight carbons or a cycloalkyl group of five to twelve carbons, R_3 is an alkyl group of four to 24 carbons, and n is 1 to 3.

In a preferred embodiment R_1 and R_2 are lower alkyl groups having 1 to 4 carbons, especially isopropyl and tert-butyl groups, and R_3 is a higher alkyl group having more than 8 carbons. The alkylthioalkanoylaminophenol compounds are prepared by the reaction between the selected alkylaminophenol and alkylthioalkanoyl chloride. The reaction is carried out in a solvent such as acetone, pyridine, dimethylformamide, water, methyl ethyl ketone, methyl isobutyl ketone, dioxane, and the like.

Stoichiometric amounts of the reactants are used and a ratio of about 1 mol of the acid chloride to 1 mol of the aminophenol is used. In the course of the reaction, hydrogen chloride is liberated forming the amine hydrochloride and consequently an alkaline material is used to neutralize the hydrogen chloride. Suitable alkaline materials which are used to neutralize the hydrogen chloride include, for example, sodium or potassium hydroxide, sodium or potassium acetate, sodium or potassium carbonate, sodium or potassium bicarbonate, and the like. Included among the acid chlorides which can be used are alkylthioacetyl chlorides, alkylthiopropionyl chlorides, alkylthiobutyryl chlorides.

Example 1: 17.9 grams (0.05 mol) β-n-octadecylthiopropionic acid was treated with 25 ml thionyl chloride and the mixture was gently heated until solution was complete. The excess thionyl chloride was stripped off and the residue dissolved in 25 ml acetone was added to 11.05 grams (0.05 mol) 4-amino-2,6-di-tert-butylphenol in 25 ml acetone. The reaction was mildly exothermic. 50 ml 1N sodium hydroxide was added, the solution was stirred for 30 minutes and then heated at 60° to 70°C for 1 hour. The reaction mixture was then allowed to cool.

The solid material was filtered off, washed with water and air dried. 27 grams of 4-(β-n-octadecylthiopropionyl)amino-2,6-di-tert-butylphenol was crystallized from methanol and there was obtained 20 grams of the desired product, melting point 74° to 82°C. The product was recrystallized from heptane and 18 grams of the substantially pure product was obtained melting between 83.5° and 86.5°C.

In general these stabilizers are used in amounts of from 0.005 to 5% by weight of the composition. A particularly advantageous range for polyolefins, such as polypropylene is from 0.05 to 2%.

Example 2: Unstabilized polypropylene powder (Hercules Profax 6501) was blended with 0.5% by weight of 4-(β-n-octadecylthiopropionyl)amino-2-6-di-tert-butylphenol, as in the oven aging test on page 1.

It was found that unstabilized polypropylene began to decompose within 3 hours. However, the polypropylene containing 0.1% of the antioxidant did not decompose for 145 hours and polypropylene containing 0.5% of the antioxidant did not decompose for 530 hours. On the addition of 0.5% dilaurylthiodipropionate, decomposition occurred at 590 hours. When 4-(β-n-dodecylthiopropionyl)amino-2,6-di-tert-butylphenol was tested under identical conditions, decomposition of the polypropylene was observed after 195 hours. On adding 0.5% dilaurylthiodipropionate, decomposition was observed at 590 hours. Similar results are obtained when in the same test 4-(α-n-butylthioacetyl)amino-2,6-di-tert-butylphenol and 4-(β-n-decylthiopropionyl)amino-2,6-dicyclohexylphenol are used as the stabilizers.

Other examples are given in the patent covering the use of these compounds in stabilizing Havea rubber, high impact polystyrene, nylon 66, mineral oil and polyethylene.

Alkylhydroxybenzylamides

Amides having a benzylamine moiety are prepared by *M. Knell; U.S. Patent 3,780,103; December 18, 1973; assigned to Ciba-Geigy Corporation.* These compounds have the formula:

where R^1 is alkyl of 1 to 30 carbons, alkenyl of 2 to 30 carbons, alkylthioethyl where the alkyl groups contain 1 to 30 carbons or the group

where R^2 is alkylene of 1 to 10 carbons or $-C_2H_4-S-C_2H_4-$; and n has a value of 0 to 6.

These compounds are conveniently prepared through condensation of an alkylhydroxy-benzyl alcohol and a mono- or dinitrile in the presence of an acid catalyst such as mineral acids. Generally the nitrile can be employed as the reaction medium. Inert organic solvents can optionally be employed. Alternatively, conventional methods of amide preparation such as the reaction of an alkylhydroxybenzylamine and an alkanoic or alkenoic acid chloride are used.

In the case of the N-(alkylhydroxybenzyl)acrylamides, the further step of addition of an alkylmercaptan can be used to yield the N-(alkylhydroxybenzyl)-3-alkylthiopropionamides. This reaction is conducted in the presence of a base catalyst such as an alkali metal alkoxide and in an inert organic solvent such as ethyl ether. Moreover, if hydrogen sulfide is used in place of the mercaptan, the coupling of two molecules of the acrylamide occurs across the thio linkage, thus yielding a bis[N-(alkylhydroxybenzyl)propionamide] sulfide. These compounds demonstrate the ability to stabilize organic material normally subject to oxidative deterioration.

In general these stabilizers are used from 0.005 to 10% by weight of the stabilized composition. A particularly advantageous range for polyolefins such as polypropylene is from 0.05% to 5%, especially from 0.1% to 1%.

The N-(alkylhydroxybenzyl)acrylamides are also useful for polymerization, both to form polymeric antioxidants and to incorporate minor yet effective amounts of antioxidant monomers into an acrylic polymer or copolymer.

Example 1: To 100 ml of acetonitrile, which is cooled in an ice bath and stirred, are added in a dropwise fashion over a period of 5 minutes, 7.5 ml of concentrated sulfuric acid. There are next added in portions, over a 20-minute period, 26.3 grams of 3,5-di-tert-butyl-4-hydroxybenzyl alcohol, maintaining the temperature below 10°C. At the end of the addition, the reaction mixture is allowed to attain room temperature, stirred for two hours and allowed to stand for 15 hours.

The reaction mixture is then poured into 200 ml of water and the solid which forms upon standing and cooling is collected by filtration, washed with 100 ml of water and dried in vacuo over phosphorus pentoxide to yield N-(3,5-di-tert-butyl-4-hydroxybenzyl)acetamide which may be further purified through recrystallization from heptane, MP 132° to 133°C.

Example 2: To a mixture of 7.5 ml of concentrated sulfuric acid and 100 ml of acrylonitrile, cooled to about 5°C, are added over a 30-minute period, 23.6 grams of 3,5-di-tert-butyl-4-hydroxybenzyl alcohol, maintaining the reaction temperatures below 10°C. Upon completion of the addition, the reaction mixture is stirred for 2½ hours at room temperature, then cooled to 5°C and filtered. The solid thus collected is washed twice with 50 ml portions of cold benzene and then air-dried to yield N-(3,5-di-tert-butyl-hydroxybenzyl)-acrylamide which is further purified through several recrystallizations from 60% aqueous ethanol, MP 114° to 116°C.

Example 3: A stream of hydrogen sulfide is passed through an ethereal solution of 5 grams of N-(3,5-di-tert-butyl-4-hydroxybenzyl)acrylamide containing 0.1 gram of sodium methoxide for five hours. The mixture is then washed three times with 75 ml portions of water, dried over magnesium sulfate and evaporated to yield bis[(3,5-di-tert-butyl-hydroxybenzyl)-propionamide] sulfide.

Example 4: Samples of compounds as prepared by the above methods were solvent blended with methylene chloride in unstabilized polypropylene flake (Hercules Profax 6501) at the indicated percentage composition. After removal of the solvent, the mixture was milled at 360°F on a 6" x 13" two-roll plastics mill for five minutes. The milled sheets were compression molded for 3 minutes at 175 lb/in^2/425°F by means of a four-cavity picture frame mold into 5" x 5" x 25 mil plaques which are cooled by immersion in cold water. Duplicate samples of ½" x 1" are aged in a forced draft oven at 149°C until the first sign of failure (crazing, embrittlement or decomposition).

Compound	Amount, percent	Hours to failure
None	---	3
N-(3,5-di-t-butyl-4-hydroxybenzyl)acetamide	0.5	60
N-(3,5-di-t-butyl-4-hydroxybenzyl)acrylamide	0.5	23
N-(3,5-di-t-butyl-4-hydroxybenzyl)dodecanamide	0.5	75
N-(3,5-di-t-butyl-4-hydroxybenzyl)-3-octylthio-propionamide	0.5	90
N-(3,5-di-t-butyl-4-hydroxybenzyl)3-octadecyl-thiopropionamide	0.1	70
	0.5	575

An example in the original patent also showed the stabilization of cyclohexene.

PHENOLIC HYDRAZIDES

Alkylhydroxyphenylalkanoyl Hydrazines

M. Dexter; U.S. Patent 3,773,772; November 20, 1973 and U.S. Patent 3,660,438; May 2, 1972; both assigned to Ciba-Geigy Corporation has prepared alkylhydroxyphenyl-alkanoyl-hydrazines useful as stabilizers of organic materials which are subject to oxidative deterioration.

These antioxidants are represented by the formula:

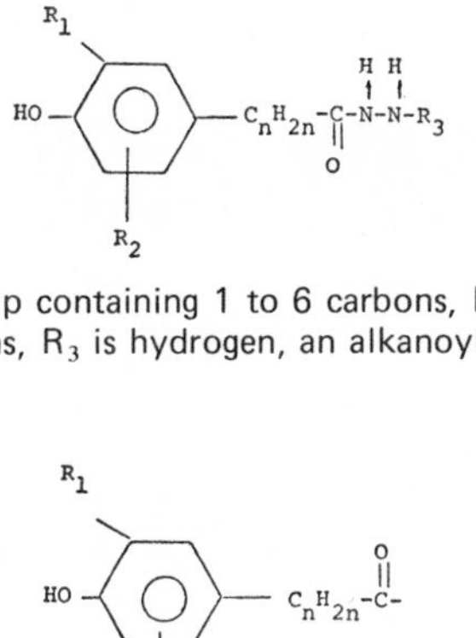

where R_1 is a lower alkyl group containing 1 to 6 carbons, R_2 is hydrogen or a lower alkyl containing 1 to 6 carbons, R_3 is hydrogen, an alkanoyl group containing 2 to 18 carbons or the group

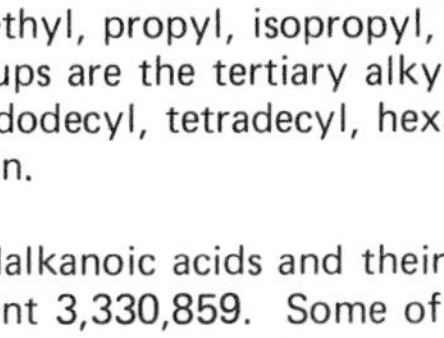

and n is an integer from 0 to 5. Examples of lower alkyl groups that are substituted on the phenyl moeity are methyl, ethyl, propyl, isopropyl, butyl, tert-butyl, pentyl, hexyl and the like. The preferred groups are the tertiary alkyls. Examples of the higher alkyl groups are heptyl, octyl, decyl, dodecyl, tetradecyl, hexadecyl, octadecyl and the like, both straight chain and branched chain.

The starting alkylhydroxyphenylalkanoic acids and their esters that are used as starting materials are described in U.S. Patent 3,330,859. Some of the procedures used in the syn-

theses of these acids and their esters include the reaction of alkali metal salts of an alkylated phenol with methyl acrylate; the reaction of alkali metal salts of alkylated phenols
with esters of α-haloalkanoic acids; the reaction of alkylhydroxybenzyl chlorides with
alkali metal cyanides to obtain alkylhydroxyphenylacetonitriles followed by hydrolysis to
the acids.

The lower alkyl esters of these alkylhydroxyphenylalkanoic acids, when reacted with hydrazine, yield a monoacylhydrazine. These esters can be hydrolyzed with a strong base,
such as sodium hydroxide, to yield the sodium salt which may be converted to the free
acid by acidification with a mineral acid, dried, and then reacted with thionyl chloride to
form the acid chloride, useful for preparing diacylhydrazines.

Monoacyl-hydrazine products can be acylated further. Illustrative acylating agents are
acetyl chlorides, propionyl chloride, octanoyl chloride, stearoyl chloride, and the like.
Since hydrogen chloride is liberated, the reaction is conducted in the presence of an acid
acceptor. The reaction can be conducted in the presence of an inert solvent. Useful solvents include, for example, methylene chloride, chloroform, benzene and the like.

Example 1: 53.8 grams (1.07 mols) of hydrazine hydrate was dissolved in 600 ml absolute methanol and to this solution was added, with stirring, 71.8 grams (0.25 mol) of
methyl β-(3,5-di-tert-butyl-4-hydroxyphenyl)propionate. The mixture was allowed to
stand at room temperature for 48 hours. The methanol was removed by distillation, under a nitrogen atmosphere, and 500 ml water was added to the residue. After stirring for
one hour, a white crystalline material was obtained and was separated by filtration. There
was obtained a yield of 71.7 grams of the product, β-(3,5-di-tert-butyl-4-hydroxyphenyl)
propionylhydrazide melting between 154° to 155.5°C. On recrystallization from a mixture
of ethanol and water, a melting point of 155.5° to 156.5°C was noted.

Example 2: 59.3 grams (0.2 mol) β-(3,5-di-tert-butyl-4-hydroxyphenyl)propionylchloride
and 500 ml benzene were placed in a reaction flask equipped with a stirrer, thermometer,
condenser and dropping funnel. To the solution were added slowly 5 grams hydrazine
hydrate (0.1 mol), 8 grams (0.2 mol) sodium hydroxide and 75 ml water at 25°C. After
one hour, a very thick precipitate was obtained. The mixture was stirred for 2½ hours
whereupon benzene was evaporated and the residue slurried up with water, filtered,
washed with water and then dried. There was obtained 55 grams of N,N'-bis-β-(3,5-di-tert-
butyl-4-hydroxyphenyl)propionylhydrazine. The white solid material was recrystallized
from an ethyl acetate/hexane mixture. A yield of 37.4 grams (67.8%) of the product was
obtained; its melting point was between 227° and 229°C.

These compounds are stated to be useful as antioxidants in a wide variety of materials
including addition and condensation polymers, synthetic and petroleum lubricants, fats,
oils and the like.

In general one or more of the stabilizers are employed in amounts, in toto, of from about
0.005 to about 5% by weight of the composition containing the organic material. A particularly advantageous range of the present stabilizers for polyolefins such as polypropylene
is from about 0.05 to about 2%. The stabilizers can be also used in combination with
other stabilizers or additives. Especially useful costabilizers are di-lauryl-β-thiodipropionate
and di-stearyl-β-thiodipropionate.

Example 3: A batch of unstabilized polypropylene powder (Hercules Profax 6501) was
thoroughly blended with 0.5% by weight of β-(3,5-di-tert-butyl-4-hydroxyphenyl)propionyl-
hydrazide and another batch with 0.5% by weight of N,N'-bis-β-(3,5-di-tert-butyl-4-hydroxy-
phenyl)propionylhydrazine.

The materials were processed and tested as in the oven aging test; see page 1. The results are set out in the table below.

[1] Distearylthiodipropionate (a synergist for phenolic anti-oxidants).

The above data clearly indicated the significant increase in the stabilization of polypropylene upon addition of the antioxidants of the process. The stabilization of cyclohexene, Havea rubber, high impact polystyrene, nylon 6,6 and polyacetal resin with these antioxidants were also covered by examples in the patents.

N-Aroyl-N'-(Alkylhydroxyphenyl)Alkanoyl Hydrazines

Similar compounds have also been prepared by *M. Dexter; U.S. Patent 3,773,830; November 20, 1973; assigned to Ciba-Geigy Corporation*, here having only one phenolic moiety in the compound. These compounds are represented by the formula:

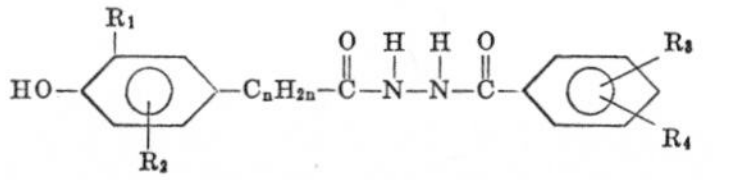

$$HO-\underset{R_2}{\overset{R_1}{\bigcirc}}-C_nH_{2n}-\overset{O}{\overset{\|}{C}}-\overset{H}{\overset{|}{N}}-\overset{H}{\overset{|}{N}}-\overset{O}{\overset{\|}{C}}-\underset{R_4}{\overset{R_3}{\bigcirc}}$$

where R_1 is an alkyl group containing 1 to 6 carbons, R_2 is hydrogen or an alkyl group containing 1 to 5 carbons, R_3 and R_4 are independently hydrogen, alkyl, alkoxy or halogen, where the alkyl group has up to 18 carbons, and n is an integer 0 to 5.

Starting materials and preparative methods are those given in the previous patents, U.S. Patent 3,660,438 and U.S. Patent 3,773,722.

Example 1: 53.8 grams (1.07 mol) of hydrazine hydrate was dissolved in 600 ml absolute methanol and to this solution was added, with stirring, 71.8 grams (0.25 mol) of methyl β-(3,5-di-tert-butyl-4-hydroxyphenyl)propionate. The mixture was allowed to stand at room temperature for 48 hours. The methanol was removed by distillation, under a nitrogen atmosphere, and 500 ml of water was added to the residue. After stirring for one hour, a white crystalline material was obtained and was separated by filtration.

There was obtained a yield of 71.7 grams of the product, β-(3,5-di-tert-butyl-4-hydroxyphenyl)propionyl hydrazide melting between 154° to 155.5°C. On recrystallization from a mixture of ethanol and water, a melting point of 155.5° to 156.5°C was noted.

8.8 grams of β-(3,5-di-tert-butyl-4-hydroxyphenyl)propionyl hydrazide was placed in a reaction vessel and dissolved with 35 ml of pyridine. To this mixture was added dropwise, 4.6 grams of benzoyl chloride. The reaction mixture was permitted to stand overnight and then filtered. To the filtrate was added 75 ml of water which caused the formation of an oil layer which, on standing, solidified. The solid was filtered and washed four times with water and dried in vacuum over P_2O_5 yielding 11.4 grams of crude product. The dried material was dissolved in 62.5 ml of 80% ethanol-water, filtered and the product, on cooling, crystallized. The purified N-benzoyl-N'-3-(3',5'-di-tert-butyl-4'-hydroxyphenyl)-propionylhydrazine was dried in vacuum over P_2O_5 yielding 9.36 grams of material melting at 169° to 170°C. NMR spectrum confirmed the structure of the product.

These stabilizers are also employed in amounts, in toto, of from about 0.005 to about 5% by weight of the composition containing the organic material. A particularly advantageous range of these stabilizers for polyolefins such as polypropylene is from about 0.05 to about 2%. The stabilizers employed in the process can be also used in combination with other stabilizers or additives. Especially useful costabilizers are dilauryl-β-thiodipropionate and di-stearyl-β-thiodipropionate.

Example 2: A batch of unstabilized polypropylene powder (Hercules Profax 6501) was thoroughly blended with 0.1% by weight of N-benzoyl-N'-(3',5'-di-tert-butyl-4'-hydroxyphenyl)propionylhydrazine and 0.3% of distearylthiodipropionate (DSTDP). The blended materials were processed and tested as in the oven aging test, page . The above stabilized composition started to decompose after 325 hours. Unstabilized polypropylene decomposes after 3 hours and polypropylene stabilized with 0.3% of DSTDP decomposes after 50 hours.

PHENOLIC IMIDES

Three series of imide compounds having the hindered phenol moiety have been prepared by the workers at Ciba-Geigy. In general, these compounds can be used as antioxidants in a wide variety of organic materials including polymers, synthetic lubricating oils, petroleum products, fats, vegetable oils and the like.

In general, one or more of these stabilizers are employed in amounts, in toto, of from 0.005 to 5% by weight of the composition to be stabilized. A particularly advantageous range is from 0.05% to 2%. The preferred range is particularly effective in polyolefins such as polypropylene.

These compounds may be incorporated in the polymer substance during the usual processing operations, for example, by hot-milling the composition then being extruded, pressed, roll-molded or the like into films, fibers, filaments, hollow-spheres and the like. The heat stabilizing properties of these compounds advantageously stabilize the polymer against degrading during such processing at the high temperatures generally encountered.

These stabilizers can also be used in combination with other stabilizers or additives. Especially useful costabilizers are dilauryl-β-thiodipropionate and distearyl-β-thiodipropionate.

Sulfur Derivatives of Alkylhydroxyphenyl Maleimides

M. Dexter, M. Knell and H.J. Peterli; U.S. Patent 3,790,597; February 5, 1974; assigned to Ciba-Geigy Corporation have prepared sulfur derivatives of alkylhydroxyphenyl maleimides which are useful as stabilizers for organic materials which are subject to thermal and oxidative deterioration. These compounds are represented by the formulas:

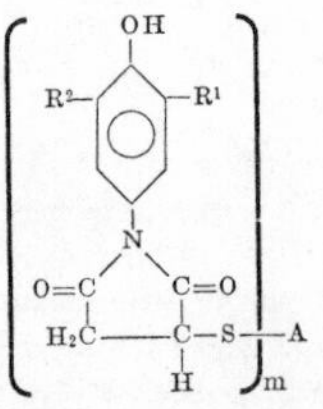

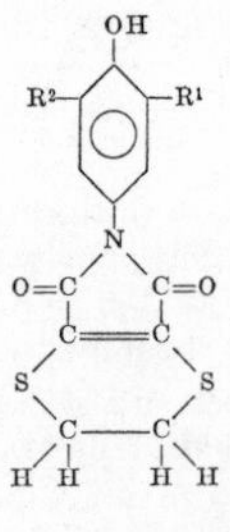

where A is alkyl of 1 to 18 carbons, ethylene-S-alkyl where alkyl contains 1 to 18 carbons benzyl when m is 1; or ethylene-S-ethylene when m is 2, each of R^1 and R^2 independently is (lower) alkyl of from 1 to 4 carbons, and m is 1 or 2. Examples of (lower) alkyl groups which are represented by R^1 and R^2 are methyl, ethyl, propyl, isopropyl, butyl, tert-butyl. The preferred groups are tert-butyl and methyl.

The compounds of Formula 1 can be prepared by reacting an alkylated hydroxyphenyl-amine in a nonaqueous, inert aprotic solvent, with maleic anhydride at room temperature to form a N(alkylhydroxyphenyl)maleamic acid. This maleamic acid is subsequently converted to the maleimide by heating at 100° in acetic anhydride catalyzed with sodium acetate.

The sulfur derivatives of the N(alkyhydroxyphenyl)maleimide are prepared by reacting the maleimide derivative with a mercaptan or dimercaptan in an inert solvent such as ether at room temperature using trimethylbenzylammonium methoxide as a catalyst. The compounds of Formula 2 can be prepared by reacting 3,6-dithia-δ-1-cyclohexene 1,2-dicarboxylic acid anhydride with an amino phenol. The anhydride can be prepared by the method described in Wolf et al, *Ang. Chem.* 72, 963 (1960).

Example 1: To a solution of 19.6 grams of maleic anhydride in 200 ml of ether was added a slurry of 44.2 grams of 4-amino-2,6-di-tert-butylphenol in 200 ml of ether with rapid stirring at room temperature. After 2 hours, the reaction mixture was cooled to 5°C, filtered and washed with petroleum ether. The N(3,5-di-tert-butyl-4-hydroxyphenyl)-maleamic acid obtained at this point was air-dried and had a melting point of 206° to 207°C.

Sodium acetate (5 grams) was slurried in 25 ml of acetic anhydride. To this slurry was added 15.95 grams of the above formed maleamic acid. The reaction mixture was then heated on a steam bath for 1 hour. After cooling to room temperature, the reaction mixture is poured into 100 ml of cold water. The product is filtered and washed with water and dried. The N(3,5-di-tert-butyl-4-hydroxyphenyl)maleimide is subsequently dissolved and recrystallized from benzene, ethanol and again from benzene to yield the desired product with the melting point of 210° to 212°C.

Example 2: To 50 ml of ether was added 9.03 grams of N(3,5-di-tert-butyl-4-hydroxy-phenyl)maleimide, 8.85 grams octadecyl mercaptan and 5 drops of trimethylbenzyl-ammonium methoxide. The reaction was mildly exothermic and the reaction was continued for about 16 hours at room temperature. The reaction mixture was washed with water and dried over magnesium sulfate. The solvent was evaporated to dryness after which the product was recrystallized first from methanol and then from hexane. The N(3,5-di-tert-butyl-4-hydroxyphenyl)-α-octadecylthiosuccinimide was air dried at room temperature and had a melting point of 76° to 77.5°C.

Example 3: A batch of unstabilized polypropylene powder (Hercules Profax 6501) was thoroughly blended with 0.5% by weight of the additives below, then processed and tested by the oven aging test, page 1. The results are set out in the table below.

Additive	Oven Aging at 150°C, hours to Failure
0.5% of N(3,5-di-tert-butyl-4-hydroxyphenyl)-α-decylthioethylthiosuccinimide	1,110
0.5% of N(3,5-di-tert-butyl-4-hydroxyphenyl)-α-octadecylthiosuccinimide	1,420
0.5% of N,N'-bis(3,5-di-tert-butyl-4-hydroxy-phenyl)thiobis(α-ethylthiosuccinimide)	663
Unstabilized polypropylene	3

The above data clearly indicates the significant increase in the stabilization of polypropylene upon addition of these antioxidants. Examples showing the stabilization of mineral oil, lubricating oil, and cyclohexene, as well as polyethylene, nylon 6,6, ABS, SBR, and high impact polystyrene are included in the patent.

Benzophenonetetracarboxylic Acid Diimides

Antioxidants are also prepared by *M. Dexter; U.S. Patent 3,734,926; May 22, 1973; assigned to Ciba-Geigy Corporation* which are benzophenone tetracarboxylic acid diimide derivatives of 3,5-dialkyl-4-hydroxyphenyl-substituted amines. These compounds are represented by the formula:

(1)

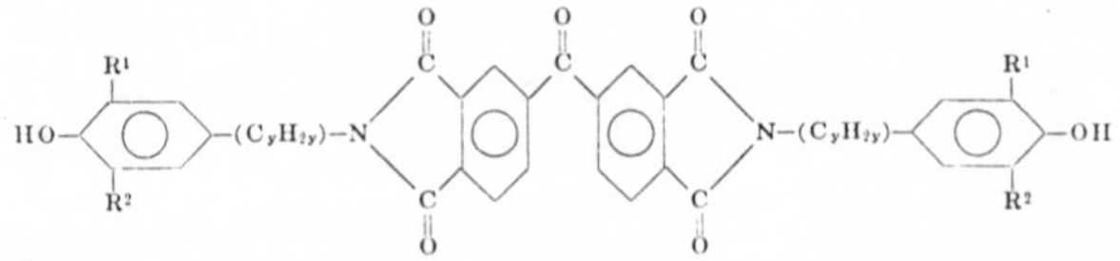

where each of R^1 and R^2 is the same or different (lower) alkyl group of 1 to 4 carbons; and y has a value of 0 to 3. Examples of (lower) alkyl groups of 1 to 4 carbons represented by R^1 and R^2 are methyl, ethyl, propyl, isopropyl, butyl and tert-butyl. The preferred groups are methyl, isopropyl and tert-butyl.

The compounds of the formula 1 where y is 0, 2 and 3, can be prepared by reacting a 3,5-dialkyl-4-hydroxyphenyl-substituted amine of the formula

(2)

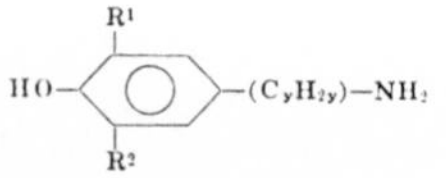

where R^1 and R^2 are as defined previously, and y is 0, 2 and 3, with benzophenone-3,4,-3',4'-tetracarboxylic acid dianhydride in an inert solvent such as dichlorobenzene at reflux temperatures.

The 3,5-dialkyl-4-hydroxyphenyl-substituted amines where y is 0 can be prepared as described in U.S. Patent 3,198,797. The amine, when y is 2 can be prepared, for example, through chloromethylation of a dialkylphenol as described in U.S. Patent 2,838,571, followed by treatment with sodium or potassium cyanide and reduction of the resultant dialkylhydroxyphenyl acetonitrile to the amine. The amine where y is 3 can be prepared by reducing 3,5-dialkyl-4-hydroxyphenyl-propylnitrile with lithium aluminum hydride to yield the corresponding amine.

The nitrile can be prepared according to the method described in U.S. Patent 3,121,732 where the appropriate dialkylhydroxyphenol is reacted with acrylonitrile. The 3,5-dialkyl-4-hydroxybenzyl dialkyl amine of formula 3 can be prepared as described by E.P. Previc et al, *Industrial and Engineering Chemistry*, Vol. 53, No. 6, page 469, June, 1961. The benzophenone-3,4,3',4'-tetracarboxylic acid diimide can be prepared by methods described in U.S. Patent 3,275,651.

The compounds of formula 1 wherein y is 1 can be prepared by reacting 3,5-dialkyl-4-hydroxybenzyldialkylamine of the formula

(3)

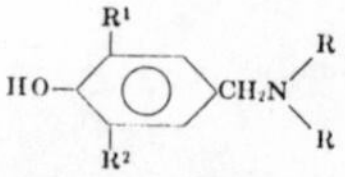

where R^1 and R^2 are as defined previously and R is an alkyl group such as methyl or ethyl, with benzophenone-3,4,3',4'-tetracarboxylic acid diimide, in an inert solvent such as dimethyl formamide at approximately 120°C.

Example 1: To 200 ml of dimethylformamide were mixed 16.0 grams of benzophenone-3,4,3',4'-tetracarboxylic acid diimide (0.05 mol) and 27.6 grams of 3,5-di-tert-butyl-4-hydroxybenzyl dimethyl amine (0.1 mol). The reaction mixture was heated under nitrogen at 120° to 125°C for 6 hours. After cooling, the reaction mixture was poured into water.

The material obtained was extracted with ether. The ether extract was washed with dilute HCl and then with water. Upon evaporation of the ether, an amorphous solid was obtained. The product was triturated with hot petroleum ether after which it was recrystallized twice from aqueous acetone. The N,N'-bis(3,5-di-tert-butyl-4-hydroxybenzyl)benzophenone-3,4,3',4'-tetracarboxylic acid diimide obtained has a melting point of 218° to 221°C.

In a similar manner, by substituting 3-methyl-5-tert-butyl-4-hydroxybenzyl-dimethylamine for 3,5-di-tert-butyl-4-hydroxybenzyl-dimethylamine there is obtained N,N'-bis(3-methyl-5-tert-butyl-4-hydroxybenzyl)benzophenone 3,4,3',4'-tetracarboxylic acid diimide.

Example 2: Unstabilized polypropylene powder (Hercules Profax 6501) was thoroughly blended with 0.2% by weight of N,N'-bis(3,5-di-tert-butyl-4-hydroxybenzyl)benzophenone-3,4,3',4'-tetracarboxylic diimide.

Also prepared were samples of polypropylene containing 0.1% by weight of the same stabilizer and 0.3% by weight of distearylthiodipropionate (DSTDP). The blended materials were processed and tested in the oven aging test, page 1, after which the stabilized polypropylene was sheeted from the mill and allowed to cool.

The milled sheets were then cut into pieces and pressed for 7 minutes on a hydraulic press at 218°C, 2,000 lb per sq in pressure. The resulting sheets of 25 mil thickness were tested for resistance to accelerated aging in a forced draft oven at 150°C. The results are set out in the table below.

Additives	Oven Aging at 150°, hours to Failure
0.2% of N,N'-bis(3,5-di-tert-butyl-4-hydroxybenzyl) benzophenone-3,4,3',4'-tetracarboxylic acid diimide	50
0.1% of N,N'-bis(3,5-di-tert-butyl-4-hydroxybenzyl) benzophenone-3,4,3',4'-tetracarboxylic acid diimide + 0.3% DSTDP	2,070
Unstabilized polypropylene	3
0.3% DSTDP* alone	<20

*Distearylthiodipropionate (a synergist for phenolic antioxidants).

Stabilized polypropylene compositions are also obtained when 0.5% of N,N'-bis[3-(3,5-di-tert-butyl-4-hydroxy-phenyl)propyl] benzophenone-3,4,3',4'- tetracarboxylic acid diimide; N,N'-bis(3-methyl-5-tert-butyl-4-hydroxybenzyl)benzophenone-3,4,3',4'-tetracarboxylic acid diimide; N,N'-bis(3,5-di-tert-butyl-4-hydroxyphenyl)-3',4'-tetracarboxylic acid diimide respectively are employed alone or in combination with DSTDP.

Nylon 6,6, SBR and linear polyethylene are also included in additional examples of the patent of the use of these compounds as antioxidants.

Aromatic Diimides

Similar diimides were also prepared by *J.F. Stephen; U.S. Patent 3,746,721; July 17, 1973; assigned to Ciba-Geigy Corporation* wherein the keto group of the benzophenone moiety of the diimide is replaced by O, SO$_2$ or alkylene group. These compounds are represented by the formula:

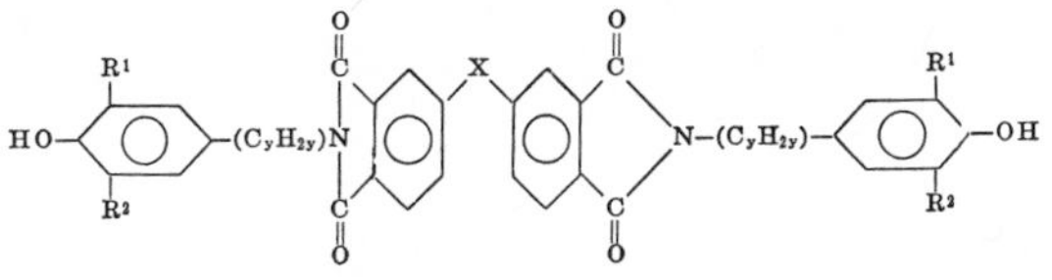

where each of R^1 and R^2 is the same or different (lower) alkyl group of from 1 to 4 carbons, X is O, SO$_2$, or an alkylene of 1 to 3 carbons; and y has a value of from 0 to 3. The phenolic starting materials are the same as those described in U.S. Patent 3,734,926. The intermediate aromatic dianhydrides and diimides can be prepared as follows:

(a) The diphenyl ether-3,4,3',4'-tetracarboxylic acid dianhydride intermediate is prepared by first preparing the corresponding tetracarboxylic acid as described by Marvel and Rassweiler, *J. Am. Chem. Sec.,* 80, 1196 (1958), followed by treatment of the tetra acid with acetic anhydride. The diphenyl ether-3,4,3',4'-tetracarboxylic acid diimide is prepared by decomposing the tetraammonium salt of diphenyl ether-3,4,3',4'-tetracarboxylic acid at 250° to 280°C as described by Marvel and Martin, *J. Am. Chem. Soc.,* 80, 6600 (1958) and in U.S. Patent 3,275,651.

(b) The diphenyl sulfone-3,4,3',4'-tetracarboxylic acid dianhydride is prepared by first preparing the corresponding tetracarboxylic acid from the nitric acid oxidation of bis(3,4-dimethylphenyl)sulfone as described in U.S. Patent 3,022,320 followed by treatment with acetic anhydride. The diphenyl sulfone 3,4,3',4'-tetracarboxylic acid diimide can be prepared from the pyrolysis of the tetraammonium salt of the corresponding tetracarboxylic acid following the procedure as outlined by Marvel and Martin, *J. Am. Chem. Soc.,* 80, 6600 (1958).

Example 1: In a nitrogen atmosphere, a stirred mixture of 4,4'-diphenylether-3,4,3',4'-tetracarboxylic acid diimide 9.5 grams and 2,6-di-tert-butyl-4-dimethylamino-methylphenol 17.9 grams in 150 ml of dimethylformamide was heated at 120°C for 23 hours. The mixture was poured into water and the solid which separated was extracted with ether. The ether extract was washed with dilute hydrochloric acid and then water. The dried (MgSO$_4$) ether solution was evaporated under reduced pressure to give 25 grams of a yellow solid. Recrystallization from 75 ml of methanol followed by a second recrystallization from ethanol-benzene mixture gave N,N'-bis(3,5-di-tert-butyl-4-hydroxybenzyl)diphenylether-3,4,3'4'-tetracarboxylic acid diimide, melting point 187° to 189°C.

Example 2: (a) The reaction flask is charged with 11.05 grams (0.05 mol) of 4-amino-2,6-di-tert-butylphenol, 8.0 grams (0.025 mol) of diphenylsulfone-3,4,3',4'-tetracarboxylic acid dianhydride and 100 ml of o-dichlorobenzene. The reaction mixture is heated to reflux until the imidization is completed. After cooling, the mixture is filtered and washed with petroleum ether. The filtrate of N,N'-bis(3,5-di-tert-butyl-4-hydroxyphenyl)-diphenylsulfone-3,4,3',4'-tetracarboxylic acid diimide is dried and recrystallized from aqueous acetone, and dried.

(b) By substituting an equivalent amount of 2-(3,5-di-tert-butyl-4-hydroxyphenyl)ethylamine for 3,5-di-tert-butyl-4-hydroxyphenylamine in the above procedure, the corresponding N,N'-bis[2-(3,5-di-tert-butyl-4-hydroxyphenyl)ethyl] diphenylsulfone-3,4,3',4'-tetracarboxylic acid diimide is obtained.

Example 3: Unstabilized polypropylene powder (Hercules Profax 6501) is thoroughly blended with 0.2% by weight of N,N'-bis(3,5-di-tert-butyl-hydroxybenzyl)diphenylsulfone-3,4,3',4'-tetracarboxylic diimide. Also prepared are samples of polypropylene containing 0.1% by weight of the same stabilizer and 0.3% by weight of distearylthiodipropionate (DSTDP).

The stabilized polypropylene has better color retention, physical integrity and less weight loss after oven aging than polypropylene which is unstabilized. Stabilized polypropylene compositions are also obtained when 0.5% of N,N'-bis(3,5-di-tert-butyl-4-hydroxyphenyl-propyl)diphenylmethane-3,4,3',4'-tetracarboxylic acid diimide and N,N'-bis(3-methyl-5-tert-butyl-4-hydroxybenzyl)diphenylsulfone-3,4,3',4'-tetracarboxylic acid diimide respectively are employed alone or in combination with DSTDP.

Other examples in the patent cover the stabilization of nylon 6,6, SBR and linear polyethylene.

AMIDES OF PHENOL SUBSTITUTED ACIDS

Water-Soluble Amides of Aminoarylsulfonic Acids

Water-soluble, noncoloring phenolic antioxidants and processes for their production are disclosed by *H.J. Peterli, E. Keller and K. Schwarzenbach; U.S. Patent 3,665,031; May 23, 1972; assigned to Ciba-Geigy Corporation.* These antioxidants are useful for stabilizing of organic polymers containing basic groups against the effect of heat and/or oxygen. Organic polymers which contain basic groups such as polyamides, polyurethanes, polyureas or basically modified acrylonitrile and polypropylene polymers, are damaged, particularly at higher temperatures, by the effect of oxygen. The damage becomes apparent in that the relative viscosity of the materials made therefrom, e.g., threads, bristles or foils, become worse. The polymers also become increasingly discolored.

Broadly, these antioxidants are compounds of the general formula:

$$(1) \qquad (A-Y-)_n Z(SO_3^- M^+)_m$$

where A is the radical of a sterically hindered phenol of the benzene series. Y is a bridge where the acylic bridging member contains a carboxylic acid amide group in the chain, Z is an aliphatic radical or a carbocyclic aromatic radical, containing at most two mono- or bi-cyclic nuclei, M^+ is one equivalent of a cation solvatizable by water, and m and n independently of each other are 1 or 2.

In Formula 1, Y represents, more particularly, a radical of the formula

$$(2) \qquad -(X)_x-\left(\!\!\begin{array}{c} R_3{'} \\ N \\ \end{array}\!\!\right)_y -\overset{\displaystyle O}{\overset{\displaystyle \|}{C}}-\overset{\displaystyle R_3}{\underset{}{N}}-(X')_{x'}--$$

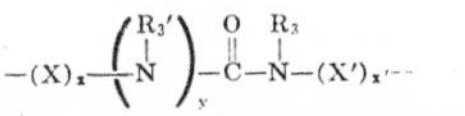

where X and X' independently of each other represent alkylene, oxaalkylene or thiaalkylene, R_3 and R_3' independently of each other represent hydrogen or an optionally substituted alkyl group, and x, x' and y independently of each other each are 0 or 1. In general, compounds in which y in Formula 2 is 0 have better stabilizing action than those compounds in which y is 1. Typical compounds are those of the formulas

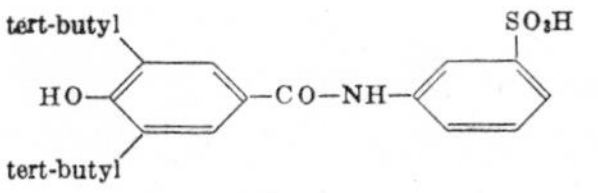

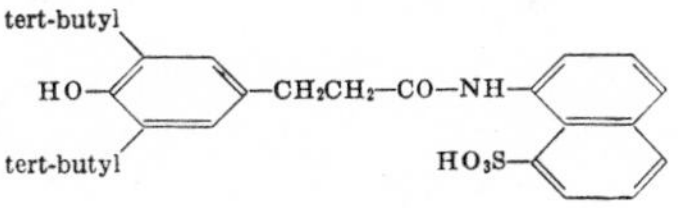

(3)   (4)

The water-soluble antioxidants of Formula 1 can be produced by known methods by reaction of reactive derivatives of corresponding acids with corresponding amino compounds to form acid amides. The following examples illustrate the synthesis of the antioxidants.

Example 1: 22.3 grams of 1-naphthylamine-4-sulfonic acid are slurried in 500 grams of N,N-dimethylacetamide and, after the addition of 20 grams of triethylamine, dissolved while stirring at 60°C. The solution is cooled to 10°C and, while continuously stirring, a solution of 31 grams of 4-hydroxy-3,5-di-tert-butylphenyl acetyl chloride, produced from 3,5-di-tert-butyl-4-hydroxyphenyl acetic acid and thionyl chloride, in 50 grams of o-di-chlorobenzene is added dropwise within 30 minutes and then 10 grams of triethylamine are added. The whole is stirred for 12 hours, precipitated triethyl ammonium chloride is filtered off under suction and the filtrate is completely evaporated in vacuo at 90° to 95°C.

The brownish syrup which remains is dissolved in 30 grams of water and about 1,000 grams of concentrated hydrochloric acid are added. A partly crystalline precipitate is formed which is filtered off under suction after 2 hours and then dried in vacuo at 100°C. The product is boiled up in a 2:1 mixture of acetic acid and water, undissolved parts are removed by filtration and the filtrate is concentrated in vacuo. The residue is recrystallized twice from a 5:2 mixture of acetic acid and 1N hydrochloric acid, a small insoluble part being filtered off hot each time. In this way, 5.8 grams of 1-N-(4-hydroxy-3,5-di-tert-butyl-phenylacetyl)-naphthylamine-4-sulfonic acid are obtained in the form of white needles which are dried in vacuo at 100°C. They are then left to stand in the open for 48 hours whereupon they contain 1 mol of crystal water. The compound melts at above 210° to 220°C with foaming. The antioxidants of this process show better stabilization of polymers with basic groups than do the formerly used Cu or Mn salts or inorganic or organic acids, phosphorus acids, aromatic amines or phenols.

Example 2: 10 grams of a nylon 6 knitted fabric are treated for 30 minutes at a constant temperature of 80°C in 250 ml of liquor which contains 100 mg of an antioxidant listed in the table below; 200 mg of a nonionic, surface active wetting and levelling agent produced from 1 mol of stearyl alcohol and 18 mols of ethylene oxide; and 2.5 ml of glacial acetic acid. The sample is then rinsed, dried and aged for 6 to 12 hours at 210°C in a circulating air oven. The tensile strength is measured on 1 cm wide strips of sample before aging and after aging for 6 or 12 hours in the oven. The results are summarized in the table below.

Antioxidant	- Tensile Strength, kg* -		- Relative Viscosity* -	
	Before	After	Before	After
1	21.0	16.5	2.35	2.20
2	21.0	8.5	2.35	1.65
3	21.0	12.5	2.35	1.95
None	21.0	6.0	2.35	1.46

*Measured before and after aging for 6 hours at 210°C.

In the table above antioxidant 1 is 1-N-(4-hydroxy-3,5-di-tert-butyl-phenylacetyl)-naphthyl-amine-4-sulfonic acid; antioxidant 2 is N-(4-hydroxy-3,5-di-tert-butyl-benzylmercapto-acetyl)-aniline-3-sulfonic acid; and antioxidant 3 is N-(4-hydroxy-3,5-di-tert-butylbenzoyl)-aniline-3-sulfonic acid. Other examples in the patent show the stabilization of nylon 6,6, polyetherurethane (Lycra) and an acrylonitrile/vinylpyridine copolymer (Acrilan) with these antioxidants.

Polyamides of Alkylhydroxyphenylalkanoic Acids

Antioxidants have also been prepared by *M. Dexter, J.D. Spivack, D.H. Steinberg; U.S. Patent 3,677,965; July 18, 1972 and U.S. Patent 3,584,047; June 8, 1971; assigned to Geigy Chemical Corporation* from hindered phenols having carboxylic acid groups. These are compounds having: (a) from 2 to 4 amide units

(1)

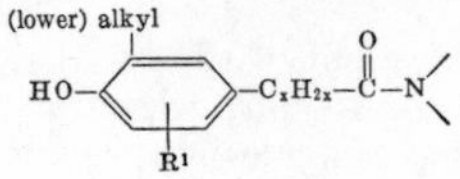

where R^1 is hydrogen or (lower)alkyl and x has a value of 0 to 6; and (b) any one of the three following sets of conditions:

1 to 3 polyvalent hydrocarbon chains having a total of 2 to 30 carbons, one of the free valences of each amide unit being satisfied by a free carbon valence of a polyvalent hydrocarbon chain and the other of the free nitrogen atom valences of the amide unit being satisfied by either a hydrogen or a free carbon valence of either the same or a second hydrocarbon chain, the total nitrogen atom valences of all amide units not satisfied by hydrogen being equal to the total free carbon atom valences on all hydrocarbon units;

a tris(polymethylene)amine group of 6 to 18 carbons, one of the free nitrogen atom valences of each of 3 of the amide units being satisfied by one of the 3 free carbon valences of the tris(polymethylene)amine and the other free nitrogen valence of each amide unit being satisfied by a hydrogen; or

an N,N,N',N'-tetra(polymethylene)alkanediamine group of 10 to 30 carbons, one of the free nitrogen valences of each of 4 of the amide units being satisfied by one of the 4 free carbon valences of the N,N,N',N'-tetrakis(polymethylene) alkanediamine and the other free nitrogen atom valence of each amide unit being satisfied by a hydrogen atom.

In Formula 1 the alkanoyl portion of these polyamides bears a phenolic group which has at least one (lower)alkyl group, in a position ortho to the hydroxy group. A second (lower)alkyl group (R^1) is optionally present either in the other position ortho to the hydroxy group or meta to the hydroxy group and para to the first (lower)alkyl group. Preferred are the di(lower)alkyl-p-phenolic groups, e.g., R^1 is (lower)alkyl, and although not so limited, the (lower)alkyl groups on the p-phenolic group are preferably branched groups such as tert-butyl. Other arrangements, however, such as for example a 3-tert-butyl-6-methyl-4-hydroxyphenyl or a 3,5-dimethyl-4-hydroxyphenyl group are included.

These compounds can be prepared via a number of conventional amidation procedures. Thus an acid moiety of Formula 1 or an alkyl ester thereof and a polyamine are heated in an inert organic solvent with the generation of water or an alcohol. Alternatively, the polyamine and the acid halide, generally the acid chloride, are allowed to react in an inert organic solvent, preferably in the presence of an organic or inorganic base which serves as an acid binding agent, with the generation of the corresponding acid halide.

Example 1: A mixture of 128.6 grams of methyl 3-(3,5-di-tert-butyl-4-hydroxyphenyl) propionate and 23.2 grams of 1,6-hexamethylenediamine are heated with stirring under nitrogen for 3.5 hours at 150° to 155°C, the methanol which is evolved being separated in moisture trap. The temperature is then raised to 160° to 190°C for 1.5 hours, the reaction going to about 86% completion. After a final heating at 200°C for 2.5 hours at 5 to 10 mm pressure, the mixture is cooled and dissolved in 550 ml of benzene.

The product 1,6-bis[3-(3,5-di-tert-butyl-4-hydroxyphenyl)propionamido]hexane solidifies, is collected by filtration and further purified through recrystallization from benzene, MP 154° to 156°C. Repeated recrystallization from 2:3 benzene:cyclohexene raises the melting point to 158° to 159°C. This product is alternatively prepared through the reaction of 1,6-hexamethylenediamine with two molar equivalent amounts of 3-(3,5-di-tert-butyl-4-hydroxyphenyl)propionyl chloride in the presence of an acid binding agent such as potassium carbonate.

Example 2: To a solution of 1.55 grams of diethylene triamine and 11 grams of potassium carbonate in 16 ml of water, cooled to 0° to 5°C is added in a dropwise fashion with stirring over a 30 minute period, a solution of 26.72 grams of 3-(3,5-di-tert-butyl-4-hydroxyphenyl)propionyl chloride in 250 ml of benzene. The mixture is stirred for approximately 15 hours, the temperature being allowed to reach 20° to 25°C. The organic phase is then separated, washed twice with water and once with saturated sodium chloride solution, dried and evaporated under reduced pressure.

The product is triturated several times with cyclohexane and heptane and then chromatographed on alumina, eluting with 1:1 benzene/chloroform. The fractions demonstrating a melting point of from 86° to 120°C are combined and recrystallized from benzene to yield N,N',N"-tris[3-(3,5-di-tert-butyl-4-hydroxyphenyl)propionyl] diethylene triamine. The following example shows the stabilization of polypropylene with various antioxidants produced by these disclosures.

Example 3: Unstabilized polypropylene powder (Hercules Profax 6501) is thoroughly blended with 0.5% by weight of stabilizer. The material is processed and tested as in the oven aging test on page 1. As shown in the table below, the composition of 0.5% by weight of stabilizer and polypropylene is stabilized against oxidative deterioration.

	Hours
Polypropylene alone	3
1,4-bis[3-(3,5-di-tert-butyl-4-hydroxyphenyl) propionamidomethyl] cyclohexane	1,340
Tetrakis[3-(3,5-di-tert-butyl-4-hydroxyphenyl) propionamidomethyl] methane	998
1,3-bis⟨N-[3-(3,5-di-tert-butyl-4-hydroxyphenyl) propionyl] piperid-4-yl⟩propane	711
N,N'-bis[3-(3,5-di-tert-butyl-4-hydroxyphenyl) propionyl] piperazine	1,285
1,2-bis[3-(3,5-di-tert-butyl-4-hydroxyphenyl) propionamido] ethane	980
1,6-bis[3-(3,5-di-tert-butyl-4-hydroxyphenyl) propionamido] hexane	380
N,N',N''-tris-[3-(3,5-di-tert-butyl-4-hydroxyphenyl) propionyl] diethylene triamine	325

All the above samples also showed excellent stability in the Fadeometer evaluation. In addition, other examples disclose the stabilization of mineral oil, lard, gasoline, paraffin wax, lubricating oil, high impact polystyrene, polyacetal (polyoxymethylene diacetate) and nylon 6,6.

CARBAMATES OF HINDERED BISPHENOLS

Compounds having antioxidant as well as insecticidal properties are disclosed by *W.E. Wright; U.S. Patent 3,632,631; January 4, 1972; assigned to Ethyl Corporation.* These are sterically hindered bisphenyl carbamates having the formula:

(1)

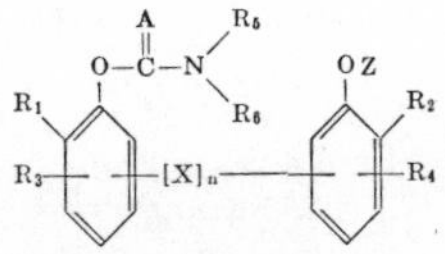

where R_1 and R_2 are α-branched C_3–C_{12} alkyl radicals, α-branched C_8–C_{12} aralkyl radicals or C_6–C_{12} cycloalkyl radicals, R_3 and R_4 are selected from hydrogen, C_1–C_{12} alkyl radicals, C_7–C_{12} aralkyl radicals and C_6–C_{12} cycloalkyl radicals, X is selected from thio-, dithio- and C_1–C_6 divalent hydrocarbon radicals, R_5 is selected from C_1–C_{20} alkyl radicals, C_6–C_{20} aryl radicals and C_7–C_{20} aralkyl radicals, R_6 is hydrogen or R_5, n is 0 or 1, A is oxygen or sulfur and Z is hydrogen or carbamyl radicals having the formula:

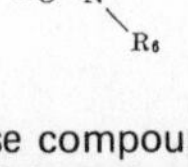

where A, R_5 and R_6 are as above. These compounds fall into three subclasses. In the first the two phenyl radicals are bonded directly to each other. The second subclass of compounds are those in which the two phenyl radicals of the bisphenyl carbamates are bonded together through a divalent hydrocarbon radical. A third subclass of hindered bisphenyl carbamates consists of those in which the two phenyl radicals are bonded together through a thio or dithio radical.

These compounds can be made by known methods. A most useful method is by the reaction of the known bisphenol compounds with an isocyanate or a carbamyl chloride. The following examples will serve to illustrate typical methods of preparation. All parts are parts by weight.

Example 1: To a reaction vessel equipped with a stirrer, thermometer, condenser and heating means add 82 parts of 4,4'-bis(2,6-di-tert-butylphenol), 22.8 parts of methylisocyanate, 1,400 parts of benzene and 0.2 part of pyridine. Heat the mixture slowly to reflux. Stir at reflux for 6 hours and then cool to room temperature. Filter off the precipitate and recrystallize it from tetrahydrofuran, which yields 4,4'-bis(2,6-di-tert-butylphenyl methylcarbamate) melting at 346° to 348°C (dec).

Example 2: To the reaction vessel of Example 1 add 80.2 parts of 4,4'-methylenebis(2,6-di-tert-butylphenol), 71 parts of toluene, 22.8 parts of methylisocyanate and 0.2 part of pyridine. Stir and heat to reflux and maintain at reflux for 48 hours. When the white precipitate that forms makes stirring difficult, add 175 parts of toluene. Evaporate off the solvent and recrystallize the remaining yellow solids from toluene, yielding 4,4'-methylene-bis(2,6-di-tert-butylphenyl methylcarbamate).

Example 3: In a reaction vessel equipped as in Example 1 place 358 parts of 4,4'-thiobis(6-tert-butyl-m-cresol), 1,500 parts of carbon tetrachloride and 215 parts of dimethylcarbamyl chloride. Heat the mixture to reflux while stirring, allowing the evolved hydrogen chloride to vent. Stir at reflux 4 hours and then wash twice with water. Evaporate off the carbon tetrachloride and recrystallize the residue from isooctane to obtain 4,4'-thiobis(6-tert-butyl-m-tolyl dimethylcarbamate).

These sterically hindered bisphenyl carbamates are useful as antioxidants in organic material normally subject to oxidative deterioration. For example, they may be employed in amounts from about 0.05 to 5 weight percent to stabilize organic material such as mineral lubricating oils, synthetic lubricating oils, natural and synthetic rubber, synthetic silicone lubricants and fats and oils of animal and vegetable origin. The hindered bisphenyl carbamates are especially useful in stabilizing homopolymers and copolymers of olefinically unsaturated monomers. The following example illustrates the stabilization of a polyolefin with these bisphenyl carbamates.

Example 4: In a mixing vessel place 1,000 parts of a high molecular weight crystalline polypropylene powder made employing a Ziegler type catalyst (diethyl aluminum chloride/titanium trichloride). To this powder is added one part of 4,4'-methylenebis(2,6-di-tert-butylphenyl methylcarbamate) and 2 parts of dilaurylthiodipropionate. The polymer is mixed until homogeneous and then used in any of the well-known methods to fabricate polypropylene articles.

AMINE AND IMINE ANTIOXIDANTS

AROMATIC SECONDARY AMINES

Tertiary-Alkylated Diarylamines

With the advent of gas turbine engines required to propel aircraft at greater speeds, has come a demand for lubricants which will function satisfactorily at higher temperatures. Dialkylated phenothiazines and dialkylated secondary amines do not pass the standard specification tests. For instance, the requirements of the Pratt and Whitney Type II oxidation corrosion tests, carried out at 425° or 450°F for 48 hr cannot be met by lubricants containing dialkylated derivatives of diphenylamine and phenothiazine.

D.R. Randell; U.S. Patent 3,696,851; October 10, 1972; assigned to Geigy Chemical Corp. and U.S. Patent 3,414,618; December 3, 1968; assigned to The Geigy Company Limited, England provides antioxidant compounds of the formula:

$$A-NH-B$$

where A and B are the same or different and each is an aryl group, and one of the aryl groups A and B contains a tertiary alkyl group having 4 to 12 carbons. Each of the aryl groups A and B may be, for example, a benzene or naphthalene nucleus otherwise unsubstituted or containing further substituents, apart from the required tertiary alkyl group; if either or both of the groups A and B is a naphthalene residue, this may be an α- or β-naphthyl group. The tertiary alkyl group contains 4 to 12 carbons and may be, for example, tert-butyl, tert-pentyl, tert-hexyl, tert-octyl, or tert-dodecyl. The tertiary alkyl substituent preferably has a tertiary carbon atom directly attached to the aryl nucleus.

If the aryl group A or B which contains the essential tertiary alkyl substituent is an unsubstituted or substituted phenyl group, the tertiary alkyl group is preferably in the 4-position relative to the carbon of the benzene directly attached to the nitrogen of the secondary amine group. If the aryl group A and B which contains the tertiary alkyl substituent is an otherwise unsubstituted or substituted naphthyl group, the tertiary alkyl group is preferably attached in the same or the analogous position as the 4-substituent in a phenyl group. Examples of such diarylamine antioxidants include:

> 4-tert-pentyl-diphenylamine
> N-p-tert-pentyl-phenyl-α-naphthylamine
> N-p-tert-pentyl-phenyl-β-naphthylamine
> 4-(1',1',3',3'-tetramethylbutyl)diphenylamine

N-p-(1,1,3,3-tetramethylbutyl)phenyl-α-naphthylamine
N-p-(1,1,3,3-tetramethylbutyl)phenyl-β-naphthylamine
4-(1',1',3',3',5',5'-hexamethylhexyl)diphenylamine
N-p-(1,1,3,3,5,5-hexamethylhexyl)phenyl-α-naphthylamine
N-p-(1,1,3,3,5,5,-hexamethylhexyl)phenyl-β-naphthylamine

These monotertiary alkyldiarylamine antioxidants are produced by contacting the corresponding diarylamine with a 1- or 2-alkylene, the total number of carbons in the alkylene being 4 to 12. The reaction with the alkylene is carried out advantageously in the presence of a Friedel-Crafts catalyst, e.g., aluminum chloride.

Example 1: 169.2 parts by weight of diphenylamine were heated with 140.3 parts by weight of diisobutylene (a mixture of 75% of 2,4,4-trimethylpentene-1 and 25% of 2,4,4-trimethylpentene-2) and with 2.2 parts by weight of anhydrous aluminum chloride for 15 hours while maintaining the temperature at 108° to 146°C.

The product was a mixture of 4- and 4,4'-tert-octyldiphenylamines with unreacted diphenylamine. The desired 4-tert-octyldiphenylamine was separated from the other constituents by fractional distillation and was recrystallized from aqueous ethanol. The 4-tert-octyldiphenylamine had melting point 48° to 49°C and boiling point 150° to 154°C at 0.22 mm of mercury pressure. The conversion was 55%.

Example 2: 657 parts by weight of N-phenyl-α-naphthylamine were heated with 673 parts by weight of diisobutylene (having the same composition as that used in Example 1), and 6.6 parts by weight of anhydrous aluminum chloride for 36 hours, while maintaining the temperature at 108° to 136°C. The product was N-p-tert-octylphenyl-α-naphthylamine, having melting point 76° to 77°C. The yield was 62% theoretical. Use of these antioxidants in synthetic lubricants is shown in the following U.S. Patents 3,536,706 and 3,642,629.

Tertiary-Alkylated Phenothiazines

D.R. Randell; U.S. Patents 3,536,706; October 27, 1970; and 3,642,629; February 15, 1972; both assigned to Geigy Chemical Corporation has also produced derivatives of the compounds disclosed in U.S. Patents 3,414,618 and 3,696,857 for use as antioxidants. These are phenothiazines having the formula

(1)

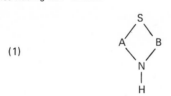

where A and B are the same or different and each is an aryl group, and one of the aryl groups A and B contains a tertiary alkyl substituent group having 4 to 12 carbons. The substitution and type of tertiary alkyl groups in Formula (1) are the same as in the previous patents cited above.

Examples of such phenothiazine compounds include 3-tert-butylphenothiazine, 3-tert-pentylphenothiazine, 3-tert-octylphenothiazine, 3-tert-dodecylphenothiazine, and analogues thereof where one or both of the benzene rings is replaced by a 1,2- or 2,1-substituted naphthalene residue.

These monotertiary alkyl substituted phenothiazine compounds are produced, for example, by thionating the corresponding monoalkyl substituted diarylamine compound. The thionation can be carried out by reacting the monoalkyl substituted diarylamine compounds with elemental sulfur, at an elevated temperature, and preferably at 100° to 250°C. If desired, the reaction can be conducted in the presence of an organic solvent inert under the reaction conditions, for instance, xylene. The reaction of the monoalkyl substituted diarylamine compound with sulfur can be carried out, if desired, in the presence of iodine or other thionation catalyst. The monoalkyl substituted diarylamine compound is preferably reacted with two atomic proportions of sulfur per molar proportion of the diarylamine compound. If desired, the monoalkylated phenothiazine compound can be isolated from the reaction mixture by conventional means, for example, by crystallization.

Example 1: 84.4 parts by weight of 4-tert-octyldiphenylamine, produced by the procedure described in Example 1 of U.S. Patents 3,414,618 and 3,696,851, were heated with 10.2 parts by weight of sulfur for 20 hr while maintaining the temperature within the range of from 200° to 220°C. The reactants were heated until the rate of evolution of hydrogen sulfide was very slow. The crude reaction product was crystallized from petroleum ether (boiling point range 60° to 80°C) to produce 3-tert-octylphenothiazine, having melting point 118°C. The yield was 72% theoretical.

Example 2: 109.4 parts by weight of N-p-tert-octylphenyl-α-naphthylamine, produced by the procedure described in Example 2 of U.S. Patents 3,414,618 and 3,696,851, were dissolved in 200 parts by volume of xylene and the solution was heated with 21.5 parts by weight of sulfur and 1.1 parts by weight of iodine as thionation catalyst. The mixture was heated at 148°C for 24 hr. The thionation product was 9-tert-octyl-12H-benzo[a]phenothiazine, having melting point 147° to 148°C. The yield was 56% theoretical.

Example 3: Synthetic ester based lubricant compositions were prepared into which were incorporated either a monotertiary alkylphenothiazine or a monotertiary alkyldiarylamine compound and subjected to an oxidation corrosion test. The base fluid in the tests was trimethylolpropane tripelargonate and each test was 6 hr at 260°C (500°F) with dry air at the rate of 5 l/hr in the presence of two mild steel specimens having ¾" outside diameter and $\frac{5}{16}$" inside diameter (British Standard Specification No. 3). To each lubricant sample had been added 1.5% by weight of a monotertiary alkyl substituted compound, based on the total weight of the lubricant composition. The results of the tests are given in the table.

Additive	Percent additive	Percent viscosity increase at 100° F.	Final acid value	Sludge	Weight change of steel specimens
None		31.7	9.9	16	+0.08; +0.07
Phenothiazine	1.0	12.9	3.7	617	+0.11; +0.16
Iminodibenzyl	1.0	4.4	3.5	Moderate	+0.22; +0.19
Diphenylamine	1.0	9.5	4.4	343	+0.08; +0.28
Di-tertiary octyl-phenothiazine	2.0	14.9	8.0	11	+0.63; +0.71
N-phenyl-α-naphthylamine	1.0	9.2	4.5	274	+0.07; +0.12
4,4'-tertiary octyldiphenylamine	2.0	19.4	6.7	10	+0.65; +0.55
10-tertiary octyl-7H-benzo[c]-phenothiamine	1.5	14.8	5.9	1	+0.10; +0.13
9-tertiary octyl-12-benzo[a] phenothiazine	1.5	24.2	7.3	24	+0.12; +0.12
3-tertiary octyl-phenothiazine	1.5	12.9	6.6	4	+0.03; +0.02
N-p-tertiary octyl-phenyl-α-naphthylamine	1.5	17.0	4.1	10	+0.19; +0.20
N-p-tertiary octyl-phenyl-β-naphthylamine	1.5	8.8	2.4	1	+0.03; +0.01

In the table the final acid value is expressed as milligrams of potassium hydroxide per gram; the sludge is expressed as milligrams; and the weight change of the steel specimens is expressed as milligrams per square centimeter. Included in the table are the results of comparative tests carried out under the same conditions but with no additive and with prior known antioxidant compounds as additives.

The results in the table demonstrate the ability of these monoalkylated compounds to protect the lubricant oil without the production of oil insolubles and magnesium attack. The dialkylated derivatives used in the comparative tests described inhibited the production of sludge but cause heavy corrosion of magnesium.

N,N'-Diaryl-1,4-Diaminonaphthalenes

Substituted 1,4-naphthadiols are used by *D.M. Fenton; U.S. Patent 3,655,763; April 11,*

1972; assigned to Union Oil Company as starting materials for producing these diaryldi-
aminonaphthalene antioxidants. These compounds produced by this process are useful as
antioxidants and in particular are useful as antioxidants in rubber compositions by incorporation in rubber in amounts from about 0.01 to about 5.0 weight percent in the conventional manner for the use of antioxidants.

The process comprises the steps of sulfonation followed by amination and desulfonation
of a 1,4-naphthadiol reactant bearing a hydrocarbyl or halo substituent in the beta position. The positions of the naphthalene ring, i.e., the 5, 6, 7 and 8 positions, can be substituted with other hydrocarbyl groups and the formula for the suitable starting material
is as follows:

where R_1 and R_2 are halo, alkyl, cycloalkyl with 5 or 6 ring carbons or monocyclic aryl
with no more than 12 carbons; and n is from 0 to 4.

Many of the diol reactants can be obtained commercially, however, these reactants can
also be obtained from naphthalene by alkylation or halogenation to substitute the naphthalene. The beta substituted naphthalene can then be reacted by suitable means to prepare
the 1,4-derivatives, e.g., oxidation by contacting chromium trioxide in acetic acid with beta
substituted naphthalenes yields the beta substituted 1,4-naphthoquinones. The quinone
can then be reduced with a suitable reducing agent, e.g., reaction with alkali metal dithionites
or with hydrazine or other reducing agents at temperatures from 25° to 200°C under liquid
conditions, e.g., with an aqueous solution of the reducing agent.

The 2-substituted-1,4-naphthadiol which is produced can then be reacted with a suitable
sulfonating agent, e.g., sulfurous acid or alkali metal bisulfites, e.g., sodium, lithium, potassium or cesium bisulfite, or metal sulfites, e.g., sodium metabisulfite, potassium metabisulfite, lithium metabisulfite or cesium metabisulfite. The concentration of the sulfonating
agent should be 0.1 to 10 molar and this treatment is performed at temperatures of 25° to
200°C. The alkali metal sulfonate salt of the 1,4-naphthadiol can be recovered from the
aqueous solution by filtration.

The alkali metal sulfonate is then mixed with an arylamine hydrohalide, optionally in the
presence of a suitable inert solvent. These reactants are heated to a temperature of 100°
to 350°C and will react with evolution of gases, chiefly sulfur dioxide with some water
vapor and hydrohalide gas. The reaction can be continued until the evolution of the gas
substantially ceases, a period of from several minutes to 12 hr, depending on the temperature of the reactants.

The crude reaction product is removed from the reaction zone and treated to recover the
desired N,N'-diaryl-1,4-diaminonaphthalene bearing a substitutent in the 2 ring position.
This amino hydrocarbon can be recovered by any suitable purification step, e.g., extraction
with solvents or by distillation. A suitable procedure comprises extraction in alcoholic solvents or other selective solvents such as ethers, esters, ketones or aromatic hydrocarbons.

The products can be further purified if necessary by liquid solid chromatography. The
arylamine hydrohalide used as the reactant can be any hydrohalide of aniline or aminonaphthalene and their alkyl derivatives containing up to 3 alkyl groups with 1 to 8 carbons
in the alkyl groups.

Example: The 1,4-naphthadiol was prepared from the 1,4-quinone by the addition of 15
grams of 2-methylnaphthaquinone, 200 ml diethyl ether and 35 g sodium hydrosulfide

and 100 ml of water to a flask which was stirred for 2 hr at room temperature. A pale yellow solution was formed which separated into distinct phases. The aqueous phase was discarded and the diethyl ether phase was then reacted by the addition of a concentrated aqueous solution containing 60 g sodium bisulfite. The mixture was heated to remove the ether and at 70°C an exothermic reaction occurred with the formation of a white precipitate comprising the sodium sulfonate of 2-methyl-1,4-naphthadiol.

The white precipitate was separated by filtration and 19 g of the separated solid was mixed with 23 g of aniline hydrochloride and the mixture was heated to 230°C and maintained at that temperature for 9 hr. A vigorous evolution of gases was observed upon heating of the reactants. After completion of the reaction period, the reactants were mixed with 500 milliliters of methanol and the methanol extract was removed and concentrated in a steam bath to 100 ml.

The concentrated extract was then contacted with 100 ml of water and 500 ml of diethyl ether and the solvents were permitted to separate into two distinct phases. The ether layer was chromatographed on activated alumina, separated into fractions and concentrated to obtain a red-purple solid, melting point 185°C. The infrared spectrum identified the product as N,N'-diphenyl-1,4-diamino-2-methylnaphthalene.

Other products prepared by this process include: N,N'-diphenyl-1,4-diamino-2-phenylnaphthalene; N,N'-di-p-tolyl-1,4-diamino-2-methylnaphthalene; N,N'-dinaphthyl-1,4-diamino-2-methylnaphthalene; and N,N'-diphenyl-1,4-diamino-2,6,7-trichloronaphthalene.

Aromatic Aliphatic Secondary Amines

Secondary aromatic aliphatic amines, and a process for their preparation are disclosed by *M.E. Cain, B. Saville and G.T. Knight; U.S. Patent 3,689,513; September 5, 1972; assigned to The Natural Rubber Producers' Research Association, England.* The conventional preparation of p-phenylenediamines involves the catalytic hydrogenation of a mixture of a p-amino-, p-nitro- or p-nitrosoaniline and an aldehyde or ketone. A disadvantage of this hydrogenation is that it is only suitable for batch operation.

By contrast, the thermal addition reaction of this process is capable of being operated continuously. Also, it may be desirable to prepare antioxidants of high molecular weights to minimize their removal from the system which they are protecting by volatilization, migration or solvent action. According to this process, p-phenylenediamine groups can advantageously be introduced into large molecules by the use of cheap and readily available unsaturated fats and oils. This process provides a method for preparing a secondary aromatic aliphatic amine by heating together (a) an aromatic nitroso compound having the formula:

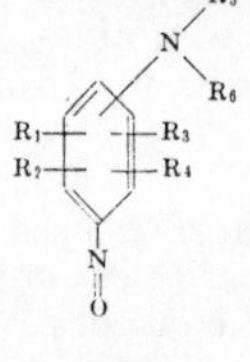

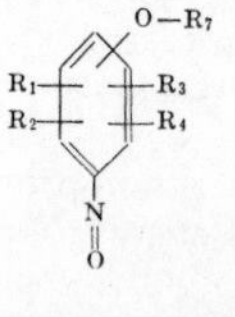

where R_1, R_2, and R_3 and R_4 may be the same or different and each represent a hydrogen, a saturated or unsaturated aliphatic (including alicyclic) group or an aryl, aralkyl or alkaryl group, which may contain one or more noncarbon atoms, or may, in Formula (1) form one or more additional aromatic rings fused to the aromatic ring, R_5, R_6 and R_7 may be the same or different and each represent a hydrogen, a saturated or unsaturated aliphatic (including alicyclic) group, or an aryl, aralkyl or alkaryl group which may contain one or more noncarbon atoms, or R_5 and R_6 together with the nitrogen form a heterocyclic ring which may contain one or more other hetero atoms; and (b) an olefin having at least one hydrogen atom attached to a carbon atom which is in the α position with respect to the carbon-

carbon double bond, i.e., having the formula:

(3) $RRC=CR-CHRR$

where R in each case is a hydrogen or a saturated or unsaturated aliphatic (including alicyclic) group or an aryl, aralkyl or alkaryl group which may contain one or more other functional groups, provided that each group R contains not more than 100 carbons. It should be noted that large substituent groups, attached to the aromatic ring of the nitroso compound, may sterically block either the nitroso group or the other functional group (e.g., amine or hydroxyl) to inhibit or prevent reaction. For example, it has been found that di-tert-butylnitrosophenol cannot easily be reacted in the manner above.

Any convenient olefin may be used provided that there is a hydrogen atom attached to the carbon atom which is alpha to the double bond. However, the rate of reaction of a specific olefin depends on its structure. Thus, trialkyl-substituted ethylenes generally react faster than di- or monoalkyl-substituted ethylenes.

The secondary aromatic aliphatic amines which are prepared by the above reaction will have one of the two formulas below, in which R, R_1, R_2, R_3, R_4, R_5, R_6 and R_7 have the significance set out above.

(4) [chemical structure: benzene ring with R_5 and R_6 on N at top; R_1, R_2 on left; R_3, R_4 on right; $NH-CRR-CR=CRR$ at bottom]   or   (5) [chemical structure: benzene ring with R_7 on O at top; R_1, R_2 on left; R_3, R_4 on right; $NH-CRR-CR=CRR$ at bottom]

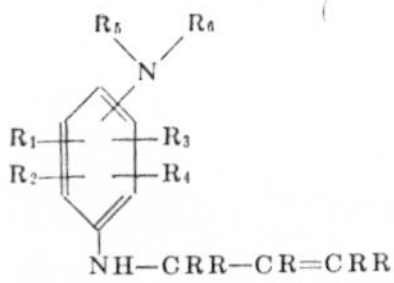

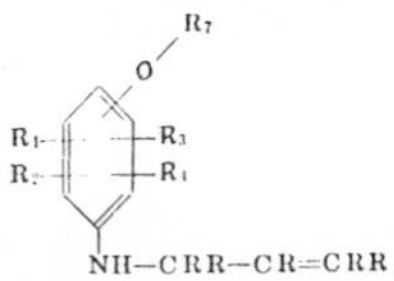

Specific compounds prepared by this process include N,N-dimethyl-N'-(1-ethyl-2-methyl-prop-2-enyl)-p-phenylenediamine; N,N-dimethyl-N'-(1-isopropenylhexyl)-p-phenylenediamine; N,N-diethyl-N'-(1-ethyl-2-methylprop-2-enyl)-p-phenylenediamine; and N-phenyl-N'-(1-iso-propenylhexyl)-p-phenylenediamine.

The reaction between the aromatic nitroso compound and the olefin is effected by heating the reactants together in the liquid phase. The olefin may constitute the liquid medium; but the aromatic nitroso compounds have only limited solubility in olefins, so a substantial excess of the olefin may have to be used. Alternatively, a nonpolar organic solvent, for example, xylene or cyclohexane, may be used; such nonpolar solvents have little effect on the rate of reaction, compared to reaction performed in the absence of solvents, but may slightly increase the yield.

To further increase the yield and reduce by-product formation, compounds capable of acting as electron transfer reductants (for example, 2 mols of zinc dimethyldithiocarbamate per mol of nitroso compound) or as hydrogen atom donors (e.g., 1 mol of hydroquinone per mol of nitroso compound) may be added as coagents to the reaction mixture either in the presence or absence of a nonpolar solvent.

Example 1: N,N-diethyl-N'-(1-ethyl-2-methylprop-2-enyl)-p-phenylenediamine was prepared by heating 8.9 g of N,N-diethyl-p-nitrosoaniline (DENA) with 16 g of 2-methyl-2-pentene in xylene (25 ml) under vacuum at 140°C for 48 hr. Removal of the solvent gave 6 g of product, boiling point 96°C/0.01 mm. Its identity was confirmed by both infrared and nuclear magnetic resonance spectroscopy.

Example 2: The antioxidant properties of four phenylenediamines of this process were evaluated in the oxygen absorption of a gum natural rubber vulcanizate using the formulation below.

Natural rubber Heveacrumb SMR5L)	100 parts by weight
Zinc oxide	5 parts by weight (continued)

Stearic acid	2 parts by weight
N-cyclohexylbenzothiazole-2-sulfen-	
amide (CBS)	0.5 parts by weight
Sulfur	2.5 parts by weight
Cure time at 140°C	40 minutes

The oxygen absorption of samples cut from 10 x 10 x 0.3 cm vulcanized sheets was meas-ured at 100°C. The results are compared in the table below with those given by three commercially available p-phenylenediamine antioxidants.

Antioxidant Activity of Substituted p-Phenylenediamines (1 pphr)

Substituents	Hours to 1% Oxygen Absorption
None	26
N-isopropyl-N'-phenyl*	60
N-(1,3-dimethylbutyl)-N'-phenyl**	51
N,N'-di-(1,4-dimethylpentyl)***	40
N,N-dimethyl-N'-(1-ethyl-2-methylprop-2-enyl)	52
N,N-dimethyl-N'-(1-isopropenylhexyl)	58
N,N-diethyl-N'-(1-ethyl-2-methylprop-2-enyl)	52
N-phenyl-N'-(isopropenylhexyl) †	45

*Commercially available as Nonex ZA
**Commercially available as Santoflex 13
***Commercially available as Santoflex 77
†75% pure

The table shows that the p-phenylenediamine antioxidants are equally as effective as the best available saturated p-phenylenediamines. The reaction may also be conducted using higher molecular weight unsaturates including naturally occuring fats and oils as the olefin to form antioxidants. Examples of such unsaturates include polybutene, palm oil, fish oil, castor oil, factice and the like. The products from these unsaturates have the advantage in that they are not readily extracted from the polymeric material they are protecting.

BENZYLATED DIPHENYLAMINE AND PHENYLNAPHTHYLAMINE DERIVATIVES

Work performed at the Uniroyal Laboratories has resulted in a complex overlapping group of seven patents. These are concerned with antioxidant derivatives of diphenylamine and the phenylnaphthylamines and their use either alone, in combination with each other, or in combination with dialkyl 3,3'-thiodipropionates, for the protection of organic materials having relatively low olefinic unsaturation. Examples of materials which are protected by the compounds of this process are alpha-olefin polymers, polyamides, polyesters, poly-acetals, acrylonitrile-butadiene-styrene thermoplastics, and lubricants of the petroleum oil type or of the synthetic type. The compounds disclosed in these processes are represented by the following formulas:

(1)

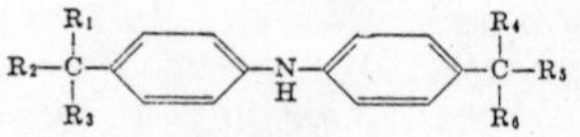

where R_1 is a phenyl or p-tolyl, R_2 and R_3 are selected from methyl, phenyl and p-tolyl, R_4 is selected from methyl, phenyl, p-tolyl and neopentyl, R_5 is selected from methyl, phenyl, p-tolyl and 2-phenylisobutyl, and R_6 is a methyl.

(2)

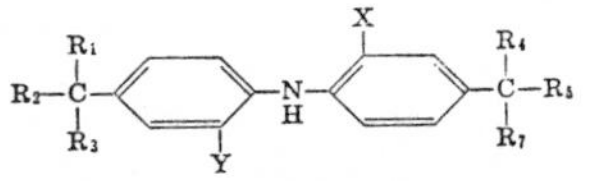

In the above formula, R_1 through R_5 are selected from the radicals shown in Formula (1) and R_7 is selected from methyl, phenyl, or p-tolyl; X is selected from methyl, ethyl, a sec-alkyl containing 3 to 10 carbons, α,α-dimethylbenzyl, α-methylbenzyl, chlorine, bromine, carboxyl, and metal salts of the carboxylic acids where the metal is zinc, cadmium, nickel, lead, tin, magnesium or copper; and Y is selected from hydrogen, methyl, ethyl, a sec-alkyl containing 3 to 10 carbons, chlorine, and bromine.

(3)

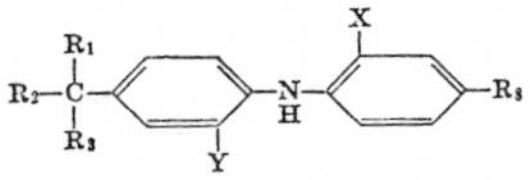

In the above formula R_1 is a phenyl or p-tolyl; R_2 and R_3 are selected from methyl, phenyl and p-tolyl; R_3 is selected from hydrogen, a primary, secondary and tertiary alkyl containing from 1 to 10 carbons, and alkoxyl containing 1 to 10 carbons which may be straight chain or branched; and X and Y are selected from hydrogen, methyl, ethyl, sec-alkyl containing 3 to 10 carbons, chlorine and bromine.

(4)

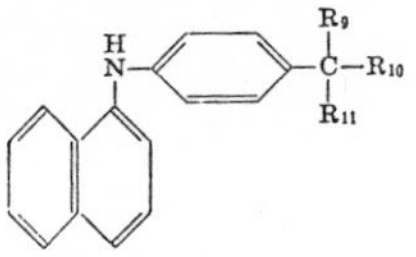

In the above formula R_9 is a phenyl or p-tolyl; R_{10} is selected from methyl, phenyl, p-tolyl and 2-phenylisobutyl; and R_{11} is selected from methyl, phenyl and p-tolyl.

(5)

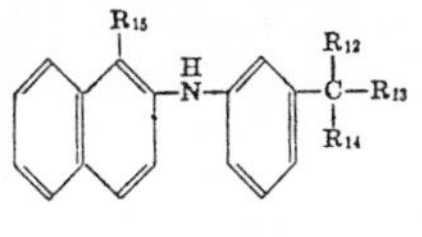

In the above formula R_{12} is a phenyl or p-tolyl; R_{13} is selected from methyl, phenyl and p-tolyl; R_{14} is selected from methyl, phenyl, p-tolyl and 2-phenylisobutyl; and R_{15} is selected from hydrogen, α,α-dimethylbenzyl, α-methylbenzhydryl, triphenylmethyl and α,α,p-trimethylbenzyl.

The compounds as shown in Formula (1) may be prepared by alkylating the appropriate diphenylamine or phenylnaphthylamine with the appropriate olefin using a suitable acid catalyst such as aluminum chloride, zinc chloride, or acid clay. Where there are two groups of different structure on the diphenylamine nucleus a stepwise alkylation may be carried out.

In the compounds which contained a trityl group, triphenylmethyl chloride may be used as the alkylating agent. The unsymmetrical diphenylamines may be prepared in two ways:

    (a)   By condensing an appropriately substituted aniline with o-chlorobenzoic acid. The carboxyl group may be removed, when desired, by thermal decarboxylation. The final unsymmetrical product may be obtained by reacting with the appropriate alkylating agent using an acid catalyst.

(b) By alkylating diphenylamine with a vinyl type olefin (i.e., butene-1, octene-1) and separating the predominant 2-alkylidiphenylamine or 2,2'-dialkyldiphenylamine. This product may then be reacted with the appropriate alkylating agent using a typical acid catalyst to obtain the final product.

These antioxidants are effective in the conventional amounts ordinarily used for protecting substrates from oxidation, usually within the range of 0.01 to 4% by weight, based on the weight of the substrate. These derivatives of diphenylamine and the phenylnaphthylamines are more effective than the parent compounds or the known 4,4'-dialkyldiphenylamines either alone, in combinations, or in combination with dialkyl 3,3'-thiodipropionates (in which the alkyl groups typically contain from 8 to 20 carbons).

Although the individual patents reviewed below contain much material included in the others of the group, the material selected for review of each patent or group of patents is based on the subject of the claims.

4,4'-Disubstituted Diphenylamines

In *E.L. Wheeler; U.S. Patents 3,505,225; April 7, 1970; 3,666,716; May 30, 1972; and N.K. Sundholm; U.S. Patents 3,452,056; June 24, 1969; 3,533,992; October 13, 1970; all assigned to Uniroyal, Inc.,* emphasis is placed on antioxidants of Formula (1) which are illustrated below.

(1)

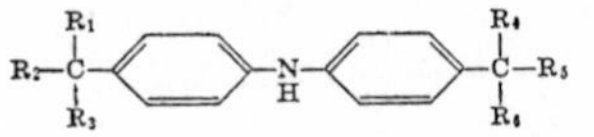

	R_1	R_2	R_3	R_4	R_5	R_6
(a)	Phenyl	Methyl	Methyl	Phenyl	Methyl	Methyl
(b)	do	Phenyl	do	do	Phenyl	Do.
(c)	do	do	Phenyl	Neopentyl	Methyl	Do.
(d)	p-Tolyl	Methyl	Methyl	p-Tolyl	do	Do.

Example 1: A mixture of 84.5 g of diphenylamine, 13 g of montmorillonite clay (Girdler Catalysts' designation KSF/O) and 100 ml of benzene was heated to the reflux temperature with stirring. Water was removed from the catalyst by azeotropic distillation of the benzene. Enough benzene was removed to allow the pot temperature to reach 130°C. 124 g of α-methylstyrene was added dropwise during 20 min and the mixture was stirred for 4 hours at 130° to 135°C.

The catalyst was removed by filtration, and the filtrate was crystallized by pouring into hexane. 152 g (75% yield) of product was obtained MP 99° to 100°C. The 4,4'-bis(α,α-dimethylbenzyl)diphenylamine was recrystallized twice from hexane, MP 101° to 102°C.

Example 2: A mixture of 7.6 g of diphenylamine, 4 g of montmorillonite clay catalyst (Girdler Catalysts' designation KSF/O) and 150 ml of toluene was heated to the reflux temperature with stirring. Water was removed by azeotropic distillation and toluene was further removed until the pot temperature reached 130°C. 24.5 g of 1,1-diphenylethylene was added dropwise during 15 min and the reaction mixture was stirred for 5 hr at 135°C.

The catalyst was removed by filtration and the product was crystallized from hexane to obtain 21 g (88%), MP 148° to 159°C. Two recrystallizations from isopropanol gave pure 4,4'-bis(α-methylbenzhydryl)diphenylamine, MP 171.0° to 171.5°C.

Example 3: A mixture of 169 g of diphenylamine and 30 g of anhydrous aluminum chloride was heated to 90°C with stirring. 112 g of diisobutylene was added dropwise over a 1 hr period. An exotherm occurred and the temperature was maintained at 115°C during the addition. The mixture was heated at 125° to 135°C for an additional hour, then cooled and poured into water. 400 ml of benzene was added and the organic layer was separated, washed and dried. The benzene was removed by distillation and the residue product was fractionally distilled under reduced pressure. The fraction boiling at 160° to 175°C (0.5 mm) was the 4-(1,1,3,3-tetramethylbutyl)diphenylamine.

A mixture of 28.1 g of 4-(1,1,3,3-tetramethylbutyl)diphenylamine, 27.9 g of triphenylmethyl chloride, 500 ml of acetic acid and 50 ml of concentrated hydrochloric acid was heated under reflux. 25 ml of acetic acid-water mixture was removed by distillation during the first hour, then the mixture was refluxed an additional 2½ hr. The reaction mixture was poured into water and the resulting solid was removed by filtration. The solid was slurried with benzene and heated under reflux, then filtered hot to remove any insoluble material. The filtrate was evaporated to dryness and the crude 4-(1,1,3,3-tetramethylbutyl)-4'-triphenylmethyldiphenylamine (27 g) recrystallized three times from hexane, MP 203° to 205°C.

Example 4: A mixture of 169 g of diphenylamine, 25 g of montmorillonite clay (Girdler Catalysts' designation KSF/O) previously dried at 120°C for 16 hr, and 150 ml of toluene was heated with stirring at 130°C. 220 g of p,α-dimethylstyrene was added over a 1 hr period and the reaction was maintained at 135°C for 4 hr. The catalyst was removed by filtration and the product 4,4'-bis(α,α,p-trimethylbenzyl)diphenylamine was crystallized from hexane, MP 102° to 103°C.

Example 5: This example demonstrates the usefulness of these compounds as stabilizers for polyethylene. The stabilizers (0.1% by weight) were milled into unstabilized polyethylene (DYNH) at 310°F for 5 to 7 min. The polymer was extruded into plates 75 ml thick. The plates were aged at 375°F and the time to resinification determined.

Compound	Minutes to Resinification (375°F)
(1) Control (unstabilized)	120
(2) 4-(1,1,3,3-tetramethylbutyl)-4'-triphenylmethyldiphenylamine	150
(3) 4,4'-bis(α-methylbenzhydryl)diphenylamine	180
(4) 4,4'-bis(α,α-dimethylbenzyl)diphenylamine	270

Examples are also included in U.S. Patents 3,505,225 and 3,666,716 on the stabilization of polypropylene, ABS, EPT (ethylene-propylene-diene terpolymer elastomer) and polyacetal resin. In U.S. Patents 3,533,992 and 3,542,056 compounds of Examples 1 and 2 are used as stabilizers for natural rubber.

Example 6: This example illustrates the use of chemicals of Examples 1 and 2 as antioxidants for natural rubber. A natural rubber composition was prepared in accordance with the following recipe.

Masterbatch Number 1

	Parts by Weight
Pale crepe	98.65
Zinc oxide	10.00
Lithopone	60.00
Whiting	60.00
Zinc laurate	0.50
Sulfur	3.00
Masterbatch number 2	1.50
	233.65

Masterbatch Number 2

	Parts by Weight
Pale crepe	90.0
Tetramethylthiuram monosulfide	10.0
	100.0

One part by weight of the antioxidants listed in the table below was then milled into 233.65 parts of masterbatch number 1 and samples were cured at 274°F for 30 min. Dumbbell shaped test specimens were prepared according to ASTM Method D412. They were aged along with specimens containing no added antioxidant in an oxygen bomb at 300 psi for 96 hr at 70°C.

In another test specimens with and without antioxidant were heated in an oven at 100°C for 24 hr. The tensile strengths of the aged and unaged specimens were determined. The greater percent retention of tensile strength of the specimens containing the compounds of this process over those containing no antioxidant demonstrates their antioxidant activity. The data are given in the following table.

	- -Percent Tensile Retained- - -	
Compound	Oxygen Bomb	Oven
None	7,19	35,47
4,4'-bis(α,α-dimethylbenzyl)diphenylamine	71	60
4,4'-bis(α-methylbenzhydryl)diphenylamine	64	62

2,4,4'-Trisubstituted Diphenylamines

Compounds of Formula (2) and (3), as shown on page 67 are covered by *E.L. Wheeler; U.S. Patent 3,751,472; August 7, 1973; assigned to Uniroyal, Inc.* Preferred compounds by these formulas are shown by the formulas below.

(2)

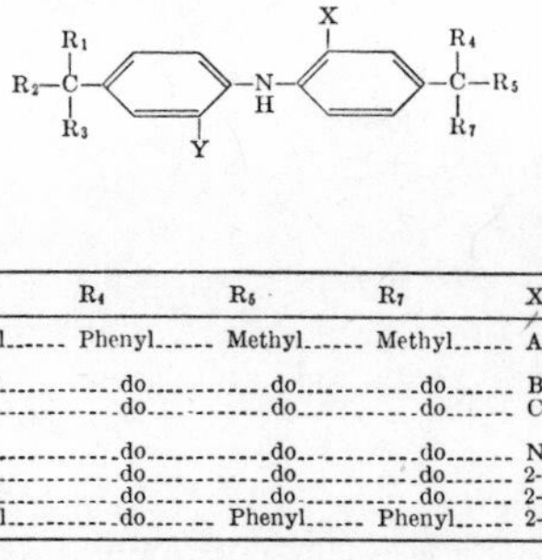

	R₁	R₂	R₃	R₄	R₅	R₇	X	Y
(1)	Phenyl	Methyl	Methyl	Phenyl	Methyl	Methyl	Alpha, alpha-dimethylbenzyl	Hydrogen.
(2)	do	do	do	do	do	do	Bromo	Bromo.
(3)	do	do	do	do	do	do	Carboxyl	Hydrogen.
(4)	do	do	do	do	do	do	Nickel carboxylate	Do.
(5)	do	do	do	do	do	do	2-butyl	Do.
(6)	do	do	do	do	do	do	2-octyl	Do.
(7)	do	Phenyl	Phenyl	do	Phenyl	Phenyl	2-hexyl	Do.

(3)

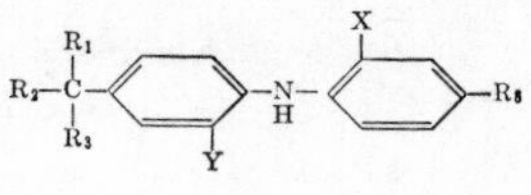

	R₁	R₂	R₃	R₈	X	Y
(1)	Phenyl	Methyl	Methyl	Isopropoxy	Hydrogen	Hydrogen.
(2)	do	do	do	Hydrogen	2-octyl	Do.
(3)	do	Phenyl	Phenyl	do	2-hexyl	Do.

Example 1: A mixture of 85 g of diphenylamine, 13.3 g of anhydrous aluminum chloride, and 200 ml of n-hexane was heated at the reflux temperature with stirring. 206 g of α-methylstyrene was added dropwise during 1½ hr, and the mixture was stirred at 80° to 85°C for 4½ hr. The reaction mixture was cooled and poured into water, the organic layer separated and washed three times with water, and the solvent was removed by distillation. The product was vacuum topped to 200°C (0.5 mm). Crystallization of the crude product (216 g) from hexane removed most of the more insoluble 4,4'-bis(α,α-dimethylbenzyl)diphenylamine.

The filtrate was evaporated to dryness and the residue product (145 g) recrystallized twice from isopropanol to obtain 49 g of 2,4,4'-tris(α,α-dimethylbenzyl)diphenylamine, MP 114° to 116°C. An analytical sample was prepared by chromatographing 10 g of the compound on 250 g of alumina using 20% benzene-80% hexane as the eluent. The first fractions obtained were evaporated and recrystallized twice from hexane, MP 121.5° to 122.5°C.

Example 2: To a stirred solution of 40 g of 4,4'-bis(α,α-dimethylbenzyl)diphenylamine in 300 ml of glacial acetic acid was added 32 g of bromine dissolved in 100 ml of glacial acetic acid at room temperature. After the addition was complete the mixture was heated at 45°C for 10 min and the product was removed by filtration. The crude dibromo derivative was dissolved in benzene and the solution extracted with dilute sodium hydroxide, then washed with water. The benzene was evaporated and the product was recrystallized from isopropanol to obtain 39 g of 2,2'-dibromo-4,4'-bis(α,α-dimethylbenzyl)diphenylamine, MP 166° to 167°C.

Example 3: A mixture of 39.5 g of 2-(α-methylheptyl)diphenylamine and 6 g of montmorillonite clay (Girdler Catalysts' designation KSF/O) was heated to 125°C and 20 g of α-methylstyrene was added over a 10 min period. The mixture was heated at 120° to 130°C for 4 hr. The reaction mixture was diluted with benzene and the catalyst was removed by filtration. The solvent was removed by distillation and the residue product was purified by fractional distillation under reduced pressure. The fraction boiling at 200°C (0.4 mm) was 2-(α-methylheptyl)-4'-(α,α-dimethylbenzyl)diphenylamine.

Example 4: This demonstrates the usefulness of the compounds as processing stabilizers for terpolymers composed of ethylene, propylene, and a small amount of nonconjugated diene. 2% by weight of the stabilizer was incorporated into unstabilized rubbery terpolymer, containing, for example, about 62% ethylene, 33% propylene and 5% dicyclopentadiene, on a mill at 150°F and the mixture subjected to milling at 300°F. After various milling times the Mooney viscosity (ML-4 at 212°F) of the polymer measured. A rise in viscosity is indicative of degenerative cross-linking of the polymer due to heat and mechanical shearing.

Compound	Mooney viscosity vs. time on 300° F. mill				
	0''	15''	30''	45''	60''
Control	53	57	74	90	97
2,2'-dibromo-4,4'-bis(alpha,alpha-dimethylbenzyl)diphenylamine	53	52.5	51	50.5	54
2,4,4'-tris(alpha,alpha-dimethylbenzyl)-diphenylamine	54	51	49.5	49	50

Other examples show the use of compounds of Formula (2) and (3) in ABS, polypropylene, polyethylene, synthetic polyester lubricants and polyacetal resins.

Phenylnaphthylamine Derivatives

Compounds of Formulas (4) and (5) as shown on page 67 are covered by *E.L. Wheeler; U.S. Patents 3,781,361; December 25, 1973; and 3,649,690; March 14, 1972; both assigned to Uniroyal, Inc.* Typical preferred compounds are shown on the following page.

(4)

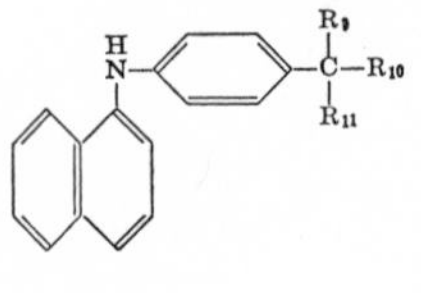

R_9 is phenyl and R_{10} and R_{11} are methyl.

(5)

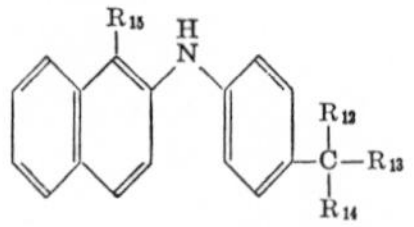

	R_{12}	R_{13}	R_{14}	R_{15}
(1).......	Phenyl	Methyl..	Methyl..	Hydrogen.
(2)...........	.do.........	.do.........	.do......	Alpha,alpha-dimethylbenzyl.

Example 1: A mixture of 219 g of N-phenyl-1-naphthylamine, 25 g of montmorillonite clay (Girdler Catalysts' designation KSF/O) and 300 ml of toluene was heated to the reflux temperature and 100 ml of toluene was distilled from the mixture. The reaction mixture was maintained at 130°C and 260 g of α-methylstyrene was added dropwise over a 1 hr period. The mixture was heated an additional 4 hr at 135°C. The catalyst was removed by filtration and the product vacuum topped to 200°C (1.0 mm).

The crude product was purified by chromatography on alumina using benzene-hexane mixtures as the eluent, followed by two recrystallizations from hexane. The pure N-(4-α,α-dimethylbenzylphenyl)-1-naphthylamine after drying under vacuum at 78°C for 6 hr melted at 91.5° to 92.5°C.

Example 2: A mixture of 219 g of N-phenyl-2-naphthylamine, 30 g of anhydrous aluminum chloride, and 250 ml of benzene was heated with stirring to 70° to 75°C. 260 g of α-methylstyrene was added dropwise during a 1 hr period and the reaction mixture was maintained at 70° to 85°C for 4 hr. The mixture was poured into water, more benzene was added and the benzene solution was washed twice with water. The benzene was removed by distillation and the crude product vacuum topped at 200°C (0.4 mm). 394 g of residue product was obtained. A pure N-(4-α,α-dimethylbenzylphenyl)-1-(α,α-dimethylbenzyl)-2-naphthylamine (MP 121.5° to 122.0°C) was obtained by two recrystallizations from a benzene-hexane mixture.

Example 3: A mixture of 110 g of N-phenyl-2-naphthylamine, 12.5 g of montmorillonite clay (Girdler Catalysts' designation KSF/O) and 150 ml of toluene was heated at the reflux temperature with stirring. Water was removed from the catalyst by azeotropic distillation along with 100 ml of toluene. 65 g of α-methylstyrene was added dropwise over a ½ hr period and the reaction mixture was maintained at 100°C for 2 hr. The catalyst was removed by filtration and the solvent removed by distillation. The N-(4-α,α-dimethylbenzylphenyl)-2-naphthylamine was crystallized from hexane and after two recrystallizations from hexane melted at 92.0° to 92.5°C.

Example 4: This example demonstrates the usefulness of the naphthyl compounds as stabilizers for polypropylene in combination with dilauryl thiodipropionate. The stabilizers were incorporated into the polypropylene (unstabilized Profax 6501) by first milling the resin at 340°F for several minutes, then adding the stabilizers to the polymer.

The milling was continued for 8 to 10 minutes. The polymer was then molded into plates 90 ml thick. Three plates of each sample of stabilized polymer were aged at 300°F in a circulating air oven. The break point was defined as the first sign of embrittlement or crumbling in two out of the three pieces.

The following table illustrates the effectiveness of the phenylnaphthylamine derivatives of the process as stabilizers for polypropylene, their synergism with dilauryl 3,3'-thiodipropionate and their superiority over chemicals of prior art.

Compound	Conc., percent	Days to break at 300° F.	Initial color	Color at break
(1)... N-phenyl 1-naphthyl-amine.[1]	0.1	1	White....	Yellow.
	0.3	1	Buff....	Dark yellow.
(2)... N-phenyl 2-naphthyl-amine.[1]	0.1	1	Off-white.	Yellow.
	0.3	1	Pink....	Dark yellow.
(3)... N-(4-alpha,alpha-di-methylbenzyl-phenyl)-1-naphthylamine.	0.1	2	White....	Tan.
	0.3	19	Tan......	Tan.
(4)... N-(4-alpha,alpha-di-methylbenzyl phenyl)-2-naphthyl-amine.	0.1	2	Off-white.	Tan.
	0.3	16	Light pink.	Tan.
(5)... {N-(4-alpha,alpha-di-methyl benzyl-phenyl)-1-naph-thylamine.	0.1	32	White....	Off-white.
Dilauryl 3,3'-thiodi-propionate.	0.4			
(6)... {N-phenyl-1-naph-thylamine.[1]	0.1	12	...do......	White.
Dilauryl 3,3'-thiodi-propionate.	0.4			
(7)... {N-phenyl-2-naph-thylamine.[1]	0.1	16	Off-white.	Off-white.
Dilauryl 3,3'-thiodi-propionate.	0.4			
(8)... {N-(4-alpha,alpha-di-methylbenzyl-phenyl)-2-naph-thylamine.	0.1	24	White....	Do.
Dilauryl 3,3'-thiodi-propionate.	0.4			

[1] Prior art.

Other examples show the stabilization of polyester lubricants, EPT, and polyacetal resins with these phenylnaphthylamine derivatives.

N-HYDROXYALKYLAMINE COMPOUNDS

Cyba has prepared a series of amines containing N-hydroxyalkyl moieties which have antioxidant properties. Borate esters of the compounds are also included in this series.

N-Hydroxyalkyl-N'-Hydrocarbylpiperazines

Piperazine derivatives are disclosed by *H.A. Cyba; U.S. Patent 3,673,186; June 27, 1972; assigned to Universal Oil Products Company* in one process. Broadly, these antioxidants encompass N-hydroxyalkyl-N'-hydrocarbylpiperazines in which the alkyl contains 1 to 10 carbons and the hydrocarbyl is preferably sec-alkyl of 3 to 40 carbons or cycloalkyl of 3 to 12 carbons.

The N-hydroxyalkyl may be replaced by an N-alkoxyalkyl in which the alkoxy moiety contains 1 to 10 carbons. Illustrative compounds in which the alkyl group preferably contains 2 carbon atoms include N-hydroxyethyl-N'-isopropylpiperazine, N-hydroxyethyl-N'-sec-butylpiperazine, etc. When the N-hydrocarbyl substituent is cycloalkyl, the cycloalkyl preferably is cyclohexyl and the compound will be N-hydroxyethyl-N'-cyclohexylpiperazine.

It is understood that hydroxyethyl group may also be replaced by hydroxymethyl, hydroxypropyl, hydroxybutyl, etc. When the N substituent is alkoxyalkyl, again preferred compounds comprise those in which the alkyl group contains 2 carbon atoms and illustrative compounds include N-methoxyethyl-N'-hydrocarbylpiperazine, N-ethoxyethyl-N'-hydrocarbylpiperazine, and the like. Preparation methods for preparing these antioxidants are disclosed in the following examples.

Example 1: N-hydroxyethyl-N'-sec-octylpiperazine was prepared as follows. Hydroxyethylpiperazine, which is commercially available, was subjected to reductive alkylation by reacting 240 g of the hydroxyethylpiperazine and 500 g of methyl hexyl ketone at 160°C in the presence of hydrogen and an alumina-platinum catalyst containing about 0.3% by weight of platinum. The resultant N-hydroxyethyl-N'-sec-octylpiperazine was analyzed and found to have a basic nitrogen of 8.27 meq/g and a basic mol combining weight of 121 which corresponds to the theoretical basic mol combining weight of 121. The product had a boiling point of 310°C at atmospheric pressure or 114°C at 0.5 mm mercury, both uncorrected.

Example 2: N-(2-hydroxypropyl)-N'-cyclohexylpiperazine is prepared by subjecting 100 g of N-(2-hydroxypropy)piperazine to reductive alkylation with 200 g of cyclohexanone at 150°C in a 1,800 liter rocking autoclave, in contact with 50 g of a sulfided alumina-platinum catalyst under an imposed hydrogen pressure of 100 atmospheres. After the theoretical amount of hydrogen is consumed, the reaction is discontinued and the reaction products are allowed to cool to room temperature. The effluent products then are filtered to remove N-(2-hydroxypropyl)-N'-cyclohexylpiperazine as a liquid product containing 8.85 meq/g of basic nitrogen.

Example 3: This example compares the effectiveness of N-(2-hydroxyethyl)-N'-sec-octylpiperazine, prepared as described in Example 1, with the N-(2-hydroxyethyl)piperazine, not subjected to reductive alkylation, in solid polypropylene. The samples were processed and tested using the Weatherometer Test given on page 2.

A sample of the polypropylene without inhibitor developed a carbonyl number of greater than 1,000 within 120 hr of exposure. Another sample of the polypropylene containing 1% by weight of N-(2-hydroxyethyl)-N'-sec-octylpiperazine, prepared as in Example 1, and 0.15% by weight of 2,6-di-tert-butyl-4-methylphenol developed a carbonyl value of 402 after 576 hr of exposure. In contrast, another sample of the polypropylene containing 1% by weight of N-(2-hydroxyethyl)piperazine, not reductively alkylated, and 0.15% by weight of 2,6-di-tert-butyl-4-methylphenol developed a carbonyl number of greater than 1,000 within 192 hr of exposure. The compound of Example 1 was also used to stabilize fuel oils in additional examples of the patent.

N-Hydroxyalkyl-N'-Hydrocarbylhexahydropyrimidines

Hexahydropyrimidine compounds similar to the piperazine compounds of the process of U.S. Patent 3,673,186 are also disclosed by *H.A. Cyba; U.S. Patent 3,787,416; January 22, 1974; assigned to Universal Oil Products Company.* Broadly these compounds are N-oxyalkyl-N'-hydrocarbylhexahydropyrimidines in which the hydrocarbyl is sec-alkyl or cycloalkyl. This encompasses the following types of compounds:

> N-hydroxyalkyl-N'-sec-alkylhexahydropyrimidines in which the alkyl contains
>   1 to 10 carbons and the sec-alkyl contains 3 to 40 carbons;
> N-hydroxyalkyl-N'-cycloalkylhexahydropyrimidines in which the cycloalkyl
>   contains 4 to 12 carbons in the ring;
> N-alkoxyalkyl-N'-sec-alkylhexahydropyrimidines in which the alkoxy contains
>   1 to 10 carbons, the alkyl contains 1 to 10 carbons, and the sec-alkyl contains 3 to 40 carbons; and
> N-alkoxyalkyl-N'-cycloalkylhexahydropyrimidines in which the alkoxy contains
>   1 to 10 carbons, the alkyl contains 1 to 10 carbons, and the cycloalkyl contains 4 to 12 carbons in the ring.

Specific compounds included in these types are the following:

> N-hydroxyethyl-N'-isopropylhexahydropyrimidine
> N-hydroxyethyl-N'-sec-butylhexahydropyrimidine
> N-hydroxyethyl-N'-cyclobutylhexahydropyrimidine
> N-hydroxyethyl-N'-cyclopentylhexahydropyrimidine
> N-methoxyethyl-N'-sec-hexylhexahydropyrimidine
> N-ethoxyethyl-N'-sec-octylhexahydropyrimidine

N-ethoxyethyl-N'-cyclohexylhexahydropyrimidine
N-propoxyethyl-N'-cyclohexylhexahydropyrimidine

The following examples illustrate the preparation and use of these antioxidants.

Example 1: N-hydroxyethyl-N'-sec-octylhexahydropyrimidine is prepared as follows. Hydroxyethylhexahydropyrimidine is subjected to reductive alkylation by reacting 240 g of the hydroxyethylhexahydropyrimidine and 500 g of methyl hexyl ketone at 160°C in the presence of 100 atmospheres of hydrogen and an alumina-platinum catalyst containing about 0.3% by weight of platinum. The resultant N-hydroxyethyl-N'-sec-octylhexahydropyrimidine is separated from excess hydrogen and unreacted products. It will have a basic mol combining weight of about 121 which corresponds to the theoretical basic mol combining weight of 121.

Example 2: Solid polypropylene is tested by the process described on page 2 for the Weatherometer Test. A sample of the polypropylene without inhibitor develops a carbonyl number of greater than 1,000 within 120 hr of exposure in the Weatherometer. In contrast, a sample of the solid polypropylene containing 1% by weight of N-(2-hydroxyethyl)-N'-sec-octylhexahydropyrimidine, prepared as in Example 1, and 0.15% by weight of 2,6-di-tert-butyl-4-methylphenol does not develop a carbonyl number of greater than 1,000 until more than 800 hr of exposure in the Weatherometer.

Other examples in the complete patent show the stabilization of fuel oils by addition of N-hydroxyethyl-N'-cyclohexylhexahydropyrimidine.

Borates of N-Hydroxyalkyl Heterocycles

Borate esters of the hydroxyalkyl compounds disclosed in U.S. Patents 3,673,186 and 3,787,416 are also disclosed by *H.A. Cyba; U.S. Patent 3,446,808; May 27, 1969; assigned to Universal Oil Products Company.* Other heterocyclic moieties which also may be used in these antioxidants include pyrrolidine, piperidine, imidazolidine, pyrazolidine, and hydrogenated or saturated derivatives of indole, carbazole, quinoline, acridine, pyridazine, triazole and phenazine. Preferred compounds are the borates of N-hydroxyalkylpiperazines and preferably of N-hydroxyalkyl-N'-alkylpiperazines. In a particularly preferred compound, the N'-alkyl substituent is of secondary alkyl configuration.

The reaction of the borylating agent and the N-hydroxyalkylheterocyclic compound is effected in any suitable manner. The orthoborates are formed by heating and stirring the reactants at a temperature up to about 100°C and thus within the range of from about 60° to 100°C when using boric acid.

The metaborates are formed at temperatures above about 100°C and thus may be within the range of from about 100° to 200°C or more. The higher temperature of from about 100° to 200°C is used when employing trialkyl borates in order to effect the transesterification reaction. In one method the reactants are refluxed in the presence of a solvent. Any suitable solvent may be used and advantageously comprises an aromatic hydrocarbon solvent including benzene, toluene, etc. Any suitable borylating agent may be used. A particularly preferred borylating agent is boric acid. Other borylating agents include trialkyl borates in which the alkyl groups preferably contain from 1 to 4 carbons each.

Example 1: Borylation of N-hydroxyethyl-N'-sec-octylpiperazine was effected by refluxing 72.6 g (4.3 mol) with 6.18 g (0.1 mol) of boric acid in 100 g of benzene at 85°C. Heating at reflux was continued until a total of about 5 cc of water was collected. Following completion of the reaction, the benzene was removed by distillation at 160°C under water pump vacuum, and the borated product recovered as a liquid which contained 1.24% by weight of boron which corresponds to a theoretical boron content of 1.47% by weight for the triester. It is believed that the triester is of the structure shown on the following page (hydrogens omitted).

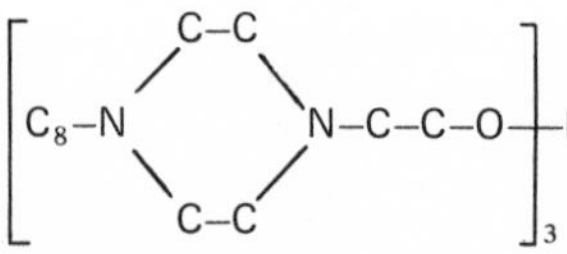

$$\left[\begin{array}{c} C_8-N \underset{C-C}{\overset{C-C}{\diagup\diagdown}} N-C-C-O \end{array} \right]_3 B$$

Example 2: A transesterification reaction is effected by heating and refluxing 3 mol proportions of N-hydroxyethyl-N'-sec-octylpiperazine and 1 mol proportion of tri-n-butyl borate at a temperature of about 160°C. The refluxing is continued until the required amount of butanol is collected, the butanol resulting from the transesterification reaction. Following completion of the reaction, the borated product is recovered as a liquid.

Example 3: Testing of these borate esters in polypropylene was also done by the Weatherometer Test described on page 2. A sample of the polypropylene without inhibitor developed a carbonyl number of greater than 1,000 within 120 hr of exposure in the Weatherometer. Another sample of the same polypropylene containing 0.15% by weight of 2,6-di-tert-butyl-4-methylphenol developed a carbonyl number over 1,000 within 360 hr of exposure.

Another sample of the solid polypropylene containing 1% by weight of the borated compound of Example 1 and 0.15% by weight of 2,6-di-tert-butyl-4-methylphenol was evaluated in the same manner. After 1,100 hr of exposure, the carbonyl number of this sample was 240. As another important advantage of the additive, the sample of polypropylene containing this additive, even after exposure in the Weatherometer for this long period of time, still remained clear and did not undergo discoloration.

Other examples of the complete patent show the preparation of borate esters of other piperazine compounds, hexahydropyrimidines, piperidines and glyoxalidines. Stabilization of polyethylene and polystyrene are also covered by other examples.

Borates of Polymeric Alkanolamines

H.A. Cyba; U.S. Patents 3,692,680; September 19, 1972; and 3,598,855; August 10, 1971; assigned to Universal Oil Products Company has also prepared cyclic borates of the following formula:

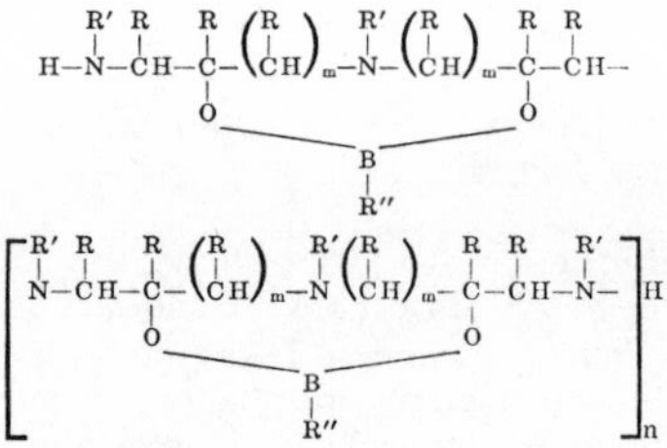

$$H-\underset{R'}{\overset{R'}{N}}-\underset{}{\overset{R}{CH}}-\underset{\underset{O}{|}}{\overset{R}{C}}-\left(CH\right)_m-\underset{}{\overset{R'}{N}}-\left(CH\right)_m-\underset{\underset{O}{|}}{\overset{R}{C}}-\underset{}{\overset{R}{CH}}-$$

$$\left[\underset{R''}{\overset{B}{|}} \right]$$

$$\left[\underset{R''}{\overset{R'}{N}}-\underset{}{\overset{R}{CH}}-\underset{\underset{O}{|}}{\overset{R}{C}}-\left(CH\right)_m-\underset{}{\overset{R'}{N}}\left(CH\right)_m-\underset{\underset{O}{|}}{\overset{R}{C}}-\underset{}{\overset{R}{CH}}-\underset{}{\overset{R'}{N}}-H \right]_n$$

where R is hydrogen, alkyl of 1 to 40 carbons, cycloalkyl, aryl or alkaryl; R' is alkyl of 1 to 40 carbons, cycloalkyl, aryl or alkaryl; R" is hydroxy, alkoxy of 1 to 40 carbons, alkyl of 1 to 40 carbons, cycloalkyl, aryl or alkaryl; n is from 1 to 100, preferably from 2 to 8 and m is 0, 1 or 2.

The cyclic borate is readily prepared by the reaction of a suitable borylating agent with a polymeric alkanolamine prepared according to U.S. Patent 3,189,652. In general, the polymeric alkanolamine is prepared by reacting a suitable amine with an epihalohydrin compound. The amine used as a reactant is selected from primary aliphatic amines containing 12 to 40 carbons and N-aliphatic polyamines including N-alkyl-1,3-diaminopropanes in which the alkyl contains at least 12 carbons, and N-aliphatic ethylenediamines, N-aliphatic aminobutanes and N-aliphatic diaminopentanes, N-aliphatic diaminohexanes, etc. in which the aliphatic group contains 12 to 40 carbons. Preferred aliphatic amines are mixtures of hydrogenated tallow amines which are available under various tradenames including Alamine H26D and Armeen HTD. These products comprise mixtures predominating in alkylamines containing 16 to 18 carbons per alkyl group. Preferred N-aliphatic-1,3-diaminopropane is a mixture available commercially as Duomeen T which is N-tallow-1,3-diaminopropane predominating in alkyl and alkenyl groups containing 16 to 18 carbons each. Other mixtures include those available commercially as N-coco-1,3-diaminopropane, N-soya-1,3-diaminopropane, etc.

In general, 1 or 2 mols of the amine are reacted with 1 or 2 mols of an epihalohydrin compound. Epichlorohydrin is preferred. The reaction generally is effected at a temperature of 20° to 100°C, preferably 50° to 75°C, although a higher temperature up to 150°C may be used, particularly when the reaction is effected at superatmospheric pressure to increase the reaction velocity. Either before or after removal of the reaction product from the reaction zone, the product is treated to remove halogen, generally in the form of an inorganic halide salt.

The polymeric alkanolamine is reacted with a suitable borylating agent to form the cyclic borate. The borylating agent is selected from boric acid, boric oxide, tri-lower-alkyl borates, in which the reaction is effected by transesterification, or a boronic acid of the formula

$$(HO)_2-B-R$$

where R is alkyl of 1 to 40 carbons, cycloalkyl, aryl and particularly phenyl, or alkaryl and particularly alkylphenyl in which the alkyl contains 1 to 30 carbons. The reaction is readily effected by refluxing the reactants, at a temperature of 60° to 200°C, in the presence of a solvent such as benzene, toluene, xylene, etc. Stoichiometric amounts of the borylating agent will be used.

Example 1: A borate of a polymeric product, as illustrated in the above formula in which R" is hydroxy and n is about 5, was prepared in the following manner. The polymeric product was prepared in the manner described in U.S. Patent 3,189,652. A mixture of 387.5 g (0.5 hydroxyl equivalent) of the polymeric product and 15.46 g (0.25 mol) of boric acid and 100 g of benzene was refluxed at a temperature of about 135°C for about 2½ hr. A total of 10 cc of water was collected. Following completion of the reaction, the product was filtered and then subjected to distillation at 150°C under water pump vacuum to remove the benzene solvent. The resultant borate had an acid number of 0.019 meq/g, a basic nitrogen equivalent of 2.54 meq/g, a mol combining weight of 394 and 0.78% by weight of boron.

Example 2: The cyclic borate prepared as described in Example 1 also was evaluated as an additive in solid polypropylene by the Weatherometer Test on page 2. A sample of the polypropylene without additive developed a carbonyl number of greater than 1,000 within 120 hr of exposure in the Fadeometer. Another sample of the same polypropylene containing 0.15% by weight of butylated hydroxytoluene (2,6-di-tert-butyl-4-methylphenol) developed a carbonyl number of over 1,000 within 360 hr of exposure in the Fadeometer. Still another sample of the polypropylene containing 1% by weight of the cyclic borate prepared according to Example 1 and 0.15% by weight of 2,6-di-tert-butyl-4-methylphenol did not reach a carbonyl number of 1,000 until 840 hr of exposure in the Fadeometer.

This shows that the cyclic borate was effective in stabilizing the polypropylene. However, still further improvements are obtained when using the cyclic borate in admixture with one or more other compounds such as 2-hydroxy-4'-octoxybenzophenone; 2,2'-dihydroxy-4-octoxybenzophenone; 2-(2'-hydroxy-5-methylphenyl)benzotriazole; phenyl salicylate; and preferably also with one or more of butylated hydroxytoluene, 1,1,3-tris(2-methyl-4-hydroxy-5-tert-butylphenyl)butane or dilaurylthiodipropionate. The borate esters were also used in other examples of the patents to stabilize fuel oil, gasoline, polyester lubricants and SBR.

1,2,3,5-TETRAMETHYLPYRAZOLIUM CHLORIDE

The preparation of various amide type compounds including amides, amidinium salts, vinylogous amidinium salts and endiamines is disclosed by *C.F. Hobbs and J.D. Wilson; U.S. Patent 3,655,690; April 11, 1972; assigned to Monsanto Company.* The compounds, prepared from carboxyl compounds by a reaction with an amine in the presence of a metal halide, have utility in the production of various nitrogen compounds and as biologically active materials, as antioxidants and acid scavengers. These compounds have the formula R–Z where Z is selected from the group consisting of

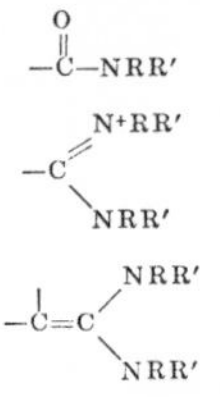

$$-\overset{\overset{\text{O}}{\|}}{\text{C}}-\text{NRR}'$$

$$-\text{C}\overset{\text{N}^+\text{RR}'}{\underset{\text{NRR}'}{\diagdown}}$$

$$-\overset{|}{\text{C}}=\text{C}\overset{\text{NRR}'}{\underset{\text{NRR}'}{\diagdown}}$$

and

$$-\overset{\overset{\text{N}^+\text{RR}'}{\|}}{\text{C}}-\left(-\underset{\overset{|}{\text{R}}\ \overset{|}{\text{R}'}}{\text{C}}=\underset{}{\text{C}}\right)_n-\underset{\overset{|}{\text{R}}}{\text{C}}=\underset{\overset{|}{\text{R}'}}{\text{C}}-\text{NRR}'$$

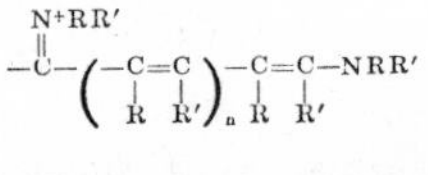

In this formula, n is a whole number from 0 to 5 and R and R' are the same or different members of the class consisting of hydrogen, alkyl and alkenyl radicals having 1 to 20 carbons, including straight chain and branched chain alkyl, alkenyl, cycloalkyl, cycloalkenyl, and aryl radicals having 6 to 30 carbons. The group of R and R' also includes the polycyclic radicals having 6 to 30 carbons. The above radicals may be unsubstituted or substituted such as with cyano or halogeno substituents.

The preparation of amide compounds, including amides, amidinium salts, vinylogous amidinium salts and endiamines, is readily carried out by reacting a carboxyl or vinylogous carboxyl compound, for example, an acid or salt with an aminating reagent providing a primary or secondary amine group, this reagent being selected from the group consisting of (a) tris(mono- or disubstituted-amino) halo metal and bis(mono- or disubstituted-amino) halo metal compounds, the halo substituent being chlorine, bromine or iodine, and (b) the combination of a metal halide (e.g., the chloride, bromide or iodide) with an amine, RR'NH, where R and R' are defined above. The carboxyl compounds have the general formula, R–Y, where Y is –C(O)–OM, or

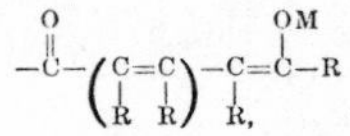

$$-\overset{\overset{\text{O}}{\|}}{\text{C}}-\left(\underset{\overset{|}{\text{R}}\ \overset{|}{\text{R}}}{\text{C}}=\text{C}\right)-\overset{\overset{\text{OM}}{|}}{\text{C}}=\overset{|}{\text{C}}-\text{R} \qquad \text{or} \qquad -\overset{\overset{\text{O}}{\|}}{\underset{\overset{|}{\text{R}}}{\text{CH}}}\text{COM}$$

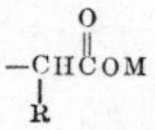

where the symbols have the meanings defined above. M is selected from the class of atoms and radicals consisting of hydrogen; positive metals, including Li, Na, K, Ca, Ba, Al, etc.; and ammonium radicals of the dialkyl, $R_2NH_2^+$; trialkyl, R_3NH^+; and tetraalkyl, R_4N^+ types.

Numerous compounds such as N,N-diethylbenzamide, tetramethyloxamide, 1-formyl-1,2-dimethylhydrazine, 1,3-dimethyl-2-phenylimidazolinium chloride, and the like are prepared in numerous examples, but the claimed product is 1,2,3,5-tetramethylpryrazolium chlorides as prepared below.

Example: To a suspension of 2.66 g (0.02 mol) 1,2-dimethylhydrazine dihydrochloride in a solution of 2.0 g (0.02 mol) acetylacetone and 10.1 g (0.1 mol) triethylamine in 100 ml

THF is added 3.8 g. TiCl$_4$, keeping the temperature of the reaction mixture below -10°C. The mixture is allowed to warm to 25°C and stir at that temperature for 4 days. The mixture is filtered, and the precipitate extracted with hot CH$_3$CN. The resulting solution is allowed to cool, is treated with a saturated aqueous K$_2$CO$_3$ solution, dried, and evaporated to dryness. From the residue 1,2,3,5-tetramethylpyrazolium chloride can be isolated by recrystallization from CH$_2$Cl$_2$, MP 255°C (dec). The NMR spectrum (CD$_3$CN solution, TMS internal standard) exhibits singlets at tau 3.6, tau 6.2, and tau 7.7 in the expected area ratio of 1:6:6, respectively.

N-(2,2-DISUBSTITUTED VINYL)ARYLIMINES

Compounds useful as metal deactivators, antiozonants, etc. are disclosed by *J.T. Arrigo; U.S. Patent 3,706,802; December 19, 1972; assigned to Universal Oil Products Company.* These compounds have the following formula:

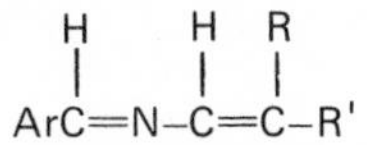

$$
\begin{array}{ccc}
H & H & R \\
| & | & | \\
\end{array}
$$
$$ArC=N-C=C-R'$$

where Ar is aryl and R and R' are hydrocarbyl containing up to 15 carbons or together form a carbocyclic ring containing up to 12 carbons. In a preferred form R and R' are independently selected from alkyl, cycloalkyl, alkenyl, cycloalkenyl, aryl, aralkyl and alkaryl. As set forth above, each of these substituents contains up to 15 carbons. These compounds are prepared by the reaction of an arylaldehyde with an N-(2,2-dihydrocarbylethylidene)-2,2-dihydrocarbylvinylamine, (referred to as an enimine) or with an N,N'-bis(2,2-dihydrocarbylethylidene)-2,2-dihydrocarbylethylidenediamine (referred to as a hydroamide).

Preferably the arylaldehyde is benzaldehyde or a substituted benzaldehyde in which the substituent group or groups are substantially inert under the reaction conditions. The enimine is an N-(2,2-dihydrocarbylethylidene)-2,2-dihydrocarbylvinylamine represented by the formula:

$$
\begin{array}{ccccc}
R & H & H & R \\
\backslash & | & | & / \\
& C=C-N=C-C-H & \\
/ & & \backslash \\
R' & & R'
\end{array}
$$

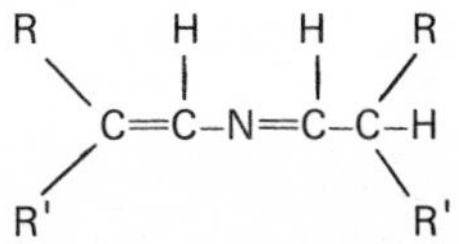

where R and R' are hydrocarbyl radicals independently selected from alkyl, cycloalkyl, alkenyl, cycloalkenyl, aryl, aralkyl and alkaryl, each containing up to 15 carbons, or R and R' attached to the same carbon may together form a carbocyclic ring containing up to 12 carbons. Illustrative N-(2,2-disubstitutedethylidene)-2,2-disubstitutedvinylamines thus include: N-(2,2-dimethylethylidene)-2,2-dimethylvinylamine; N-(2-methyl-2-ethylethylidene)-2-methyl-2-ethylvinylamine; etc. The hydroamide are N,N'-bis(2,2-dihydrocarbylethylidene)-2,2-dihydrocarbylethylidenediamines represented by the formula:

$$
\begin{array}{ccccc}
R & H & H & H & R \\
| & | & | & | & | \\
H-C-C=N-C-N=C-C-H & & \\
| & & | & & | \\
R' & & R-C-R' & & R' \\
& & | & \\
& & H
\end{array}
$$

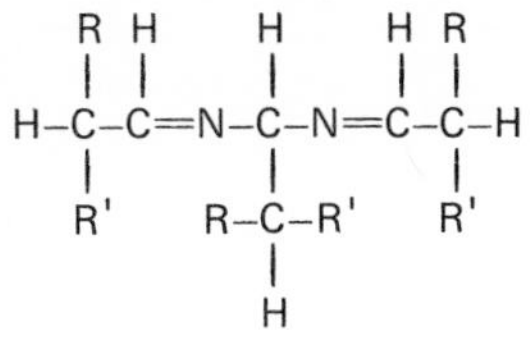

where R and R' have the same designations as in the description of the enimine. Illustrative N,N'-bis(2,2-disubstitutedethylidene)-2,2-disubstitutedethylidenediamines thus include: N,N'-bis(2,2-dimethylethylidene)-2,2-dimethylethylidenediamine; N,N'-bis(2-methyl-2-ethylethylidene)-2-methyl-2-ethylethylidenediamine; etc.

The reactions may be illustrated by the following equations. For simplification purposes, R and R' in the formula are methyl radicals and hydrogen atoms are omitted. When employing an enimine as the reactant, the equation is illustrated as follows:

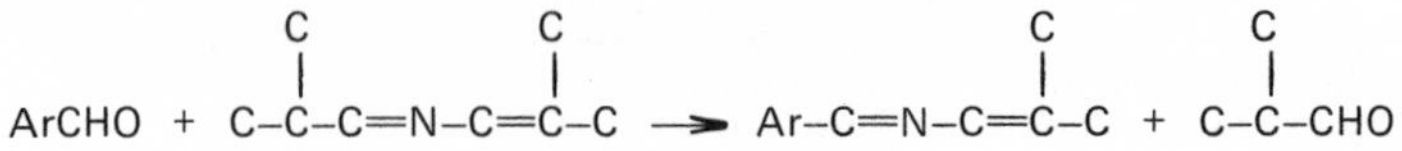

$$\underset{\displaystyle \text{ArCHO}}{} + \underset{\displaystyle \overset{\textstyle C}{|}}{\text{C–C–C}} = \text{N–}\underset{\displaystyle \overset{\textstyle C}{|}}{\text{C}} = \text{C–C} \longrightarrow \text{Ar–}\underset{\displaystyle \overset{\textstyle C}{|}}{\text{C}} = \text{N–}\underset{\displaystyle \overset{\textstyle C}{|}}{\text{C}} = \text{C–C} + \text{C–C–CHO}$$

When employing a hydroamide, the reaction may be illustrated by the following equation:

$$2\text{ArCHO} + \underset{\displaystyle \overset{\textstyle C}{|}}{\text{C–C–C}}\left(\text{N}=\underset{\displaystyle \overset{\textstyle C}{|}}{\text{C}}\text{–C–C}\right)_2 \longrightarrow 2\text{ArC}=\text{N–}\underset{\displaystyle \overset{\textstyle C}{|}}{\text{C}}=\text{C–C} + \text{C–C–CHO}$$

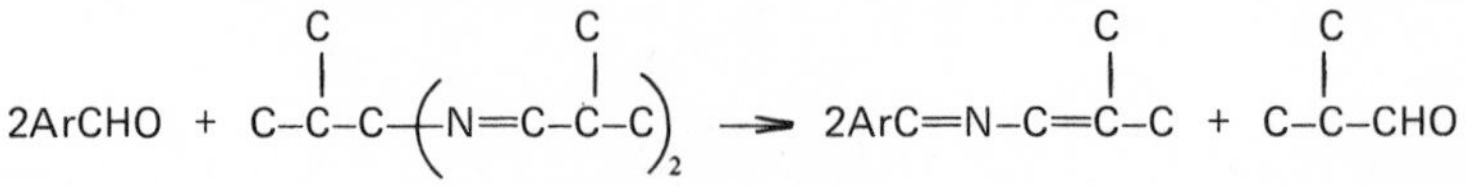

The above compounds will have varied utility. These compounds are useful as metal deactivators and will form chelates with metals and particularly copper in organic substrates such as gasoline, solvent oil, fatty material, etc. These compounds also will serve as antioxidants to retard deterioration of various organic materials such as hydrocarbon distillates, plastics or other organic substrates which are normally subject to oxidative deterioration, either as such or induced by ultraviolet light. These compounds also will serve as antiozonants to retard deterioration of materials normally subject to ozone induced reactions.

Example 1: This example describes the reaction of benzaldehyde and N-(2,2-dimethylethylidene)-2,2-dimethylvinylamine, the latter referred to herein as EI. The reaction was effected as follows. Benzaldehyde (21.8 g, 0.20 mol) and EI (25.1 g, 0.20 mol) were mixed and refluxed for 3 hr at 140° to 260°C with isobutyraldehyde (90% of theoretical) being distilled off as formed. The remainder of the reaction mixture was distilled through a 10" Vigreux column and appropriate cuts were combined and vacuum fractionated through a Minical spinning band column to afford 14.3 g (45% yield) of deep yellow product, BP 56°C at 0.3 mm. The product was identified as N-benzal-2-methylpropenylamine.

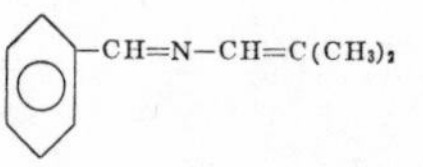

Example 2: N-benzal-2-methylpropenylamine, prepared as described in Example 1, is used as an antiozonant in butadiene-styrene rubber. The additive is incorporated in a concentration of 4 parts/100 parts of rubber hydrocarbon and serves to retard cracking of the rubber which otherwise occurs upon exposure to ozone.

TRIAZINE AND CYANURATE ANTIOXIDANTS

TRIAZINE DERIVATIVES WITH HINDERED PHENOL MOIETIES

Tris(m-Hydroxybenzylthio)-s-Triazines

Triazine compounds having hindered meta-hydroxybenzyl moieties have been prepared by *J. Song; U.S. Patent 3,723,428; March 27, 1973; assigned to American Cyanamid Co.* These compounds have the formula

(1)

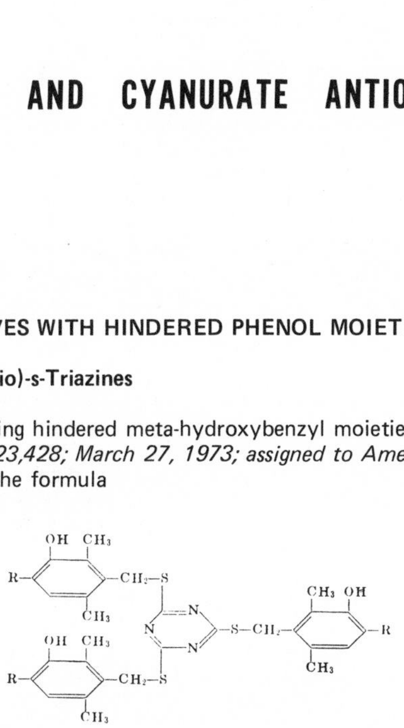

where R is a branched chain alkyl group containing 3 to 12 carbons. This process also relates to the use of such compounds to inhibit oxidative degradation of organic materials such as polyolefins, ABS resins, polyamides, polyacetals, polystyrene, high impact polystyrene, natural and synthetic rubbers including ethylene-propylene copolymers and carboxylated latices, fats, oils, greases, gasoline, etc.

The compounds, as defined in Formula 1, in addition to inhibiting oxidation of organic materials, possess outstanding resistance to extraction by boiling water, a property which has considerable importance when used in plastic materials in applications such as fibers, washing machine agitators, dishwasher parts, and the like, where contact with hot water is likely.

In these compounds, the three nitrogens of the s-triazine are each connected to a hindered phenolic moiety through a thiomethylene group. It will be noted that the hydroxyl group of each phenolic moiety is meta with respect to the thiomethylene group attaching the phenolic moiety to the s-triazine. It is critical that this hydroxyl group be in the meta position to avoid discoloration of the substrate in which these compounds are used and to provide a high degree of antioxidant protection. It will also be noted that all positions ortho and para to the hydroxyl group are substituted, one ortho position with a branched chain alkyl group and the other two such positions with methyl groups. Thus, this phenolic moiety is hindered by the branched chain alkyl substituent adjacent to the hydroxyl group.

Illustrative of the branched chain alkyl groups represented by R in the position ortho to the phenolic hydroxy group in these compounds of Formula 1 are isopropyl, tert-butyl, sec-butyl, tert-amyl, sec-heptyl, sec-octyl, tert-octyl, tert-nonyl (1,1-dimethylheptyl), α,α-dimethylbenzyl, methylcyclopentyl, methyl cyclohexyl, and the like. These compounds are readily prepared by known procedures, such as the reaction of 1 mol of 2,4,6-tri-mercapto-s-triazine with 3 mols of an appropriate 4-alkyl-3-hydroxy-2,6-dimethylbenzyl chloride or the reaction of 1 mol of cyanuric chloride with 3 mols of an appropriate 4-alkyl-3-hydroxy-2,6-dimethylbenzyl mercaptan.

Example 1: 4-tert-butyl-3-hydroxy-2,6-dimethylbenzyl mercaptan (22.4 grams, 0.1 mol) was added to 5.6 grams (0.1 mol) of potassium hydroxide in 125 ml ethanol. Cyanuric chloride (5.5 grams, 0.03 mol) was added, the mixture heated to reflux for a period of 4 hours, cooled, and 6.65 grams of potassium chloride filtered off. The filtrate afforded 23 grams of semisolid residue which, on treatment with acetone, gave 9.3 grams of product, MP 123° to 128°C. Further purification from acetone, followed by recrystallization from 300 ml methanol-water (2:1) gave 5 grams of colorless crystals, MP 130° to 133°C. The infrared spectrum was identical with a sample of 2,4,6-tris(4-tert-butyl-3-hydroxy-2,6-dimethylbenzylthio)-s-triazine prepared from reacting 2,4,6-trimercapto-s-triazine with 4-tert-butyl-3-hydroxy-2,6-dimethylbenzyl chloride.

Example 2: Sample preparation — Antioxidants were incorporated into unstabilized polypropylene at concentrations shown in the following table by milling at 170° to 180°C on a two-roll laboratory mill. As indicated, some samples also contained distearyl thiodipropionate (STDP). The milled samples were then compression molded into films 15 mils thick. Oven aging — The films were aged in a forced draft oven at 150°C and the time (hours) to embrittlement recorded. Extractability — Films containing the antioxidant were refluxed in 200 ml water for 7 hours (1 cycle). The water was replaced at the end of each cycle until 6 cycles (42 hours) of boiling water extractions was completed. The films were then aged as described above.

A second set of films was exposed to 15 cycles (105 hours) of boiling water and oven aged as above. The oven aged stability of the films after boiling water treatment is a measure of the extractability of the compound.

| Process Conditions* | -----Oven Aging at 150°C** ----- | |
	Example 1	Control***
None	<4	<4
0.05	27–31	50–96
0.10	552–536	545–553
0.20	839–855	833–841
0.02 + 0.25 STDP	1,360–1,381	385–432
0.10 + 0.25 STDP	2,345–2,353	1,331–1,344
0.2, 6 cycles	797–813	227–269
0.2, 15 cycles	583–597	64–75
0.1 + 0.25 STDP, 6 cycles	1,643–1,651	0–47
0.1 + 0.25 STDP, 15 cycles	503–519	8–10

*Additive concentration (%) and number of cycles of boiling water extractions
**Hours to embrittlement
***2,4,6-tris(3,5-di-tert-butyl-4-hydroxybenzylthio)-s-triazine

The data shown in the above table indicate that the compound of Example 1 when used alone in polypropylene is about equivalent in activity to the prior art compound which is closest in structure. When tested in combination with distearylthiodipropionate, the compound of Example 1 is superior. Of considerable significance, however, is the fact that after treatment in boiling water, samples containing the compound of Example 1 retain much of their resistance to oxidation whereas the samples containing the prior art compound lose nearly all their protection.

Tris(3,5-Dialkyl-4-Hydroxyphenyl)-s-Triazines

The hindered phenol moiety also appears in the antioxidants prepared by *M. Dexter and M. Knell; U.S. Patent 3,706,740; December 19, 1972; assigned to Ciba-Geigy Corporation.* These are compounds of the formula

(1)

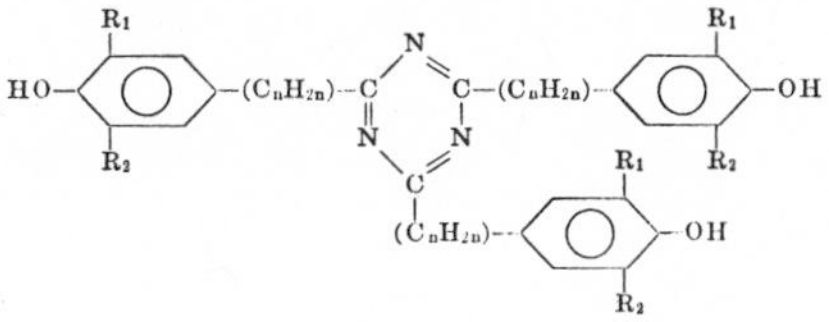

where each R_1 and R_2 is a (lower)alkyl group of 1 to 6 carbons; and n has a value of 0, 1 or 2.

The compounds where n of Formula 1 is 0 are prepared by reacting cyanuric chloride in an nonaqueous aprotic solvent such as tetrachlorethane with 2,6-dialkylphenol having the formula

(2)

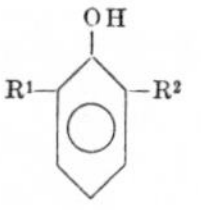

where R^1 and R^2 are the same as R_1 and R_2, the reaction being carried out at room temperature and catalyzed with aluminum chloride.

The compounds where n of Formula 1 is 1 or greater, are prepared by first forming a dialkyl-4-hydroxyphenyl alkyliminoester hydrochloride by reacting methanol and HCl in an inert solvent with a 3,5-dialkyl-4-hydroxyphenylalkyl nitrile derivative of the formula

(3)

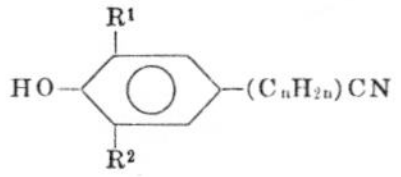

where R^1, R^2 and n are previously defined. The dialkyl-4-hydroxyphenyl alkyliminoester hydrochloride is then cyclized by treating the compound with sodium acetate in ethyl alcohol.

Example 1: A mixture of 18.5 grams of cyanuric chloride and 40 grams of aluminum chloride in 700 grams of tetrachloroethylene were stirred for 40 minutes at room temperature. To this mixture was added 73 grams of 2,6-dimethylphenol. The reaction continued with stirring at room temperature for an additional 93 hours. The crude 2,4,6-tris-(3',5'-dimethyl-4'-hydroxyphenyl)-1,3,5-triazine was separated by filtration and washed with 1,000 grams of 1 N HCl. Purification was accomplished by recrystallization from 100 grams of hot dimethylformamide. The recrystallized product had a MP of 311° to 315°C. The pure product showed only one spot by TLC analysis and had the expected NMR spectrum.

By following essentially the same procedure 2,4,6-tris(3',5'-di-tert-butyl-4'-hydroxyphenyl)-1,3,5-triazine is prepared by substituting 2,6-dimethylphenol with an equivalent amount of 2,6-di-tert-butylphenol.

Example 2: To 150 ml of benzene was added 21.95 grams of 3,5-di-tert-butyl-4-hydroxy-phenylpropionitrile, and 4 ml of methanol. The reaction was cooled to about 0°C and HCl was bubbled through the reaction mixture for 1 hour. The reaction was allowed to stir at 0° to 5°C for several hours followed by refluxing for 16 hours. The product was filtered and vacuum dried over KOH to yield the corresponding iminoester hydrochloride.

To 16.47 grams of the iminoester hydrochloride thus formed was added 4.16 grams of sodium acetate and 20 ml of methanol. The mixture was allowed to react for approximately 16 hours at room temperature. 50 ml of water was added to the reaction mixture after which the alcohol was removed by heating on a steam-bath. A water-benzene mixture was added to the resulting slurry and after an ether extraction, the organic layer was concentrated on a steam-bath till incipient crystallization occurred. The 2,4,6-tris-[2'-(3'',5''-di-tert-butyl-4''-hydroxyphenyl)-ethyl]-1,3,5-triazine thus obtained was recrystallized twice from acetic acid and had a melting point of 208.5° to 209.5°C.

Example 3: A batch of unstabilized polypropylene powder (Hercules Profax 6501) was thoroughly blended with 0.5% by weight of various antioxidants of Formula 1 and processed and tested as by the Oven Aging Test on page 1. The results are set out in the table below:

Additive(s)	Oven aging at 150° C., hours to failure
0.5% of 2,4,6-tris(3',5'-dimethyl-4'-hydroxyphenyl)-1,3,5-triazine	15
0.1% of 2,4,6-tris(3',5'-dimethyl-4'-hydroxyphenyl)-1,3,5-triazine plus 0.5% DLTDP¹	1,028
0.5% of 2,4,6-tris[2'-(3'',5''-di-t-butyl-4''-hydroxyphenyl)ethyl]-1,3,5-triazine	1,120
0.1% of 2,4,6-tris[2'-(3'',5''-di-t-butyl-4''-hydroxyphenyl)ethyl]-1,3,5-triazine plus 0.5% DLTDP¹	955
0.5% of DLTDP¹	300
Unstabilized polypropylene	3

¹ Dilaurylthiodipropionate (a synergist for phenolic antioxidants).

The above data clearly indicates the significant increase in the stabilization of polypropylene upon addition of these antioxidants.

The complete patent also includes examples of the stabilization of nylon 6, nylon 6,6, SBR, high impact polystyrene, cyclohexane, mineral oil, polyester lubricant, linear polyethylene, ABS and polyacetal resin.

Hindered Bisphenol Derivatives

M. Robin and S.R. Schulte; U.S. Patent 3,729,471; April 24, 1973; assigned to Ashland Oil, Inc. has disclosed antioxidants of substituted triazines in which at least one of the carbons in the triazine ring is connected to a hindered phenol through the oxygen of a phenolic hydroxyl group.

The hindered phenol is a hindered bisphenol with the two phenolic rings bridged through a saturated aliphatic hydrocarbon linkage, and with at least one position ortho to the hydroxyl group on each ring substituted with a bulky hydrocarbon group, other than the hydrocarbon linkage, of at least one carbon. Preferably all three of the carbons in the triazine ring are connected to a hindered phenol through the oxygen remaining after the removal of the hydrogen of a phenolic hydroxyl group.

These compounds unexpectedly exhibit superior antioxidant and ultraviolet light stabilization properties as compared to substituted triazines where the phenolic compound precursor contains only a single phenolic ring. Furthermore, these compounds may stabilize as much as 10 times as effectively as the parent phenolic compounds from which they are obtained. Briefly, these compounds are prepared by reacting a triazine compound and a hindered bisphenol in methyl ethyl ketone and/or diethyl ketone as a diluent. The triazine compounds used in preparing these compounds can be any of the triazine compounds having reactive groups. Examples of such compounds are the halide substituted triazines. The preferred triazine compounds are the trihalide triazines, such as the chlorides, bromides, and iodides. The bisphenol compounds are represented by the following formula:

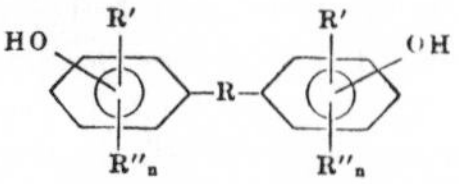

R is a saturated aliphatic hydrocarbon (alkylidenes and alkylenes) having 1 to 8 carbons, preferably 1 to 5 carbons. The preferred R group is methylene. The OH group on each ring can be in any position but preferably is either ortho or para to the hydrocarbon linkage and is most preferably in the ortho position. Each R' individually is a bulky hydrocarbon group of at least one carbon and is ortho to the OH group on each ring. Usually the bulky hydrocarbon group is free of nonbenzenoid unsaturation. R' is preferably a bulky hydrocarbon group of 1 to 22 carbons, more preferably 1 to 12 carbons. It is especially preferred that the bulky hydrocarbon group is an alkyl group. The most preferred bulky hydrocarbon group is tert-butyl.

Each R" individually is any substituent which can be attached to the ring. R" advantageously is, but is not limited to: a hydrocarbon group such as the hydrocarbon groups set forth above for R'; or a halide group such as chlorine or bromine; or $-NO_2$; or $-SR'''$; or $-OR'''$; or $-COOR'''$; or $-NR''R'''$; or $-NHR''''NH_2$; or $-NHOH$; or $-NHR''''OH$; where R''' is H or a hydrocarbon group as defined above for R', and R'''' is an alkylene group of 1 to 22 carbons and preferably of 1 to 12 carbons.

Specific examples of suitable bisphenols are 4,4'-methylenebis-(2,6-dimethylphenol); 2,2'-methylenebis-(6-tert-butyl-4-methylphenol); 2,2'-methylenebis-(4-chloro-6-tert-butylphenol); 4,4'-methylenebis-(2-tert-butylphenol); 2,2'-methylenebis-(6-tert-butylphenol); 2,2'-methylenebis-(4,6-di-tert-butylphenol); 2,2'-isopropylidenebis-(4,6-di-tert-butylphenol); and 2,2'-ethylidenebis-(4,6-di-tert-butylphenol). The preferred hindered bisphenol is 2,2'-methylenebis-(4-methyl-6-tert-butylphenol).

Unexpectedly, it was found that an improved process is achieved when using methyl ethyl ketone and/or diethyl ketone as the diluent as compared with other similar diluents. It was discovered that when using as reaction diluents, compounds other than methyl ethyl ketone and diethyl ketone it was necessary to use at least one purification, such as recrystallization, in addition to the initial isolation step and washing, if any, to obtain a product of comparable purity.

Preferably the amount of diluent is between 0.5 and 1.5 parts per part of reactants. The process is not limited to specific reaction temperatures, since the reaction can be carried out over a wide range of temperatures. For example, the process can be carried out at 0° to 250°C. The preferred temperature range varies from 15° to 100°C, and the most preferred is between 15° and 75°C. Also the process is not limited to any specific reaction time, since the time required will vary, primarily dependent upon the particular reactants, temperatures, and reaction environment. Preferably the reaction time varies from 1 to 6 hours. About 4 hours is the reaction time which is most commonly used.

Atmospheric pressure is the most commonly used pressure for carrying out the process. Of course, higher or lower pressures can be employed when desired. Usually the reaction is conducted under alkaline and in particular, caustic conditions. It is understood that it is not necessary to employ caustic conditions, particularly when temperatures at the upper end of the disclosed range are used.

The products obtained are substituted triazines where each H attached to the C atoms is

replaced by an —OH group or the oxygen of a phenol group of bisphenol. Cyclic derivatives are also possible where both phenolic groups of a bisphenol are united to a single
triazine molecule. In the following examples, all parts are by weight unless the contary
is stated.

Example 1: To a mixture of 1 mol of cyanuric chloride (2,4,6-trichloro-1,3,5-triazine)
dissolved in 2,000 parts of acetone, at ambient temperature are added all at once and with
agitation, 3 mols of 2,2'-methylenebis-(6-tert-butyl-4-methylphenol). While maintaining
the temperature of the mixture at about room temperature, 3 mols of NaOH as a 25%
aqueous caustic soda solution are slowly added with agitation over approximately 1 hour.
While stirring, the mixture is heated at 60°C for 30 minutes, at which time 1,000 parts of
water are added. The mixture is heated while stirring at 70°C for 1 hour, and then cooled
to ambient temperature. The product is isolated from the reaction medium by filtration,
washing with acetone and then with water, and then recrystallizing from benzene. The recrystallized product, 2,4,6-tris[2-(2-hydroxy-3-tert-butyl-5-methylbenzyl)-4-methyl-6-tert-
butylphenyl] cyanurate, is a white solid melting at about 230°C.

Other compounds which are prepared by similar methods include 2,4,6-tris-[2-(2-hydroxy-
3,5-di-tert-butylbenzyl)-4,6-di-tert-butylphenyl] cyanurate; 2,4,6-tris-[2-(2-hydroxy-3-nonyl-
5-methylbenzyl)-4-methyl-6-nonylphenyl] cyanurate; 2,4,6-tris-[2-(2-hydroxy-3,5-di-tert-
butylmethylbenzyl)-4,6-di-tert-butylphenyl] cyanurate; 2,4,6-tris-[2-(2-hydroxy-2-tert-
butyl-5-chlorobenzyl)- 4 -chloro-6-tert-butylphenyl] cyanurate; and 2,4,6-tris-[2-(2-hydroxy-
3,5-di-methylbenzyl)-4,6-di-methylphenyl] cyanurate.

Example 2: The product of Example 1 is admixed with a polypropylene of 0.90 density
and approximately 325,000 molecular weight in a steel container and the mixture is extruded twice at 380°F. The resulting polypropylene compositions containing 0.5% by
weight of the product of Example 1 are then pressed into a 6 to 6.5 mil film at 350°F
and 1,280 psi on a 10" hydraulic ram press. Likewise, a film of the same polypropylene
without any antioxidant and a film of the same polypropylene containing 0.5% of 2,2'-
methylenebis-(6-tert-butyl-4-methylphenol) are prepared by the method set forth above.
The resulting 3 films are then subjected to 150° ± 1°C in a forced draft oven. The absorbance in the carbonyl region of the IR Spectrum (5.8 microns) is then recorded after periods
of exposure. When absorbance reaches 94% the sample is considered to be oxidized, and
the time of exposure to reach this point is recorded.

Additive	Amount, percent	Time in hours to reach 94% absorbance
None		2
2,2'-methylenebis-(6-tert-butyl-4-methylphenol)	0.5	20
Product of Example 1	0.5	140

Polyethylene is also stabilized with the same stabilizer as used for polypropylene in another example of the original patent.

Derivatives of Thiobisphenols

Similar derivatives of triazines have also been produced by *M. Robin and S.R. Schulte;
U.S. Patent 3,700,666; October 24, 1972; assigned to Ashland Oil & Refining Company*.
The method of proparation and use are the same as the bisphenol derivatives of U.S.
Patent 3,729,471. Here the thiobisphenols which can be used in the process are: 2,2'-
thiobis-(4,6-di-tert-butylphenol); 2,2'-dithiobis-(4,6-di-tert-butylphenol); 2,2'-thiobis-(6-tert-
butyl-4-methylphenol); 2,2'-thiobis-(4-methyl-6-nonylphenol); 4,4'-thiobis-(5-tert-butyl-2-
methylphenol); 4,4'-thiobis-(6-tert-butyl-3-methylphenol); bis-(3-tert-butyl-2-hydroxy-5-
methyl) sulfone; bis-(3-tert-butyl-2-hydroxy-5-methyl) sulfoxide; 2,2'-dithiobis-(4-methyl-
6-nonylphenol); and 2,2'-trithiobis-(4,6-di-tert-butylphenol). The most preferred hindered
thiobisphenol is 2,2'-thiobis-(6-tert-butyl-4-methylphenol).

Example 1: To a mixture of 1 mol of cyanuric chloride (2,4,6-trichloro-1,3,5-triazine) dissolved in 2,000 parts of acetone, at room temperature are added all at once with agitation, 2 mols of 2,2'-thiobis(6-tert-butyl-4-methylphenol) while maintaining the temperature at about room temperature. 2 mols of a 25% aqueous caustic soda solution are then slowly added with agitation over approximately 1 hour. The reaction mixture is then agitated at room temperature for 1 hour. While stirring, the mixture is heated at 60°C for 30 minutes, at which time 1,000 parts of water are added. The mixture is heated while stirring at 70°C for 1 hour, and then cooled to ambient temperature. The reaction product is isolated from the reaction medium by filtration, washing with acetone and then with water, and then recrystallizing from benzene. The product is a white solid melting at 193° to 196°C and has the following structure as determined by elemental analysis, nuclear magnetic resonance (NMR) and IR spectra:

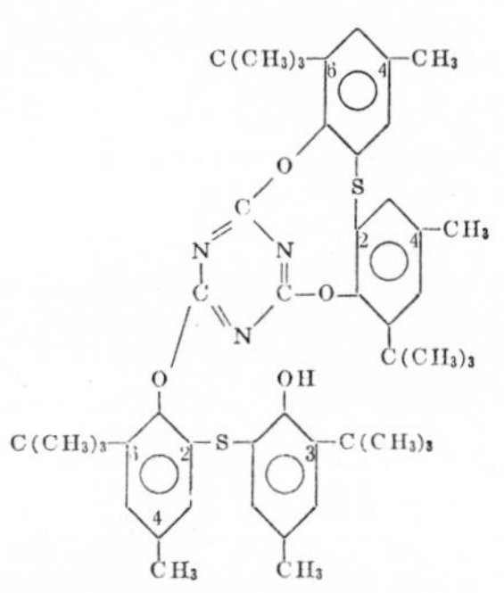

2-[2-(2-hydroxy-3-tert-butyl-5-methylphenylthio)-4-methyl-6-tert-butylphenoxy]-4,6-[2,2'-thiobis-(4-methyl-6-tert-butylphenoxy)]-s-triazine

Other compounds prepared by the process include 2-[2-(2-hydroxy-3,5-di-tert-butylphenyl-thio)-4,6-di-tert-butylphenoxy]-4,6-[2,2'-thiobis-(4,6-di-tert-butylphenoxy)]-s-triazine, 2,4,6-tris[2-(2-hydroxy-3-tert-butyl-5-methylphenyldithio)-4-methyl-6-tert-butylphenyl] cyanurate, 2,4,6-tris[2-(2-hydroxy-3-nonyl-5-methylphenylthio)-4-methyl-6-nonylphenyl] cyanurate, and 2,4,6-tris[2-(2-hydroxy-3,5-di-tert-butylphenyltrithio)-4,6-di-tert-butylphenyl] cyanurate.

Example 2: The product of Example 1 is mixed with a polypropylene of 0.90 density and approximately 325,000 molecular weight as in U.S. Patent 3,729,471. The data are given below.

Additive	Amount, percent	Time in hours to reach 95% absorbance
None		2
2,2' thiobis-(4-methyl-6-tert.-butylphenol)	0.1	6
Reaction product of Example 1	0.1	23

The original patent also includes an example of the stabilization of polyethylene.

2,4-Bisphenolic Triazine Derivatives

Phenolic derivatives useful as antioxidants for organic materials, particularly polymers, are disclosed by *H. Brunetti; U.S. Patent 3,775,411; November 27, 1973.* Here the derivatives have the formula shown of the following page

(1)

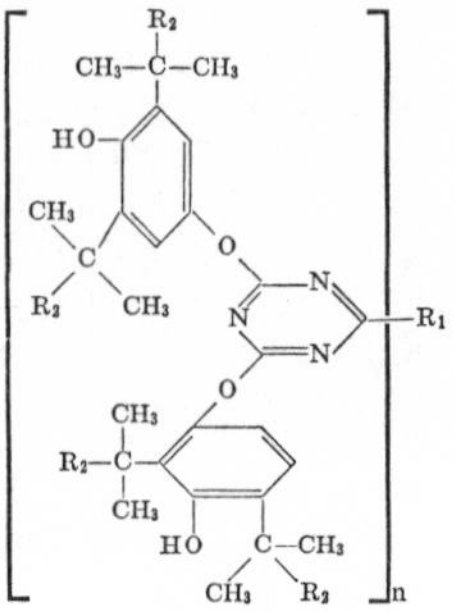

in which R_1 denotes hydrogen, alkyl with 1 to 17 carbons, alkenyl with 2 to 4 carbons, thiaalkyl with 3 to 20 carbons, cyclohexyl, benzyl, alkylene with 4 to 8 carbons or the radical

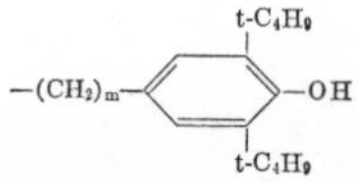

R_2 denotes methyl or ethyl and m and n denote 1 or 2. They are prepared by reacting the bis-[imino-carbonic acid-(3,5-di-tert-butyl-4-hydroxyphenyl)ester]-imide with a corresponding carboxylic acid chloride.

The compounds of the Formula 1 are incorporated into the substrates at a concentration of 0.01 to 5% by weight, calculated relative to the material to be stabilized. Preferably, 0.05 to 1.5, and particularly preferably 0.1 to 0.8% by weight of the compounds, calculated relative to the material to be stabilized, are incorporated into the latter. The incorporation into polymers can take place before or after polymerization, or before or after shaping, for example by mixing the compounds of the Formula 1, and optionally further additives, into the melt or solution of the polymers in accordance with the methods customary in the art. It can also be effected by applying the dissolved or dispersed compounds to the polymer, where necessary with subsequent evaporation of the solvent.

Example 1: Compounds of Formula 1 are prepared as follows.

Stage 1 — 111 grams of 3,5-di-tert-butyl-4-hydroxyphenyl-cyanate are first introduced into 500 ml of hexane. Ammonia gas is passed over the surface of the stirred solution, at 0° to 5°C, until the precipitate which has formed no longer increases. The bis-[imino-carbonic acid-(3,5-di-tert-butyl-4-hydroxyphenyl)-ester]-imide is filtered off and dried in vacuo. 128 grams of melting point 188° to 190°C (Kofler bench) are thus obtained.

Stage 2 — 10.2 grams of bis-[imino-carbonic acid-(3,5-di-tert-butyl-4-hydroxyphenyl)-ester]-imide are suspended in 40 ml of toluene. 4.8 grams of lauric acid chloride are added dropwise at 0° to 5°C over the course of 15 minutes, followed by 2.2 grams of triethylamine added dropwise. The temperature is raised to 50°C and maintained thereat for 1 hour, the mixture is filtered, the residue is washed with toluene, and the entire filtrate is evaporated in vacuo. The residue is dissolved in petroleum ether. On cooling the solution to ~0°C, the product crystallizes out. It is filtered off, rinsed with cold petroleum ether and recrystallized from hexane. 10.5 grams of 2,4-bis-(3,5-di-tert-butyl-4-hydroxyphenoxy)-6-undecyl-s-triazine (Stabilizer 8) of MP 58° to 60°C are thus obtained.

If the lauric acid chloride in the preceding example is replaced by an equivalent amount of the corresponding acid chloride, the stabilizers indicated in the table below are obtained under the same reaction conditions. Working up has to be varied slightly from case to case, and this is recorded very briefly in the table. Stabilizer 1 was obtained if, in the above method of manufacture, the lauric acid chloride was replaced by an excess amount of orthoformic acid triethyl ester and the triethylamine was omitted.

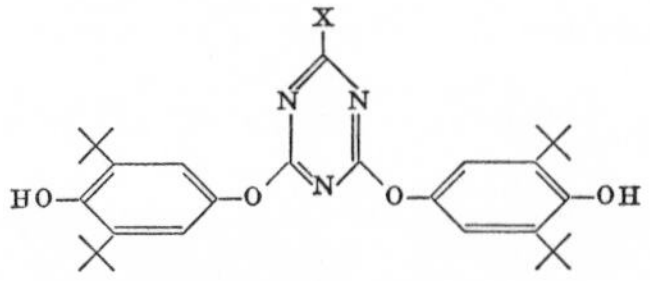

Stabilizer	X	Working up	Melting point, ° C.
1	H	Recrystallised from hexane	214
2	—CH₃	do	186
3	—C₂H₅	Recrystallised from ligroin	180
4	—C₅H₁₁	do	180
5	—C₇H₁₅	do	163
6	$-CH_2-CH-CH_2-C-CH_3$ with CH₃, CH₃, CH₃ groups	do	207
7	—C₉H₁₉	Chromatographed (toluene/silica gel)	~50
9	—C₁₇H₃₅	Chromatographed (toluene/silica gel) and recrystallised from acetonitrile	<50
10	—CH=CH₂	Recrystallised from ligroin	196
11	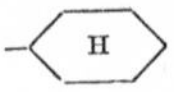 (cyclohexyl with H)	Recrystallised from methanol/water	205
12	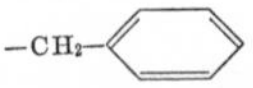 —CH₂—(phenyl)	Recrystallised from isopropanol	165
13	—CH₂—S—C₄H₉	Recrystallised from hexane	172
14	—CH₂CH₂—S—C₄H₉	do	132
15	—CH₂CH₂—S—C₈H₁₇—(n)	Chromatographed (toluene/silica gel)	98
16	—CH₂CH₂—S—C₈H₁₇(tert.)	do	63–65
17	—CH₂CH₂—S—C₁₂H₂₅	do	113
18	—CH₂CH₂—S—C₁₈H₃₇	Recrystallised from acetonitrile (cooling with CO₂)	(¹)
19	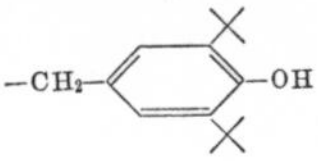 —CH₂—(phenol —OH)	Recrystallised from ligroin	226
20	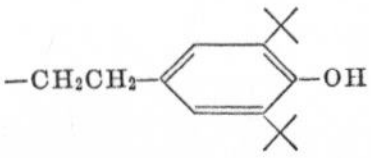 —CH₂CH₂—(phenol —OH)	do	185
21	—(CH₂)₄—²	Recrystallised from toluene	206
22	—(CH₂)₈—²	Recrystallised from ligroin	157

¹ Below room temperature (oil).
² In this case, 1 mol of imide was reacted with ½ mol of dicarboxylic acid chloride and 1 mol of triethylamine.

Example 2: Stabilization of Polypropylene — Manufacture of the test specimens: 100 parts of polypropylene (melt index 3.2) are kneaded in a Brabender plastograph for 10 minutes at 200°C with the stabilizers listed in the table below. This ensures homogeneous distribution of the stabilizers. The composition thus obtained is subsequently pressed in a platen press at 260°C platen temperature to give 1 mm thick sheets from which strips 1 cm wide and 17 cm long are punched. The effectiveness of the stabilizers added to the test sheets is tested by heat aging the sheets in a circulating air oven at 135°C and 149°C. The incipient visible decomposition of the test specimen is regarded as the end point. For results, see the table below.

	Time up to decomposition, in days at—	
	135° C.	149° C.
Without stabilizer	1	<1
0.2% of stabilizer No. 8	162	35
0.2% of stabilizer No. 9	158	31
0.2% of stabilizer No. 20	176	53
0.2% of stabilizer No. 21	175	45
0.2% of stabilizer No. 22	173	45

Hindered Phenolcarboxylate Esters of Alkanolaminotriazines

3,5-Dialkyl-4-hydroxyphenylalkanoic acid esters of 2,4,6-tris-(alkanolamino) derivatives of s-triazine are also disclosed by *M. Dexter and D.H. Steinberg; U.S. Patent 3,709,884; January 9, 1973; assigned to Ciba-Geigy Corporation*. These compounds are useful as stabilizers of organic substrates subject to oxidative and thermal degradation. •

Broadly these compounds are represented by the generic formula

(1)

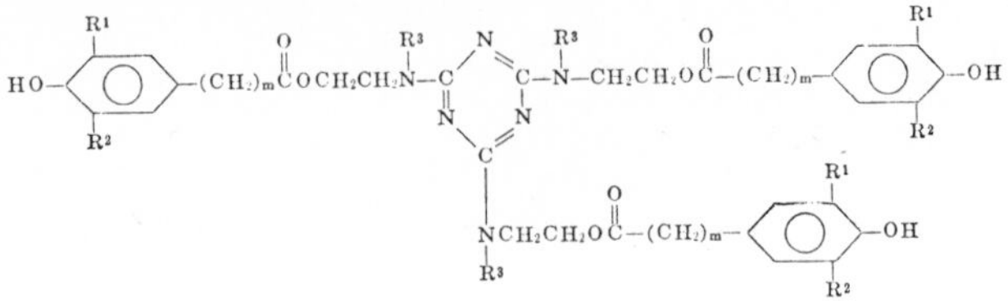

where each of R^1 and R^2 is a (lower)alkyl group of 1 to 4 carbons, R^3 is an alkyl of 1 to 8 carbons or hydrogen, and m is 1 or 2.

In general, these stabilizers are used from 0.005% to 10% by weight of the stabilized composition, although this will vary with the particular substrate. An advantageous range is from 0.05 to 5% and especially 0.05% to 2%. These compounds are particularly useful for the stabilization of polyolefins such as polypropylene and polyethylene.

These compounds can be prepared through esterification procedures known in the art. Thus, the triesters can be prepared by reacting a 3,5-dialkyl-4-hydroxyphenylalkanoic acid or acid halide with the appropriate 2,4,6-tris-(alkanolamino) derivative of triazine.

Example 1: 2,4,6-Tris-[3'-(3",5"-Di-tert-Butyl-4"-Hydroxyphenyl)Propionoxyethylamino]-1,3,5-Triazine — A mixture consisting of 38.6 grams of methyl-3,5-di-tert-butyl-4-hydroxyphenylpropionate, 10.34 grams of 2,4,6-tris-(2-hydroxyethylamino)-1,2,3-triazine and 100 mg of lithium hydride were heated under a nitrogen atmosphere for 5½ hours at 120°C at atmospheric pressure followed by 2½ hours at 130°C at 30 mm pressure. The methanol distillate was collected in a Dean-Stark trap connected to a Dry Ice cooled condenser. The crude product was dissolved in 75 ml of hot benzene and 0.8 ml of acetic acid and the mixture filtered.

The solvent was evaporated under vacuum and the product redissolved in 135 ml of benzene. The benzene solution containing the product was passed through an alumina column (670 grams of Woelm, neutral, activity II) and eluted first with benzene, then with a 1:1 ratio of benzene and chloroform and finally with chloroform. The product fractions were combined and the solvent evaporated under vacuum. The pure product was dried under vacuum at 80° to 90°C to constant weight and had a MP of 70° to 80°C.

In a similar manner, by substituting an equivalent amount of 2,4,6-tris-(N-methyl-2-hydroxyethylamino)-1,3,5-triazine for 2,4,6-tris-(2-hydroxyethylamino)-1,2,3-triazine in the above procedure there is obtained 2,4,6-tris-[3',5'-di-tert-butyl-4'-hydroxyphenyl)acetoxy-N-methylethylamino]-1,3,5-triazine.

Example 2: Unstabilized polypropylene powder (Hercules Profax 6501) was thoroughly blended with 0.25% by weight of 2,4,6-tris[3'-(3",5"-di-tert-butyl-4"-hydroxyphenyl)propionoxyethylamino]-1,3,5-triazine and 0.5% by weight of a UV stabilizer 2-(3',5'-di-tert-butyl-2'-hydroxyphenyl)-5'-chlorobenzotriazole (Tinuvin 327). Also prepared were samples of polypropylene containing 0.1% by weight of the same stabilizer and 0.3% by weight of DSTDP (distearyl-β-thiodipropionate). The blended materials were processed and tested as in the Oven Aging Test on page 1. The results are set out in the table on the following page.

Additive(s)	Hours to Failure*
0.25% of 2,4,6-tris[3'-(3'',5''-di-tert-butyl-4''-hydroxyphenyl)propionoxyethylamino]-1,3,5-triazine + 0.25% Tinuvin 327	160
0.1% of 2,4,6-tris[3'-(3'',5''-di-tert-butyl-4''-hydroxyphenyl)propionoxyethylamino]-1,3,5-triazine + 0.3% DSTDP** + 0.25% Tinuvin 327	340
Unstabilized polypropylene	3
0.3% DSTDP** alone	<20
0.5% Tinuvin 327 alone	3

*Oven aging at 150°C
**Distearylthiodipropionate (a synergist for phenolic antioxidants)

Other materials stabilized with antioxidants of Formula 1 in the original patent include nylon 6,6, mineral oil, high impact polystyrene, SBR, polyacetal resin, linear polyethylene, cyclohexane, and a polyester lubricant.

HEXAHYDROTRIAZINE DERIVATIVES WITH HINDERED PHENOL MOIETIES

Thiopropionylhexahydrotriazine Derivatives

Organic materials normally subject to oxidative and/or thermal degradation, for example, synthetic polymers such as polyolefins, mineral and synthetic lubricating oils and the like, are stabilized against degradation by incorporating in such compositions tris(alkylhydroxyphenyl) derivatives of thiopropionylhexahydrotriazines.

These compounds disclosed by *M. Knell and D.H. Steinberg; U.S. Patent 3,763,094; Oct. 2, 1973; and U.S. Patent 3,694,440; September 26, 1972; both assigned to Ciba-Geigy Corp.* can be represented by the generic formula

(1)

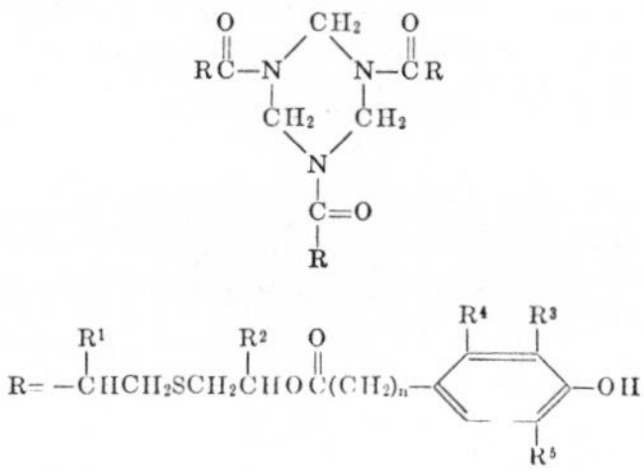

$$
\begin{array}{c}
RC-N \quad CH_2 \quad N-CR \\
\quad CH_2 \quad CH_2 \\
\quad N \\
\quad C=O \\
\quad R
\end{array}
$$

$$R= -CHCH_2SCH_2CH_2OC(CH_2)_n- \text{(hydroxyphenyl)} -OH$$
(with substituents R^1, R^2, R^3, R^4, R^5)

where R^1, R^2 and R^4 are independently hydrogen or methyl, R^3 and R^5 are independently hydrogen or (lower)alkyl, and n is 0 to 2. The groups R^1, R^2 and R^4 are preferably hydrogen. The groups R^3 and R^5 besides hydrogen can be (lower)alkyl groups having 1 to 6 carbons. Preferably, those groups are methyl or tert-alkyl groups such as tert-butyl, tert-pentyl, and tert-hexyl. The value of n is preferably 2.

These antioxidants are prepared by reacting the following materials: (1) an acrylonitrile and (2) formaldehyde to form the tris-acrylylhexahydrotriazine; (3) mercaptoethanol to form the hydroxyethylthiopropionyl moieties of the compound; and (4) an hydroxyphenylcarboxylic acid for esterifying the hydroxyethyl groups. The above constituents can be combined in various sequences to form the final compound 1.

Example 1: To a methanol solution of 1 mol of 1,3,5-triacrylylhexahydro-1,3,5-triazine containing 3 mol percent of trimethylbenzylammonium hydroxide is added dropwise with stirring a solution of 3 mols of 2-mercaptoethanol in methanol. After the addition, the reaction mixture is kept at 35°C until TLC indicates the reaction is complete, after which it is cooled, filtered from a small amount of insoluble and the solvent stripped under vacuum. The residue is dissolved in water and extracted into isobutyl alcohol. After washing with saturated sodium chloride solution, the solvent is removed under vacuum, leaving a solid residue which is then washed with ether to give the product, 1,3,5-tris(hydroxyethyl-thiopropionyl)hexahydro-1,3,5-triazine which melts at 52° to 54°C.

Example 2: To a mixture of 0.1 mol of 1,3,5-tris(hydroxyethylthiopropionyl)-hexahydro-1,3,5-triazine in 100 ml of dry benzene is added a solution of 0.33 mol of 4-hydroxy-3,5-di-tert-butylphenylpropionyl chloride in benzene. Pyridine (0.33 mol) is then added dropwise and the reaction mixture is stirred overnight. After filtering off the solid, the filtrate is washed successively with water, 2 N sodium hydroxide and again with water. The product, 1,3,5-tri(4'-hydroxy-3',5'-di-tert-butylphenylpropionyloxyethylthiopropionyl)-hexahydro-1,3,5-triazine is purified by elution chromatography from a silica gel column using benzene-heptane (1:1). After drying the product is obtained as a glass which softens at 55°C.

Example 3: Following the procedures of Examples 1 and 2, only using 1-mercapto-2-propanol and 4-hydroxy-3,5-di-tert-butylbenzoyl chloride, there is obtained 1,3,5-tris[2'(4"-hydroxy-3",5"-di-tert-butylbenzoyloxy)propylthiopropionyl]-hexahydro-1,3,5-triazine.

Example 4: The Oven Aging Test was conducted on polypropylene powder (Hercules Profax 6501) thoroughly blended with 0.5% by weight of 1,3,5-tris(4'-hydroxy-3',5'-di-tert-butylphenylpropionyloxyethylthiopropionyl)-hexahydro-1,3,5-triazine. The stabilized polypropylene is found to be much more stable compared to the unstabilized composition. Stabilized polypropylene compositions are also obtained when 0.05% of the above compound is employed.

Other materials stabilized by these materials in examples of the complete patents include nylon 6,6, high impact polystyrene, and polyacetal resin (U.S. Patent 3,763,094 only).

1,3,5-Tris(4-Hydroxyphenylalkanoyl)-Hexahydro-s-Triazines

Antioxidants have been prepared by *W.L. Beears; U.S. Patents 3,639,336; February 1, 1972; and 3,567,724; March 2, 1971; both assigned to B.F. Goodrich Company* which consist of a symmetrical hexahydro-1,3,5-triazine nucleus containing 3 hindered phenolic moieties attached through carbonyl linkages.

These compounds are especially useful as stabilizers for α-monoolefin homopolymers and copolymers particularly polyethylene, polypropylene and ethylene-propylene copolymers and terpolymer, polyacetal homopolymers and copolymers, polyamides, polyesters and polyurethanes. These hexahydrotriazines are represented by the structural formula

where R_1 and R_2 are tertiary alkyl groups containing 4 to 18 carbons, R_3 is hydrogen or alkyl group containing 1 to 18 carbons, R_4 is hydrogen or an alkyl group containing 1 to 4 carbons, and m is an integer from 2 to 5. Preferred compounds have the formula on the following page where R_6 is hydrogen or methyl and n is an integer between 4 to 12. Although these compounds are high molecular weight materials, the weight ratio of the phenol moiety to the total weight of the molecule remains high. Accordingly, effective stabilization of organic materials with low levels of these compounds is possible. This results in a significant economic advantage to the user. These compounds are also effective stabilizers for high temperature applications due to their extremely low volatility.

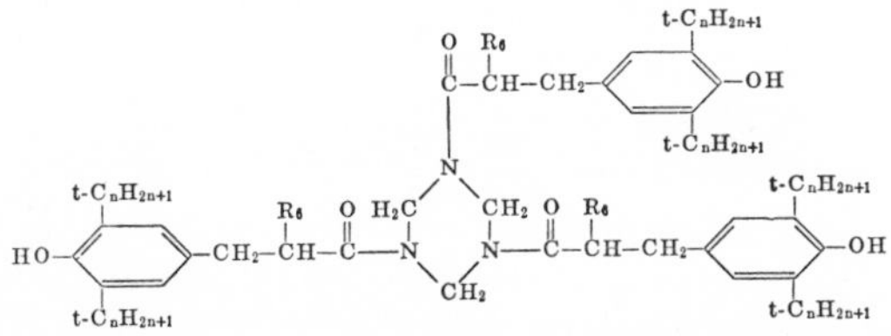

These antioxidants are prepared by combining 3 mols of the appropriate hindered phenol with 1 mol of a hexahydro-s-triazine of the formula

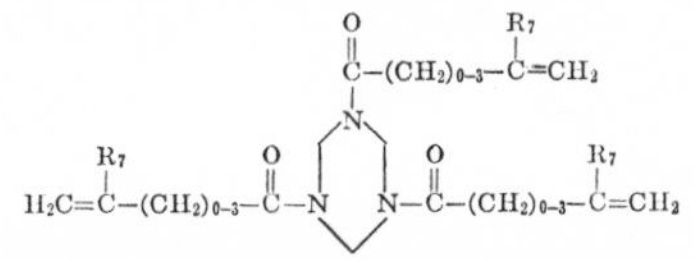

where R_7 is hydrogen or an alkyl group containing 1 to 4 carbons. A metal salt of the hindered phenol, formed by the action of a base on the phenol, is reacted with the above hexahydro-s-triazine compound.

Example 1: A glass reactor equipped with a stirrer, condenser and dropping funnel was charged with 21.6 grams (0.4 mol) powdered sodium methoxide and 785 grams of N,N-dimethylformamide previously dried and distilled over calcium hydride. To this was added 453.2 grams (2.2 mols) of redistilled 2,6-di-tert-butylphenol and the resulting mixture heated with stirring under nitrogen to distill off methanol. The distillation was terminated when the temperature reached 149°C. The reaction was then allowed to cool to room temperature and 116 grams (0.666 mol) 1,3,5-triacryl-perhydro-s-triazine dissolved in 785 grams of N,N-dimethylformamide containing about 2 grams of 2,6-di-tert-butyl-p-cresol added. The resulting mixture was then heated at 135°C for 3 hours maintaining the nitrogen blanket. 80 grams of 1:1 hydrochloric acid was then charged to the cooled reaction mixture.

The sodium chloride formed was removed by filtration and 10.9 grams of sodium hydrosulfite added to the filtrate. The N,N-dimethylformamide was then partially removed under vacuum and the resulting mass heated to approximately 80°C and 154 grams of distilled water added with rapid stirring. This mixture was allowed to cool to 20°C with continuous stirring. The resulting cream colored solid was collected by filtration and washed successively with 10% aqueous ethanol and 70% aqueous ethanol. The white crystalline solid obtained upon recrystallization from chloroform-hexane melted at 237° to 239°C on a melting block.

A sample nine times recrystallized from chloroform-hexane had a MP, determined in a capillary, of 228° to 229°C (uncorrected). Elemental analysis of this product agreed with the calculated values for 1,3,5-tris-β-(3,5-di-tert-butyl-4-hydroxyphenyl)propionylhexahydro-s-triazine.

Example 2: 1,3,5-Tris-β-(3,5-di-tert-butyl-4-hydroxyphenyl)propionylhexahydro-s-triazine was incorporated in polypropylene by itself and in combination with β-dialkylthiodipropionates as set forth below in the table. The additives were incorporated into the polypropylene by dissolving them in acetone, suspending the polypropylene therein, and then removing the acetone under vacuum. The stabilized polypropylene was hot milled (290° to 300°F) for 5 minutes, sheeted off, placed in a 4-cavity ACS mold shimmed to the desired thickness and heated at 400°F and 4,000 psi for 2 minutes. The samples were then transferred to a cold press maintained at 4,000 psi for a 2 minute cooling period. 25 mil samples were aged in an air-circulating oven at 140°C. The polypropylene samples were deemed to have failed at the first signs of crazing. Test results are also tabulated in the table below.

Sample	1	2	3	4	5	6	7	8	9
Polypropylene*	100	100	100	100	100	100	100	100	100
1,3,5-Tris-β-(3,5-di-tert-butyl-4-hydroxyphenyl)-hexahydro-s-triazine*	–	0.1	0.25	0.5	0.25	0.5	0.1	0.25	0.5
β-dilaurylthiodipropionate*	–	–	–	–	0.2	1.0	–	–	–
β-distearylthiodipropionate*	–	–	–	–	–	–	0.25	0.25	0.25
Hours to crazing	1	960	1,500	1,728	2,322	3,498	1,720	2,148	2,232

*Parts

Examples were also included in the complete patent on the use of these compounds in the stabilization of polyethylene, a blend of polyvinyl chloride with methyl methacrylate/butadiene/styrene terpolymer, EPT, ABS, polystyrene, nylon 6, polyethylene terephthalate, polyoxymethylene, mineral oil, synthetic lubricants, NR, polybutadiene, SBR, polystyrene and cyclohexane.

OTHER TRIAZINE DERIVATIVES

2,4,6-Tris(Alkylthioalkylthio)-1,3,5-Triazines

M. Dexter and M. Knell; U.S. Patent 3,652,561; March 28, 1972 have also prepared antioxidant triazine derivatives by reacting cyanuric chloride, an alkylthioalkylmercaptan and a base. These compounds are useful as stabilizers of organic material subject to oxidative deterioration and particularly as synergists in combination with other stabilizers.

In particular these compounds have the following formula:

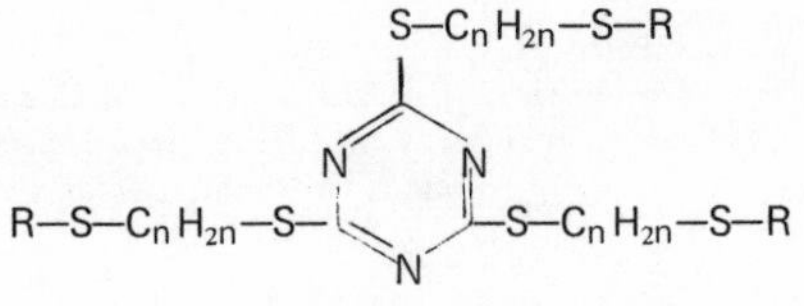

$$R-S-C_nH_{2n}-S-\underset{N}{\overset{S-C_nH_{2n}-S-R}{\underset{\displaystyle\bigg|}{\bigvee_{N}^{N}}}}-S-C_nH_{2n}-S-R$$

where R is alkyl group having up to 24 carbons and n is an integer of 2 to 18. By $-C_nH_{2n}-$ is meant a straight chain or a branched chain alkylene group having 2 to 18 carbons. The alkylene groups can be attached to the sulfur atoms either through carbons which are adjacent to each other or through any other 2 nonadjacent carbons. The preferred group are those having 2 to 6 carbons and the most preferred is ethylene. The R group in the above formula is an alkyl group having 6 to 24 carbons or an alkylthioalkane group, i.e., $-C_mH_{2m}-S-R'$ where the integer m is 1 to 6 and R' is an alkyl group having 6 to 24 carbons. The alkyl groups in R and R' preferably have 8 to 18 carbons.

In general these stabilizers are used from 0.005% to 10% by weight of the stabilized composition. A particularly advantageous range for polyolefins, such as polypropylene is from 0.1 to 1%. Although these compounds are useful as stabilizers per se, their greatest importance is the ability to improve the effectiveness of numerous other compounds especially phenolic compounds, which are used as stabilizers for organic materials normally subject to deterioration. Thus, the compounds of this disclosure may be classified as synergists since when they are combined with stabilizers they exhibit the ability to increase the total stabilization to a degree far exceeding that which could be expected from the additive properties of the individual components. The stabilizers with which these compounds may be combined are, generally, phenolic triazines, phenolic phosphonates, phenolic esters and phenolic hydrocarbons.

Example 1: A reaction vessel was charged with 9.2 grams of cyanuric chloride in 100 ml of ethanol and 30.9 grams of n-octylthioethyl mercaptan. The vessel was flushed with nitrogen and cooled to 0°C. While stirring 3.45 grams of sodium metal dissolved in 200 ml of ethanol were added to the reaction mixture. About 30 minutes after the addition had been completed, the reaction mixture was allowed to warm to 20°C and then flooded with water. On standing and cooling the reaction product solidified and was extracted with ether. The ether extract was dried over magnesium sulfate, filtered and the ether stripped, yielding an almost colorless viscous liquid weighing 31.3 grams. The 2,4,6-tris-(n-octyl-thioethylthio)-1,3,5-triazine was redissolved in ether, dried, filtered and stripped again yielding 30.7 grams of viscous liquid which crystallized on standing. This material had a MP of 32°C.

Other compounds which can be prepared by this process include: 2,4,6-tris-(n-dodecyl-thioethylthio)-1,3,5-triazine; 2,4,6-tris-(n-tetradecylthioethylthio)-1,3,5-triazine; 2,4,6-tris-(n-octadecylthioethylthio)-1,3,5-triazine; and 2,4,6-tris-(n-octylthioethylthioethyl)-1,3,5-triazine.

Unstabilized polypropylene powder (Hercules Profax 6501) is thoroughly blended with the antioxidant and processed and tested as in the Oven Aging Test on page 1. When unstabilized polypropylene is tested as described above, its oven life is about 3 hours. The example below shows the effectiveness of the stabilizers as well as the unusually high synergistic activity of these stabilizers when employed in combination with other stabilizers.

Example 2: Effectiveness of Stabilizers —

	Hours
0.1% Compound (A): Dioctadecyl 3,5-di-tert-butyl-4-hydroxybenzylphosphonate	50
0.1% Compound (B): 2,4-bis-(3',5'-di-tert-butyl-4'-hydroxyphenoxy)-6-(n-octylthio)-1,3,5-triazine	120
0.1% Compound (C): 2,4-bis-(n-octylthio)-6-(3',5'-di-tert-butyl-4'-hydroxyanilino)-1,3,5-triazine	120
0.1% Compound (D): Tetra-[3-(3',5'-di-tert-butyl-4'-hydroxyphenyl)propionyloxymethyl] methane	600

The combinations of stabilizers gave the following results.

	Hours
0.5% 2,4,6-tris-(n-octylthioethylthio)-1,3,5-triazine	35
0.1% Compound (A):0.5% 2,4,6-tris-(n-octylthio-ethylthio)-1,3,5-triazine	1,960
0.1% Compound (C):0.5% 2,4,6-tris-(n-octylthio-ethylthio)-1,3,5-triazine	1,735

Additional examples in the original patent include the stabilization of the following with these compounds (or synergistic mixtures containing these compounds): ABS; high impact polystyrene; polyethylene; lard; cottonseed oil; paraffin; mineral oil; gasoline; and polyester lubricants.

Substituted Hydroxylamine Stabilizers

P. Klemchuk; U.S. Patent 3,644,278; February 22, 1972; assigned to Ciba-Geigy Corp.; and U.S. Patent 3,778,464; December 11, 1973 has found that substituted hydroxyl-amines exhibit activity as antioxidants for a diverse group of substrate materials under specific conditions of exposure to an oxidizing environment. Illustrative embodiments of substituted hydroxylamine antioxidants are bis(p-nitrobenzyl)hydroxylamine, 2-diethyl-amino-4,6-bis(N-n-propyl-N-hydroxyamino)-s-triazine, and didodecyl-β,β'-hydroxyimino-dipropionate.

Included in this category of antioxidants are compounds represented by the formulas listed on the following page.

(1)

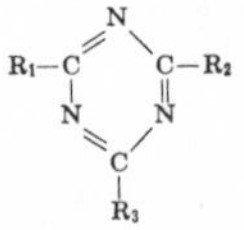

$$R_1-C \overset{\displaystyle N}{\underset{N}{\diagup}} \overset{\diagdown}{\underset{N}{\diagup}} C-R_2$$

$$\underset{R_3}{\overset{|}{C}}$$

where R_1, R_2 and R_3 are alkyl, dialkylamino, monoalkylamino, hydroxylamino, alkylthio, alkoxy, phenoxy or alkylphenoxy, the alkyl and alkoxy groups containing from 1 to 12 carbons, with the proviso that at least one of R_1, R_2 and R_3 is a hydroxylamino or alkyl hydroxylamino group;

(2)

$$R_4[(CH_2)n-\overset{\displaystyle O}{\overset{\|}{C}}-X]_m$$

where R_4 is HON, HONH or HONR$_5$, where R_5 is alkyl or phenylalkyl, the alkyl groups containing 1 to 3 carbons, m and n are 1 or 2, X is amino, monoalkylamino, dialkylamino or alkoxy, the alkyl and alkoxy groups containing 1 to 12 carbons;

(3)

$$\underset{\displaystyle OH}{[R_6N(CH_2)nSO_3]_mM}$$

where R_6 is alkyl or phenylalkyl, the alkyl groups containing 1 to 3 carbons, n is an integer from 1 to 4, m is an integer from 1 or 2 and M is a metal cation such as an alkali metal or alkaline earth metal, and

(4)

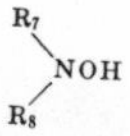

$$\underset{\displaystyle R_8}{\overset{\displaystyle R_7}{\diagdown}} NOH$$

where R_7 or R_8 is alkyl containing 1 to 3 carbons, benzyl, chlorobenzyl, nitrobenzyl, benzhydryl or triphenylmethyl with the proviso that only one of R_7 or R_8 is alkyl and that R_8 is hydrogen when R_7 is benzhydryl or triphenylmethyl, or R_7 and R_8 taken together with the nitrogen atom form a heterocyclic group such as morpholino, piperidino or piperazino.

These hydroxylamine compounds are prepared by a variety of conventional procedures. In one procedure, cyanuric chloride or a substituted mono- or dialkylamino-chloro-s-triazine is reacted with hydroxylamine or alkylhydroxylamine. An alternative procedure involves the reaction of a benzyl halide with hydroxylamine or alkylhydroxylamine. Another procedure involves reaction of a di-substituted amine that is, a dialkylamine, with methyl acrylate to form a tertiary amine which is then oxidized, as, for example, with peracetic acid and the resulting amine oxide is then treated with alkali such as sodium hydroxide, ammonium hydroxide, sodium carbonate and the like, to form the desired hydroxylamine product. Still another procedure involves the reaction of hydroxylamine or monoalkyl hydroxylamine with an acrylic acid ester or amide such as, for example, ethyl acrylate, lauryl acrylate or acrylamide. A further procedure for preparing hydroxylamines of this process involves reacting a monoalkyl hydroxylamine with a sultone, i.e., a cyclic sulfonate ester.

Example 1: Hydroxylamine hydrochloride (31.5 grams, 0.45 mol) was dissolved in 75 ml of water and the solution was then cooled to a temperature of 0°C. Sodium hydroxide (18.6 grams, 0.45 mol) in 75 ml water was then added at a temperature of 0° to 5°C. A solution of 51.5 grams of 4-nitrobenzyl chloride (0.3 mol) in 500 ml was added and the mixture was then heated to reflux for 4 hours. There was some precipitate formed which was filtered off while hot. The solution was then cooled and the product filtered and washed with water. The product weighed about 23 grams (slightly moist). On recrystallization from methyl cellosolve/water, yellow crystals of bis-(p-nitrobenzyl hydroxylamine) were obtained, 18.4 grams melting between 159° and 161°C.

Example 2: 1 mol of aqueous diethylamine was added over 30 minutes to 1 mol of cyanuric chloride, at a temperature of 0° to 5°C in aqueous acetone. Aqueous sodium carbonate solution (0.5 mol) was added in 20 minutes at a temperature of 0° to 5°C. The slurry was stirred at 0° to 5°C for 1¼ hours, and filtered. The filter cake was washed twice with cold water, and dried under vacuum. The yield of colorless crystalline 2-diethylamino-4,6-dichloro-s-triazine was 83.8 grams (75.7%); MP 74° to 77°C. On recrystallization from n-heptane, the MP was found to be between 76.5° and 78.5°C.

To a solution of 15.0 grams (0.20 mol) of n-propylhydroxylamine in 60 ml of 1:1 dioxane/water was added, over a 30 minute period at 0° to 5°C, a solution of 2-diethylamino-4,6-dichloro-s-triazine in 75 ml of dioxane. The mixture was heated at 55° to 60°C for 90 minutes, and refluxed for 30 minutes. A solution of 4.0 grams (0.10 mol) of sodium hydroxide was added, bringing the pH to a slight pink color with phenolphthalein. The reaction product was refluxed for 3 hours more and then poured into 1 liter of cold water. After standing, the reaction product solidified. This product was filtered, washed with water and then dried. The crude product (13.9 grams, 93.3% yield) was recrystallized 3 times from petroleum ether. The colorless needles of 2-diethylamino-4,6-bis-(N-n-propyl-N-hydroxyamino)-s-triazine obtained had a MP of 84.0° to 86.0°C.

Example 3: Hydroxylamine hydrochloride (4.0 grams) was dissolved in 100 ml of methanol and the resulting solution was added, at a temperature of 10°C to 2.7 grams of sodium methoxide in 50 ml methanol. A solution of 24.0 grams of lauryl acrylate in 100 ml of methanol was added at 5°C and the temperature was allowed to rise slowly. At 15°C, the reaction was noticeably strongly exothermic and needed cooling. At the same time, the reaction mixture thickened and 100 ml of ether was added to keep it mobile. The mixture was stirred overnight. The solvent was evaporated, the residue taken into 600 ml of ether and the organic solution was extracted with a concentrated sodium chloride solution, dried, filtered and evaporated. The white amorphous residue was recrystallized from alcohol (200 ml). There was obtained a yield of 18.0 grams of didodecyl-β,β'-hydroxyiminodipropionate melting between 55° and 57°C.

The tests given in the table below show that the subject hydroxylamines exhibit a remarkable light stabilization when incorporated in polypropylene.

Performance of 0.5% Hydroxylamine Antioxidants in Polypropylene

Antioxidant	Fadeometer Failure Time, hr
- - - - - - - -Antioxidants Incorporated by Milling - - - - - - - - - - - -	
None	100
2-Diethylamino-4,6-bis-(N-methyl-N-hydroxyamino)-s-triazine	900
2,4-Bis(dibutylamino)-6-N-hydroxyamino-s-triazine	700
- - - - Antioxidants Incorporated by Powder Pressing- - - - - - - - - -	
None	60
2-Diethylamino-4,6-bis-(N-methyl-N-hydroxyamino)-s-triazine	780
2-Octylthio-4,6-bis-(N-hydroxyamino)-s-triazine	280
2,4-Bis(octylthio)-6-N-hydroxyamino-s-triazine	480
2,4-Bis(dodecylamino)-6-N-hydroxyamino-s-triazine	660

Other tables in the complete patent show the stabilization of cyclohexene, lard, mineral oil and ABS resin by these hydroxylamine compounds, particularly the triazine derivatives.

ISOCYANURATE DERIVATIVES WITH HINDERED PHENOL MOIETIES

Tris(p-Hydroxybenzyl)Isocyanurates

The disclosure by *J.C. Gilles; U.S. Patent 3,531,483; September 29, 1970; assigned to The B.F. Goodrich Company* covers compounds of the general formula

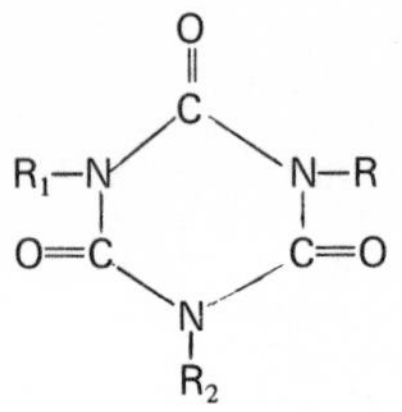

$$
\begin{array}{c}
\text{O} \\
\|\\
\text{C} \\
R_1\!-\!N \diagup \quad \diagdown N\!-\!R \\
O\!=\!C \diagdown \quad \diagup C\!=\!O \\
N \\
|\\
R_2
\end{array}
$$

where R is a hydroxyphenylalkyleneyl radical having the formula

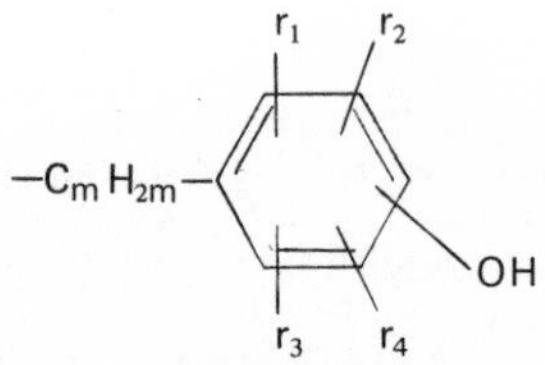

$$
-C_m H_{2m}-
\begin{array}{c}
r_1 \quad r_2 \\
\bigcirc \\
r_3 \quad r_4
\end{array}
OH
$$

where m is an integer from 1 to 4, r_1 is an alkyl group, either aliphatic or cycloaliphatic, containing 1 to 18 carbons and positioned immediately adjacent to the hydroxyl group on the ring, and r_2, r_3 and r_4 are hydrogen or an aliphatic or cycloaliphatic group containing 1 to 18 carbons; and R_1 and R_2 are hydrogen or the same as R above.

The symmetrical tris-(3,5-di-tert-alkyl-4-hydroxybenzyl)isocyanurates are a preferred class of compounds represented by the formula

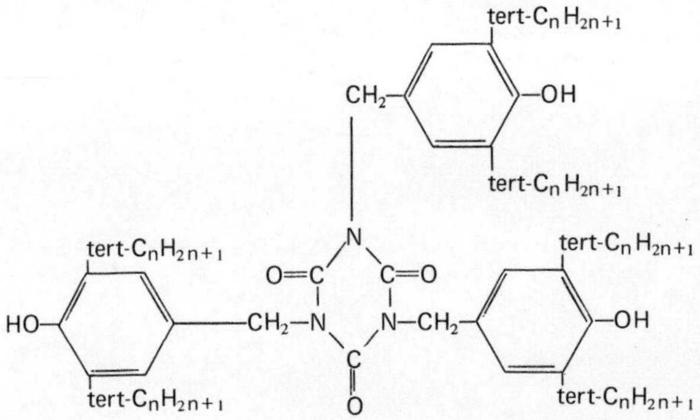

$$
\text{tert-}C_n H_{2n+1}
$$
$$
CH_2\!-\!\bigcirc\!-\!OH
$$
$$
\text{tert-}C_n H_{2n+1}
$$

$$
\text{tert-}C_n H_{2n+1} \qquad\qquad \text{tert-}C_n H_{2n+1}
$$
$$
HO\!-\!\bigcirc\!-\!CH_2\!-\!N\quad\begin{array}{c}O\!=\!C\quad C\!=\!O\\ N\\ C\\ \|\\ O\end{array}\quad N\!-\!CH_2\!-\!\bigcirc\!-\!OH
$$
$$
\text{tert-}C_n H_{2n+1} \qquad\qquad \text{tert-}C_n H_{2n+1}
$$

where n is an integer from 4 to 8. These compounds are excellent stabilizers for organic materials which are subject to oxidative, thermal and ultraviolet degradation, such as for example, natural rubber and olefin homopolymers and copolymers. They possess a good balance of properties useful for many stabilizing applications. It is most significant with these tris-(3,5-di-tert-alkyl-4-hydroxybenzyl)isocyanurates that although they are high molecular weight, a necessary requirement if low volatility is to be achieved, the concentration of the hindered phenol grouping has nevertheless been maintained at a high level (3 hindered phenol groups/molecule). This permits lower levels of stabilizer to be employed which results in a considerable economic advantage for the user.

To obtain the 4-hydroxybenzyl isocyanurates an alkali metal cyanate is reacted with a tertiary alkyl hindered p-hydroxybenzyl halide in an aprotic solvent, such as dimethyl sulfoxide or N,N-dimethylformamide, and at a temperature of about 100° to 130°C it is essential that the alkali metal cyanate and the 4-hydroxybenzyl halide be employed in equimolar amounts if the tris-(4-hydroxybenzyl)isocyanurate is to be obtained. The mono- and di-substituted isocyanurates can be obtained when excess alkali metal cyanate is employed for the reaction. Other preparative techniques may also be employed to obtain the compounds, such as for example, the process described in U.S. Patent 3,075,979.

Organic materials which are stabilized by these compounds include both natural and synthetic polymers. In addition to polymeric materials, the compounds act to stabilize a wide variety of other organic materials. Such compounds include: waxes, synthetic and petroleum derived lubricating oils and greases; animal oils such as, for example, fat, tallow, lard, cod-liver oil, sperm oil; vegetable oils such as castor, linseed, peanut, palm, cottonseed and the like; fuel oil; diesel oil; gasoline; and the like. The 4-hydroxybenzyl isocyanurates are especially useful for the stabilization of α-monoolefin homopolymers and copolymers.

Generally, for the effective stabilization of organic materials an amount of the 4-hydroxybenzyl isocyanurate ranges from 0.001% to 10% by weight based on the weight of the organic material to be employed. In most applications the amount of the compounds of this process will vary between about 0.01 and about 5% by weight. With the poly(α-monoolefin) homopolymers and copolymers about 0.01 to about 1.5% by weight of the stabilizer based on the weight of the olefin polymer will be employed.

Example 1: A glass reactor equipped with a stirrer, condenser and dropping funnel was charged with 200 ml of anhydrous N,N-dimethylformamide and 16.2 grams (0.2 mol) anhydrous potassium cyanate suspended therein. The reactor and dropping funnel were maintained under a nitrogen blanket throughout the run. The suspension was heated to 130°C and 51 grams (0.2 mol) 3,5-di-tert-butyl-4-hydroxybenzyl chloride dissolved in 50 ml dry N,N-dimethylformamide added dropwise over a two hour period. The reaction mixture was heated with stirring for an additional hour, allowed to cool and poured into ice water. The crude reaction product was recovered by filtration.

Purification of the tris-(3,5-di-tert-butyl-4-hydroxybenzyl)isocyanurate was achieved by multiple extraction of an ether solution of the crude product with 5% aqueous sodium hydrosulfite, water and saturated salt solution. The ether was removed by evaporation and the product recrystallized from methanol and water. 25 grams of tris-3,5-di-tert-butyl-4-hydroxybenzyl)isocyanurate melting at 213° to 215°C was obtained. Infrared analysis showed a single carbonyl peak at 1,710 cm^{-1} and no nitrogen-hydrogen linkages. Elemental analysis of the product agreed with values calculated for tris-(3,5-di-tert-butyl-4-hydroxybenzyl)isocyanurate. Tris-(3,5-di-tert-amyl-4-hydroxybenzyl)isocyanurate was prepared following this procedure.

Example 2: Tris-(3,5-di-tert-butyl-4-hydroxybenzyl)isocyanurate was incorporated in polypropylene by dissolving the additive in acetone, suspending the polypropylene in the solvent and then removing the acetone with a rotary evaporator. The stabilized polypropylene was hot-milled (290° to 300°F) for 5 minutes, sheeted off and placed in a warm 4-cavity ACS mold, shimmed to the desired thickness. The test samples were prepared by molding the stabilized polymer at 400°F and 4,000 psi. Ten mil samples are heated for 1 minute and 25 mil samples for 2 minutes before transferring to a cold press maintained at 4,000 psi for a 2 minute cooling period. Twenty-five mil samples were aged in an air-circulating oven at 140°C. Samples were deemed to have failed at the first sign of crazing. The following table sets forth the results obtained at several levels of stabilizer. Unstabilized polypropylene crazed within 1 hour under these same test conditions.

Sample	1	2	3	4
Stabilizer level (parts per hundred parts polypropylene)	0.1	0.25	0.5	1.0
Hours to crazing	120	192	1,320	1,400*

*Test terminated at this point with no sample failure

The complete patent also includes examples of the stabilization of polyethylene, 4-methyl-1-pentene/1-hexane copolymer, natural rubber, cis-polyisoprene, PVC, ABS, elastomeric polyurethane, ethyl acrylate/acrylonitrile copolymer, EPT, SBR, epichlorohydrin/ethylene oxide copolymer.

Tris(m-Hydroxybenzyl)Isocyanurates

Similar compounds having a m-hydroxy group rather than a p-hydroxy group in the phenolic moiety are disclosed by *P.V. Susi; U.S. Patent 3,723,427; March 27, 1973; assigned to American Cyanamid Company.* These compounds have the formula:

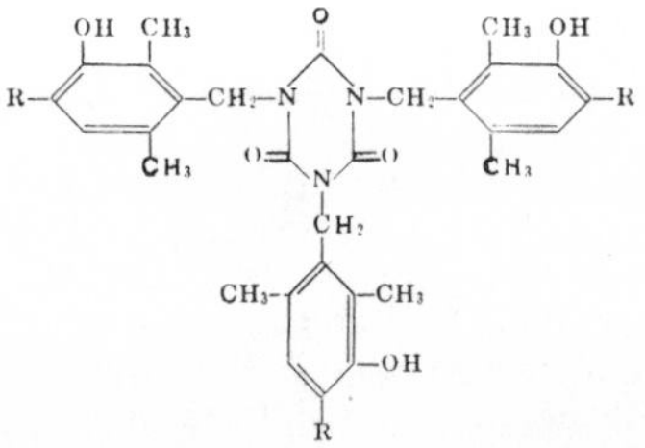

where R is a branched chain alkyl group containing 3 to 12 carbons. These compounds, as defined in the above formula, in addition to inhibiting oxidation of organic materials, possess outstanding resistance to extraction by boiling water, a property which has considerable importance when used in plastic materials in applications such as fibers, washing machine agitators, dishwasher parts, and the like, where contact with hot water is likely. In addition, these compounds are useful processing antioxidants for polyolefins; that is, they protect the polymer against breakdown during milling, extrusion, and other high-temperature processing operations.

These compounds are readily prepared by known procedures, such as the reaction of 1 mol of cyanuric acid with 3 mols of an appropriate 4-alkyl-3-hydroxy-2,6-dimethylbenzyl chloride. The benzyl chloride utilized can be prepared from the corresponding 2,4-dimethyl-6-alkylphenol by introducing the chloromethyl group into the 3-position by reaction with hydrochloric acid and formaldehyde or by reaction with methylal in the presence of hydrochloric acid and sulfuric acid.

Example 1: To a stirred mixture of 3.23 grams (0.025 mol) of cyanuric acid and 16.9 grams (0.075 mol) of 4-tert-butyl-3-hydroxy-2,6-dimethylbenzyl chloride in 50 ml dimethylformamide at 40°C was added dropwise 12 ml (0.08 mol) of triethylamine. The reaction mixture was stirred for 18 hours; 50 ml water and 50 ml benzene were added and the two liquid layers separated. The benzene phase was washed twice with 50 ml portions of water, the remaining water azeotropically removed, and the benzene solution clarified with 50 grams Superfiltrol. The benzene was removed and replaced with 50 ml methanol. After decolorizing with 10 grams of activated charcoal and cooling there was obtained 12 grams (78%) of the above identified product, MP 150°C. Recrystallization from methanol gave an analytical sample of 1,3,5-tris(4-tert-butyl-3-hydroxy-2,6-dimethylbenzyl)-s-triazine-2,4,6-(1H,3H,5H)trione melting at 154° to 155°C.

Compounds prepared in a similar way include: 1,3,5-tris(4-sec-butyl-3-hydroxy-2,6-dimethylbenzyl)-s-triazine-2,4,6(1H,3H,5H)trione; 1,3,5-tris(4-tert-amyl-3-hydroxy-2,6-dimethylbenzyl)-s-triazine-2,4,6(1H,3H,5H)trione; and 1,3,5-tris(4-tert-octyl-3-hydroxy-2,6-dimethyl-benzyl)-s-triazine-2,4,6(1H,3H,5H)trione.

Example 2: Evaluation in Polypropylene — The compound of Example 1 was incorporated into Avisun unstabilized polypropylene at the designated concentration using the process and test methods of the Oven Aging Test on page 1. Similar films were prepared containing the closest prior art compound: 1,3,5-tris(3,5-di-tert-butyl-4-hydroxybenzyl)-s-triazine-2,4,6(1H,3H,5H)trione, disclosed in U.S. Patent 3,531,483, which will be identified as control compound. The films were aged in a forced-draft oven at 140°C and the time (hours) to embrittlement recorded in the table below.

Compression molded films containing the antioxidants were refluxed in 200 ml water for 7 hours (1 cycle). The water was replaced at the end of each cycle until 15 cycles (105 hours) of boiling water extractions were completed. The films were then aged as above at 150°C in a forced-draft oven and hours to embrittlement noted (the table below). The oven-aged stability of the films after boiling water treatment is a measure of the extractability of the antioxidants.

	- - - - - - - Hours to Embrittlement - - - - - - - - -		
	Compound in Example 1*	Control Compound*	No Additive
Oven aging at 150°C	970–980	360–370	4
Oven aging at 150°C after 15 cycles boiling water	215–255	23–39	–

*Additive (used at 0.2% concentration)

This data shows that the m-hydroxy compound is much superior in antioxidant activity as compared to the control compound. Of particular significance is the startling resistance to extraction by hot water, a most important property with respect to materials which are laundered or used immersed in water.

Phenolic Carboxylates of Tris(Hydroxyalkyl)Isocyanurates

Esters of tris(hydroxyalkyl)isocyanurates with hindered hydroxyphenylcarboxylates are stabilizers of organic materials which are otherwise subject to thermooxidative and/or actinic deterioration. Thus, through the incorporation in various substrates of from 0.005 to 5% (by weight) of one or more of these compounds, either alone or in combination with other stabilizers such as dilaurylthiodipropionate, distearylthiodipropionate, ultraviolet light absorbers, and the like, there is observed a significant increase in the stability of the substrate. Such substrates include synthetic organic polymeric substances, such as vinyl resins, polyolefins, polyisoprene, polyurethanes, polyamides, polyesters, polycarbonates, polyacetals, polystyrene, polyethyleneoxide, and copolymers of the foregoing such as those of high impact polystyrene containing copolymers of butadiene and styrene and those formed by the copolymerization of acrylonitrile, butadiene and/or styrene.

These triesters can be prepared through esterification of tris(hydroxyalkyl)isocyanurate with a dialkyl-4-hydroxyphenylcarboxylic acid derivative such as the free acid, an acid halide thereof such as the acid chloride or acid bromide, or an acid anhydride thereof. When the free acid is employed, the esterification is preferably conducted in an inert nonaqueous organic solvent in the presence of an acid catalyst. An inert nonaqueous organic solvent is also preferably employed when the acid halide or anhydride is utilized, together with an acid acceptor such as triethylamine or dimethylaniline. Other esterification techniques, such as transesterification or utilization of an alkali metal salt of these derivatives with a tris(haloalkyl)isocyanurate in a manner known per se can also be employed.

In the first disclosure by *D.H. Steinberg and M. Dexter; U.S. Patent 3,707,542; Dec. 26, 1972; assigned to Ciba-Geigy Corporation,* these esters have the formula on the following page:

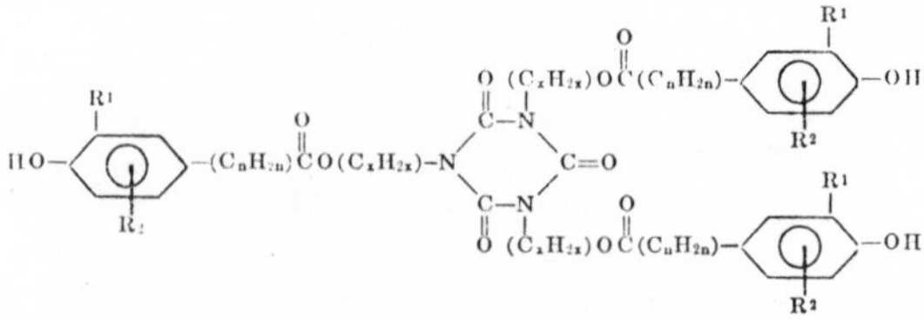

where each of R^1 and R^2 is the same or different alkyl group of 1 to 4 carbons, i.e., methyl, ethyl, n-propyl, isopropyl, n-butyl, sec-butyl or tert-butyl. The symbol n may be 1 or 2, thus embracing the appropriately substituted phenylacetic acid and phenylpropionic acid esters of tris(hydroxyalkyl)isocyanurate. The symbol x is an integer from 1 to 6.

Example: A mixture of 48.3 grams (0.165 mol) of methyl-3-(3,5-di-tert-butyl-4-hydroxyphenyl)propionate, 13.06 grams (0.05 mol) of tris(2-hydroxyethyl)isocyanurate and 1.87 grams (0.0075 mol) of dibutyltin oxide is first heated at 135° to 140°C under nitrogen for 4 hours, and then at 130°C/0.1 to 0.2 mm for 3 hours. The cooled reaction mixture is next dissolved in 100 ml of dry benzene, filtered through 600 grams of alumina, and washed with about 1 liter of benzene. The combined filtrate and washings are evaporated under vacuum and the product (48.3 grams) is further purified through several recrystallizations from heptane. The tris(2-[3-(3,5-di-tert-butyl-4-hydroxyphenyl)propionyloxy] ethyl)isocyanate melts in the range of 101° to 106°C.

In a similar fashion utilizing 46 grams of methyl-3,5-di-tert-butyl-4-hydroxyphenylacetate in the above procedure in place of the designated quantity of methyl-3-(3,5-di-tert-butyl-4-hydroxyphenyl)propionate, there is obtained tris[2-(3,5-di-tert-butyl-4-hydroxyphenylacetoxy)ethyl] isocyanurate.

D.H. Steinberg and M. Dexter; U.S. Patent 3,707,543; December 26, 1972; assigned to Ciba-Geigy Corporation have also prepared the benzoate esters having the formula

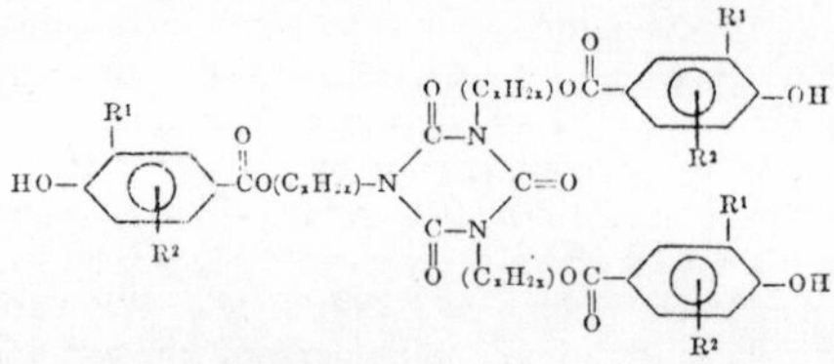

where each of R^1 and R^2 is the same or different butyl group, such as n-butyl, sec-butyl or tert-butyl. The preferred group is tert-butyl. The symbol x is an integer from 1 to 6.

Example: Tris[2-(3,5-Di-tert-Butyl-4-Hydroxybenzoyloxy)Ethyl] Isocyanurate — A solution consisting of 10.45 grams (0.040 mol) of tris(2-hydroxyethyl)isocyanurate, 18.18 grams (0.15 mol) dimethylaniline and 250 ml toluene is stirred under nitrogen at room temperature. To this is added in a dropwise fashion, a solution of 45.7 grams (0.17 mol) of 3,5-di-tert-butyl-4-hydroxybenzoyl chloride in 250 ml of toluene over an interval of 2.5 hours. The resulting mixture is then stirred and heated at 90°C for an additional 3 hours. After cooling, the mixture is filtered and the filtrate washed successively with water, 1 N hydrochloric acid, water, 2 N sodium hydroxide, water and saturated sodium chloride solution. The washed solution is dried over molecular sieves. Filtration, followed by removal of the solvent yields 29.9 grams of product which is crystallized from heptane-toluene and recrystallized from heptane-cyclohexane. The product is a white crystalline solid having a MP of 169° to 172°C.

Alkylhydroxyphenylcarboalkoxy-Substituted Nitrogen Heterocycles

Antioxidant compounds containing one or more alkylhydroxyphenyl groups bonded through carboalkoxy linkages to a nitrogen atom of a heterocyclic nucleus containing an imidodi-carbonyl group or an imidodithiocarbonyl group have been prepared by G. *Kletecka and P.D. Smith; U.S. Patents 3,763,093; October 2, 1973; and 3,678,047; July 18, 1972; assigned to The B.F. Goodrich Company.*

These compounds are represented by the general formula

(1)

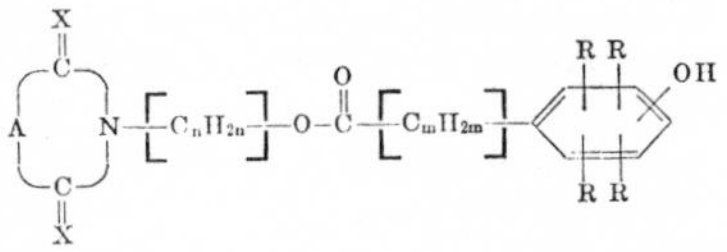

where n is an integer from 1 to 12, m is an integer from 0 to 8, R is hydrogen or a hydrocarbon radical containing 1 to 12 carbons, X is oxygen or sulfur and A is a bivalent molecular grouping. The bivalent radical A may be a hydrocarbon radical, such as alkylene or phenylene, or may contain one or more heteroatoms or other functional groups, such as $>NH$, $>C=S$, $>C=O$ or the like. Compounds of Formula 1 which are especially useful are those where X is oxygen, n is an integer from 1 to 8, m is an integer from 1 to 4 and the hydroxyl group is in the 4-position on the ring and is hindered, i.e., has positioned on the ring immediately adjacent thereto at least one alkyl group containing from 1 to 12 carbons.

A useful class of compounds for use as stabilizers for organic materials, particularly polymeric materials, are the derivatives of isocyanuric acid. These compounds contain one or more alkylhydroxyphenyl groups bonded to the isocyanuric acid nucleus through a carboalkoxy linkage and have the structural formula

(2)

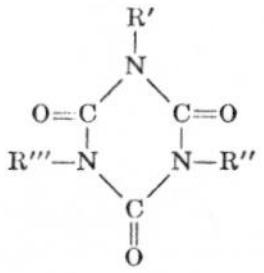

where R' is an alkylhydroxyphenylcarboalkoxy group having the formula

(3)

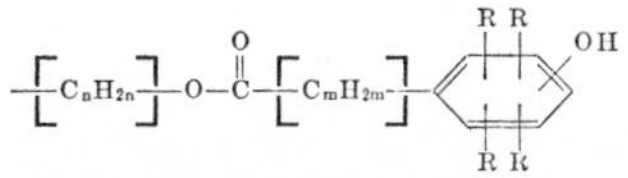

where n, m and R are the same as defined for Formula 1 above; and R" and R''' are the same as R' or are hydrogen, a hydrocarbon radical containing from 1 to 20 carbons such as alkyl, cycloalkyl, aryl, alkaryl or aralkyl, a hydroxyalkyl group containing from 1 to 12 carbons or an alkylcarboalkoxy group containing from 2 to 20 carbons. Especially useful derivatives of isocyanuric acid are those compounds where two, and more preferably all, of the nitrogens of the ring are substituted with radicals of the Formula 3.

To obtain the alkylhydroxyphenylcarboalkoxy-substituted nitrogen heterocycles any number of reaction schemes may be employed. Esterification of a hydroxyalkyl-substituted nitrogen heterocycle with an acid of the formula on the following page:

$$\text{HO} \underset{R_1 \ R_1}{\overset{R_1 \ R_1}{\diamondsuit}} \left[C_mH_{2m} \right] - COOH$$

where R_1 and m are the same as defined above in Formula 1, is particularly convenient to prepare these compounds. The esterification reaction will generally be conducted with an acidic catalyst in an inert solvent. The amounts of reactants employed will be determined by the degree of substitution desired and the particular nitrogen heterocycle to be substituted. For example, if a tris(hydroxyalkyl)isocyanurate is to be completely substituted, 3 mols of the acid will be employed per mol of the isocyanuric acid derivative. If partial substitution of the nitrogen heterocycle is desired, the amount of the acid reacted therewith will be decreased proportionately in accordance with the desired degree of substitution.

The acid to be reacted may be obtained by any of the conventional methods including hydrolysis of an ester precursor. Similarly, the hydroxyalkyl-substituted nitrogen heterocycle may be obtained by a variety of methods depending on the particular hydroxyalkyl group to be substituted. For example, hydroxymethyl groups may be substituted on isocyanuric acid or other nitrogen heterocycle by reaction with formaldehyde. 3 mols of formaldehyde would be reacted with 1 mol of cyanuric acid at an elevated temperature to obtain tris(hydroxymethyl)isocyanurate. Tris(2-hydroxyethyl)isocyanurate may be obtained by the reaction of ethylene oxide and cyanuric acid in dimethylformamide or dimethylacetamide. If long chain hydroxyalkyl groups are to be substituted they may be prepared by the procedure described in U.S. Patent 3,249,607.

Example 1: Esterification of 3-(3,5-di-tert-butyl-4-hydroxyphenyl)propanoic acid with tris-(2-hydroxyethyl)isocyanurate, obtained by the reaction of cyanuric acid with ethylene oxide in N,N-dimethylformamide as described by R.W. Cummins, *J. Amer. Chem. Soc.,* 28, 85 (1963), gives THPI, 2,2',2"-tris[3-(3,5-di-tert-butyl-4-hydroxyphenyl)propionyloxy]- ethylisocyanurate, in good yield. The reaction was conducted in a 12 liter glass reactor equipped with a Dean-Stark water trap by combining 157 grams (0.6 mol) tris-(2-hydroxyethyl)isocyanurate and 552 grams (1.98 mols; 10% molar excess) 3-(3,5-di-tert-butyl-4-hydroxyphenyl)propanoic acid in 3 liters dry xylene. Hydrogen chloride was then bubbled into the reaction mixture until it was saturated and 5.53 grams p-toluene sulfonic acid charged.

The reaction mixture was then heated to reflux for about 6 hours during which time about 33 ml water was removed by azeotropic distillation, allowed to cool and the catalyst residues removed by filtration. The xylene was removed under reduced pressure to obtain a glass-like crude product. This crude product was dissolved in about 2 liters of diethyl ether and washed with several portions of 0.5% aqueous sodium hydroxide until the wash has a pH of 10 or greater and then with water. After drying the ether was stripped under vacuum and about 95% yield THPI obtained as a crude glassy material having a softening point of about 67°C. This material was further purified by dissolving at 65° to 70°C in about 5 liters heptane and allowing the solution to cool to room temperature with vigorous agitation.

By recrystallization from isopropanol THPI is obtained as a colorless crystalline material melting at 127° to 128°C. The product was identified as THPI by infrared spectroscopy and nuclear magnetic resonance spectroscopy.

Example 2: An alkylhydroxyphenylcarboalkoxy-substituted derivative of phthalimide was prepared in accordance with the procedure of Example 1 by the reaction of 28.6 grams (0.16 mol) of N-(2-hydroxyethyl)phthalimide and 41.7 grams (0.15 mol) 3-(3,5-di-tert-butyl-4-hydroxyphenyl)propanoic acid in 250 ml dry xylene with 0.42 gram p-toluene sulfonic acid. A 65% yield of N-2-[3-(3,5-di-tert-butyl-4-hydroxyphenyl)propionyloxy] ethylphthalimide melting at 107° to 109°C was obtained. The structure was confirmed by nuclear magnetic resonance spectroscopy and infrared spectroscopic analysis.

Example 3: Polypropylene samples stabilized with THPI were subjected to long-term oven aging to demonstrate the effectiveness of the stabilizer compounds by themselves and in combination with sulfur-containing synergist compounds such as distearylthiodipropionate. To prepare the test samples polypropylene was dry blended with the stabilizers and then fluxed in an extruder at 450°F. The extrudate was pelletized and hot pressed at 420°F into 10 mil thick specimens which were aged in an air-circulating oven at 150°C. The samples were deemed to have failed at the first sign of crazing. Test results for the various samples are tabulated below:

	Sample					
	a	b	c	d	e	f
Polypropylene	100	100	100	100	100	100
THPI		0.10	0.25	0.10	0.25	
Distearylthiodipropionate				0.25	0.25	0.25
Days to failure	<1	20	45	45	59	<1

Materials stabilized in other examples of the complete patent include polyethylene, polystyrene, acrylic latexes, natural rubber, neoprene, cis-polyisoprene, ethylene-propylene terpolymers, ABS, PVC, polyurethanes, polyacetals, nylon 6, ethylene oxide/epichlorohydrin copolymers and turbine oil.

PHOSPHORUS-CONTAINING ANTIOXIDANTS

PHOSPHATE ESTERS

Antioxidants containing the phosphate group have been disclosed in the following four patents.

Esters of Hindered Phenols

The preparation and use of tris(3,5-dihydrocarbyl-4-hydroxyphenyl)phosphate antioxidants have been described by *B.R. Meltsner; U.S. Patent 3,716,603; February 13, 1973; assigned to Ethyl Corporation.* These phosphates have the formula:

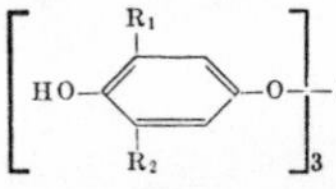

$$\left[HO-\underset{R_2}{\overset{R_1}{\diamondsuit}}-O-P=O \right]_3$$

where R_1 is alpha-branched alkyl containing 3 to 18 carbons, alpha-branched aralkyl containing 8 to 18 carbons or cycloalkyl containing 6 to 18 carbons and R_2 is alkyl containing 1 to 18 carbons, aralkyl containing 7 to 18 carbons, aryl containing 6 to 18 carbons or cycloalkyl containing 6 to 18 carbons.

It is preferred that R_1 and R_2 be alpha-branched hydrocarbyl radicals, more preferably that both be tertiary alkyl radicals. Preferred compounds include tris(3,5-di-tert-butyl-4-hydroxyphenyl)phosphate, tris(3,5-di-tert-amyl-4-hydroxyphenyl)phosphate, tris(3,5-di-tert-octyl-4-hydroxyphenyl)phosphate, tris(3,5-di-tert-dodecyl-4-hydroxyphenyl)phosphate, and the like.

These phosphate compounds are readily prepared by reacting a 2,6-dihydrocarbyl-p-hydroquinone with a phosphorus oxyhalide. Although any of the phosphorus oxyhalides may be used, the preferred reactants are phosphorus oxybromide and phosphorus oxychloride and especially phosphorus oxychloride because of its low cost, availability and excellent results obtained with its use. The following example will illustrate the preparation and use of these phosphates.

Example: To a reaction vessel fitted with stirrer, thermometer, liquid addition means and cooling means were added 8.6 parts of 2,6-di-tert-butyl-p-hydroquinone, 3.9 parts of triethylamine and 70 parts of diethyl ether. The vapor space above the liquid was displaced with nitrogen which was maintained during reaction. A solution of 1.99 parts of phosphorus oxychloride in 18 parts of diethyl ether was added with stirring. The reaction temperature was maintained at about 30°C during this addition. The reaction was then stirred for about 12 hours, during which a triethylamine hydrochloride precipitate formed.

This precipitate was filtered off and the ether solvent removed from the filtrate by evaporation under vacuum (about 20 mm Hg). The residue was recrystallized from a methanol-water mixture, giving white crystals melting at 201° to 204°C. The infrared spectrum was consistent with that for tris(3,5-di-tert-butyl-4-hydroxyphenyl)phosphate. Results of testing the compound of the example are shown in the following table where data from the standard oven-aging test (page 1) are recorded for polypropylene.

Additive	Concentration (weight percent)	Sample thickness, mils	Hours to failure
None		25	2.5
2,6-di-tert-butyl-4-methylphenol	0.3	25	16
2,2'-methylenebis-(4-methyl-6-tert-butylphenol)	0.3	25	112
4,4'-thiobis(2-tert-butyl-5-methylphenol)	0.3	25	96
Tris(3,5-di-tert-butyl-4-hydroxyphenyl)-phosphate	0.3	25	1,648
Tris(3,5-di-tert-butyl-4-hydroxyphenyl)-phosphate	0.3	62	1,760

Examples are included in the complete patent on the stabilization of the following with these phosphate esters: elastomers (natural rubber, SBR, NBR, EPT); polyethylene; petroleum products (gasoline, antiknock formulations, diesel fuel, petroleum and synthetic polyester lubricants); and foods (coconut oil and lard).

Esters of Hindered Thiobisphenols

M. Robin and S.R. Schulte; U.S. Patent 3,676,530; July 11, 1972; assigned to Ashland Oil & Refining Company has prepared phosphate esters in which at least one of the available bonds on the phosphorus is connected to a hindered phenol through the oxygen remaining after removal of the hydrogen of a phenolic hydroxyl group. The hindered phenol is a thiobisphenol represented by the formula:

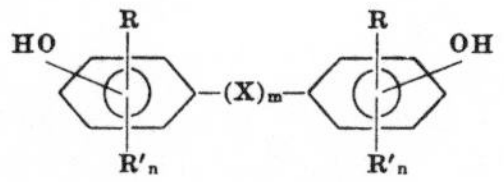

The X is a sulfur linkage, and can be, for example:

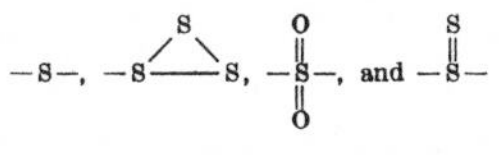

and preferably is S.

The m is an integer of at least 1, and preferably is 1 to 3, and most preferably is 1. The OH group on each ring can be in any position but is preferably para to the sulfur linkage. Each R individually is a bulky hydrocarbon of at least 1 carbon and is ortho to the OH on each ring. Usually the bulky hydrocarbon is free of nonbenzenoid unsaturation. R is preferably a bulky hydrocarbon of 1 to 22 carbons, more preferably of 3 to 12 carbons, and even more preferably is an alkyl containing 1 to 22 carbons. Especially preferable is an alkyl group containing 3 to 12 carbons of which tert-butyl is the most preferred. Each R' individually is a hydrocarbon such as set forth above for R; or a halide group such as chlorine or bromine; or $-NO_2$; $-SR''$; or $-OR''$; $-COOR''$; $-NR''R'''$; $-NHR'''NH_2$; $-NHOH$; or $NHR'''OH$; where R'' is H or a hydrocarbon as defined above for R, and R''' is an alkylene group of 1 to 22 carbons and preferably of 1 to 12 carbons.

These compounds may constitute, for instance, the reaction products from 1 reacted mol of a phosphate ester-forming phosphorous compound and at least 1 reacted mol and preferably 3 reacted mols of a hindered phenol, and if necessary, at least 1 other phenolic compound in an amount so that each of the available bonds on the phosphorus atom is connected to a phenol through the oxygen remaining after the removal of the hydrogen of a phenolic hydroxyl group.

The reaction products are formed by using conventional phosphate ester-forming conditions such as time, temperature and catalyst. The production of these compounds was unexpected since attempts to prepare phosphite esters of the same hindered thiobisphenols by using phosphorous trichloride were not successful.

Example 1: To a mixture of 3 mols of 4,4'-thiobis(6-tert-butyl-3-methylphenol), 4,000 parts of o-dichlorobenzene as an inert solvent and 0.4 mol of a magnesium metal catalyst in a glass lined container equipped with a glass surfaced stirrer is added all at once and with agitation, 1 mol of phosphorous oxychloride. The resultant mixture is agitated for 24 hours at a pressure of about 1 atmosphere with the temperature maintained between 165° and 175°C. Hydrogen chloride gas evolves as the reaction proceeds and is neutralized in a scrubbing device. The reaction mixture is cooled, 1,000 parts of water added and the magnesium catalyst separated by filtration.

The clarified mixture is then neutralized to a pH between 6 and 8 by use of an aqueous sodium carbonate solution. The organic portion of the mixture is then washed with 1,000 parts of water, and an organic layer is separated from the aqueous portion of the mixture. The reaction product and inert solvent are then separated by vacuum distillation. The reaction product, tris[2-tert-butyl-4-(2-methyl-4-hydroxy-5-tert-butylphenylthio)-5-methylphenyl] phosphate is a clear friable glass melting between 62° and 67°C and has the following structure as determined by elemental analysis and IR spectra.

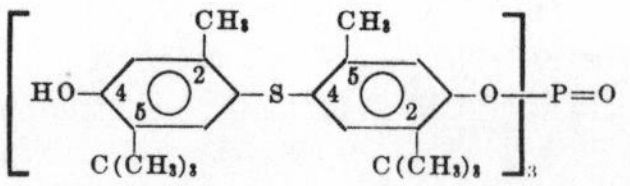

Example 2: The product of Example 1 is mixed with a polypropylene of 0.90 density and approximately 325,000 molecular weight in a steel container and the mixture is extruded twice at 380°F. The resulting polypropylene compositions containing 0.5% by weight of the product of Example 1 are then pressed into a 6 to 6.5 mil film at 350°F and 1,280 psi on a 10 inch hydraulic ram press.

Likewise a film of the same polypropylene without any antioxidant and a film of the same polypropylene containing 0.5% of 2,2'-methylenebis(6-tert-butyl-4-methylphenol) are prepared by the above method. The resulting 3 films are then subjected to 150° ± 1°C in a forced draft oven. The absorbance in the carbonyl region of the IR spectrum (5.8 Angstroms) is then recorded after periods of exposure. When absorbance reaches 94%, the sample is considered to be oxidized, and the time of exposure to reach this point is recorded in the table below.

Additive	Amount	Time in hrs. to reach 94% Absorbances
NONE		4
2,2'-thiobis-(6-tertiary-butyl-4-methyl phenol)	0.5	6
Reaction Product of Example 1	0.5	166

Polyethylene is also stabilized in an example in the original patent.

Cyclic Phosphates

Compounds containing 2-hydroxybenzophenone residues and cyclic phosphate groups have been prepared by *R. Cowling; U.S. Patent 3,686,367; August 22, 1972; assigned to Imperial Chemical Industries, Ltd., England* as stabilizers for organic materials against degradation by light, heat and oxidation. These are compounds of the formula:

where R is a 3-hydroxy-4-benzoylphenyl group and A is ethylene, 1,2-propylene, 1,3-propylene and 1-methyl-1,3-propylene, 2,2-dimethoxymethyl-1,3-propylene, phenylethylene, tetradecylethylene, 1,2-bis-ethoxycarbonyl-ethylene, o-phenylene, 1,8-naphthylene and 2,3-naphthylene, 4-methyl-1,2-phenylene, 4-chloro-1,2-phenylene, 3-nitro-1,2-phenylene, 1,1'-tolylene and 4-chloro and 4-methyl substituted derivatives.

These phosphates may be prepared in any conventional manner. For example, a monochlorocyclic phosphate ester may be reacted with a dihydroxybenzophenone, such as 2,4-dihydroxybenzophenone, or with a compound of 2-hydroxylbenzophenone having a linking group containing a reactive hydroxyl group. Alternatively, for example, a dichlorophosphate ester in which the esterifying group is or contains a 2-hydroxybenzophenone residue is reacted with a dihydroxy compound where the hydroxyl groups are so positioned that a cyclic phosphate ester is formed.

These reactions may be carried out by well known procedures for similar reactions, for example, by mixing the reactants optionally in a solvent at room temperature or at a higher temperature. If necessary, an acid binding agent such as pyridine, methylamine, dimethylaniline or sodium carbonate is added.

Example 1: A solution of 32.1 parts of 2,4-dihydroxybenzophenone and 11.8 parts of pyridine in 143 parts of ether is stirred at 20°C under a slow stream of nitrogen and there is added over 1 hour a solution of 25.6 parts of 2-chloro-2-oxo-4-methyl-1,3,2-dioxaphosphorinane in 21 parts of ether. After completion of the addition, the reaction mixture is stirred at room temperature for 1 hour, at the boiling point for 30 minutes.

After cooling to room temperature there is added 285 parts of ether and the mixture is stirred overnight. The ether layer is removed by decantation and the residue further extracted with 4 x 353 parts of ether. The combined ether extracts are filtered and evaporated under reduced pressure.

The residue, after evaporation of the ether, is dissolved in 440 parts of benzene and the solution is extracted with 4 x 500 parts of 5% aqueous sodium carbonate solution. After drying, the solvent is evaporated under reduced pressure to give 2-oxo-2-[3-hydroxy-4-benzoylphenoxy]-4-methyl-1,3,2-dioxaphosphorinane as a white solid.

Example 2: 2-Oxo-2-[3-hydroxy-4-benzoylphenoxy]-4-methyl-1,3,2-dioxaphosphorinane (A) is well mixed with polypropylene powder together with a commercial antioxidant, 1,1,3-tris[2-methyl-4-hydroxy-5-tert-butylphenyl]butane (B), and dilauryl thiodipropionate (C). A portion of this mixture is pressed onto 0.75 mm film using a steam heated press at 185°C. A second portion is extruded from a screw extruder with a melt temperature of 250°C and the extrudate is then pressed into 0.75 mm film as before. Both films are exposed to UV irradiation in a Xenon arc type of light aging apparatus designed to simulate daylight conditions and the time to film embrittlement is noted.

A commercial stabilizer, 2-hydroxy-4-octyloxybenzophenone (D) is similarly incorporated into polypropylene and the films formed are simultaneously tested in the same manner. The results, shown in the table on the following page, illustrate the superiority of 2-oxo-2-[3-hydroxy-4-benzoylphenoxy]-1,3,2-dioxaphosphorinane.

Film Formed From:	Percent Additives in Polypropylene				Embrittlement Time (hours)
	A	B	C	D	
Pressed	0.5	0.1	0.25	-----	775
Powder	-----	0.1	0.25	0.5	333
Pressed	0.5	0.1	0.25	-----	775
Extrudate	-----	0.1	0.25	0.5	429

S-Allylic and S-Vinylic O,S'-Dialkyl Dithiophosphates

Dealkylation of alkyl dithiophosphates having no olefinic unsaturation is old, having been discovered by Carius more than a hundred years ago: L. Carius, *Ann. Chem. Pharm.* 112, 190 (1859). However, none of the prior thiophosphate ester products has ever had any allylic or vinylic substituents. The apparent reason for this is that successful dealkylation of allylic esters was not expected in view of the fact that allylic cations are much more stable than the alkyl cations; hence, owing to their stability, allylic cations would be expected to undergo elimination in preference to alkyl cations from such esters.

However, *A.A. Oswald and P.L. Valint, Jr.; U.S. Patent 3,662,034; May 9, 1972; assigned to Esso Research and Engineering Company* have found that S-allylic and S-vinylic O,O'-dialkyldithiophosphates can be selectively dealkylated to form their corresponding salts, which then can be reacted with alkyl halides to form S-allylic and S-vinylic O,S'-dialkyl-dithiophosphates. Both the dealkylated products and the alkylated products are useful as pesticides, especially as insecticides, and as antioxidants, lubricating oil additives, etc.

The dealkylation of S-alkenyl, i.e., S-allylic and S-vinylic dialkyldithiophosphates occurs selectively, without a significant elimination of the S-alkenyl groups. The dealkylation is depicted by the following general scheme:

$$
\begin{array}{c} R'O \\ \diagdown \\ \diagup \\ R''O \end{array} \!\!\! \underset{S}{\overset{}{P}} - S - \left[\underset{R_2}{\overset{R_1}{C}} \right]_{0\text{-}1} \!\!\! \underset{R_5}{\overset{R_3}{C}} \!\!=\!\! \underset{}{\overset{R_4}{C}} \;\; \xrightarrow{\;D\;} \;\; \begin{array}{c} R'O \\ \diagdown \\ \diagup \\ O^{(-)}S \end{array} \!\!\! P \!-\! \left[\underset{R_2}{\overset{R_1}{C}} \right]_{0\text{-}1} \!\!\! \underset{R_5}{\overset{R_3}{C}} \!\!=\!\! \underset{}{\overset{R_4}{C}}
$$

where R' and R'' are each C_1 to C_{30} monovalent aliphatic hydrocarbyl radicals, e.g., alkyl, alkenyl, alicyclic, aralkyl, and substituted derivatives thereof, which substituted derivatives may contain halogen, nitrogen, alkylmercapto, carbalkoxy groups, etc., preferably R' and R'' are C_1 to C_{16} alkyls, most preferably C_1 to C_6 alkyls; R_1 to R_5 are hydrogen, chlorine, cyano, C_1 to C_3 acyl, C_1 to C_6 carbalkoxy, C_1 to C_3 alkylmercapto, or C_1 to C_{16} unsubstituted or substituted hydrocarbyl radicals, preferably alkyl and/or aryl, and substituted derivatives thereof containing halogen, nitrogen, alkylmercapto, carbalkoxy groups, etc. R_1 to R_5 are most preferably C_1 to C_4 unsubstituted, monosubstituted, or disubstituted alkyls; D is a dealkylating agent such as a nitrogen base such as ammonia, amines, etc.; a thiolate salt, such as the sodium salts of hydrocarbyl thiols and thiol acids; or an inorganic salt such as lithium chloride, sodium iodide, calcium chloride, etc.

Dealkylation may occur with the elimination of either R' or R''. If R' and R'' are different n-alkyl groups, dealkylation involving the smaller alkyl group may preferably occur. The dealkylated product is a partial ester of dithiophosphoric acid, i.e., an S-alkenyl-O-alkyl dithiophosphate. As such, it may exist either as an ionic salt or a hydrogen bonded complex of the corresponding acid. The composition of the salt or complex formed is dependent on the dealkylation agent used.

It has been found that the alkylation of the S-allylic and S-vinylic O-alkyl dithiophosphate salts is highly selective since it occurs exclusively on the sulfur. These alkylation reactions all involve the ambient S-alkenyl O-alkyl dithiophosphate anion as a common intermediate.

This anion can, of course, be derived from an amine-acid complex or from a salt. It will displace the halide, sulfate, or sulfonate group of the alkylating agent. It is, of course, possible by this process to use a mol of alkylene dihalide in place of 2 mols of alkyl monohalide.

Additive uses of phosphorus compounds as antioxidants, antiwear agents, extreme pressure agents, etc. are well known. These compounds of the present process, however, are of special interest because they are more thermally stable than the corresponding nonisomerized compounds. Also, the presence of the S-alkenyl groups provides special benefits as far as high level additive action and low level toxicity to warm blooded animals are concerned.

Example: The dealkylation of S-crotyl O,O'-dimethyl dithiophosphate with ammonia and its subsequent alkylation with methyl bromide is effected as follows. Into an evacuated Pyrex pressure tube, equipped with a magnetic stirrer and containing 42.4 grams (0.2 mol) of S-crotyl O,O'-dimethyl dithiophosphate, 6.8 grams (0.4 mol) of ammonia were condensed using a Dry Ice-isopropanol cooling bath. The sealed contents were then thoroughly mixed and placed into a water bath at ambient temperature. Transient blue coloration of the reaction mixture during the first hour indicated the reaction.

After standing 3 days, all the volatile components were removed from the mixture at 0.5 millimeter pressure. The weight loss corresponded to the 3.4 grams (0.2 mol) excess of ammonia. A nuclear magnetic resonance (NMR) spectrum of the liquid residue indicated that the dealkylation product was methyl ammonium S-crotyl O-methyl dithiophosphate.

The above intermediate was dissolved in 100 ml of acetonitrile. To the solution 25.5 grams (0.27 mol) of methyl bromide were condensed. The sealed mixture was then heated at 60°C for 4 hours. The resulting crude mixture was diluted with 500 ml of water and the neutral ester phase separated. The water phase was washed with 300 ml ether. The combined organic phases were diluted with 200 ml ether, washed, in turn, with 200 ml water and 100 ml 5% aqueous sodium hydrogen carbonate solution. The ether solution was then dried and fractionally distilled. Vacuum distillation yielded 90.0 grams (41.5%) of S-crotyl O,S'-dimethyl dithiophosphate as a colorless liquid boiling at 91° to 93°C at 0.3 millimeter. The structure of the product was confirmed by its NMR spectrum.

Other compounds prepared by this method include S-allyl O,S'-diethyl dithiophosphate, S-vinyl O,S'-dimethyl dithiophosphate and S-propenyl O,S'-diethyl dithiophosphate. Examples in the original patent showing use of these compounds were limited to their use as pesticides.

PHOSPHITE ANTIOXIDANTS

Workers at the Weston Chemical Corporation have developed several classes of organophosphite stabilizers and antioxidants as shown in the first of three disclosures.

Hydrogenated Bisphenol Diphosphites

L. Friedman, K.H. Rattenbury and A. Guttag; U.S. Patent 3,641,218; February 8, 1972; assigned to Weston Chemical Corporation have prepared phosphites having the formula:

$$(1) \qquad \begin{array}{c} R_1O \\ \diagdown \\ R_2O \diagup \end{array} P-O-Z-O-P \begin{array}{c} OR_3 \\ \diagup \\ \diagdown \\ OR_4 \end{array}$$

where R_1, R_2, R_3 and R_4 are selected from alkyl, aryl, alkenyl, haloalkyl, haloaryl or the monovalent residue of a hydrogenated dihydric phenol, Z is the residue of a dihydric alcohol or a hydrogenated dihydric phenol and at least one of R_1, R_2, R_3 and R_4 is a residue of a hydrogenated dihydric phenol. Preferably at least three of R_1, R_2, R_3 and R_4 are hydrogenated dihydric phenol residues. A particularly preferred compound has all of R_1, R_2, R_3, R_4 and Z as residues of a hydrogenated dihydric phenol.

When R_1, R_2, R_3 and R_4 are the residues of a hydrogenated dihydric phenol, they have the formula:

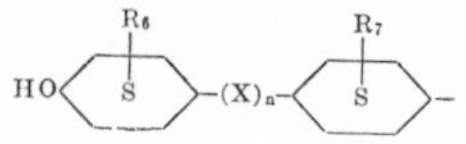

$$HO\!-\!\underset{R_6}{\bigcirc}\!-\!(X)_n\!-\!\underset{R_7}{\bigcirc}\!-$$

where R_6 and R_7 are hydrogen or alkyl, X is O, S or SO_2 or:

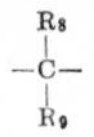

$$-\!\underset{R_9}{\overset{R_8}{C}}\!-$$

where R_8 and R_9 are hydrogen or lower alkyl and n is O or 1.

Typical examples of Z are $-(CH_2)_n-$ where n is an integer from 2 to 20 or more, $-(C_xH_{2x}O)_yC_xH_{2x}-$ where x is an integer of 2 to 6 and y is an integer of 1 to 100 or even more, $-C_xH_{2x}SC_xH_{2x}-$,

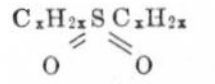

$$C_xH_{2x}\overset{\Vert}{\underset{O}{S}}C_xH_{2x}$$

and the residue of a hydrogenated dihydric phenol having the formula:

$$-\underset{R_6}{\bigcirc}\!-\!\underset{R_7}{\bigcirc}- \qquad\qquad -\underset{R_6}{\bigcirc}\!-\!O\!-\!\underset{R_7}{\bigcirc}-$$

$$-\underset{R_6}{\bigcirc}\!-\!S\!-\!\underset{R_7}{\bigcirc}- \qquad\qquad -\underset{R_6}{\bigcirc}\!-\!SO_2\!-\!\underset{R_7}{\bigcirc}-$$

where R_6 and R_7 are hydrogen or alkyl.

These compounds are useful as high molecular weight stabilizers for halogen containing resins such as vinyl chloride resins, hydrocarbon polymers such as monoolefin polymers including polypropylene, polyethylene, ethylene-propylene copolymers and terpolymers, natural rubber, synthetic rubbers, e.g., cis-isoprene polymer, butadiene styrene copolymer (SBR rubber) and rubbery and resinous acrylonitrile-butadiene-styrene copolymers. They are also useful for stabilizing hydrocarbon oils and foodstuffs. The compounds having free hydroxyl groups can be used as reactants in making polyurethanes and polyesters. They also impart heat and light stability to such polymers.

These compounds can be prepared by ester interchange of a compound of Formula (1) where all the R_1, R_2, R_3 and R_4 are alkyl, aryl, alkenyl or haloaryl with 1 to 4 mols of a hydrogenated dihydric phenol and removing 1 to 4 mols of the displaced alcohol. When R_1, R_2, R_3, R_4 and Z are all residues of a hydrogenated dihydric phenol, the compounds can be formed by reacting 5 mols of the hydrogenated dihydric phenol with 2 mols of a phosphite having the formula:

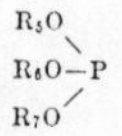

$$\begin{array}{l} R_5O \\ R_6O\!-\!P \\ R_7O \end{array}$$

and removing 6 mols of R_5OH, R_6OH and R_7OH. The R_5OH, R_6OH, R_7OH and R_8OH phenol or alcohol which is to be removed should be lower boiling than the hydrogenated dihydric phenol and preferably does not boil substantially above $200°C$. The transesterification reactions are preferably catalyzed with 0.1 to 5% based on the weight of the phosphite reactant or reactants of a catalyst which usually is a phosphite, e.g., a dialkyl phosphite, a diaryl phosphite or a dihaloaryl phosphite or an alkaline catalyst.

Example 1: Five mols of hydrogenated bisphenol A, 2 mols of triphenyl phosphite and 10 grams of diphenyl phosphite were subjected to vacuum distillation at 10 mm until 6 mols of phenol were removed. The product remaining in the pot was tetra(hydrogenated bisphenol A) hydrogenated bisphenol A diphosphite, a solid.

Example 2: Five mols of di(4-hydroxycyclohexyl) methyl ethyl methane, 2 mols of tris-isodecyl phosphite and 9 grams of diisodecyl phosphite were subjected to vacuum distillation at 10 mm until 6 mols of isodecyl alcohol were removed. The solid product remaining in the pot after cooling was tetra(4-hydroxycyclohexyl sec-butylidene cyclohexyl) bis-(cyclohexylene) methyl ethyl methane diphosphite.

These phosphate esters are useful as heat and light stabilizers and antioxidants. They can be readily ground for incorporation in an amount of 0.01 to 20% into various polymers such as halogen containing resins, e.g., vinyl chloride resins, as stabilizers against heat and light or as antioxidants. They are particularly useful in stabilizing rigid polyvinyl chloride resins where many other phosphites are unsuitable.

Example 3:

	Parts
Type 1 rigid polyvinyl chloride (QYSJ)	100
Calcium-zinc stearate (1:1 mixture)	2
Epoxidized soybean	3
Stearic acid (processing acid)	0.5
Phosphite of Example 1	0.8

This mixture was extruded in the form of a parison and a bottle blow molded therefrom. The bottle was water white and perfectly clear and showed good heat and light stability.

Example 4: Two parts of the phosphite prepared in Example 1, 1 part of dioleyl thiodipropionate and 1 part of 2,2-methylene bis(4-methyl-6-tert-butylphenol) were mixed with 100 parts of polypropylene (melt index 0.8) to give a stabilized product.

Example 5: Two parts of the phosphite prepared in Example 1 and 1 part of 4,4'-isopropylidene diphenol were milled into 100 parts of SBR rubber (60% butadiene, 40% styrene) to give a product stabilized against oxidation.

Polymercapto Polyphosphites

Thiophosphites have been prepared by *K.H. Rattenbury; U.S. Patent 3,666,837; May 30, 1972; assigned to Weston Chemical Corporation* which are useful as antioxidants and defoliants. Thiophosphates may also be prepared by this process but these phosphates find use as plasticizers and defoliants.

The thiophosphites are useful as antioxidants, e.g., for polyethylene, polypropylene, EPDM rubber, vinyl chloride resins, foods, lubricating oils, natural rubber, butadiene-styrene copolymer, butadiene-acrylonitrile copolymer, acrylonitrile-butadiene-styrene (ABS), poly cis-isoprene, polyesters, etc. These compounds have the formula:

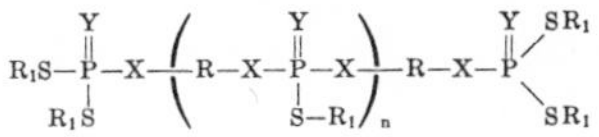

$$R_1S-\overset{\overset{Y}{\|}}{\underset{\underset{R_1S}{|}}{P}}-X-\left(R-X-\overset{\overset{Y}{\|}}{\underset{\underset{S-R_1}{|}}{P}}-X\right)_n-R-X-\overset{\overset{Y}{\|}}{P}\overset{SR_1}{\underset{SR_1}{<}}$$

where n is 0 or an integer, preferably not over 9, R is a divalent aromatic, aliphatic or cycloaliphatic group, R is alkyl, haloalkyl, aryl, haloaryl, alkenyl, haloalkenyl, cycloalkyl or aralkyl, X is S, and Y is nothing or oxygen. Preferably Y is nothing. The R_1 groups can be the same or different. In one form of the process, R is $-(R_2Z)_m R_2-$ where R_2 is alkylene of at least 2 carbons, Z is oxygen or sulfur and m is an integer of at least 1.

The thiophosphite products are conveniently prepared by reacting phosphorus trichloride with a compound R_1SH and a compound HXRXH. When n is 0, there is employed 1 mol of PCl_3, 4 mols of R_1SH and 0.5 mol of HXRXH. A slight excess of R_1SH can be used if desired. When n is 1, there is employed 3 mols of PCl_3, 5 mols of R_1SH and 2 mols of HXRXH. Preferably a slight excess of PCl_3 is employed. When n is 2 to 9, the following mol ratios should be used.

n	PCl_3	R_1SH	HXRXH
2	4	6	3
3	5	7	4
4	6	8	5
5	7	9	6
6	8	10	7
7	9	11	8
8	10	12	9
9	11	13	10

To prepare the corresponding thiophosphates, air or oxygen can be passed through the thiophosphite. If a mixture of R_1SH compound is used, then the product will have mixed R_1 groups; while if a single R_1SH compound is used, the product will have only one type of R_1 group. Examples of thiophosphite compounds as prepared by this process are tetrakis(mercaptoethyl) 1,2-dimercaptoethylene diphosphite, tetrakis(mercaptohexyl) 1,2-dimercaptoethylene diphosphite, tetrakis(mercaptolauryl) 1,2-dimercaptoethylene diphosphite, etc.

Example 1: Preparation of Tetrakis(Mercapto Lauryl) 1,6-Dimercaptohexylene Diphosphite — To a mixture consisting of 37.5 grams of 1,6-hexanedithiol (0.25 mol) and 212 grams of n-dodecyl-mercaptan (1.04 mols) was added 68 grams of phosphorus trichloride during a 25 minute period. The temperature during the addition was 25° to 50°C. HCl was evolved rapidly during the addition. After the PCl_3 had been added, the temperature of the reaction mass was raised to 145°C during a 2½ hour interval. HCl evolution had substantially ceased at the termination of this heating period. The pressure was then reduced to 25 torr while heating and stirring for an additional 2 hour interval. Then the pressure was reduced to 2 torr and the temperature increased to 190°C. Vacuum was released by a nonoxidizing gas (nitrogen). The liquid product (flask residue) was stirred with 5 grams of dry soda ash and 10 grams of Hy-flo and filtered at 130°C. The properties of the filtrate were:

RI n_D^{25}	1.5217
Specific gravity, 25°C/25°C	0.955
Acid number, milligrams KOH per gram	0.05
Color, APHA	0
Phosphorus, percent	6.2
Sulfur, percent	18.7

These phosphites are normally employed in an amount of at least 0.01% and usually 0.1 to 10% by weight of the polymer they are intended to stabilize. They can also be used as synergistic stabilizers with other sulfur containing compounds. Thus, they can be used with neutral sulfur compounds having a thio linkage beta to a carbon atom having both a hydrogen atom and a carboxyl group. Such compounds are used in an amount of 0.01 to 10%, preferably 0.1 to 5%.

Example 2: One hundred parts of polypropylene (melt index 0.4) was mixed with a stabilizer consisting of 0.2 part of the product of Example 1, 0.2 part dilaurylthiodipropionate and 0.2 part of calcium stearate to give a polypropylene of improved heat stability, e.g., at 133°C. Other examples in the complete patent showed similar qualitative examples of the stabilization of PVC, natural rubber, and EPDM rubber.

Thiodiphosphites

K.H. Rattenbury and M.S. Larrison; U.S. Patent 3,692,879; September 19, 1972; assigned to Weston Chemical Corporation have also prepared antioxidant compounds of the general formula:

$$\begin{array}{ccc} R_1SP{-}SR_2S{-}P{-}SR_3 \\ | & \ | \\ O & \ O \\ | & \ | \\ R_4 & \ R_5 \end{array}$$

(1)

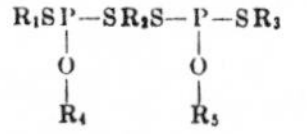

where R_1 and R_3 are alkyl, haloalkyl, aryl, haloaryl, alkenyl, aralkyl, haloalkenyl, cycloalkyl, R_2 is a divalent aromatic, aliphatic or cycloaliphatic group and R_4 and R_5 are aryl or haloaryl. Preferably R_2 is alkylene of at least 2 carbons, cycloalkylene or arylene.

These compounds are conveniently made by reacting 1 mol of a phenol, 1 mol of a mercaptan (including thiophenols), 0.5 mol of a dimercaptan and 1 mol of phosphorus trichloride and removing the HCl formula. Preferably a slight excess of the phenol is employed. The formula set forth above is for only one of the possible isomers. Actually the mercaptan and phenol react at random so that some molecules will have the formula:

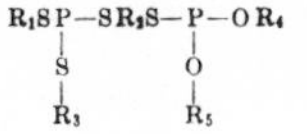

$$\begin{array}{ccc} R_1SP{-}SR_2S{-}P{-}OR_4 \\ | & \ | \\ S & \ O \\ | & \ | \\ R_3 & \ R_5 \end{array}$$

while others will have Formula 1. There can also be used mixtures of mercaptans and mixtures of phenols rather than a single mercaptan or phenol. Examples of these thiophosphites include diphenyl di(mercaptoethyl) 1,2-dimercaptoethylene diphosphite having the formula:

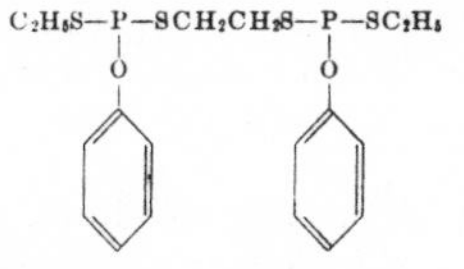

$$C_2H_5S{-}P{-}SCH_2CH_2S{-}P{-}SC_2H_5$$

diphenyl di(mercaptohexyl) 1,2-dimercaptoethylene diphosphite, diphenyl di(mercaptolauryl) 1,2-dimercaptoethylene diphosphite, and the like.

These compounds are normally employed in an amount of at least 0.01% and usually 0.1 to 10% by weight of the polymer they are intended to stabilize. They can also be used as synergistic stabilizers with other sulfur containing compounds.

Example 1: 47.0 grams (0.5 mol) of ethanedithiol, 202 grams (1.0 mol) of n-dodecyl mercaptan and 104 grams (1.1 mols) of phenol were placed in a 3-necked, 1-liter flask. The mixture was heated to 45°C and then 137 grams (1.0 mol) of PCl_3 were added dropwise at 45° to 80°C while continuously evolving HCl. The crude product was then heated to 140°C at atmospheric pressure followed by placing the system under vacuum (25 torr) to remove residual HCl. Excess phenol was then removed to 210°C at a pressure of 2 mm. The liquid product, diphenyl di(mercaptolauryl) 1,2-dimercaptoethylene diphosphite, weighed 355 grams and contained 8.3% P and 8.6% S.

Example 2: One hundred parts of propylene (melt index 0.4) was mixed with a stabilizer consisting of 0.2 part of the product of Example 1, 0.2 part of dilaurylthiodipropionate and 0.2 part of calcium stearate to give a polypropylene of improved heat stability, e.g., at 133°C. Other qualitative examples in the patent show the stabilization of EPDM rubber, natural rubber and polyvinyl chloride.

N,N-Disubstituted Aminoalkyl Phosphites

Phosphite stabilizers have been developed also by *H.A. Cyba; U.S. Patents 3,637,587; January 25, 1972; and 3,480,698; November 25, 1969; both assigned to Universal Oil Products Company* which comprise an N,N-dialkylaminoalkyl phosphite or N,N-dicyclo-alkyl-aminoalkyl phosphite. These additives have the following formula:

$$(A) \qquad [O_y{=}]P{-}(X{-}R{-}\overset{\displaystyle R'}{\underset{\displaystyle R'''_n}{N}}{-}R'')_m$$

where n ranges from 0 to 2, m ranges from 1 to 3, the sum of m + n is 3, y is 0 or 1, X is oxygen or sulfur, R is alkylene of 1 to 4 carbons, R' and R" are alkyl or cycloalkyl, and R''' is hydrogen, alkyl, aryl or cycloalkyl, R''' being hydrogen when y is 1.

The additives are prepared in any suitable manner. For example, referring to Formula A, when X is oxygen and n is 0, the compounds are preferably prepared by the reaction of a trialkyl phosphite or triphenyl phosphite with a dialkylaminoalkanol or a dicycloalkyl-aminoalkanol. These compounds are named as N,N-disubstituted-aminoalkyl phosphites. This is a transesterification reaction and, accordingly, the alkyl groups in the trialkyl phosphite preferably contain from 1 to 4 carbons each.

The reaction is effected in the presence of a basic catalyst including sodium carbonate, potassium carbonate and trialkyl amines by heating and refluxing the trialkyl or triphenyl phosphite and N,N-disubstituted aminoalkanol to form the desired product. The temperature used will be sufficient to vaporize the alcohol resulting from the transesterification and will be selected with reference to the particular phosphite used as a reactant.

In another method of preparation, the dialkylaminoalkanol is reacted with phosphorus trichloride, phosphorus oxytrichloride or alkyl, aryl or alkaryl phosphorus dichloride. This reaction is also effected by heating and mixing the reactants in the presence of a basic hydrogen halide acceptor in substantially the same manner as described above.

When n is 1 and R''' is H in Formula (A), the compounds are named as N,N-disubstituted aminoalkyl hydrogen phosphites. These compounds are prepared using a dialkyl phosphonate in a transesterification reaction. The following examples will illustrate the preparation and use of these stabilizers.

Example 1: The additive compound of this example was prepared by charging 53.7 grams (0.1 mol) of N,N-di-tallow-aminoethanol, 20.2 grams (0.2 mol) of triethylamine as catalyst and 200 grams of anhydrous ether into a 1-liter, 3-necked reaction flask. The mixture was heated to 35°C with continuous stirring. Nitrogen was also blown into the reaction flask. A calcium chloride tube was attached to the condensor to prevent intake of moisture. Upon heating and stirring, the mixture formed a homogeneous solution.

Then 4.5 grams (0.03 mol) of phosphorus trichloride were dissolved in 50 grams of ether and added dropwise to the heated and stirred mixture. This precipitated triethylamine hydrochloride. The heating and stirring were continued for 4 hours, after which the white precipitate was vacuum filtered and washed with 200 grams of hexane. The filtrate was air dried and 18 grams were recovered. The main portion of the desired product was contained in the triethylamine hydrochloride and was recovered by suspending it in warm benzene, purifying by mixing with activated charcoal, filtering and distilling off the benzene and ether. The crude product was distilled and the β-N,N-di-tallow-aminoethyl phosphite was recovered as a solid in a 57.4% yield.

Example 2: Deterioration of the polyolefin exposed outdoors increases rapidly during the late spring, summer and early fall months. A standard placque of polypropylene was placed outdoors about the middle of May and by the end of the month it had increased from an initial carbonyl number of 144 to a carbonyl number of 764. Another sample of the solid polypropylene was placed outdoors on October 6 and increased to a carbonyl number of greater than 1,000 within 15 days. It is apparent that this polypropylene, without additive, was undergoing rapid deterioration. A sample of the polyolefin containing 1% by weight of β-N,N-ditallow-aminoethyl phosphite, prepared as described in Example 1, was placed outdoors on September 21 and increased from an initial carbonyl number of 237 to a carbonyl number of 458 after 184 days of outdoor exposure. Also of importance is the fact that the polypropylene did not undergo discoloration. Examples were also included in the complete patents on the addition of these stabilizers to polyethylene, polystyrene, ABS (only in U.S. Patent 3,637,587), fuel oil, petroleum lubricant and grease and polyester lubricants.

PHOSPHINIC ACID DERIVATIVES

J.V. Spivack of the Geigy Chemical Corporation has four disclosures on preparing phosphinic acid derivatives and their use as antioxidants and stabilizers. These active compounds contain a hindered phenol moiety.

Preparative Methods

Details of the preparation of these compounds are given by *J.D. Spivack, U.S. Patent 3,534,127; October 13, 1970; assigned to Geigy Chemical Corporation.* An alkylated hydroxyphenylalkyl halide of the formula:

(1)

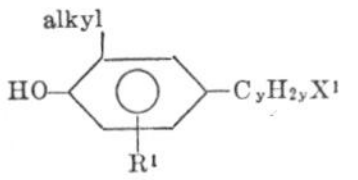

where R^1 is hydrogen or alkyl, X^1 is chloro, bromo or iodo, and y has a value of 1 to 18, is treated in a nonaqueous inert aprotic solvent, with a phosphorus halide (alternatively named as a halophosphine) of the formula:

(2)

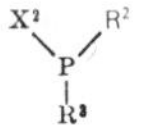

where X^2 is chloro, bromo or iodo and each of R^2 and R^3 is chloro, bromo, iodo, alkyl, aryl, alkoxy or aryloxy, in the presence of a complexing metal halide Lewis acid. The resultant reaction complex is then treated with a quantity of a compound of the formula H_2Z in which Z is O or S, sufficient to dissociate the reaction complex and liberate the phosphoryl or thiophosphoryl compound. When the phosphorus halide reactant of Formula (2) is a trihalophosphine and the quantity of H_2Z used is just sufficient to dissociate the reaction complex, the product will be a phosphoryl or thiophosphoryl dihalide where if an excess of H_2Z is used, the product will be the corresponding phosphonic or thiophosphonic acid. If the phosphorus halide is a dihalophosphine and the quantity of H_2Z used is just sufficient to dissociate the reaction complex, the phosphoryl or thiophosphoryl monohalide results; if an excess of H_2Z is used, the product will be the corresponding phosphinic or thiophosphinic acid. If the phosphorus halide is a monohalophosphine, the product will be a phosphine oxide or phosphine sulfide whether or not an excess of H_2Z is employed. These reactions are as follows.

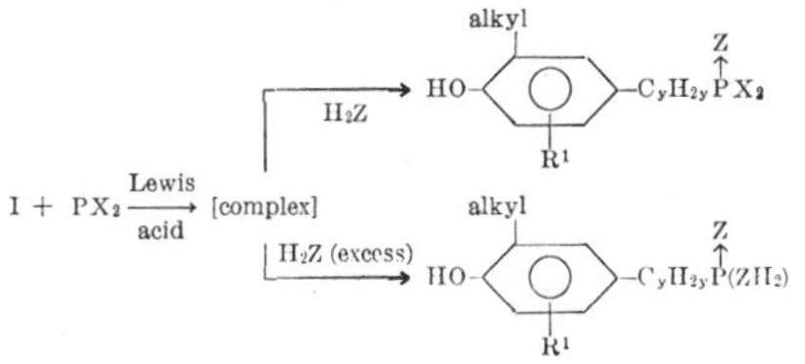

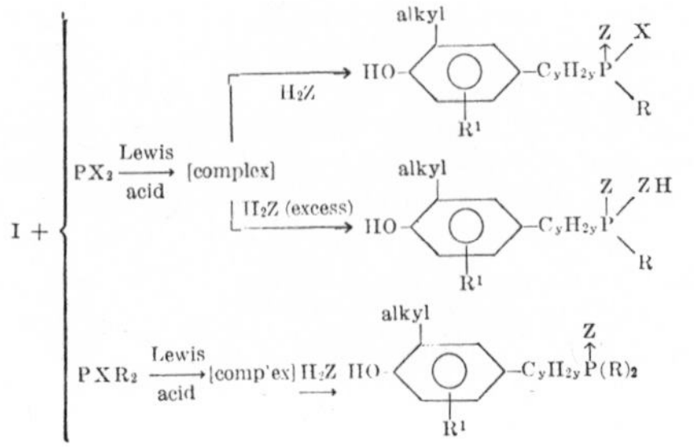

In the foregoing R^1, Z and y are previously defined, X is chloro, bromo or iodo and R is alkyl, aryl, alkoxy or aryloxy. The reaction complex obtained when the phosphorus halide reactant is a dihalo or trihalophosphine may also be treated prior to the dissociation step with an alcohol or mercaptan of the formula HZR^4 where R^4 is alkyl, haloalkyl, hydryoxyalkyl, aryl or aralkyl, and then dissociated through treatment with H_2Z as previously described. If the phosphorus halide reactant is a phosphorus trihalide, the product will be a phosphonate or thiophosphonate whereas if the phosphorus halide is a dihalophosphine, the product will be a phosphinate or thiophosphinate. These reactions may be represented as follows.

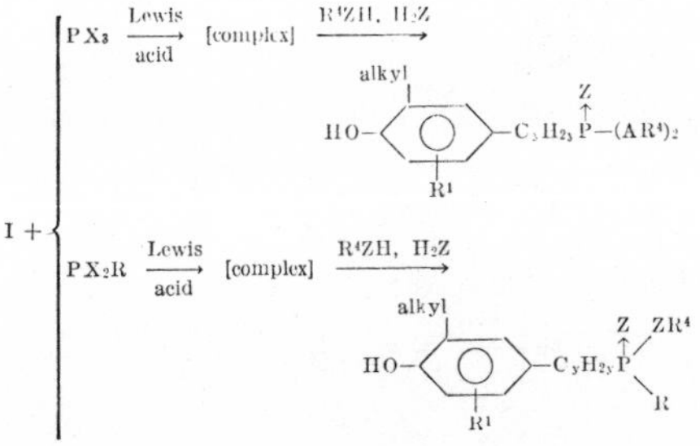

In the foregoing R, R^1, R^4, Z and y are as previously defined. The atom represented by Z need not be the same in R^4ZH and in H_2Z. Thus one can employ either an alcohol or a mercaptan with either water or hydrogen sulfide. Examples of the preparation of the phosphinic and phosphonic acids are given below.

Example 1: A solution of 14.7 grams of anhydrous aluminum chloride in 50 milliliters of nitromethane is prepared under nitrogen at -9°C, the temperature of the solution rising to 20°C. The solution is then added to a solution of 25.4 grams of 3,5-di-tert-butyl-4-hydroxy-benzyl chloride and 18.7 grams of phenylphosphonous dichloride in 50 milliliters of nitro-methane over a period of 15 minutes at a temperature of -12° to -10°C. The reaction mixture is stirred at -15° to -12°C for 40 minutes. One hundred milliliters of water are then added dropwise at a temperature of from 0° to +10°C, the dispersion being stirred for 20 minutes and then extracted twice with 125 milliliter portions of diethyl ether.

After drying these extracts over anhydrous sodium sulfate, the solvents are removed through evaporation under vacuum, initially at 20 mm Hg and finally at 1 mm Hg. The solid is triturated with 200 milliliters of n-hexane to give white crystalline 3,5-di-tert-butyl-4-hydroxybenzyl benzenephosphinic acid, melting point 179° to 182°C. After crystallization from nitromethane, the melting point is raised to 183° to 185°C.

Example 2: A solution of 15.2 grams of anhydrous aluminum chloride (0.114 mol) in 50 milliliters of nitromethane is added dropwise at -15°C and under a nitrogen atmosphere to a solution of 25.4 grams of 3,5-di-tert-butyl-4-hydroxybenzyl chloride (0.100 mol) and 16.7 grams of phosphorus trichloride (0.125 mol) in 50 milliliters of nitromethane over a period of 15 minutes. The resultant complex is stirred for 30 minutes, poured with stirring into about 1,000 grams of ice and 100 milliliters of water, stirred at 0°C for 1 hour and extracted with two 300 milliliter portions of ether. The aqueous phase is extracted with an additional 300 milliliters of ether and the combined ether extracts are dried over anhydrous sodium sulfate and evaporated under vaccum to yield 3,5-di-tert-butyl-4-hydroxybenzylphosphonic acid which is further purified through crystallization from n-heptane and recrystallization from acetonitrile, melting point 200°C (dec).

Metal Alkylhydroxyphenylalkylphosphinates

Salts of the phosphinic acids are prepared by *J.D. Spivack; U.S. Patent 3,488,368; January 6, 1970; assigned to Geigy Chemical Corporation.* The compounds have the following formula:

$$
\left[\begin{array}{c} \text{(lower) alkyl} \\ \\ \text{HO} - \hspace{-0.5em}\bigcirc\hspace{-0.5em} - C_yH_{2y} - \overset{\overset{O}{\uparrow}}{\underset{R}{P}} - O - \\ \\ H - (C_zH_{2z}) \end{array} \right]_n M
$$

where M is a metal or metal complex cation having an available valence of 1 to 4, R is an aliphatic, cycloaliphatic or aromatic hydrocarbon of 12 carbons or less, z has a value of 0 to 6, y has a value of 1 to 4 and n has a value of 1 to 4, the value of n being the same as the available valence of M.

The group M consists of a metal cation in a free valence state such as the cation form of lithium, sodium, potassium, copper, magnesium, calcium, zinc, strontium, cadmium, barium, aluminum, titanium, zirconium, tin, vanadium, antimony, chromium, molybdenum, manganese, iron, cobalt and the like, that is, a metal having an atomic number of up to 56. Alternatively, the group M may be a metal complex in which part but not all of the free valence state of the metal is satisfied by one or more organic or inorganic anions.

Illustrative of such organic anions are the acyloxy group derived from carboxylic acids containing from 1 to 30 carbons, preferably 2 to 18 carbons, e.g., acetoxy, lauroyloxy, stearoyloxy, benzoyloxy, malonoyloxy, succinoyloxy, and the like; phenoxy including alkylphenoxy; alkyl; alkyl- and arylsulfates and -sulfonates; alkyl- and arylphosphates and -phosphonates and the like. Suitable inorganic anions include chloides, bromides, iodide, fluoride, nitrate, cyanide, cyanate, thiocyanate, sulfate and the like. Of these metal complexes, particularly useful species are represented by dialkyltin and nickel monoacetate.

The phenylalkyl group of phosphinic acid moiety is substituted in the aromatic ring by a hydroxy group and one (z = 0) or two (z = 1 to 6) lower alkyl groups. These substituents may be located on the phenylalkyl group in a number of ways. From the standpoint of maximizing the antioxidant properties, it is generally desirable to use a 3,5-dialkyl-4-hydroxyphenylalkyl arrangement, e.g., 3,5-di-tert-butyl-4-hydroxybenzylphosphinate. However, other arrangements such as 2-hydroxy-5-(lower)alkylphenylalkyl are also within the scope of the process.

The alkylhydroxyphenyl group is linked to the phosphinic acid group through a straight or branched chained alkylene group of 1 to 4 carbons, the number of carbons being shown by the designation y. In addition to the alkylhydroxyphenylalkyl group, the phosphorus atom of the phosphinic acid group bears a hydrocarbon group of 1 to 12 carbons. This hydrocarbon group may be an aliphatic hydrocarbon group, notably alkyl and preferably lower alkyl, a cycloalkyl group, such as cyclopentyl, or cyclohexyl, or an aryl group such as phenyl, naphthyl, xylyl and the like. In addition to their use as antioxidants and stabilizers, these salts may be used as dyeing aids for polyolefins such as polypropylene and polyethylene.

The preparation of the compounds is realized through treatment of the appropriate alkyl-hydroxyphenylphosphinic acid with a reactant form of the metal or metal complex, e.g., sodium hydroxide, lithium hydroxide, potassium hydroxide or the like. Alternatively, and preferably in the case of metal complexes and metals other than the alkali metals, a double decomposition is used. Thus, for example, a sodium salt of the acid is treated with nickel chloride.

Use of equimolar amounts yields the nickel phosphinate chloride which itself may be further treated such as with an alkali metal alkanoate, e.g., sodium propionate, to yield the corresponding nickel phosphinate alkanoate. Alternatively, use of a two or more molar quantity of the sodium phosphinate results in formation of the nickel biphosphinate. In a similar fashion, use of other halides such as aluminum chloride, barium chloride and the like results in formation of the corresponding metal derivative. A third method uses the reaction of the free phosphinic acid and a metal or metal complex oxide, such as stannous oxide.

Example 1: A dispersion of 1.7 grams of (3,5-di-tert-butyl-4-hydroxybenzyl)benzenephos-phinic acid in 46.5 milliliters of 0.965 N aqueous sodium hydroxide and 40 milliliters of isopropanol is heated at 45°C for 30 minutes. The mixture of water and isopropanol is next removed by distillation in vacuum at an initial pressure of 25 millimeters Hg and finally at 14 millimeters Hg. 250 milliliters of n-heptane are then added and the traces of moisture are next removed by azeotropic distillation at atmospheric pressure. The insoluble sodium salt is collected by filtration, washed with heptane and dried in vacuum at 40°C and 0.20 millimeters Hg. The dried sodium (3,5-di-tert-butyl-4-hydroxybenzyl)benzenephosphinate does not melt or decompose when heated up to a temperature of 310°C.

Example 2: A solution of 7.65 grams of the sodium salt described in Example 1 (0.02 mol) in 30 milliliters of methanol and 40 milliliters of isopropanol is added dropwise at 27° to 31°C over 6 minutes to 2.37 grams of nickel chloride hexahydrate (0.01 mol). The turbid yellowish-green reaction mixture is then allowed to stand at 30°C for 20 minutes and at 45° to 50°C for 1¾ hours. The precipitated sodium chloride is separated by centrifugation and the clear yellow centrifugate is concentrated by distillation at 45° to 50°C at an initial pressure of 20 millimeters Hg and a final pressure of 0.5 millimeter Hg. The brown residue of nickel bis[(3,5-di-tert-butyl-4-hydroxybenzyl)benzenephosphinate] is dissolved in 125 milliliters of n-heptane, a slight turbidity removed by filtration and the solution concentrated to dryness by distillation of the solvent at an initial pressure of 20 millimeters Hg and a final pressure of 0.20 millimeter Hg.

Example 3: Various metal salts and complexes as prepared by this process are milled into polypropylene at 0.5% by weight concentration (except as otherwise noted). Plaques of 25 mil thickness are molded and exposed to oven aging at 300°F and the time for embrittle-ment is noted. Polypropylene compositions with the indicated extended aging times are obtained:

Sodium (3,5-di-tert-butyl-4-hydroxybenzyl)benzenephosphinate	20 hours
Barium bis[(3,5-di-tert-butyl-4-hydroxybenzyl)benzenephosphinate]	20 hours
Nickel bis[(3,5-di-tert-butyl-4-hydroxybenzyl)benzenephosphinate]	745 hours
Aluminum tris[(3,5-di-tert-butyl-4-hydroxybenzyl)benzenephosphinate]	185 hours
Tin bis[(3,5-di-tert-butyl-4-hydroxybenzyl)benzenephosphinate]	86 hours
Dibutyltin bis[(3,5-di-tert-butyl-4-hydroxybenzyl)benzenephosphinate]	64 hours
Nickel [(3,5-di-tert-butyl-4-hydroxybenzyl)benzenephosphinate] acetate	91 hours
Calcium bis[(3,5-di-tert-butyl-4-hydroxybenzyl)benzenephosphinate]	84 hours
Zinc bis[(3,5-di-tert-butyl-4-hydroxybenzyl)benzenephosphinate]	53 hours

Unstabilized polypropylene failed in less than 3 hours. Other examples of the complete patent show the stabilization of polyethylene, nylon 6, PVC, ABS, polyurethane, gasoline, lard, polyester lubricants, heptaldehyde, and paraffin wax.

Alkyl p-Hydroxyphenylphosphinates

Alkylated hydroxyphenylalkylphosphinates as disclosed by *J.D. Spivack; U.S. Patent 3,742,096; June 26, 1973; assigned to Ciba-Geigy Corporation* are useful as stabilizers of organic materials normally subject to oxidative deterioration. Such organic materials include synthetic organic polymeric substances such as vinyl resins, polyolefins, polyurethanes, polyamides, polyesters, polycarbonates, polyacetals, polystyrene, polyethyleneoxide, and copolymers of such materials. These alkylated hydroxyphenylalkylphosphinic acid esters are represented by the formula:

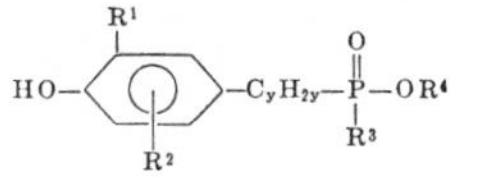

where R^1 is a lower alkyl group of 1 to 6 carbons, R^2 is alkyl, ortho or meta to the hydroxy group and having up to 6 carbons, R^3 is alkyl of 1 to 18 carbons or aryl, R^4 is hydrogen, hydroxy(lower)alkyl, alkenyl of 3 to 6 carbons, halo(lower)alkyl or alkyl of 1 to 18 carbons, provided that R^3 is not phenyl when R^4 is alkyl or hydrogen, and y is 1 to 3.

Examples of such compounds include (3,5-di-tert-butyl-4-hydroxybenzyl)ethanephosphinic acid, 2,2-dimethyl-3-hydroxypropyl-(3,5-di-tert-butyl-4-hydroxybenzyl)benzenephosphinate, allyl-(3,5-di-tert-butyl-4-hydroxybenzyl)benzenephosphinate and 2-chloroethyl-(3,5-di-tert-butyl-4-hydroxybenzyl)benzenephosphinate. Using the processes given in U.S. Patent 3,534,124, the esters can be prepared as shown in Example 1.

Example 1: 5.7 grams of (3,5-di-tert-butyl-4-hydroxybenzyl)ethanephosphinic acid were dissolved in 100 milliliters of toluene. 2.1 grams of thionyl chloride were added to the toluene solution, followed by 2 drops of dimethylformamide, the reaction mixture being stirred for about 16 hours at room temperature. 1.9 grams of triethylamine were added followed by the dropwise addition of 4.9 grams of n-octadecanol dissolved in 20 milliliters of toluene. The reaction mixture was then stirred at room temperature for 3 hours followed by 30 minutes at 90°C. The reaction mixture was cooled to 25°C and the precipitated triethylamine hydrochloride filtered.

The resulting product, n-octadecyl(3,4-di-tert-butyl-4-hydroxybenzyl)ethanephosphinate, was recovered by removing the toluene by distillation at reduced pressure, the residual oil being recrystallized twice from nitromethane and finally from a mixture of 200 milliliters of nitromethane and 25 milliliters acetone. After drying, the white crystals melt at 63° to 65°C.

Example 2: Unstabilized polypropylene powder (Hercules Profax 6501) was thoroughly blended with 0.5% by weight of n-octadecyl(3,5-di-tert-butyl-4-hydroxybenzyl)ethanephosphinate and another batch with 0.1% by weight of n-octadecyl(3,5-di-tert-butyl-4-hydroxybenzyl)ethanephosphinate plus 0.3% by weight of DSTDP as in the Oven Aging Test (page 1). DSTDP is distearylthiodipropionate. Results of the test are shown below.

Concentration of Stabilizer (percent)	Oven Aging Test (hours)
0.5	185
0.1 + 0.3 DSTDP	500
0	3

The above data clearly shows the significant stabilization of polypropylene upon the addition of this antioxidant. Lubricating oil of the aliphatic ester type, animal and vegetable derived oils, hydrocarbon materials such as gasoline, mineral oil, fuel oil, drying oil, cutting fluids, waxes, resins, and the like as well as nylon 6.6 are also stabilized by these esters.

Polyol Esters of Phosphinic Acids

In another disclosure *J.D. Spivack; U.S. Patent 3,769,372; October 30, 1973; assigned to Ciba-Geigy Corporation* prepared similar antioxidants which are alkylated-4-hydroxybenzyl-phosphinic acid esters of organic polyols. The esters are useful as stabilizers of organic materials which are subject to thermal and oxidative deterioration caused by heat and/or light. These polyol esters of alkylated-4-hydroxybenzyl phosphinic acids are represented by the formula:

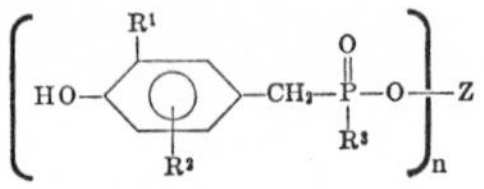

where R^1 is a lower alkyl group of 1 to 4 carbons, R^2 is hydrogen or a lower alkyl of 1 to 4 carbons, R^3 is alkyl of 1 to 4 carbons or phenyl, n has a value of 2 to 4, and Z is a cycloalkylene of 4 to 8 carbons, alkylenephenylenealkylene of 8 to 12 carbons, cyclo-alkylenealkylenecycloalkylene of 13 to 18 carbons, phenylenealkylenephenylene of 13 to 15 carbons or an aliphatic hydrocarbon

$$C_y H_{2y + 2n}$$

in which y has a value of 2 to 12 when n is 2 and a value of 3 to 7 when n is greater than 2, the value of y in all cases being equal to or greater than that of n. These compounds exhibit one alkyl group (R^1) in a position ortho to the hydroxy group. A second like or different alkyl group (R^2) is optionally present either in the other position ortho to the hydroxy group or meta to the hydroxy group and para to the first alkyl group.

These esters are prepared by transesterifying a phenyl alkylated-4-hydroxybenzyl phosphinate with the appropriate polyol using conventional techniques or by reacting an acid halide of an alkylated-4-hydroxybenzyl phosphinic acid with the appropriate polyol in the presence of a tertiary amine.

Example 1: Phenyl(3,5-Di-tert-Butyl-4-Hydroxybenzyl)Benzenephosphinate – 117.8 grams of 3,5-di-tert-butyl-4-hydroxybenzyl chloride (0.456 mol) dissolved in 130 milliliters of heptane were added dropwise to a solution of 147 grams of diphenyl phenyl phosphonite in 100 milliliters of heptane at 85° to 90°C over a period of 45 minutes in a nitrogen atmosphere. The reaction solution becomes turbid, an oily product appears and becomes crystalline as the addition proceeds. After the addition was completed, the thick slurry was stirred at reflux for 5½ hours and then allowed to cool to room temperature. 175 milliliters of methanol was added and the clear reaction mixture heated at reflux for 2.5 hours.

The solvent was then removed by distillation at atmospheric pressure, the by-product phenol being removed at reduced pressure. 250 milliliters of heptane were slowly added to the residue and heated at reflux for 30 minutes and cooled to about 150°C. The precipitate was filtered and triturated with boiling heptane. The white crystals were filtered and recrystallized from cyclohexane, melting at 132° to 134°C after drying.

Example 2: 2,2-Dimethyl-1,3-Propanediol-Bis[(3,5-Di-tert-Butyl-4-Hydroxybenzyl)Benzene-phosphinate] – 2.16 grams of 2,2-dimethyl-1,3-propanediol (0.02 mol) and 18.30 grams of phenyl (3,5-di-tert-butyl-4-hydroxybenzyl)benzenephosphinate (0.042 mol) of Example 1 were melted together at about 150°C under a nitrogen atmosphere. 0.26 gram of sodium methylate was then added and the pink melt heated at 150°C for 1 hour. Vacuum was then applied and the reaction mixture heated at 150° to 160°C for 7 hours under 12 mm Hg nitrogen pressure while the evolved phenol was collected in a cooled receiver. The reaction mixture was finally heated for 20 minutes at 0.70 mm Hg of nitrogen pressure. In this manner, 3.50 grams of phenol were collected.

After cooling the reaction mixture to room temperature, the vacuum was released and the product dissolved in 100 milliliters of benzene and the benzene solution successively washed with 2 N sodium bicarbonate and hot water. The clear light yellow benzene solution was dried over anhydrous sodium sulfate and evaporated under vacuum. The residue was then crystallized from a solvent mixture of benzene and heptane yielding white crystals melting at 175° to 177°C to a turbid melt. The following example illustrates the stabilization of polypropylene with compounds prepared by this process.

Example 3: A batch of unstabilized polypropylene powder (Hercules Profax 6501) was thoroughly blended with 0.5% by weight of various compounds of this process. Also prepared were samples of polypropylene containing 0.1% by weight of the compounds of this process and 0.3% by weight of DSTDP. The process used was the Oven Aging Test on page 1. The results are set out in the following table.

Additives	Oven aging at 150° C. hours to failure
0.5% of 2, 2-dimethyl-1, 3-propandiol-bis-[(3, 5-di-t-butyl-4-hydroxybenzyl)-benzenephosphinate]	730
0.5% of 2-methyl-2-ethyl-1, 3-propandiol-bis-[(3, 5-di-t-butyl-4-hydroxybenzyl)-benzenephosphinate]	905
0.5% of 2, 2-diethyl-1, 3-propandiol-bis-[(3, 5-di-t-butyl-4-hydroxybenzyl)benzenephosphinate]	520
0.5% of 2-ethyl-2-butyl-1, 3-propandiol-bis[(3, 5-di-t-butyl-4-hydroxybenzyl)-benzenephosphinate]	690
0.5% of 1, 4-dimethylolbenzene-bis[(3, 5-di-t-butyl-4-hydroxybenzyl)benzenephosphinate]	165
0.5% of 2, 2, 4, 4-tetramethyl-1, 3-cyclobutanediol-bis-[(3, 5-di-t-butyl-4-hydroxybenzyl)-benzenephosphinate]	755
0.1% of 2, 2, 4, 4-tetramethyl-1, 3-cyclobutanediol-bis-[(3, 5-di-t-butyl-4-hydroxybenzyl)-benzenephosphinate plus 0.3% DSTDP [1]	1,455
0.1% of 1, 1, 1-trimethylolethane-tris-[(3, 5-di-t-butyl-4-hydroxybenzyl)benzenephosphinate] plus 0.3% DSTDP [1]	335
0.5% of 1, 1, 1-trimethylolpropane-tris-[(3, 5-di-t-butyl-4-hydroxbenzyl) benzenephosphinate]	480
0.1% of 1, 1, 1-trimethylolpropane-tris-[(3, 5-di-t-butyl-4-hydroxybenzyl)-benzenephosphinate] plus 0.3% DSTDP [1]	495
0.1% of 1, 1, 1-trimethylolbutane-tris-[(3, 5-di-t-butyl-4-hydroxybenzyl)benzenephosphinate] plus 0.3% DSTDP [1]	695
0.1% of pentaerythritol-tetrakis-[(3, 5-di-t-butyl-4-hydroxy-benzyl)benzenephosphinate plus 0.3% DSTDP [1]	670
0.1% of 4, 4'-isopropylidenedicyclohexano-[(3, 5-di-t-butyl-4-hydroxybenzyl)benzenephosphinate] plus 0.3% DSTDP [1]	280
0.1% of 2, 2, 4-trimethyl-1, 3-pentanediol-bis-[(3, 5-di-t-butyl-4-hydroxybenzyl)-benzenephosphinate] plus 0.3% DSTDP [1]	210
0.1% isopropylidenediphenol-bis[(3, 5-di-t-butyl-4-hydroxy-benzyl)benzenephosphinate] plus 0.3% DSTDP [1]	430
0.5% of 1, 6-hexanediol-bis[(3, 5-di-t-butyl-4-hydroxy-benzyl)benzenephosphinate]	408
Unstabilized polypropylene	3
0.3% DSTDP alone	20

[1] Distearylthiodipropionate (a synergist for phenolic antioxidants).

The above data clearly indicates the significant increase in the stabilization of polypropylene upon addition of these antioxidants. The stabilization of nylon 6.6, mineral oil, high impact polystyrene, SBR, polyacetal resins, polyethylene, cyclohexene and synthetic polyester lubricants were also covered by examples in the original patent.

PHOSPHONATE COMPOUNDS

Two similar series of compounds having phosphonate groups and hindered phenol moieties are disclosed by J.D. Spivack of Ciba Geigy Corporation as stabilizers for organic polymers, petroleum products and the like. In general, these stabilizers are employed from 0.005 to 10% by weight of the stabilized composition. A particularly advantageous range for polyolefins such as polypropylene is from 0.01 to 5%. These stabilizers may be used alone or in combination with other stabilizers or additive materials. Especially useful in certain cases is a composition containing an active phosphonate with the stabilizer dilauryl β-thiodipropionate or distearyl β-thiodipropionate.

Bis(Hindered Phenol)Alkane Phosphonates

In the first disclosure, *J.D. Spivack; U.S. Patent 3,676,531; July 11, 1972; assigned to*

Ciba-Geigy Corporation has prepared bis(hindered phenol)alkane phosphonates having the formula:

where R, R^1, R^2 and R^3 are hydrogen, alkyl groups having 1 to 18 carbons, or cycloalkyl having 5 to 12 carbons; R^4 is hydrogen or alkyl having up to 18 carbons; R^5 is alkyl, alkaryl or aralkyl having up to 30 carbons or alkylthio (lower) alkyl where the alkyl has up to 30 and (lower) alkyl up to 6 carbons; G is alkylene group having from 1 to 6 carbons; m is 0 or 1.

In a preferred embodiment, R, R^1 R^2 and R^3 are lower alkyl groups having up to 8 carbons, especially tertiary alkyl groups such as tert-butyl, tert-amyl, tert-octyl and the like. Group G is preferably methylene and m can be 0 or 1. R^4 is preferably an alkyl group having 4 to 24 carbons and most preferably 8 to 24 carbons when the integer m is 0. However, when the integer m is 1, R^4 is an alkyl group having from 1 to 24 carbons; R^5 groups are alkyl or alkaryl groups having up to 30 carbons.

The bis(hindered phenol)alkane phosphonates can be prepared by a variety of condensation procedures. One method is to condense a haloalkyl ketone with a phenol or a hindered phenol in the presence of a Lewis acid. The resulting 2,2-bis(hindered phenol)alkyl halide is reacted with trialkyl phosphite or sodium dialkyl phosphonate to yield the corresponding bis(hindered phenol)alkane phosphonate. Another method is to condense directly a keto-phosphonate with a hindered phenol in the presence of a Lewis acid.

Example 1: To a solution containing 46.1 parts of chloroacetone, 206 parts of 2,6-di-tert-butylphenol and 200 parts by volume of ethylene chloride, was added 98 parts of sulfuric acid. The reaction mixture was stirred for 2 hours at –15° to –10°C and poured into a cooling mixture of 300 parts of ice and 300 parts of water. The resulting dispersion was diluted with 3 liters of ethanol and allowed to stand overnight. The precipitate was filtered, dried, triturated in hexane and the resulting solid 2,2-bis(3',5'-di-tert-butyl-4'-hydroxyphenyl)-1-chloropropane (A) was recrystallized from n-hexane yielding the product melting at 151° to 153°C.

To 2.76 parts of diethyl phosphite dissolved in 100 parts by volume of xylene was added 0.46 part sodium. The reaction mixture was heated at 110°C until all of the sodium was reacted. The product (A) above was then dissolved in 25 parts by volume of xylene and added slowly at 45° to 50°C to the reaction mixture. The resulting reaction mixture was heated at 50°C for 3 hours and then evaporated to dryness under a reduced pressure. The residue was dissolved in 50 parts by volume of methanol, water was added to the methanol solution to the point of turbidity and the solution was then filtered. The filtrate was concentrated to dryness and the residue was recrystallized from heptane yielding diethyl 2,2-bis(3',5'-di-tert-butyl-4'-hydroxyphenyl)-1-propanephosphonate melting at 156° to 158°C.

Other compounds which may be prepared by this process include dimethyl 2,2-bis(3',5'-di-tert-butyl-4'-hydroxyphenyl)-1-nonadecanephosphonate, di-p-tert-octylphenyl-2,2-bis-(3',5'-di-tert-butyl-4'-hydroxyphenyl)-1-hexanephosphonate and ditriacontyl-5,5-bis(3',5'-di-tert-butyl-4'-hydroxyphenyl)-n-hexanephosphonate.

Example 2: Polypropylene (Hercules Profax 6501) was thoroughly blended with antioxidant. When polypropylene was stabilized with 0.5% by weight of diethyl 1,2-bis-(3,5-di-tert-butyl-4-hydroxyphenyl)ethanephosphonate, the stabilized polypropylene had the oven aging life of 120 hours. Comparable stabilization is obtained when the stabilizer is employed in the amount of 0.01% by weight of polypropylene.

When the stabilizer was used in the amount of 0.1% by weight in combination with 0.5% by weight of dilaurylthiodipropionate, the following results were obtained: Oven Aging Test, 275 hours; Fadeometer Test, 240 hours. The unstabilized polypropylene had an oven aging life of less than 3 hours and failed in the Fadeometer after 40 to 60 hours. Other examples in the complete patent include stabilization of gasoline, paraffin wax, polyester lubricants, high impact polystyrene, nylon 66 and polyacetal resins.

Bis(Hindered Phenol)Alkylene Diphosphonates or Phosphonoacetates

J.D. Spivack; U.S. Patent 3,714,300; January 30, 1973; assigned to Ciba-Geigy Corporation also prepared the compounds having the formula:

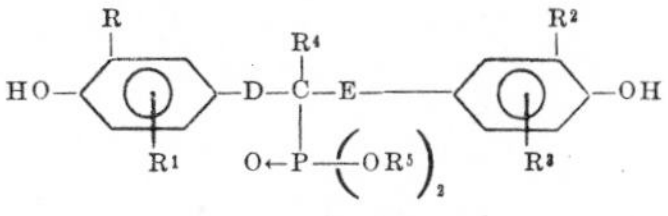

where R, R^1, R^2 and R^3 are alkyl groups having 1 to 18 carbons or cycloalkyl having 5 to 12 carbons, R^4 is a phosphoryl group of the formula:

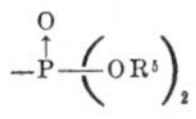

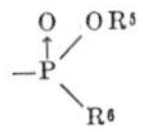

or carbalkoxy of the formula:

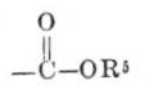

where R^6 is alkyl, phenyl or alkylphenyl of up to 18 carbons, R^5 is alkyl, alkaryl or aralkyl having up to 30 carbons or alkylthio (lower) alkyl where the alkyl has up to 30 and the (lower) alkyl up to 6 carbons, D and E are alkylene groups independently having from 1 to 6 carbons.

There are a number of applicable methods of the preparation of these compounds. For example, in preparing bis(hindered hydroxybenzyl)phosphonoalkanoates, a hindered hydroxybenzyl halide is reacted with a phosphonoalkanoate to give the desired product. Similarly, in preparing bis(hindered hydroxybenzyl)phosphonates, a hindered hydroxybenzyl halide is reacted with the desired bis-phosphonate. The various preparations are described in greater detail in the following examples.

Example 1: In 200 parts by volume of tert-butanol was dissolved 3.9 parts of potassium. Half of this solution was added at room temperature to 11.2 parts of triethylphosphono-acetate, followed by the dropwise addition of 14.5 parts of 3,5-di-tert-butyl-4-hydroxy-benzyl chloride dissolved in 50 parts by volume of toluene. Thereafter, the remaining portion of the potassium solution was added followed by the addition of 14.5 parts of 3,5-di-tert-butyl-4-hydroxybenzyl chloride. Then 300 parts of water were added to the reaction mixture and the product was extracted with benzene. After drying, benzene was stripped under reduced pressure yielding 33 parts of the crude product. Upon recrystal-lization from a 1:1 mixture of n-hexane and petroleum ether and from n-heptane, triethyl-bis(3,5-di-tert-butyl-4-hydroxybenzyl)phosphonoacetate was obtained, melting point 156° to 158°C.

Example 2: To a solution of 4 parts of potassium in 200 parts by volume of tert-butanol prepared as in Example 1 were added 14.5 parts of tetraethyl methylene-bis-phosphonate. While maintaining the reaction mixture at a temperature of about 50°C, 29 parts of

3,5-di-tert-butyl-4-hydroxybenzyl chloride was added dropwise. The reaction mixture was then stirred at room temperature for 2 hours and acidified with 5 parts of glacial acetic acid. 500 parts of water were then added and the product extracted with ether and benzene. The combined extracts were washed with water, dried and the solvent evaporated under reduced pressure. The residue was triturated with petroleum ether and recrystallized from methanol yielding the product, tetraethyl methylene-α,α-bis(3,5-di-tert-butyl-4-hydroxy-benzyl)methylenediphosphonate.

Example 3: Using the procedure described on page 1 polypropylene was stabilized with 0.5% by weight of triethyl-bis(3,5-di-tert-butyl-4-hydroxybenzyl)phosphonoacetate. The thus stabilized polypropylene was submitted to the Oven Aging Test and the Fadeometer Test yielding the following results: Oven Aging, 175 hours; Fadeometer, 160 hours. This example was repeated in which polypropylene was stabilized with 0.1% by weight of the above stabilizer and 0.5% by weight of dilaurylthiodipropionate. This composition in an Oven Aging Test had a life of 525 hours.

Example 4: Using the same procedure, polypropylene was stabilized with 0.5% by weight of tetraethyl methylene-bis(3,5-di-tert-butyl-4-hydroxybenzyl)phosphonate. On testing, the following results were obtained: Oven Aging Test, 300 hours; Fadeometer Test, 180 hours. Other materials stabilized by these materials in examples of the complete patent include polyisoprene, polyurethane, polymethylene, terephthalate, polyacetal, polyethylene oxide, gasoline, paraffin wax, polyester lubricating oil, high impact polystyrene, polyoxymethylene diacetate and nylon 66.

OTHER PHOSPHORUS COMPOUNDS

Arylene Phosphinites

L. Maier; U.S. Patent 3,632,689; January 4, 1972; assigned to Monsanto Company has described arylene phosphinites of the general formula $R(OPR'_2)_n$ in which R signifies a possibly substituted and/or ethylenically or acetylenically unsaturated arylene group which is at least divalent. R' signifies a possibly substituted and/or ethylenically or acetylenically unsaturated hydrocarbon group or a heterocyclic group and n stands for a number from 2 to 10.

The process is characterized in that a hydroxyl compound, having at least 2 aromatically linked hydroxyl groups of the general formula $R(OH)_n$ in which R and n are defined as above, and an amino-phosphine of the general formula $R'_2PNR''_2$ in which R' is defined as above and NR''_2 signifies an amino group which is derived from ammonia, a primary amine or a secondary amine having a lower boiling point than the hydroxyl compound to be reacted, are heated until substantially no more ammonia or amine evolves from the reaction mixture.

The alkylene diphosphinite rearrange on heating to the corresponding ditertiary alkylene diphosphine dioxides; however, it has been found that arylene diphosphinites, undiscovered up to now, are very temperature resistant compounds possessing a relatively wide liquid range. They are consequently well suited as noncombustible hydraulic oils, heat transfer agents, lubricants and additives to lubricants, such as antioxidants.

In practicing the reaction, a mixture of the amino phosphine and the hydroxyl compound in the calculated proportion is heated until no more substantial amount of ammonia or amine evolves. The temperature is increased from room temperature up to such a temperature at which the evolution of ammonia or amine is considered to be sufficiently great. Temperatures of about 100°C and more are expediently employed. The reaction time can be several minutes to several hours according to the kind of amine to be cleaved and to the temperature employed. The reaction may also be carried out in an inert solvent; however, it is preferred that the cleaved amine escapes as fast as possible and completely from the reaction mixture. Many end products are distillable in vacuo. Others can be purified by crystallization or by using extraction methods.

Example 1: A mixture of 21.7 grams (0.1 mol) of $(n\text{-}C_4H_9)_2PN(C_2H_5)_2$ and 5.5 grams (0.05 mol) of hydroquinone is heated at 140°C for 2 hours. 6.1 grams (83.5%) of diethylamine distill off within fifteen minutes. After a small forerun of starting material (0.3 gram, boiling point 65° to 72°C/0.1 mm) there are obtained 17 grams (83.5%) of phenylene-1,4-bis(di-n-butylphosphinite); boiling point 180° to 183°C/0.1 mm, P^{31} chemical shift, 134.6 ppm.

Example 2: A mixture of 21.7 grams (0.1 mol) of diethylamino-di-n-butylphosphine and 9.9 grams (0.05 mol) of 4,4'-dihydroxy-biphenyl is heated at 140°C for 2 hours. 6.4 grams (87.5%) of diethylamine escape. The reaction mixture is distilled. After a forerun (3.6 grams, boiling point 72° to 130°C/0.1 mm), there are obtained 15.1 grams (62.4%) of biphenylene-4,4'-bis(di-n-butylphosphinite); boiling point 240° to 245°C/0.1 mm, P^{31} chemical shift, 132.7 ppm (impurities at –181.8 ppm).

Phenylphosphine Dichloride-Malonic Ester Reactants

A phenyl substituted phosphorous compound is produced by *G. Bergerhoff, B. Tihanyi, J. Falbe and J. Weber; U.S. Patent 3,681,435; August 1, 1972; assigned to Ruhrchemie AG, Germany* by the reaction of malonic acid diethylester with phenylphosphine dichloride. Apparently, 2 mols of each of the reactants, under elimination of 4 mols of hydrogen chloride, form the compound. The compound is useful as pest control agents and antioxidants.

Example: 17.9 grams phenyl-phosphine dichloride (0.1 mol) and 16.0 grams malonic acid diethylester (0.1 mol) are dissolved in 250 ml benzene and heated to 50°C under a nitrogen atmosphere. 20.2 grams (0.2 mol) triethylamine dissolved in 100 ml benzene are added dropwise under stirring. Precipitated triethylamine hydrochloride is separated by filtration and washed with benzene. The benzene filtrate together with the washing solution is concentrated to about one third of its volume by evaporation at 40° to 50°C under water-jet vacuum. Thereby a colorless crystal sludge is precipitated which is sucked off and washed with ether. This product can be purified by recrystallization from benzene followed by washing with alcohol and ether. The pure compound has a melting point of 114°C. The entire yield amounts to 70 to 80% by theory.

The following data could be determined. Melting point, 114°C; molecular weight, 532. The compound is soluble in benzene, acetone, acetic acid ethylester, but difficult to dissolve in benzene, ether, alcohol.

Of particular importance is the oxidation inhibiting efficacy of the compound, as is seen from the following comparison. Through 159.5 grams n-butyraldehyde were passed 31 liters air during 30 minutes, whereby 15.6 grams butyric acid were formed. Under similar conditions but with addition of 3.2 grams of the phosphorous compound, only 2 grams butyric acid were formed.

Phosphorus Derivatives of Hindered Phenol Substituted Alkanols

Phosphorus containing derivatives of ω-(3,5-dialkyl-4-hydroxyphenyl) alkanols, e.g., phosphites, phosphates, phosphonates, thiophosphates and thiophosphonates thereof are described by *M.E. Chiddix and D.J. Tracy; U.S. Patent 3,763,287; October 2, 1973; assigned to GAF Corporation* together with methods for their preparation and their use as antioxidants. These products are represented by the following formula:

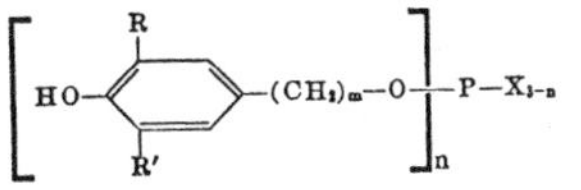

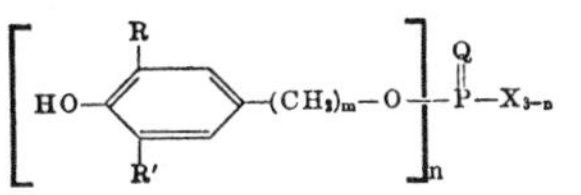

where R and R' are alkyl of 1 to 18 carbons, arylalkyl of 7 to 18 carbons and cycloalkyl of 6 to 18 carbons; m is 1 to 4; n is 1 to 3; Q is O or S and X is alkyl of 1 to 24 carbons, aryl of 6 to 18 carbons, arylalkyl of 7 to 18 carbons, cycloalkyl of 6 to 18 carbons, phenoxy, alkoxy, alkylphenoxy, thioalkyl, thiophenyl, haloalkyl or alkylcarboxyl of the formula:

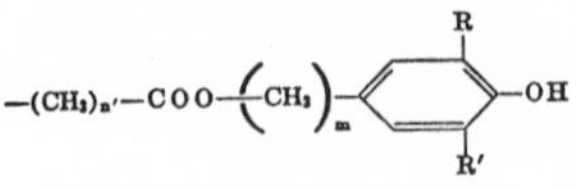

$$-(CH_2)_{n'}-COO-(CH_2)_m-\underset{R'}{\overset{R}{\diamondsuit}}-OH$$

where n' is 1 to 4 and R, R' and m are as defined above.

These compounds may be prepared from ω-(3,5-dialkyl-4-hydroxyphenyl) alkanols of the formula:

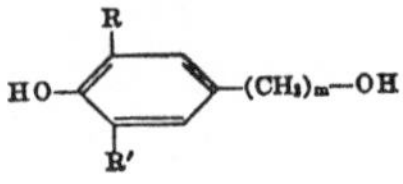

$$HO-\underset{R'}{\overset{R}{\diamondsuit}}-(CH_2)_m-OH$$

where R, R' and m are as defined above, by known synthetic methods for producing phosphites, phosphates, phosphonates, thiophosphates and thiophosphonates of other alkanols. The ω-(3,5-dialkyl-4-hydroxyphenyl) alkanols which are useful as intermediates for the production of these esters include known 3,5-dialkyl-4-hydroxy-benzyl alcohols, e.g., those described in U.S. Patent 3,116,305. As specific examples of suitable ω-(3,5-dialkyl-4-hydroxyphenyl) alkanols may be mentioned 3,5-dimethyl-4-hydroxybenzyl alcohol, 3-ethyl-5-methyl-4-hydroxybenzyl alcohol and 3-isopropyl-5-methyl-4-hydroxybenzyl alcohol.

Instead of the benzyl alcohols, higher alkanols having corresponding 3,5-dialkyl-4-hydroxyphenyl substituents on their carbon atoms may be used. As examples thereof may be mentioned 2-(3,5-dimethyl-4-hydroxyphenyl) ethanol, 2-(3,5-di-tert-butyl-4-hydroxyphenyl) ethanol, 3-(3,5-di-tert-butyl-4-hydroxyphenyl) propanol and 3-(3-tert-octyl-5-isopropyl-4-hydroxyphenyl) propanol.

The phosphites may be prepared by an ester interchange reaction with a trialkyl phosphite (preferably a tri-lower alkylphosphite), such as trimethylphosphite or triethylphosphite, or a triarylphosphite, such as triphenylphosphite or tricresylphosphite, as illustrated in Equation 1 below or by reaction with phosphorus trichloride as illustrated in Equation 2. In the following reactions Z = ω(3,5-dialkyl-4-hydroxyphenyl)alkyl radical and X and n are as defined above.

(1)　$nZOH + PX_3 \longrightarrow (ZO)_nP-X_{3-n} + 3-n(XOH)$　　(2)　$3ZOH + PCl_3 \longrightarrow (ZO)_3P + 3HCl$

The phosphates may be prepared by reaction with phosphorus oxychloride, as illustrated in Equation 3 or by oxidation of the corresponding phosphite, (e.g., with hydrogen peroxide) as illustrated in Equation 4.

(3)　$3ZOH + POCl_3 \longrightarrow (ZO)_3P=O + 3HCl$　　(4)　$(ZO-)_nP-X_{3-n} + H_2O_2 \longrightarrow (ZO-)_n\overset{O}{\overset{\|}{P}}-X_{3-n}$

The phosphonates can be prepared by reaction with an alkyl or phenyl phosphonyl dichloride as illustrated in Equation 5 where R" represents alkyl (including haloalkyl) of 1 to 24 carbons, aryl (C_6 to C_{18}), arylalkyl (C_7 to C_{18}) or cycloalkyl.

(5)　$2ZOH + R''-\overset{O}{\overset{\|}{P}}-Cl_2 \longrightarrow (ZO-)_2\overset{O}{\overset{\|}{P}}-R'' + 2HCl$

By reaction with dichloro-alkyl or phenyl-phosphines, such as dichloro-phenylphosphine, phosphinates may be prepared as illustrated in Equation 6.

(6)　$2ZOH + R''-P-Cl_2 \longrightarrow (ZO-)_2P-R'' + 2HCl$

The thiophosphates may be prepared by reacting the phosphites (prepared as outlined in Equation 1 or Equation 2 above) by heating with sulfur as illustrated in Equation 7.

$$(7) \qquad 2ZOH \ + \ R''-\overset{\overset{S}{\|}}{P}-Cl_2 \ \longrightarrow \ (ZO)_2\overset{\overset{S}{\|}}{P}-R'' \ + \ 2HCl$$

The thiophosphonates may be prepared by reaction with an alkyl- or phenyl-thiophosphonyl dichloride as illustrated in Equation 8.

$$(8) \qquad (ZO-)_nP-X_{3-n} \ + \ S \ \overset{\Delta}{\longrightarrow} \ (ZO-)_n\overset{\overset{S}{\|}}{P}-X_{3-n}$$

The following example shows the stabilization of polypropylene with some of the compounds prepared by examples included in the original patent.

Example: To illustrate the effectiveness of the compounds of this process as antioxidants in protecting polypropylene, the standard oven oxidation test was used. The antioxidant compound under test is compounded into unstabilized polypropylene on a Banbury type laboratory mill (Brabender Plastograph) at 183°C for 10 minutes. A 40 mil thick sheet of compounded material is compression molded on a laboratory press (Carver) using 245°C platen temperatures, 10,000 pounds pressure on the 2¼ inch diameter ram, and a dwell time of 2 minutes.

The sheets are air cooled under pressure before removal from the press. Standard micro-dumbbell specimens (ASTM D 1708-59T) are die cut from the sheet. The specimens are suspended vertically in an air circulating oven operating at 300°F. Time to failure is noted as the exposure time required to produce breaking of the specimen when flicked with the finger. The results obtained in this test when using the antioxidants at a concentration of 0.5 part thereof per 100 parts of polypropylene are summarized in the following table.

Additive	Concentration (phr)	Hours to Failure
Product of:		
Di-3-(3,5-di-tert-butyl-4-hydroxyphenyl)-propyl phenyl phosphonate	0.5	1,140
Tris-3-(3,5-di-tert-butyl-4-hydroxyphenyl)-propyl phosphate	0.5	950
Di-3-(3,5-di-tert-butyl-4-hydroxyphenyl)-propyl-β-chloro-ethyl-phosphonate	0.5	732
Tris-3-(3,5-di-tert-butyl-4-hydroxyphenyl)-propyl phosphite	0.5	904
Tris-(3,5-di-tert-butyl-4-hydroxybenzyl)-phosphite	0.5	411

Mineral oil and gasoline were also stabilized with the compounds of this process in additional examples of the complete patent.

OTHER ANTIOXIDANT COMPOUNDS

THIOETHERS AND THIOESTERS

Bis(Hydroxyalkyl)Sulfides

W. Umbach, R. Mehren and W. Stein; U.S. Patent 3,637,864; January 25, 1972; assigned to Henkel & Cie, GmbH, Germany has developed a method for the production of bis(hydroxyalkyl)sulfides in a single step from epoxides and hydrogen sulfide.

This method comprises reacting an epoxide selected from mono-vicinal-epoxy-epoxide compounds and poly-vicinal-epoxy-epoxide compounds with substantially the stoichiometric amount of hydrogen sulfide, in the absence of solvents at a temperature between 40° and 200°C and normal pressures in the presence of 0.01 to 10% by weight, based on the epoxide, of a strongly basic catalyst. Broadly, these bis(hydroxyalkyl)sulfides have the formula:

$$\left(R_1 - \overset{\overset{\text{H}}{|}}{\underset{\underset{\text{HO}}{|}}{C}} - \overset{\overset{\text{H}}{|}}{\underset{\underset{\text{R}_2}{|}}{C}} - \right)_2 S$$

where R_1 is a C_{1-22} alkyl or alkylol, R_2 is hydrogen, alkyl having 1 to 21 carbons or alkylol having 1 to 21 carbons with the proviso that the sum of the carbons in R_1 and R_2 is between 6 and 22. The compounds are useful as antioxidants (particularly for rubber), insecticides, fungicides and intermediates.

The strongly basic catalysts are added in an amount of 0.01 to 10%, preferably 0.05 to 7% by weight, based on the weight of the epoxide. These strongly basic catalysts may be inorganic, such as alkali metal or alkaline earth metal hydroxides or organic such as alkali metal lower alcoholates; alkali metal phenolates, tertiary onium bases; quaternary onium bases; and the dimethylates of the product obtained of the reaction in a methanolic solution of 1 mol of N,N,N',N'-tetramethylhexamethylenediamine with 3 mols of propyleneoxide. Weak bases, such as hydrazines or amines are less suitable as catalysts due to their lower basicities.

In carrying out the reaction, the epoxide is preferably charged into the reactor and then the catalyst in the amount necessary is added. The mixture is then heated to the reaction temperature desired. Then the hydrogen sulfide is slowly introduced under agitation, so that the hydrogen sulfide is completely absorbed by the reaction mixture. The end of the reaction is determined by the decrease of the heat of the reaction, and is completed the moment the reaction mixture does not accept any further hydrogen sulfide. Generally, the reaction period lasts 3 to 4 hours. The working up of the reaction products can be effected in the usual manner. For instance, the raw product can be introduced into ice water. After neutralization of the catalyst the separated product can be isolated. If need be, the product can be purified by recrystallization. Where bis(hydroxyalkyl)sulfides with a low melting point are produced, they can be worked up by distillation. In this method, the catalyst is neutralized by treating the raw products with diluted acid. A water-immiscible solvent is then added, the aqueous phase is separated, and the organic phase is fractionally distilled.

Example: 55.3 grams (0.3 mol) of n-dodecene-oxide-1,2 were mixed with 3.7 grams of sodium ethylate (6.7% by weight of catalyst with reference to the amount of epoxide used). The mixture was then heated at 52°C. Subsequently, hydrogen sulfide was introduced under agitation in a slow manner, so that the temperature of the reaction mixture remained constant, and the amount of hydrogen sulfide introduced was completely absorbed. The hydrogen sulfide absorption was controlled by means of a bubble counter disposed downstream of the reactor.

After 3 hours, the reaction mixture did not accept any further hydrogen sulfide. The colorless, solid raw product was introduced into ice water and neutralized with diluted sulfuric acid. The product was then recovered by filtration. The yield obtained was quantitative. After recrystallization from ethanol, the melting point was 82° to 83°C. The analysis data obtained and the molecular weight estimated osmometrically in benzene were in good accordance with the values calculated for bis(2-hydroxydodecyl)sulfide. The structural formula was confirmed by the nuclear resonance spectra.

Bis(Tetrahydropyranyl) Sulfides, Sulfones and Sulfoxides

P.R. Stapp; U.S. Patent 3,651,093; March 21, 1972; assigned to Phillips Petroleum Company has prepared bis(tetrahydropyranyl)sulfides by reacting a halo-tetrahydropyran with an alkali metal or an alkaline earth metal sulfide. Bis(tetrahydropyranyl)sulfones and sulfoxides can be prepared by oxidizing the bis(tetrahydropyranyl)sulfide with hydrogen peroxide. The bis(tetrahydropyranyl)sulfides that can be prepared according to this process include the compounds represented by the structures I through VI below:

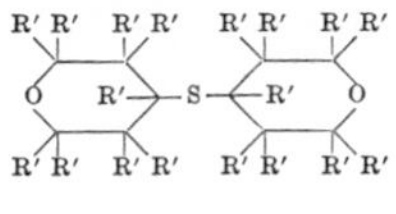

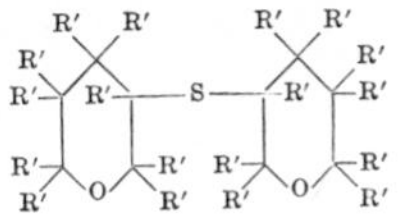

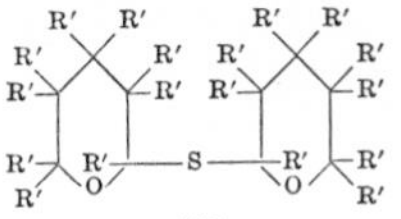

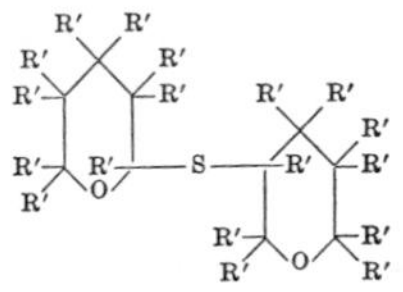

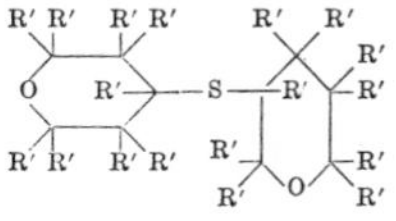

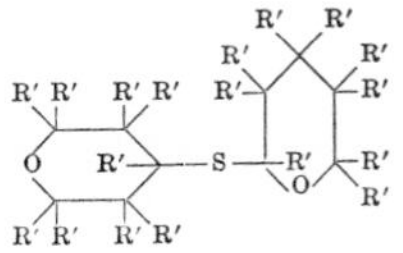

where R' is hydrogen or an alkyl group having not more than 6 carbons per R' group, and where there are not more than 10 carbons in all R' groups on each ring.

In the synthesis of a bis(tetrahydropyranyl)sulfide, an alkali metal or alkaline earth metal sulfide is mixed with a halo-tetrahydropyran under reaction conditions that can vary widely. Preferably, the mol ratio of alkali or alkaline earth sulfide to halo-tetrahydropyran is within the range of 0.05:1 to 5:1. Generally, the reaction is carried out for a time from 10 seconds to 24 hours, at a temperature from 50° to 250°C, and under a pressure sufficient to maintain the reactants in a substantially liquid phase. A substantially nonreactive diluent can be employed, if desired. Specific examples of such diluents are hexane, benzene, N-methylpyrrolidone, ethanol, 2-butanol, methoxyethanol, tetrahydropyran, toluene, sulfolane, and the like. The diluents can comprise from 1 to 95 weight percent of the reaction mixture.

The bis(tetrahydropyranyl)sulfides can be converted to bis(tetrahydropyranyl)sulfoxides by oxidizing the sulfides with a peroxide. The equivalent ratio of peroxide to bis(tetrahydropyranyl)sulfide is in the range of 0.8:1 to 1.2:1. The bis(tetrahydropyranyl)sulfides also can be converted to bis(tetrahydropyranyl)sulfones by oxidizing the sulfides with a peroxide. Here, the equivalent ratio of peroxide to bis(tetrahydropyranyl)sulfide is in the range of 1.8:1 to 2.2:1.

Example 1: Under a nitrogen atmosphere, 180 grams of sodium sulfide nonahydrate and 850 ml of N-methylpyrrolidone were charged to a stirred reactor. Water was driven off by raising the temperature to 200°C. After the reactor temperature was lowered to 140° to 150°C, 192.8 grams of 4-chlorotetrahydropyran were added and the temperature was maintained at 140° to 150°C for about 4 hours. Upon cooling, the reaction mixture was diluted with water and extracted with ether. The ether extract was washed with water and dried over magnesium sulfate. Volatiles were stripped from the ether extract on a rotary evaporator and the residue was distilled under reduced pressure. A yield of 53.4 grams of bis-4-tetrahydropyranyl sulfide was the product. IR analysis showed absorption bands for the sulfides that were consistent with the expected absorption bands for tetrahydropyran.

Example 2: To a stirred reactor containing 10 grams of bis(tetrahydropyranyl)sulfide, prepared as above, and 100 ml of glacial acetic acid, was added 13 ml of 30% hydrogen peroxide over a period of 13 minutes at a temperature of 80°C. The exothermic reaction increased the reactor temperature to reflux temperature. The reaction mixture was stirred and cooled to room temperature for 2 hours. A small amount of palladium on carbon was added to decompose any excess hydrogen peroxide. The reaction mixture was filtered, and the filtrate was stripped of volatiles on a rotary evaporator. The residue weighed 18 grams and was recrystallized from 95% (vol) ethanol to yield 11.1 grams of purified bis(tetrahydropyranyl)sulfone. This product comprised a 95% mol yield based on the charged bis-4-tetrahydropyranyl sulfide. The melting point of the bis(tetrahydropyranyl)sulfone was 156° to 157°C.

Example 3: The procedure of Example 2 was repeated, except that 6.6, rather than 13 ml of hydrogen peroxide were employed. The product was 12.9 grams of bis-4-tetrahydropyranyl sulfoxide. Upon recrystallization from ethanol, a yield of 8.7 grams of purified bis-4-tetrahydropyranyl sulfoxide was recovered. This product comprised an 80 mol percent yield based on the charged bis-4-tetrahydropyranyl sulfide. The melting point of the bis(tetrahydropyranyl)sulfoxide was 140° to 142°C. IR analysis showed sulfoxide bands and bands that were consistent with the bands of tetrahydropyran.

These bis(tetrahydropyranyl)sulfones and sulfoxides can be used as antioxidants for polymers such as polybutadiene, polyisoprene, polypropylene, and the like. The compounds may also be used in lubricants as shown in the following example.

Example 4: A lubricant was prepared by admixing two parts of bis-4-tetrahydropyranyl sulfide, prepared as above, with 98 parts of SAE-10 Mid Continent base oil. Comparative runs were made with a Shell 4 ball machine and method. The data are shown in the following table.

Material	Scar Size in Microns
Base oil plus 2% bis-4-tetrahydropyranyl sulfide	2,475, 2,451
Base oil above	3,975, 3,474
Percent decrease in scar size, 37%, 29%.	

This example demonstrates the usefulness of bis(tetrahydropyranyl)sulfide in preparing antiwear lubricants.

Synergistic Polyol Esters of Alkylthioalkanoic Acids

Esters to be used with phenolic antioxidants to stabilize organic materials have been developed by *M. Dexter and D. Steinberg; U.S. Patent 3,758,549; September 11, 1973; assigned to Ciba-Geigy Corporation.* These esters include compounds of the formula:

$$\left(R{-}S{-}CH_2CH_2\overset{\displaystyle O}{\overset{\|}{C}}O \right)_n Z$$

where R is an alkyl group of 1 to 18 carbons, n has a value of 2 to 4, and Z is an aliphatic hydrocarbon of the formula: C_yH_{2y+2-n} in which y has a value of 2 to 18 when n is 2 and a value of 3 to 6 when n is greater than 2, the value of y in all cases being equal to or greater than that of n.

These alkylthioalkanoic acids esters of alkane polyols have the ability to vastly improve the effect of numerous other compounds which are used as stabilizers for organic material normally subject to thermal and oxidative deterioration. Thus while these compounds may be considered as stabilizers in their own right, their properties are such that they would be more conventionally classified as synergists in that when combined with known stabilizers, they exhibit the ability to increase stabilization to a degree far exceeding that which would be expected from the additive properties of the inidividual components.

The alkyl alkylthioalkanoic acid esters are preferably used in a concentration of 0.005 to 10% by weight of the total composition with 1 or more of the following: Phenolic antioxidants, ultraviolet light absorbers and/or phosphite stabilizers. These are particularly useful in synthetic organic polymeric substances such as polypropylene, polyethylene, polystyrene and the like to protect such substances from deterioration both during use and during processing such as milling polypropylene or blow molding polyethylene. These esters exhibit superior compatability in diverse substances with little or no odor formation.

They are particularly useful in organic polymeric fibers because of their extraction resistance and low volatility. The compounds of the above formula may be prepared by reacting an alkyl mercaptan with methyl acrylate as described by Stevens et al, *J. Am. Chem. Soc.* 73, Vol 50 (1951). The monoester obtained is reacted with an alkane polyol via a standard transesterification reaction. The transesterification reaction involves a treatment of the polyol with up to a 15% excess, preferably from 5 to 10% excess, over the stoichiometric amount of the ester.

This reaction is catalyzed with a hydride or lower alkoxide of an alkaline metal such as lithium hydride, lithium methoxide or sodium methoxide. These catalysts are employed in an amount from 0.01 to 0.30 mol equivalents per mol of polyol. The reaction is conducted at elevated temperatures and under reduced pressure, the lower alkanol which is formed being removed by distillation.

Example 1: Methyl acrylate, 86.1 parts, was added to a cold mixture of n-dodecyl mercaptan, 123 parts, and sodium methylate, 0.5 parts, over a 50 minute interval. The temperature of the reaction was kept at 25° to 30°C by means of an ice-bath. After all the reactants were combined, the reaction mixture was stirred at the ambient temperature for about 17 hours. After this time, about 1 part of filtercel was added and the resulting slurry filtered through a sintered glass funnel. The product was purified by vacuum distillation. There was obtained 125.8 parts of methyl-3-n-dodecylthiopropionate having boiling point 152° to 153.5°C, 0.3 to 0.4 mm.

Example 2: A mixture consisting of 31.74 parts of methyl 3-n-dodecylthiopropionate and 3.10 parts of ethylene glycol was stirred and 0.14 parts of sodium methylate added. The reaction mixture was heated for about 6.5 hours at 100 ± 5°C in a nitrogen atmosphere. After cooling to room temperature, the reaction mixture was dissolved in 1:1 benzene-heptane and passed through a bed of alumina. After removing impurities in the early fractions, the pure ethylene bis(3-n-dodecylthiopropionate) was obtained as a white solid having melting point 50° to 52°C.

Example 3: Unstabilized polypropylene powder (Hercules Profax 6501) was thoroughly blended with 0.3% by weight of various alkylthioesters prepared by this process and 0.1% by weight various phenolic antioxidants. The blended materials were then milled on a two-roll mill at 182°C for 10 minutes, after which time the stabilized polypropylene was sheeted from the mill and allowed to cool. The milled polypropylene sheets were then cut into pieces and pressed for 7 minutes on an hydraulic press at 218°C and at 500 psi and then transferred to a cold press at 500 psi. Samples of the resulting 25 mil sheet were tested for resistance to accelerated aging in a forced draft oven at 150°C. The results are given in the following table.

Additive(s)	Hours to Failure
0.3% pentaerythritol tetrakis(3-n-dodecyl-thiopropionate) + 0.1% pentaerythritol tetrakis[3-(3,5-di-tert-butyl-4-hydroxy-phenyl)propionate]	3,170
0.3% 1,1,1-trimethylolethane tris(3-n-do-decylthiopropionate) + 0.1% pentaerythritol tetrakis[3-(3,5-di-tert-butyl-4-hydroxyphenyl)propionate]	3,200
0.3% pentaerythritol tetrakis(3-n-dodecyl-thiopropionate) + 0.1% 1,1,3-tris(3-tert-butyl-4-hydroxy-6-methylphenyl)butane	970
0.3% 1,1,1-trimethylolethane tris(3-n-do-decylthiopropionate) + 0.1% 1,1,3-tris-(3-tert-butyl-4-hydroxy-6-methylphenyl)-butane	1,120
0.3% ethylene bis(3-n-dodecylthiopropion-ate) + 0.1% 1,1,3-tris(3-tert-butyl-4-hy-droxy-6-methylphenyl)butane	660
0.1% 1,1,1-trimethylolethane tris(3-n-do-decylthiopropionate) + 0.3% di-n-octyl-(3,5-di-tert-butyl-4-hydroxybenzyl)phos-phonate	850
0.3% pentaerythritol tetrakis[3-(3,5-di-tert-butyl-4-hydroxyphenyl)propionate]	1,170
0.3 di-n-octyl(3,5-di-tert-butyl-4-hydroxy-benzyl)phosphonate	245
0.3% 1,1,3-tris(3-tert-butyl-4-hydroxy-6-methylphenyl)butane	40
Unstabilized polypropylene	3

The above data clearly indicates the significant increase in the stabilization of polypropylene upon the addition of the alkyl esters of alkylthioalkanoic acids. Mineral oil, high impact polystyrene, SBR, linear polyethylene, cyclohexane and polyester lubricant were also stabilized in additional examples of the patent.

MISCELLANEOUS CYCLIC ANTIOXIDANTS

Substituted 1,2,4-Thiadiazole Sulfenyl Halides

It has been found by *W.A. Thaler; U.S. Patent 3,691,183; September 12, 1972; assigned to Esso Research and Engineering Company* that contacting cyanodithioimidocarbonate anion with halogen under reaction conditions results in the formation of 3-halo-1,2-4-thiadiazole-5-sulfenyl halide. This reaction occurs according to the following formula:

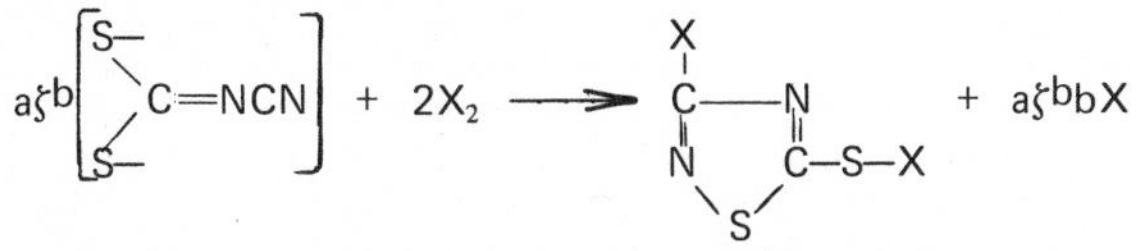

$$a\zeta b \begin{bmatrix} S- \\ C=NCN \\ S- \end{bmatrix} + 2X_2 \longrightarrow \begin{matrix} X \\ | \\ C-N \\ \| \quad \diagdown \\ N \quad C-S-X \\ \diagdown S \diagup \end{matrix} + a\zeta bbX$$

where a is the number of mols of neutralizing cation required to form the salt of cyanodithioimidocarbonate and is usually 1 or 2; b is the valence of the neutralizing cation, and also the number of mols of halogen per mol of salt reaction product, preferably 1 or 2; X is halogen, usually Cl or Br, with Cl most preferred, (X_2 will thus usually relate to Br_2 or Cl_2, but also includes BrCl, ICl and other halogenating compounds. In general, any compound which provides a source of positive halogen, such as sulfuryl and thionyl chloride is useful in the reaction, although Br_2 and Cl_2 are preferred, and Cl_2 most preferred); ζ equals any neutralizing cation, chosen from Groups Ia, IIa and IIIa of the Periodic Table, and usually Na, K, Li, Ca or Mg, with Na and K preferred, and K most preferred. The cyanodithioimidocarbonate is easily synthesized from cyanamide and carbon disulfide by the addition of a base to a solution of the above in absolute alcohol.

The above reactions are preferably run with the cyanodithioimidocarbonate salt dissolved or slurried in a solvent. The preferential solvents are those that are capable of dissolving some amount of the cyanodithioimidocarbonate and yet are substantially inert to the halogenating compound.

The halogen is usually added continuously to the cyanodithioimidocarbonate solvent blend with agitation. The reaction is exothermic, thus the halogen is added slowly to control the temperature rise. The temperature of the reaction can vary from −100° to +100°C, with a preferable range of −50° to +50°C, and −50° to 0°C most preferred. The reaction can be run under subatmospheric or superatmospheric pressure, but usually ambient pressure conditions are obtained.

The 3-halo-1,2,4-thiadiazol-5-yl sulfenyl halides can be further reacted to give other products, which also show utility as pesticides, antioxidants, anticorrosion additives, UV stabilizers, and additives for increasing the load-carrying capacity of mineral oil lubricants. The 3-halo-1,2,4-thiadiazol-5-yl sulfenyl halides can be reacted with olefins to give 5-(halo-hydrocarbyl-thio)-3-halo-1,2,4-thiadiazoles. This reaction is illustrated by the following equation:

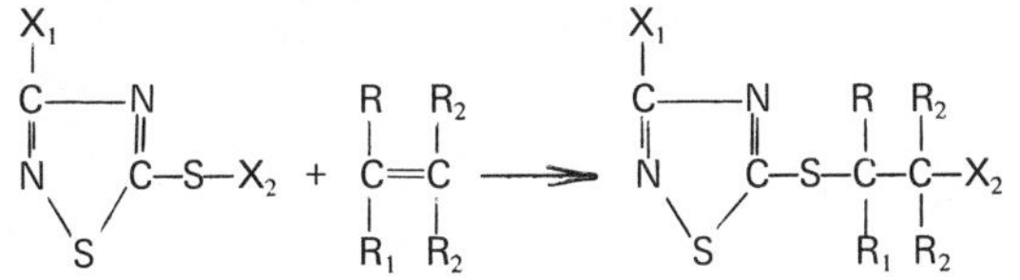

$$\begin{matrix} X_1 \\ | \\ C-N \\ \| \quad \diagdown \\ N \quad C-S-X_2 \\ \diagdown S \diagup \end{matrix} + \begin{matrix} R \quad R_2 \\ | \quad | \\ C=C \\ | \quad | \\ R_1 \quad R_2 \end{matrix} \longrightarrow \begin{matrix} X_1 \\ | \\ C-N \quad\quad R \quad R_2 \\ \| \quad \diagdown \quad\quad | \quad | \\ N \quad C-S-C-C-X_2 \\ \diagdown S \diagup \quad\quad | \quad | \\ \quad\quad\quad R_1 \quad R_2 \end{matrix}$$

where X_1 and X_2 are independently selected from the halogen group, preferably Cl, or Br, and most preferably Cl. R, R_1, R_2 and R_3 are hydrocarbon radicals independently selected from hydrogen, alkyl, alkenyl, aryl, aralkyl or cycloalkyl.

The 5-(halo-hydrocarbylthio)-3-halo-1,2,4-thiadiazoles may be further reacted with thiophosphate salts to give further products. For example, the reaction product of 5-(2-chloro-ethylthio)-3-chloro-1,2,4-thiadiazole and the ammonium salt of diethyl dithiophosphate is a compound which has demonstrated utility as a soil fungicide. The 3-chloro-1,2,4-thiadia-zol-5-sulfenyl halide may be converted to di(3-chloro-1,2,4-thiadiazol-5-yl)disulfide, by con-tacting with Cu_2Cl_2 in tetrahydrofuran at room temperature. The disulfide form is also use-ful as a pesticide, an antioxidant, a vulcanizing aid and a lubricating oil additive.

Example 1: To a stirred solution of 100 grams (2.38 mols) of cyanamide dissolved in 250 ml of absolute alcohol was added 199 grams (2.62 mols) carbon disulfide. The mix-ture was placed in a round bottom Pyrex flask fitted with an automatic stirrer and kept below 20°C while a solution of 314 grams of 85% potassium hydroxide in 600 ml of absol-ute alcohol was added over a period of 30 minutes. The mixture was stirred for an addi-tional 45 minutes and then suction filtered, washed with tetrahydrofuran and dried in a vacuum oven at 50°C yielding 416 grams (90% yield based on cyanamide) of dipotassium cyanodithioimidocarbonate. A slurry of 103 grams (0.53 mol) of potassium cyanodithio-imidocarbonate in 750 ml methylene chloride was placed in a round bottom flask equipped with an automatic stirrer and a chlorine inlet tube and cooled to –40°C. 75.3 grams (1.06 mol) of chlorine was slowly added to the stirred mixture.

The reaction mixture was then mechanically stirred at 0°C for 1 hour, suction filtered under dry nitrogen, and the methylene chloride evaporated under reduced pressure yielding 85 grams (86% yield) of a yellow solid. Infrared and ultraviolet spectral studies confirm that 3-chloro-1,2,4-thiadiazol-5-yl sulfenyl chloride was formed.

Example 2: A solution of 9.35 grams (0.05 mol) of 3-chloro-1,2,4-thiadiazol-5-yl sulfenyl chloride in 100 ml dry tetrahydrofuran was stirred with 4.9 grams (0.025 mol) Cu_2Cl_2 for 1 hour at room temperature, during which time the green cuprous chloride changed to the brown cupric chloride. The solid was filtered off, the solution evaporated, redissolved in methylene chloride and filtered again. Evaporation of the methylene chloride yielded 7.6 grams (100% yield) of the disulfide product which was recrystallized from CH_2Cl_2-methanol giving 5.0 grams of a pale yellow solid, di(3-chloro-1,2,4-thiadiazol-5-yl)disulfide with a melt-ing point of 118° to 120°C.

2,3-Dihydro-p-Oxathiins and Their Sulfoxides and Sulfones

An improved process for the preparation of these oxathiins is disclosed by *F. Asinger, P. Scherberich and H. Offermanns; U.S. Patent 3,793,344; February 19, 1974; assigned to Deutsche Gold- und Silber-Scheideanstalt, Germany.* These compounds are useful as anti-oxidants in synthetic materials and elastomers.

The process involves the reaction between an α-mercaptooxo compound and an oxirane followed by dehydration of the formed alkoxylated α-mercaptooxo compound. The reac-tion preferably is carried out at a temperature between 25° and 30°C. It is not necessary in all cases to isolate the obtained alkoxylated α-mercaptooxo compound. However, this may be done and the product may be subjected to a purification prior to the subsequent cyclization. The process permits one to obtain 2,3-dihydro-p-oxathiins and the correspond-ing sulfones and sulfoxides, all of which are illustrated by the following formulas.

The products are obtained at a high yield and with a high degree of purity. The inert sol-vents for the reaction may for instance be hydrocarbons such as benzene, toluene, xylene, furthermore dioxane, tetrahydrofuran, chloroform, ether, dimethylformamide, etc. The use of alcohols is particularly desirable. Among them methanol is preferred. The basic catalysts used in the alkoxylation may be alkali hydroxides, particularly potassium hydroxide, alcoholates, carbonates, bicarbonates, organic bases such as tertiary amines or pyridine or quaternary nitrogen bases. These catalysts may be used in amounts from 0.5 to 10% by weight, preferably from 1 to 2% by weight relative to the α-mercaptooxo compound. As α-mercaptooxo compounds all compounds can be used in the process which include the structural element:

$$-C=O$$
$$|$$
$$-CH-SH$$

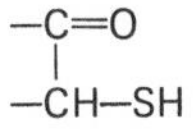

These may in particular be compounds of the formula:

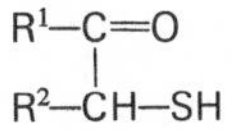

$$R^1-C=O$$
$$|$$
$$R^2-CH-SH$$

R^1 and R^2 in this formula are the same or different and are hydrogen, alkyl of 1 to 18 carbons, aryl, aralkyl, heteroalkyl, $-COOH$ or $-COOR$. R^1 may also form a ring with R^2 of 4 to 12 members which may in addition include an O, S, N or P atom. The groups just listed may also be substituted by halogen, particularly chlorine, or $-CN$, $-COOR$, $-OR$, $-SR$, $-NR_2$ or $-OH$ groups. In all these groups R may be alkyl with 1 to 12 carbons. R^1 and R^2 may also be $-COOMe$, $-CONRR$, $-CONHR$ and $-CONH_2$ in which case Me is an alkali metal atom, particularly sodium. Examples of these α-mercaptooxo compounds include: mercaptobutanones, mercaptopentanones, mercaptoacetone, mercaptocyclohexanone, and the like. As oxiranes all compounds may be used which include the structural elements:

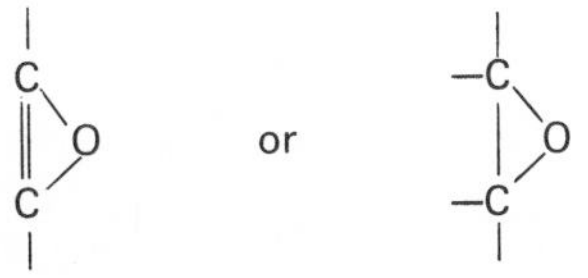

Examples of these oxiranes include the following: ethylene oxide, propylene oxide, 1,2-butylene oxide(ethylethylene oxide), hydroxymethylethylene oxide (glycidol), 1,1-dimethylethylene oxide, trimethylethylene oxide, tetramethylethylene oxide, and the like.

The reaction in the first stage is preferably carried out by placing the α-mercaptooxo compound and the base into the reactor whereupon the oxirane is added dropwise while stirring and, if desired, upon cooling so as to obtain the reaction temperature within the above-stated range. There is obtained an intermediate addition product which has the following structure:

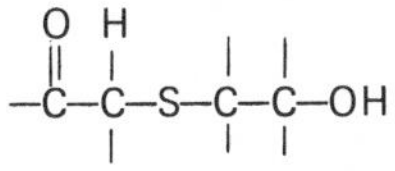

This intermediate in most cases has such a high degree of purity that the product may be directly passed into the cyclization operation, after distilling off the solvent. The cyclization is preferably effected by heating in an organic solvent such as benzene, toluene, xylene, chloroform or carbon tetrachloride and in the presence of an acid catalyst such as p-toluenesulfonic acid, methanesulfonic acid, orthophosphoric acid, mineral acids, Lewis acids, acid salts such as alkali hydrogen sulfates or acid-exchange resins, molecular sieves while employing a water trap. It is also possible to effect the cyclization with an equimolar amount of anhydrous zinc chloride or phosphorus pentoxide in an inert organic solvent at room temperature. The conversion of the 2,3-dihydro-p-oxathiins into the corresponding sulfones or sulfoxides, can be carried out by subjecting the compound to an oxidizing agent such as H_2O_2, hydroperoxides, peracids, permanganate in acetic acid ester, acetone, or preferably, glacial acetic acid.

Example 1: Ethylene oxide was passed at room temperature into a solution of 23.6 grams (0.2 mol) 2-mercaptopentanone-(3) in 50 ml methanol after adding 0.5 gram potassium hydroxide and upon vigorous stirring. A strongly exothermic reaction took place. By cooling with a water bath and adjusting the ethylene oxide current, the temperature was kept between 25° and 30°C. The introduction of ethylene oxide was continued until an exothermic reaction was no longer noticeable. Subsequently, stirring was continued at room temperature for another 30 minutes. After distilling off the solvent in a vacuum, the crude 2-(β-hydroxyethyl)mercaptopentanone-(3) added dropwise to a boiling solution of 2 grams of p-toluenesulfonic acid in 250 ml toluene during 1 hour while stirring.

After about 1.5 hours the condensation was complete. 3.6 ml water were collected in a water trap. The reaction mixture was then cooled and washed with water. The solvent was distilled off in a vacuum. Fractionation of the residue in a vacuum furnished 26 grams of 2,3-dihydro-5-methyl-6-ethyl-p-oxathiin (90% of the theoretical value, related to the α-mercaptoketone used as starting product). The product was in the form of a colorless liquid having a boiling point of 44°C/1.5 mm and n_D^{20} 1.5132.

Example 2: 28.8 grams (0.2 mol) of 2,3-dihydro-5-methyl-6-ethyl-p-oxathiin were dissolved in a small amount of acetone and were slowly reacted at 0°C with 23.5 grams (0.2 mol) of a 30% aqueous solution of hydrogen peroxide. After completion of the reaction the mass was heated to room temperature and about 200 ml of an inert organic solvent were added. After washing of the organic phase and drying of Na_2SO_4, the solvent was removed in a vacuum. The thus-obtained residue was distilled in a vacuum. There were obtained 22.4 grams (70% of the theoretical value) of 2,3-dihydro-5-methyl-6-ethyl-p-oxathiin-oxide, $BP_{0.1}$ 76°C; n_D^{20} 1.5272.

Thiourazole Derivatives

Adducts formed by reacting an α,β-unsaturated compound with a thiourazole are described by *J.W. Gates, Jr., A.W. Wise, D.J. Beavers and P.E. Miller; U.S. Patent 3,641,046; Feb. 8, 1972; assigned to Eastman Kodak Company.* Generally, the process involves the reaction of an α,β-unsaturated compound with a thiourazole of the following formula or a tautomer thereof:

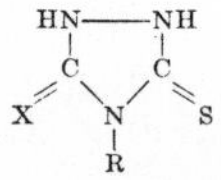

where X is an oxygen atom, sulfur atom or imino group and R is hydrogen or an alkyl group having 1 to 8 carbons such as methyl, ethyl, propyl, isopropyl, butyl, isobutyl and the like, or an aryl group such as a phenyl group and the like. The α,β-unsaturated organic compounds preferably have the formula:

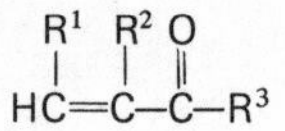

where R^1, R^2 can be hydrogen or an alkyl group containing 1 to 4 carbons, R^3 can be hydrogen, an hydroxyl group, an amine group, an alkyl ether group or an alkyl group containing 1 to 10 carbons. In one embodiment where R is a hydrogen atom and an α,β-unsaturated organic aldehyde is reacted with a thiourazole, it is believed that the reaction product is bicyclic and represented by the formula or a tautomer thereof:

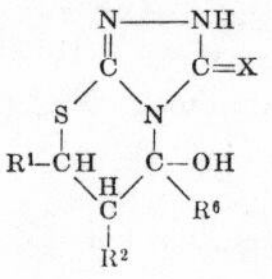

In the formula, X is oxygen, sulfur, or imino group, and R^1 and R^2 are as represented above and R^6 can be hydrogen or an alkyl group containing 1 to 10 carbons. In another embodiment where an α,β-unsaturated acid, ester, amide or ketone is reacted with a thiourazole, the product is believed to be as follows or a tautomer thereof:

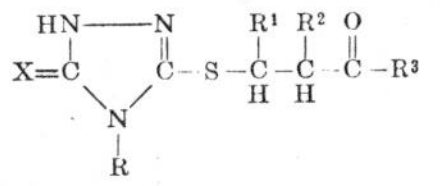

$$
\begin{array}{c}
HN\!-\!-\!-\!N \qquad R^1\ R^2\ O \\
\quad \parallel \qquad\qquad |\ \ |\ \ \parallel \\
X\!=\!C \qquad C\!-\!S\!-\!C\!-\!C\!-\!C\!-\!R^3 \\
\quad\backslash\ \ \diagup \qquad H\ \ H \\
\qquad N \\
\qquad | \\
\qquad R
\end{array}
$$

where R, R^1, R^2, R^3 and X are as described above. Where a dithiourazole with an R represented by a hydrogen atom is reacted with the α,β-unsaturated aldehyde or ketone, it is believed that a bicyclic compound is formed when 2 molar equivalents of the α,β-unsaturated compound are used. The reaction product is believed to be as follows:

$$
\begin{array}{c}
N\!-\!-\!-\!N \qquad R^4\ R^5\ O \\
\parallel \qquad \parallel \qquad |\ \ |\ \ \parallel \\
C \qquad C\!-\!S\!-\!C\!-\!C\!-\!C\!-\!R^7 \\
\diagup\ \ \backslash\ N \qquad H\ \ H \\
S \qquad | \\
R^1\!-\!CH \quad C\!-\!OH \\
\quad\backslash H\diagup\ \ \backslash \\
R^2\!-\!C \qquad R^6
\end{array}
$$

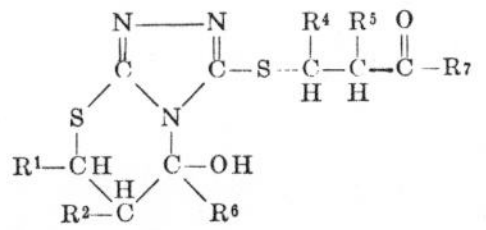

where R^1, R^2, R^4, R^5 and R^6 are as described above and R^7 is an alkyl group having 1 to 10 carbons, a hydroxyl, an amine, or an alkyl ether. It is understood that R^1, R^2, R^4 and R^5 can each be different groups from the others. These compounds are very useful as additives to photographic compositions as well as other applications such as corrosion inhibitors, fuel additives, antioxidants and plasticizers of polymeric compositions and the like. An example of the preparation of these compounds is given in the following example.

Example: 3-[β-Carboxyethylthio]-1,2,4-Triazoline-5-Thione — To a stirred suspension of 6.65 grams of 1,2,4-triazolidine-3,5-dithione in 50 ml of water is added 3.6 grams of acrylic acid. Within 15 minutes the solids dissolve, and after ½ hour a precipitate forms. After stirring ½ hour longer and chilling, the precipitate is collected. The crude product (11 grams) is recrystallized from dilute alcohol to produce a yield of 84%, MP 204° to 205°C.

Dibenzopyrans, Fluorenols and Dibenzothiopyrans

Dibenzopyrans and dibenzothiopyrans are disclosed by *W.L. Hall and J.L. Webb; U.S. Patent 3,723,465; March 27, 1973; assigned to General Electric Company.* The dibenzopyrans and dibenzothiopyrans have the formula:

(1)

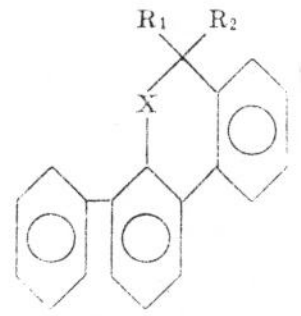

and the fluorenol isomers of the dibenzopyrans have the formula:

(2)

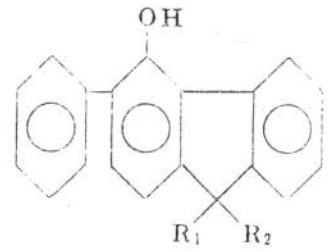

X is oxygen or sulfur, R_1 and R_2, taken together with the carbon to which both are attached form a cyclohexyl ring, including a lower alkyl substituted cyclohexyl ring and, in addition, separately, R_1 is hydrogen or lower alkyl free of a tertiary α-carbon and R_2 is lower alkyl free of a tertiary α-carbon, phenyl, lower alkyl substituted phenyl and, when X is sulfur and R_1 is hydrogen, carboxyl. In strongly acidic liquid media, 2,6-diphenylphenol and 2,6-diphenylthiophenol react with most aldehydes and ketones to produce dibenzopyrans or dibenzothiopyrans. Both the pyran and thiopyran ring as intermediates can be cleaved to phenols which differ from starting phenols because one of the o-phenyl substituents, itself, now has an ortho substituent characteristic of the aldehyde or ketone reactant. Both these phenols and the fluorenols are useful as antioxidants, stabilizers, etc.

It was found that 2,6-diphenylphenol, unlike almost all other phenols, did not react with aldehydes or ketones in the presence of the usual mineral acid catalysts to form bisphenols. Both 2,6-diphenylphenol and its thio isologue yield dibenzopyrans or dibenzothiopyrans with other aldehydes and ketones except for all-aromatic ketones which do not react at all. In general, the compounds of Formulas (1) and (2) are made by reacting 2,6-diphenylphenol or 2,6-diphenylthiophenol with the desired aldehyde or ketone in an acidic liquid phase in which the reactants are soluble and which is nonreactive with the other components, containing no more than 5% water and whose acid strength, as measured on the Hammett H_0 scale, is at least as strong as trifluoroacetic acid.

Preferably, the liquid phase should be a solvent in which the amount of both reactants used are completely soluble. However, this is not a requisite, and heterogeneous reaction mixtures can be used when the reactants are sufficiently soluble in the liquid phase to give a reasonable reaction rate. Preferably, any inert organic liquid used as a diluent and solvent for the acid should be aprotic and should have a high dielectric constant since such a solution will have a higher negative Hammett H_0 activity function for a given acid than a solvent having a lower dielectric constant.

Typical examples of acids that are readily available and which can be used to provide the required acidity are: hydrogen fluoride, trifluoracetic acid, mono-, di- and hexafluorophosphoric acids, fluoboric acid, methanesulfonic acid, trifluoromethanesulfonic acid, etc. Mixtures of these acids can be used but offer no advantage over the use of a single acid.

Example: A solution of 370 grams of 2,6-diphenylphenol in 2 liters of trifluoroacetic acid was heated to reflux and 174 grams of acetone was added over a 10 minute period. After refluxing for 5.5 hours an additional 87 grams of acetone was added and reflux continued for an additional 0.5 hour. On cooling to room temperature, the crude 4-phenyl-6,6-dimethyl-4-phenyl-6H-dibenzo[b,d]pyran, corresponding to Formula (1) where X is oxygen and R_1 and R_2 are each methyl, precipitated as a crystalline material which was filtered, washed with water and air dried. The product was dissolved in one liter of heptane containing 150 ml of toluene. The solution was extracted three times with 300 ml portions of Claisen's alkali to remove any phenolic bodies.

After washing with water and drying with anhydrous magnesium sulfate, the solvent was removed under vacuum from the extracted heptane-toluene solution leaving a solid residue which was recrystallized from methanol to yield 281 grams of the purified dibenzopyran as white crystals having a melting point of 79°C, whose structure was confirmed by infrared, nmr and mass spectrometry.

Cyclo-Substituted Gamma-Butyrolactones

Lactones are disclosed by *E.A.I. Heiba and R.M. Dessau; U.S. Patent 3,758,513; Sept. 11, 1973; assigned to Mobil Oil Corporation* which are precursors for the preparation of antioxidants for hydrocarbon fuels and lubricants. The lactones themselves are useful as antiwear additives for lubricants and anticorrosion agents for iron. These lactones have the formula

(1)

$$\begin{array}{c} \gamma \quad \overset{R}{\diagup} \quad \beta \\ HC \text{——} CH \\ \overset{\displaystyle O}{} \quad \overset{\displaystyle C}{\diagup} \overset{\displaystyle -R_1}{\underset{R_2}{}} \; \alpha \\ \overset{\displaystyle C}{\underset{\displaystyle O}{\parallel}} \end{array}$$

where R may be $-(CH_2)_n-$ when n is at least 6 but not greater than 15, an alkylene group containing at least 3 but not more than 10 carbons, or butyrolactone connected through its beta and gamma carbons with 1 to 8 $-CH_2-$ groups interposed between either or both its beta or gamma carbons. R_1 and R_2 may be hydrogen or chlorine or a hydrocarbyl, carboxyl, amido, cyano, isocyano, or nitro group. They may also be an alkyl group containing as a substituent a carboxyl, amido, cyano, isocyano, or nitro group. Where R_1 and R_2 are groups containing carbon, they may contain between 1 and 16 carbons. R_1 may be the same as or different from R_2. In the formula above, the alpha, beta and gamma carbons are labeled.

These lactones can be prepared whereby a solution containing an olefin is heated for a period of time with a carboxylic acid in the presence of a metal ion of higher valent form such as trivalent manganese ion. The carboxylic acid must contain at least one hydrogen atom on the alpha carbon atom. The reaction may be carried out by heating between 80° and 100°C. The time of reaction may be an hour or less to 5 or 10 hours or more. An inert atmosphere, such as nitrogen, carbon dioxide, helium, and the like, is desirably maintained over the reaction mixture to lessen or avoid oxidation by air.

The solvent, in which the compound of the metal must also be soluble, is preferably an alpha-hydrogen-containing aliphatic carboxylic acid of which acetic acid is preferred, but which may also be propionic, butanoic, pentanoic, or other higher molecular weight acid. Besides manganese, other higher valent metal ions such as cerium, vanadium, and nickel may be used. In the reaction mixture, the concentration of the olefin may range from 0.01 to 3 mols, preferably 0.25 to 1 mol, per mol of metal compound.

The nature of the R group in the lactone will be determined by the olefin that is used, i.e., whether a cyclomonoolefin or a cyclopolyolefin is employed. Where R is to be $-(CH_2)_n-$, a cyclomonoolefin will be employed. Where R is to be an alkylene group, a cyclopolyolefin will be used. Where R is to be a butyrolactone group, a cyclopolyolefin will also be employed. Cyclomonoolefins which may be employed are cyclooctene, cyclononene, cyclodecene, cycloundecene, cyclododecene, cyclotridecene, cyclotetradecene, cyclopentadecene, cyclohexadecene, and cycloheptadecene.

Example: Cyclooctene is dissolved in glacial acetic acid to form a solution approximately 0.1 molar with respect to the olefin. To such a solution there are added 2 mol equivalents of manganic acetate dihydrate, $Mn(C_2H_3O_2)_3 \cdot 2H_2O$ and about 300 g/l of anhydrous potassium acetate; the latter serves to suppress any undesired side product. The resulting solution is then heated to reflux under a nitrogen atmosphere until the brown manganic color disappears. Thereafter the resulting reaction mixture is analyzed for lactone content by means of vapor phase chromatography. The following lactone is obtained in a yield of 65% by weight:

(2)

$$\begin{array}{c} \overset{H_2}{C} \text{——} \overset{H_2}{C} \\ H_2C \diagup \quad \diagdown CH_2 \\ H_2C \quad \quad \quad CH_2 \\ HC \text{——} CH \\ \overset{\displaystyle O}{} \quad CH_3 \\ \diagdown C \diagup \\ \overset{\displaystyle}{\underset{\displaystyle O}{\parallel}} \end{array}$$

Such lactones may be used to prepare compounds which, when added to hydrocarbon fuels and lubricants, effectively reduce such oxidative deterioration. For example, the lactones may be reacted with an amine such as CH_3NH_2 to form:

(3)

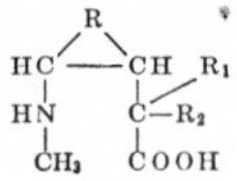

$$
\begin{array}{c}
R \\
HC\!-\!-\!CH\quad R_1 \\
HN\qquad C\!-\!R_2 \\
CH_3\quad COOH
\end{array}
$$

and   (4)

$$
\begin{array}{c}
R \\
HC\!-\!-\!CH \\
CH_3N\qquad C\!-\!R_1 \\
C\quad R_2 \\
O
\end{array}
$$

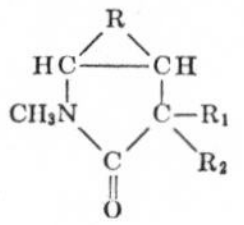

By further treatment of (3) with an amine CH_3NH_2, there may be formed:

(5)

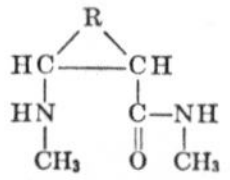

$$
\begin{array}{c}
R \\
HC\!-\!-\!CH \\
HN\qquad C\!-\!NH \\
CH_3\quad O\quad CH_3
\end{array}
$$

Compounds (3), (4) and (5) are effective antioxidants for hydrocarbon fuels and lubricants. A specific lactone which can be used for preparing these antioxidants is the lactone of the example.

5,7-Diisopropyl-1,1-Dimethyl-6-Hydroxyindan

T.F. Wood and G.H. Goodwin; U.S. Patent 3,644,540; February 22, 1972; assigned to Givaudan Corporation have prepared the title compound by reacting 2,6-diisopropylphenol and isoprene, in the presence of a protonic acid catalyst, at temperatures from -20° to 150°C. This compound may be represented by its skeletal formula as follows:

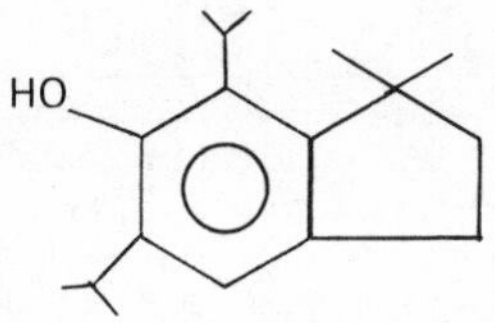

The preparation of this compound may be represented by the following equation:

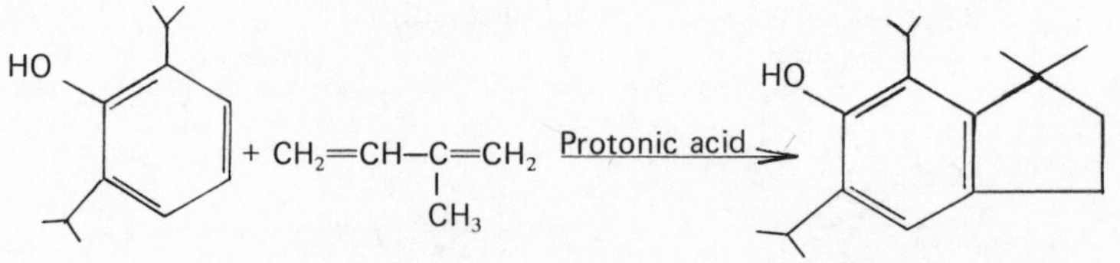

In general, a mixture of the phenol and isoprene is slowly fed into a mixture of more of the starting phenol and the catalyst employed. If desired where a mild protonic acid catalyst is used, a stronger protonic acid catalyst may also be added at any desired stage of the reaction, to bring the reaction to the desired completion more quickly.

In carrying out the cyclo-addition reaction protonic acidic condensing agents, such as sulfuric acid, phosphoric acid, hydrofluoric acid, boron trifluoride-water adduct, sometimes described as monohydroxyfluoroboric acid, etc., may be used. Sulfuric acid of 75% strength and stronger has been found effective in the process. When the strength of the sulfuric acid is 85 to 88%, the process is operable between 5° and 50°C. At sulfuric acid strengths of 93 to 96%, the process is operable between –20° and +35°C. When a milder alkylating catalyst, such as phosphoric acid, is used, higher temperatures may be employed such as 40° to 150°C. An especially effective catalyst is phosphoric acid of 95% concentration. Anhydrous hydrogen fluoride is an efficient alkylating catalyst within the temperature range of –10° to 50°C.

In general, it has been found that reaction times between 3 and 6 hours give the desired results. About 3 to 4 hours are required to feed the phenol-isoprene mixture into the phenol-catalyst mixture. Stirring is then continued for 10 minutes to 2 hours. In general, equimolecular amounts of the starting phenol and isoprene give excellent results. While a slight molar excess of isoprene may be used, this is not recommended because the excess will be lost through polymerization. If desired, the phenol may be employed in a molar excess of 3 to 1 of isoprene. An excess of phenol may be desirable when a strong alkylating catalyst, such as sulfuric acid, is used. With respect to the alkylating catalyst, amounts from 5 to 55%, based on the total amount of 2,6-diisopropylphenol may be used with satisfactory results; but larger or smaller amounts may be employed, if desired.

Since the catalysts are mainly insoluble in the reaction mixture, stirring is provided. When the reaction is complete, stirring is discontinued and the catalyst allowed to separate. It is run off and discarded or reused in the process. In order to obtain efficient separation at this stage it is sometimes necessary to add a suitable solvent, such as benzene or ethylene dichloride, which can be recovered by distillation. Alternatively, the reaction contents may be quenched in ice water after the stirring is discontinued, then allowed to settle and the lower aqueous layer containing the catalyst is removed and discarded.

In addition to its use in perfume formulation, this indan has been found to be an effective and useful antioxidant for the stabilization of unsaturated acids, such as oleic acid and aldehyde compounds as, for example: p-isopropyl-2-methyl-hydrocinnamaldehyde, nonanal and p-isopropylbenzaldehyde. In addition, the compound is a good stabilizer for olefins as, for example, for myrcene.

Example 1: A solution of 68 grams (1 mol) of isoprene in 100 grams of 2,6-diisopropylphenol was fed over a 3 hour period into a rapidly-stirred mixture of 240 grams of 2,6-diisopropylphenol and 120 grams of 93% sulfuric acid while the reaction temperature was maintained at 25° to 30°C. The resulting thick reaction mixture was stirred 10 minutes longer and quenched by addition of 300 grams of ice-water. 200 ml of benzene was stirred in to facilitate separation. After settling, the lower acid layer was withdrawn and discarded.

The remaining benzene solution was washed successively with water and 10% sodium bicarbonate solution and distilled for removal of the benzene solvent. The residual liquid was vacuum distilled and the fraction boiling from 127° to 132°C at 2 mm collected as a colorless solid amounting to 46 grams. After crystallization, first from petroleum ether and then from 90% aqueous ethanol, the product was obtained as colorless crystals, MP 99° to 100°C, having a strong and pleasant musk odor.

Example 2: The antioxidant activity of 5,7-diisopropyl-1,1-dimethyl-6-hydroxyindan (DDHI) was demonstrated in oleic acid. The oleic acid used was representative of commercially available material except that no stabilizer was present. Samples of oleic acid with and without 0.01% DDHI were agitated in open Erlenmeyer flasks on a rotary shaker at ambient temperatures. Periodically small aliquots (ca 0.2 gram) were removed and analyzed for peroxide content by standard iodometric procedures. Results were as follows:

Peroxide Values

Days	7	20	46
DDHI	0	6.0	8.9
No additive	69.0	430.0	625.0

Additional examples in the patent show the stabilization of several unsaturated aldehydes and myrcene.

Dihydro- and Tetrahydroimidazoles

A large group of imidazoles have been prepared by *E.F. Ullman, L. Call, R.K. Leute and J.H. Osiecki; U.S. Patent 3,740,412; June 19, 1973; assigned to Synvar Associates.* These have the following formulas:

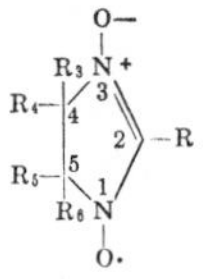

(I) 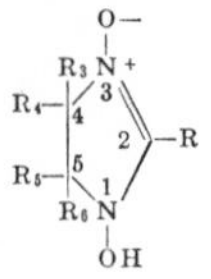   (II) 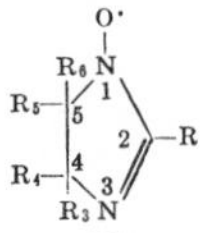   (III)

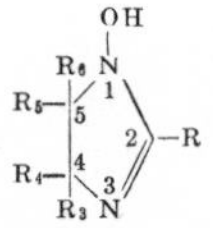

(IV) 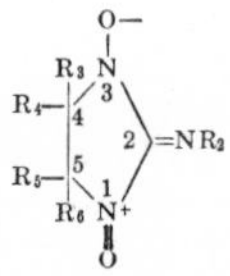   (V)

where R is generally $-NR_1R_2$, $-NR_2^-$, $-S^-$, $-SR_1$, or $-OR_1$. More particularly, R in Formula (I) is $-NR_1R_2$, $-NR_2^-$, $-S^-$, or $-SR_1$; in Formula (II), $-NR_1R_2$, or $-SR_1$; in Formula (III), NR_1R_2, $-SR$, or $-OR_1$; and in Formula (IV), $-NR_1R_2$, $-SR_1$, or $-OR_1$. The R_1 group is hydrogen, alkyl, aryl, alkenyl, alkynyl, cycloalkyl, and substituted derivatives thereof, and the R_2 group is hydrogen, alkyl, aryl, alkenyl, alkynyl, cycloalkyl,

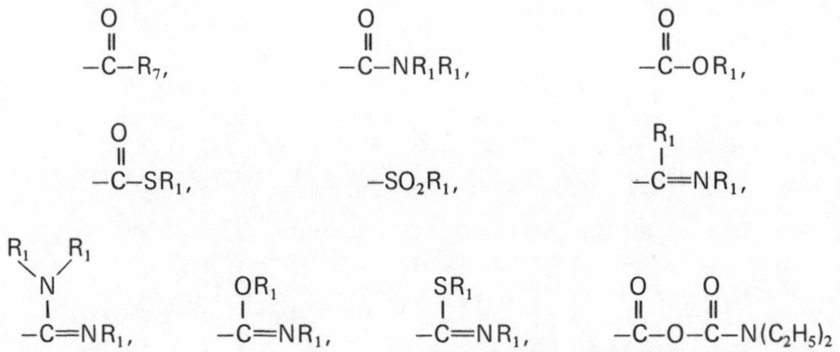

$$\underset{\text{O}}{\overset{\text{O}}{\|}}\quad -C-R_7,$$

$$-C-NR_1R_1,$$

$$-C-OR_1,$$

$$-C-SR_1,$$

$$-SO_2R_1,$$

$$\overset{R_1}{\underset{}{|}}-C=NR_1,$$

$$\underset{N}{\overset{R_1\quad R_1}{\diagdown \diagup}}\ -C=NR_1,$$

$$\overset{OR_1}{\underset{}{|}}-C=NR_1,$$

$$\overset{SR_1}{\underset{}{|}}-C=NR_1,$$

$$-C-O-C-N(C_2H_5)_2$$

and substituted derivatives thereof. The R_1 groups may be the same or different. Two R_1 groups or an R_1 and R_2 group may form part of a common ring. Each of R_3, R_4, R_5 and R_6 are an alkyl group, an alkenyl group, an alkynyl group, an aryl group, each of 1 to 12 carbons or form part of an alkylene or alkenylene group R_3-R_4 or R_5-R_6, the alkylene and alkenylene groups each containing from 3 to 10 carbons.

In general, the compounds of Formula (V) and the compounds of Formulas (I), (II), (III) and (IV) where R is $-NR_1R_2$ and $-NR_2^-$ (R_1 and R_2 are as defined above), may be prepared from 2-bromoimidazoline-1-oxide-3-oxyls according to the following reaction sequence.

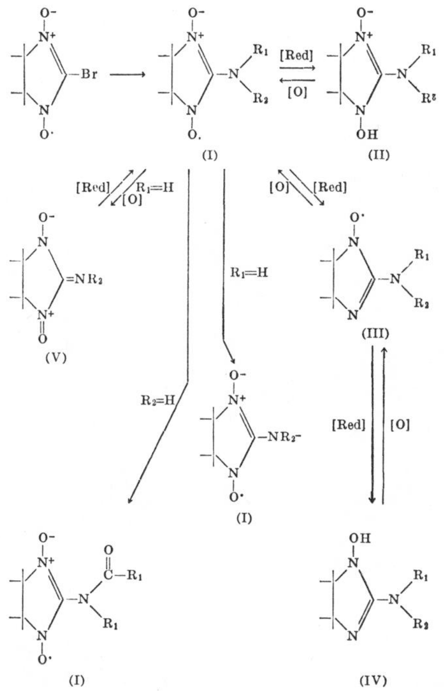

(I)   (II)

[Red]/[O]   R₁=H   [O]   [Red]

(V)   R₁=H   (III)

R₂=H   (I)   [Red]   [O]

(I)   (IV)

In the above amino reaction sequence the Roman numerals near the formula correspond with the formula described earlier so that one method for preparation of each of the types of the molecules within the scope of the process can be appreciated. The symbol (Red) stands for reduction, and the symbol (O) stands for oxidation.

Compositions in accordance with Formula (V) are useful as oxidizing agents because of their very powerful oxidizing properties. The compounds of Formula (I) where R is $-NR_2^-$ are very good infrared absorbers. The remaining compositions included within the scope of Formulas (I), (II), (III) and (IV) are useful as antioxidants. In general, the free radical structures of Formulas (I) and (III) are useful for the measurement of weak magnetic fields by known techniques. In addition, because of their free radical structure, the compound Formulas (I) and (III) exhibit electron spin resonance (ESR) and can be used as spin labels for attachment to biologically active molecules. A large number of preparative examples are given in the original patent, but no examples of application of the compounds as antioxidant were given.

SYNERGIST MIXTURES OF NON-NITROGEN BORON COMPOUNDS

Borates of nitrogen-containing compounds and synergistic mixtures of these compounds have been used as stabilizers for plastics. *H.A. Cyba; U.S. Patent 3,644,217; February 22, 1972; assigned to Universal Oil Products Company* has found that useful synergistic stabilizers are also obtained from boron compounds free of nitrogen. This comprises a synergistic mixture of a boron compound devoid of nitrogen and at least one of a hydroxyphenone, an N-hydroxyphenylbenzotriazole and a salicylic acid ester.

Any suitable boron compound devoid of nitrogen is used as one component of the synergistic mixture. The boron compound may be represented by the formula $B-(OR)_3$, $R-B-(OR)_2$, R_2-B-OR or R_3-B, where R is hydrogen except in the case of R_3-B, alkyl, aralkyl, aryl, alkaryl, cycloalkyl, alkcycloalkyl or cycloalkalkyl, which may in turn be sub-stituted with non-nitrogen-containing groups such as alkoxy, thioalkoxy, halogen, etc., or R may comprise carbons of the same or different cyclic structure. Any suitable hydroxy-phenone is used in the synergistic mixture. The hydroxyphenone is of the following struc-tural formula:

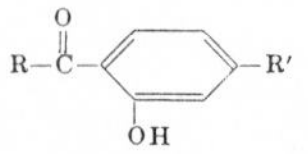

where R is aryl, alkyl, alkylene or cycloalkyl and R' is hydrogen, alkyl, alkylene, aryl, cy-cloalkyl, hydroxy, alkoxy, alkyleneoxy, aryloxy, cycloalkoxy, hydroxyalkyloxy or carboxy-alkyloxy. Where R is aryl, the hydroxyphenone is a hydroxybenzophenone which may con-tain one or more hydroxy groups. In fact, a preferred hydroxybenzophenone is 2,2'-dihy-droxybenzophenone. The N-hydroxyphenylbenzotriazole for use in the synergistic mix-ture is illustrated by the following formula:

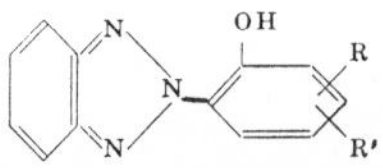

where R and R' are independently hydrogen, alkyl of 1 to 30 carbons or alkoxy of 1 to 30 carbons.

Any suitable salicylic acid ester may be used in the synergistic mixture. Preferred esters are phenyl salicylate (Salol), p-alkylphenyl salicylates in which the alkyl contains 1 to 30 car-bons including p-tert-butylphenyl salicylate or the corresponding n or sec-alkyl counterparts, polyalkylphenyl salicylates, in which each alkyl contains 1 to 30 carbons and salicylates in which the ester portion is derived from terpenic moieties, such as homomenthyl, carboxy-phenyl salicylate, strontium, calicum or barium salicylates, etc.

The synergistic mixture comprises 10 to 90% by weight of the boron compound and 10 to 90% by weight of at least one of the hydroxyphenone, N-hydroxyphenylbenzotriazole and salicylic acid ester, exclusive of other ingredients included in the mixture. Generally, it is preferred that the boron compound is in a proportion of from 50 to 90% by weight and the other component is in a proportion of from 10 to 50% by weight. The synergistic mixture may also contain one or more additional additives and more particularly at least one phenolic antioxidant, e.g., a trialkylphenol.

Example: This example describes the use of a synergistic mixture in solid polypropyl-ene exposed to carbon arc rays in a Fadeometer. The polypropylene without additive de-veloped a carbonyl number of greater than 1,000 within 120 hours of exposure in the Fadeo-meter. Another sample of the same polypropylene containing 0.15% by weight of butylated hydroxytoluene (2,6-di-tert-butyl-4-methylphenol) also developed a carbonyl number of over 1,000 within 120 hours of exposure in the Fadeometer.

Still another sample of the polypropylene was prepared to contain 1% by weight of tri-m, p-cresyl borate, available commercially as Borester 8, and 0.15% by weight of butylated hydroxytoluene. This sample reached a carbonyl number of over 1,000 within 200 hours of exposure in the Fadeometer. In contrast to the above, another sample of the polypropyl-ene is prepared to contain 0.5% by weight of the tri-m, p-cresyl borate, 0.5% by weight of 2-hydroxy-4-octoxy-benzophenone, available commercially as Cyanosorb 531, and 0.15% by weight of butylated hydroxytoluene. These components are incorporated into the poly-propylene by milling at a temperature of 375°F for 5 minutes. After 480 hours of expos-ure in the Fadeometer, the carbonyl number is below 400.

Other examples in the patent showed the use of synergistic mixtures containing B-nonyl-bis(octylphenol)sulfide in polystyrene, the borate of 2,2'-dihydroxy-3,3'-di-tert-butyl-5,5'-dimethyldiphenyl sulfide in ABS, and other borates in polyesters, nylon 6, and polyacetal.

REDOX POLYMERS

Redox polymers containing the hydroquinone-quinone system have been prepared (H.G. Cassidy and K.A. Kun *Oxidation-Reduction Polymers,* Interscience Publishers, Inc., New York, N.Y., 1965). Vinylhydroquinone cannot be successfully polymerized since the free hydroquinone group is a strong inhibitor for both radical and ion-induced polymerization. This difficulty has been overcome to some extent by blocking one or both of the phenolic hydroxyl groups by ester or ether formation prior to polymerization.

Careful removal of blocking groups yields the redox polymer. Such methods have the twin disadvantages of requiring the extra steps of introducing and removing the blocking groups. Moreover, the polymer obtained, apparently as a result of side reactions, has redox properties differing somewhat from these of the reversible hydroquinone-quinone system.

H.G. Cassidy, G. Wegner and N. Nakabayashi; U.S. Patent 3,600,411; August 17, 1971 and U.S. Patent 3,707,488; December 26, 1972; both assigned to Research Corporation have developed the process whereby redox polymers useful as antioxidants are prepared by the direct condensation of a quinone-diol with a diacyl chloride, phosgene or a diisocyanate.

The redox polymers of this process are particularly useful in the treatment of boiler feedwaters, as antioxidant stabilizers in various industrial products, in battery cells, and as photographic chemicals where their low diffusability is of advantage. The process uses the following quinone-diol intermediates in the preparation of the polyester, polycarbonate and polyurethane redox polymers: 2,5-bis(2'-hydroxyethyl)-1,4-benzoquinone, 2,5-bis(3'-hydroxypropyl)-1,4-benzoquinone, and 2-(duroquinonyl)propan-1,3-diol.

The benzoquinone-diol intermediates are most conveniently made by oxidation of the corresponding hydroquinones. The hydroquinones, in turn, are made by reduction of the diesters of the diols as shown in Example 1.

Example 1: 2,5-Bis(2'-Hydroxyethyl)Hydroquinone — This example illustrates the general procedure for the preparation of bis(hydroxyalkyl)hydroquinones by reduction of the corresponding esters. A solution of 0.02 mol of diethyl 3,6-dihydroxy-1,4-benzenedicarboxylate in 50 ml of dry tetrahydrofuran was added dropwise to a well-stirred slurry of 3.0 grams (0.079 mol) of lithium aluminum hydride in 40 ml of dry tetrahydrofuran and heated with stirring for 1 hour at reflux. The reaction mixture was then cooled in an ice bath and excess lithium aluminum hydride destroyed by careful addition of 5 ml of cold water.

Two layers formed on addition of 40 ml of 50% sulfuric acid and 40 ml of saturated ammonium chloride. The organic layer was separated and the aqueous layer further extracted with four 80 ml portions of tetrahydrofuran. The combined extracts were shaken with anhydrous magnesium sulfate, filtered, and concentrated in vacuo at room temperature to about 50 ml. The crystals obtained on cooling to –20°C were separated, washed with a small amount of solvent and dried in vacuo. The product was recrystallized from a small amount of hot water to give long white needles, MP 184°C, yield 76.5%.

Example 2: 2,5-Bis(2'-Hydroxyethyl)-1,4-Benzoquinone — This example illustrates the general procedure for the preparation of bis(hydroxyalkyl)hydroquinones. 2.0 mols of 2,5-bis(2'-hydroxyethyl)hydroquinone in 40 ml of dry tetrahydrofuran was treated with 0.6 gram of silver oxide and 1.0 gram of magnesium sulfate. The reaction mixture was stirred at room temperature for 30 minutes, filtered and the filtrate evaporated in vacuo at room temperature to a yellow, crystalline solid. The product was recrystallized from tetrahydrofuran-pentane to give yellow needles, MP 77°C in 95% yield.

The redox polyesters, polycarbonates, and polyurethanes are conveniently prepared by condensation of the quinone-diol reactants with equivalent quantities of a diacyl chloride, phosgene or diisocyanate, respectively. Mixed polycarbonates or polyurethanes are prepared by reacting benzoquinone-diol and phosgene or diisocyanate precondensate with a second quinone-diol. Extended polycarbonates are prepared by the condensation of the quinone-diol reactant with equivalent quantities of a glycol bischloroformate, prepared by the reaction of a monomeric or polymeric glycol with phosgene.

Generally speaking, the quinone and hydroquinone forms of the redox polymers are reversibly interconvertible. The yellow quinone form, as produced by condensation, exhibits typical carbonyl absorption in the infrared at 1,650 cm^{-1} and in the ultraviolet at 250 to 260 millimicrons. These disappear completely on reduction and the white hydroquinone form is characterized by absorption in the ultraviolet at about 300 mμ. Solutions of the hydroquinone form are more viscous, presumably due to an increase in hydrogen bonding.

The hydroquinone form of the duroquinonyl-based polymers is readily oxidized in air to the quinone form. A stable red quinhydrone-like product is obtained when mixed 2-(duroquinonyl)propan-1,3-diol and 2,5-bis(hydroxyalkyl)-1,4-benzoquinone based polymers are exposed to air. Examples are given in the complete patents on the preparation of the redox polyester, polycarbonate and polyurethane resins from these intermediates.

STABILIZED PETROLEUM PRODUCTS

Chemical additives are incorporated into most petroleum products. Antioxidants have been added to gasolines since the late twenties. Lubricants and greases which must withstand the increasingly higher temperatures and pressures of today's engines and machinery create the need for compositions having stronger and longer lasting antioxidant acitivity.

In addition to the antioxidants reviewed in this section, most lubricants contain other additives such as rust inhibitors, antiwear agents, detergents and/or dispersants, pour-point depressants, viscosity-index improvers and foam inhibitors. The interaction of the numerous additives makes the formulation of a high temperature lubricant a highly complex science.

ANTIOXIDANTS WITH HINDERED PHENOL MOIETIES

Dialkyl-4-Hydroxybenzyl Alkylates of Aryl Amines or Carbazole

W.F. Werzner and J.R. Miller; U.S. Patent 3,673,091; June 27, 1972; assigned to Shell Oil Company have found that the reaction products of various aryl amines or carbazole and 3,5-di-tert-butyl-4-hydroxybenzyl alcohol have good oxidation inhibition characteristics when added to mineral oils and other lubricants. A broad range of aryl amines are contemplated for use in these antioxidants. Those considered most suitable are diaryl or secondary aromatic amines, i.e., amines having two aromatic groups attached to the nitrogen atom. However, primary and tertiary aromatic amines are also within the scope of the process. Representative of such amines are aniline and triphenylamine. The aryl groups can have one, two or more rings, e.g., they can be phenyl, naphthyl, etc., and can be substituted or unsubstituted.

Each aryl group can have 6 to 30 or more carbons depending upon the nature and degree of substitution although generally they will have 6 to 18 carbons. Especially suitable are diphenylamine and substituted diphenylamines such as p,p'-dioctyl-diphenylamine, phenyl-α-naphthylamine, and phenyl-β-naphthylamine. The amine group can also have both alkyl and aryl substituents. Also useful as reactants are materials in which the nitrogen is contained within the ring structure, i.e., heterocyclic amines, such as carbazole, phenazines and acridines. Carbazole, however, is the most advantageous.

Preparation of the antioxidants can be carried out in an acetic acid medium using sulfuric acid as a catalyst. The reaction can take place from 20° to 120°C or higher. At 25°C, the reaction proceeds slowly requiring about 10 hours for completion; at 50°C the reaction proceeds more rapidly and the reaction period is reduced to about 3 hours. The reaction can result in alkylation of the rings and/or of the nitrogen atoms. Thus, the alkylation of diphenylamine with 3,5-di-tert-butyl-4-hydroxybenzyl alcohol produces a mixture of alkylated products in which any or most of the available ortho and para positions of the two aryl groups of the amine are substituted with the 3,5-di-tert-butyl-4-hydroxybenzyl group. If equal molar quantities of the amine and the hindered phenolic compound are reacted, the product mixture, although it cannot be completely resolved, consists principally of a mixture of two materials having a hydroxybenzyl group on the 2 or 4 position. Small quantities of materials are also obtained having the hydroxybenzyl group on the nitrogen.

By increasing the amount of the phenolic compound relative to the amine, the formation of the polyalkylated material is accentuated. Thus compounds having the hydroxybenzyl group substituted at any of the positions numbered 2,2',4,4',6,6' are probably produced when high ratios of the phenolic compound to the amine are used in the synthesis. Carbazole also gives a variety of substituted products. Monoalkylation occurs at the 1, 3 or 9 position. Dialkylation occurs at any combination of positions numbered 1,3,6,8 and 9. The alkylated amines are added to an appropriate oil base in an amount sufficient to inhibit oxidation, usually in a concentration of 0.01 to 5% by weight and preferably from 0.1 to 1% by weight.

The lubricating oil can be mineral, synthetic, or a blend of mineral and/or synthetic lubricating oils. While synthetic lubricating oils can be used with these antioxidants, high viscosity index (HVI) mineral oils are preferred, i.e., oils having a viscosity index (VI) of about 80 or higher. Paraffinic base oils are especially exemplary since they characteristically have a high viscosity index, although methods of refinement along with suitable VI improvers can approximate the same objective with other type oils. The following example illustrates the preparation and use of these compounds.

Example: The alkylation of carbazole by 3,5-di-tert-butyl-4-hydroxybenzyl alcohol was conducted as follows. To a 1-liter flask equipped with a magnetic stirring bar, 300 ml glacial acetic acid, 0.1 mol (16.7 grams) carbazole and 0.5 ml concentrated sulfuric acid were added. One-tenth mol of 3,5-di-tert-butyl-4-hydroxybenzyl alcohol dissolved in 250 ml glacial acetic acid was added dropwise from a separatory funnel to the carbazole-acetic acid slurry over a 10-hour period (about 1 drop every 10 seconds). The reaction mixture was kept at 30° to 35°C and agitation maintained for 3 hours after addition of the alcohol and then allowed to stand undisturbed for 48 hours. The reaction products included mono- and polyalkylated carbazole.

The mixture was decanted into a separatory funnel containing 200 ml benzene, subsequently a 500 ml saturated sodium chloride aqueous solution was added. The organic layer was washed further with 200 ml saturated sodium chloride solution followed by extractions with aqueous sodium bicarbonate until the washings became neutral or slightly alkaline. To reduce the possibility of forming HCl the mixture may be washed with an aqueous solution of sodium sulfate. The combined aqueous fractions were extracted with 300 ml benzene, then washed and neutralized with sodium bicarbonate as before. The combined benzene fractions were washed with 200 ml of water and dried over sodium sulfate. The volume was reduced by evaporation to 150 ml and 300 ml of hexane added.

A white residue which formed was separated from the hexane and fractionally crystallized from an ethanol-water solvent system. The white crystals (Product 1) were identified as a mixture of the ring monoalkylated carbazole, 1- and 3-(3,5-di-tert-butyl-4-hydroxybenzyl) carbazole, the major portion being the 3-substituted isomer. Other forms of alkylated carbazole including N-alkylated forms were contained in the hexane and in the alcohol from which the white crystals were fractionally precipitated. A ring polyalkylated product (Product 2) 3,6-bis(3,5-di-tert-butyl-4-hydroxybenzyl) carbazole was obtained from the hexane solution by solvent evaporation.

The reaction products were subjected to a Micro Air Oxidation Test (MAOT) to determine their oxidation inhibition properties. The MAOT was conducted at 300°F, using 20 gram oil samples, an air flow of 4.2 liters per hour, and 20 ppm Fe/Cu catalyst in the form of naphthenates to accelerate oxidation. The table below gives the test results.

Micro Air Oxidation Test Results

Oil Sample		Hours for 1 mmol O_2 Uptake per Gram of Oil
A	Base oil consisting of	1.4
	50% by volume high viscosity index 100 neutral	
	50% by volume high viscosity index 250 neutral	
	0.04% by weight C_{22} (average) alkylated derivative of succinic acid	
B	A + 1% by weight Product 1	126
C	A + 1% by weight Product 2	87
D	A + 1% by weight of a 1:2 molar mixture of carbazole and 3,5-di-tert-butyl-4-hydroxyphenyl alcohol	31

If carbazole is dissolved in benzene to which an equal volume of glacial acetic acid is added, the reaction products recovered will consist of about 22% N-alkylated carbazole, about 25% ring monoalkylated carbazole and the remainder being a mixture of polyalkylated compounds and starting material.

Mixtures of Secondary Trialkylphenols

Liquid hydrocarbons in the form of fuel oils or lubricating oils accumulate considerable quantities of water when maintained for long periods in storage vessels; and when subsequently brought into contact with metal surfaces, deterioration of equipment as a result of corrosion occurs. In addition, where such lubricating oils are incorporated into solid lubricants such as greases, similar deleterious results are encountered.

It has been found by *H.J. Andress, Jr.; U.S. Patents 3,759,831; September 18, 1973; and 3,609,081; September 28, 1971; both assigned to Mobil Oil Corporation* that the oxidative and corrosive properties of fuels, lubricants, heat exchange fluids, automatic transmission fluids, polymers such as rubber, plastics and the like, can be overcome by incorporating as antioxidant and anticorrosion agent, small amounts, sufficient to inhibit deterioration, of a secondary trialkylphenol having 6 to 9 carbons per alkyl group. In general, the organic compositions contain a small amount of the secondary trialkylphenols usually from 0.001 to 10% by weight, of the total weight of such compositions. When these secondary trialkylphenols are incorporated into liquid hydrocarbons such as gasolines, jet fuels and the like, or in lubricating oils, they are preferably used from 0.001 to 0.01% by weight, of the total weight of the composition. When incorporated into an organic grease composition, they are preferably employed from 0.1 to 5% by weight, of the total weight of the grease.

The secondary trialkylphenols may be prepared, in general, by reacting an olefin having 6 to 9 carbons per molecule, or mixtures of such olefins, with phenol to obtain the corresponding secondary trialkylphenol. The reaction is, in general, carried out at 75° to 100°C, and preferably 85° to 95°C. The details of the preparation and use of these compounds is given in the following examples.

Example 1: A mixture of 252 grams (3 mols) of 1-hexene, 94 grams (1 mol) of phenol and 20 grams of boron trifluoride ethyletherate was stirred at a temperature of 85° to 90°C for about 6 hours. The reaction mixture was then washed with hot water until the washings were neutral to litmus. Topping at a reduced pressure produced secondary trihexylphenol.

Examples 2 and 3: Secondary triheptylphenol and mixed secondary C_{7-8}-trialkylphenols were made by substituting 1-heptene and a 1:1 mixture of 1-hexene and 1-heptene for the 1-hexene of Example 1. In order to determine the sedimentation characteristics of fuel oils in which these trialkylphenols are incorporated, the 110°F Fuel Oil Storage Test was employed. In this test a 500 ml sample of the fuel oil is placed in a convection oven maintained at 110°F for 16 weeks. Thereafter, the sample is removed from the oven, cooled, and filtered through a tared asbestos filter (Gooch crucible) to remove insoluble matter. The weight of such matter in milligrams is reported as the amount of sediment.

A sample of the base uninhibited oil is run along with a fuel oil blend under test. The secondary trialkylphenols of Examples 1, 2, and 3 were individually incorporated in a gasoline blend comprising 100% catalytically cracked component, and boiling from 100° to 400°F, and containing 3 cc of tetraethyl lead, and 1 pound per 1,000 barrels of a metal deactivator comprising the di-salicylaldimine of 1,2-propanediamine. The test results are given in the table below.

Compound	Conc. lbs./ 1,000 bbls.	Gum formation, mg./100 ml.
Base fuel	0	15.4
Base fuel plus Example 1	5	11.3
Do	10	10.0
Base fuel plus Example 2	5	10.5
Do	10	10.5
Base fuel plus Example 3	5	12.1
Do	10	11.2

It will be seen from the table that a marked decrease in ASTM gum content is observed in fuel blends containing these secondary trialkylphenols.

Derivatives of 4-Hydroxy- and 4-Thiolbenzenecarbodithioic Acids

Esters of 4-hydroxy- and 4-thiolbenzenecarbodithioic acids, 1,4-dihydro-1-oxo-4-dithiomethylenebenzenes and 1,4-dihydro-1-oxo-4-(dithiacyclopent-2-ylidene)-benzenes in which the hydroxy, thiol and oxo groups are sterically hindered are disclosed by *B.R. Kennedy and L. deVries; U.S. Patent 3,778,370; December 11, 1973; assigned to Chevron Research Co.*

These compounds and their mixtures are useful as additives for lubricating oils providing such oils with high resistance to oxidative change. In addition, oils containing certain of the esters, particular bis-alkylene esters, and certain of the dithiacyclopentylidene benzenes and their mixtures show superior extreme pressure lubricating properties. Preferred compounds include esters of 4-hydroxy- and 4-thiolbenzenecarbodithioic acids having formulas 1 and 2;

(1)   and   (2)

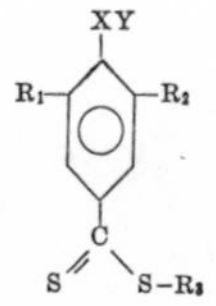

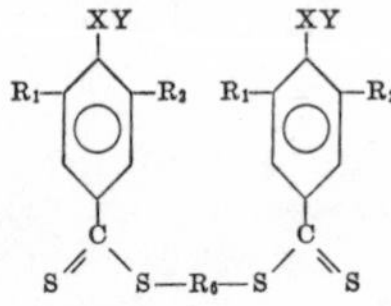

1,4-dihydro-1-oxo-4-dithiomethylenebenzenes having formula 3; and 1,4-dihydro-1-oxo-4-(1,3-dithiacyclopent-2-ylidene)-benzenes having formula 4.

(3)   and   (4)

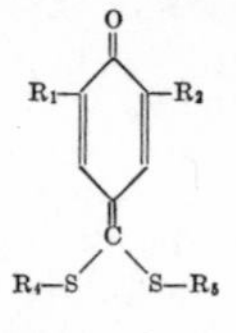

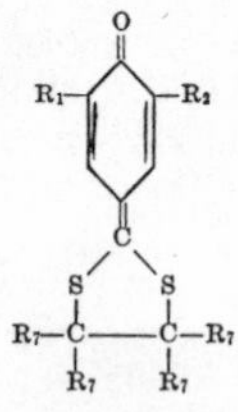

In the above formulas, R_1 and R_2 each is an alkyl group, which sterically hinders the adjacent hydroxy, thiol, or oxo group, containing 4 or more carbons desirably 4 to 9 carbons in a branched chain. R_3, R_4 and R_5 each represent alkyl containing 1 to 20 carbons such as methyl, ethyl, isobutyl, tert-butyl and the like; hydroxyalkyl, e.g., —R—OH, hydroxyalkyloxyalkyl, e.g., —R—O—R—OH, or hydroxyalkyl poly(oxyalkyl), e.g., —(R—O)$_n$R—OH in which the alkylene moieties R contain 2 to 5 carbons and can be straight or branched chain such as ethylene, 1,2-propylene, 1,2-butylene, and the like and n is 2 to 6; aralkyl such as benzyl, p-xylyl, and the like; or aryl such as phenyl, 4-tolyl and the like; R_6 is an alkylene group containing 1 to 8 carbons such as methylene, tetramethylene, pentamethylene, and the like. Each R_7 is hydrogen, alkyl such as defined above for R_3 or aryl such as phenyl, tolyl, and the like, and preferably R_7 is hydrogen. X is oxygen or sulfur and preferably oxygen. Y is hydrogen or a metallic cation such as derived from alkali metal such as sodium and potassium and those derived from alkali earth metals, such as calcium and barium, preferably Y is hydrogen. Preparative methods are shown by the following examples.

Example 1: The intermediate 3,5-di-tert-butyl-4-hydroxybenzenecarbodithioic acid is prepared in the following manner. To a 500 ml 3-neck flask equipped with stirrer, thermometer, nitrogen bleed, dropping funnel and condenser is added 2,6-di-tert-butylphenol (20.6 grams, 0.1 mol) in dimethyl sulfoxide (50 ml). A solution of potassium hydroxide (13.2 grams, 0.2 mol) in water (15 ml) is prepared, cooled and diluted with dimethyl sulfoxide. This solution is added to the phenolic solution above with stirring under a nitrogen blanket. The solution is cooled to $10° \pm 5°C$ with an ice-water bath and carbon disulfide (7.6 grams, 0.1 mol) is added to the stirred solution while maintaining the temperature at $10°C$. Stirring is continued at $10°C$ for 30 minutes after addition is complete. Cooling is discontinued and the temperature of the stirred solution is allowed to rise to room temperature.

Example 2: To the nonisolated intermediate prepared according to Example 1 is added concentrated hydrochloric acid (10 ml) slowly with stirring followed by the addition of 1-bromooctane (19.3 grams, 0.1 mol). Stirring is continued for 1 hour at room temperature. The temperature is raised to $70° \pm 10°C$ for 1 hour. The reaction mixture is then cooled and poured into ice water (500 ml) with stirring to yield a liquid product. The aqueous mixture is extracted three times with 200 ml of ether. The combined organic phases are dried over anhydrous sodium sulfate and the solvent is removed under vacuum on a rotary evaporator to yield 35.4 grams n-octyl 3,5-di-tert-butyl-4-hydroxybenzenecarbodithioate suitable for use without further purification. Recrystallization of a portion of the product from mixed hexanes yields a red crystalline solid.

Example 3: To the nonisolated intermediate obtained from the general preparation above is added iodomethane (28.4 grams, 0.2 mol) slowly with stirring. Stirring is continued at room temperature for 1 hour followed by heating to $70° \pm 10°C$ for 1 hour. The reaction mixture is cooled to room temperature and 200 ml of water is added followed by stirring for an additional 15 minutes. The aqueous mixture is extracted with ether (250 ml) three times. The combined organic phases are dried over anhydrous sodium sulfate and the solvent is removed on a rotary evaporator to yield 24.4 grams of 1,4-dihydro-1-oxo-2,6-di-tert-butyl-4-dimethylthiomethylenebenzene suitable for use without further purification.

Lubricating oils containing these esters as shown in Formulas 1 through 4 were tested in an oxidation test along with other lubricant additives. These compounds of Formulas 1 through 4 exhibited at least as much and generally greater resistance to oxidative change than the reference compound bis(3,5-di-tert-butyl-4-hydroxyphenyl) methylene.

NITROGEN-CONTAINING ANTIOXIDANTS

Guanidinium Salts

Phenoxide and naphthoxide salts of guanidine and hydrocarbon substituted guanidine are disclosed by *N.L. Allphin, Jr. and B.W. Hotten; U.S. Patent 3,740,338; June 19, 1973; assigned to Chevron Research Company.* Also disclosed are automatic transmission fluids and other functional fluids containing these salts as base reserve additives and antioxidants. Broadly, these compounds have the formulas:

In the above formulas, R^1, R^2, R^3, and R^4 each represents a hydrogen, C_1 to C_{20} alkyl, or C_6 to C_{10} aryl radical, and R^5 represents 1 or 2, preferably 1, hydrocarbon radicals having a total of 8 to 50, and preferably 8 to 30, carbons. Because of oil solubility requirements, at least one of the radicals R^1 to R^5 must be a C_{10} to C_{20} alkyl when any one or more of R^1 to R^4 is a C_6 to C_{10} aryl. Formulas 1 and 2 are meant to include both the α-naphthol and β-naphthol derivatives; the structure shown indicates that the oxygen atom may be at either the α- or β-position.

The basic additives are prepared by reacting guanidine or one of the guanidine derivatives described above with an alkyl-substituted phenol or naphthol. There may be one or two, preferably one, alkyl substituents on the aromatic rings of the phenol or naphthol. Total carbon content of the substituted phenol or naphthol should not exceed 50, preferably 30, carbons. At least one of the substituents must contain at least eight, and preferably at least twelve carbons. Preferably, these substituents have a linear structure or a linear structure with short side chains of 1 to 2 carbons, such as that obtained by the polymerization or copolymerization of lower alkenes such as ethylene, propylene, and isobutylene. The following examples will illustrate the preparation of typical guanidine additives. Polypropylene indicates a mixture of C_{12} to C_{14} alkyl groups derived from propylene monomer.

Example 1: One mol of a commercial guanidine hydrochloride was dissolved in a 5:6 volumetric mix of methanol and ethanol. This was then reacted with 1 mol of p-polypropylenephenol and 1 mol of potassium hydroxide as a 40% solution in methanol. The reaction took place at ambient temperature. Guanidinium p-polypropenyl phenate was recovered.

Example 2: One-half mol of N,N',N'-tetramethylguanidine was reacted with one-half mol of p-polypropylene phenol. During the exothermic reaction, the temperature rose from ambient to 54°C. N,N,N',N'-tetramethylguanidinium p-polypropylene phenate was recovered.

Example 3: A solution of 0.1 mol of p-polypropylene phenol in methanol was reacted with 0.1 mol of N,N'-di-o-tolylguanidine at a temperature of 50°C. N,N'-di-o-tolylguanidinium p-polypropylene phenate was recovered. The base reserve additives described above were incorporated into a conventional automatic transmission fluid having the formulation:

	Volume Percent
Blend of neutral and pale hydrocarbon oils	90.4
Alkyl methacrylate/vinyl pyrrolidone polymer	3.0
High molecular weight polyisobutylene	3.0
Diisobornyl diphenylamine	1.0
Zinc dioctyl dithiophosphate	0.5
Calcium sulfonate	2.1

Each fluid described in the table below was tested in an oxidation test to determine its viscosity increase under the test conditions. In this test, the samples were placed in glass tubes containing coils of steel and copper wire as catalysts, and air was bubbled through the solutions. The test was continued for 350 hours at 325°F. The concentration of the guanidine or calcium base reserve agent was 200 meq/kg in each case. Data from these tests are presented in the table below.

Base reserve agent	Concentration, weight percent	Viscosity at 210° F., SUS Before	Viscosity at 210° F., SUS After	Viscosity increase, percent
None		51	ª +205	ª +300
Calcium polypropylene phenate	10	50	ᵇ 194	290
Guanidinium polypropylene phenate (Ex. 1)	6.4	54	61	14
N,N,N',N'-tetramethyl guanidinium polypropylene phenate (Ex. 2)	7.2	50	164	230
N,N'-di-o-tolyl guanidinium polypropylene phenate (Ex. 3)	10	50	69	38

ª Stopped at 230 hours because of excessive viscosity increase.
ᵇ Gelatinous at room temperature.

Aminoguanidine Derivatives

Derivatives of aminoguanidine are prepared and used by *H.J. Andress, Jr.; U.S. Patents 3,809,719; May 7, 1974; and 3,655,560; April 11, 1972; both assigned to Mobil Oil Corp.* for the prevention of gum deposits in fuel oils, lubricating oils and greases. These antioxidants include ketimines of aminoguanidine, aldimines of ketimines of aminoguanidine and aldimines of amides of aminoguanidines.

These antioxidants may be prepared, in general, by reacting an aminoguanidine salt with a ketone to produce the ketimine of aminoguanidine; or the ketimine of aminoguanidine thus produced may be further reacted with an aldehyde to produce the aldimine of the ketimine of aminoguanidine. Each of these reactions can be carried out at 100° to 200°C and in a mol ratio of 1:1. It is also within the scope of the process to react an aminoguanidine salt, an organic acid and an aldehyde, at the above temperature range and in a mol ratio of 1:1:1, to produce the corresponding aldimine of the amide of aminoguanidine. For the above reactions, a wide variety of aminoguanidine salts, ketones, aldehydes, acids and derivatives thereof may be successfully employed. The following examples will illustrate the preparation of the antioxidants and their use as improving agents in organic compositions.

Example 1: A mixture of 68 grams (0.5 mol) aminoguanidine bicarbonate, 110 grams (0.5 mol) methyl coco ketone and 100 grams of benzene diluent was refluxed to a temperature of about 175°C over a period of about 8 hours to produce the methyl coco ketimine of aminoguanidine.

Example 2: To 159 grams (0.5 mol) of the product prepared in Example 1 were added 61 grams (0.5 mol) salicylaldehyde and 100 grams of toluene. The resulting mixture was stirred at a temperature of 175°C for a period of about 3 hours to produce the salicylaldimine of the methyl coco ketimine of aminoguanidine.

Example 3: The salicylaldimine of methyl nonyl ketimine of aminoguanidine was prepared as in Examples 1 and 2 replacing the methyl coco ketone with methyl nonyl ketone.

Example 4: A mixture of 68 grams (0.5 mol) aminoguanidine bicarbonate, 100 grams (0.5 mol) phenylstearic acid and 100 grams benzene was refluxed to a temperature of about 177°C over a period of about 8 hours. The resulting mixture was cooled to 80°C and 61 grams (0.5 mol) salicylaldehyde and 100 grams toluene were added. The resulting mixture was then refluxed to a temperature of about 178°C over a 6-hour period to produce the salicylaldimine of phenylstearyl amide of aminoguanidine.

The oxidation stability of a fuel in the form of gasoline using these aminoguanidine compounds was tested by the Induction Period Method, in accordance with ASTM Test D525. The inhibitor agents as set forth in the table below were blended in a full boiling range catalytically cracked gasoline containing 3 cc of uninhibited tetraethyl lead fluid per gallon within a 100° to 400°F boiling range.

		Induction period in seconds	
Compound	Conc., lbs./ 1,000 bbls.	No added copper	With 0.2 mg. 1 liter copper as copper naphthenate
Base gasoline	0	509	331
Base gasoline plus—			
Ex. 1	10	905	374
Ex. 2	10	>1,200	>1,200
Ex. 3	10	>1,200	>1,200
Ex. 4	10	1,122	893

Unsaturated Polynitriles

S.N. Massie; U.S. Patent 3,723,316; March 27, 1973; assigned to Universal Oil Products Co. has found that undesired oxidation is inhibited by incorporating an alpha, beta-unsaturated polynitrile in an organic substance normally subject to oxidative deterioration. These alpha, beta-unsaturated nitriles may be illustrated by the formula shown on the following page.

$$R_1-\overset{\overset{\displaystyle R_2}{|}}{C}=\overset{\overset{\displaystyle R_3}{|}}{C}-C\equiv N$$

where R_1, R_2 and R_3 are independently selected from hydrogen, alkyl, cyano and cyano-alkyl, at least one being cyano or cyanoalkyl. In a preferred antioxidant, the alkyl groups contain 1 to 10 carbons each. A particularly preferred nitrile is tetracyanoethylene where R_1, R_2 and R_3 are cyano groups in the above formula. Other tetracyano compounds include 1,1,3,3-tetracyano-1-propene, 1,1,6,6-tetracyano-1-hexene, 1,1,3,3-tetracyano-2-methyl-1-propene, etc. Illustrative compounds containing three cyano groups include tricyanoethylene, 1,1,2- and 1,1,3-tricyano-1-propene, 1,1,4-tricyano-2-methyl-1-butene, 1,1,2-tricyano-1-decene, etc. Illustrative dicyano compounds include 1,1- and 1,2-dicyanoethylene (cis and trans), 1,1-, 1,2- and 1,4-dicyano-1-butene, 10,11-dicyano-10-eicosene, etc., as well as dicyano compounds containing branching in the aliphatic chain.

The alpha, beta-unsaturated polynitrile may be used to stabilize any organic substance normally subject to oxidative deterioration. This includes petroleum products, animal and vegetable oils, synthetic polyester lubricants, plastics, resins and elastomers.

Example: This example illustrates the use of tetracyanoethylene as an oxidation inhibitor in cracked gasoline. The gasoline has a boiling range of from 27° to 210°C and contains unsaturated compounds. Upon exposure to air, the gasoline tends to form gum and undergo discoloration. To stabilize the gasoline against such deterioration, 0.005% by weight of tetracyanoethylene is incorporated in the gasoline, and the gasoline is transported and stored in conventional manner. The stabilization of lithium grease, lard and toluene was also covered by other examples in the complete patent.

Polyamide and/or Polyimide Stabilizers

Polymeric stabilizers are disclosed by *H.A. Cyba; U.S. Patent 3,660,289; May 2, 1972; assigned to Universal Oil Products Company* for use in plastics, petroleum lubricants and polyester lubricants. These stabilizers are condensates formed at 175° to 500°F of (a) a polyamine containing at least two primary nitrogens, at least two secondary nitrogens or a mixture thereof, (b) a polyhalopolyhydropolycyclicdicarboxylic acid, corresponding anhydride or ester of the acid and (c) a halogen-free dicarboxylic acid, corresponding anhydride or ester of this second acid.

The polyamine may contain any suitable number of nitrogen atoms and generally will contain 2 to 6 nitrogens per molecule. Illustrative polyamines include ethylenediamine, diethylenetriamine, triethylenetetramine, tetraethylenepentamine, pentaethylenehexamine, and these polyamines in which one or more of the nitrogens is substituted with a hydrocarbon group, which may be aliphatic and particularly alkyl of 1 to 25 or more carbons, aryl and particularly phenyl or naphthyl and/or cycloalkyl containing 4 to 12 carbons in the ring.

Examples of diamines containing one primary and one secondary nitrogen atom are N-alkyl-diaminoalkanes. A particularly preferred amine in this class is N-alkyl-1,3-diaminopropane in which the alkyl group is derived from a fatty acid and contains 8 to 25 carbons. A number of N-alkyl-diaminoalkanes in this class are available commercially, such as Duomeen T and Diam 26 in which the alkyl group is derived from tallow and contains about 12 to 20 carbons per group, mostly 16 to 18 carbons per group.

Another reactant used in preparing the reaction product is a polyhalopolyhydropolycyclic dicarboxylic acid or derivative. In a preferred embodiment the acid or anhydride is used. In one embodiment the acid or anhydride is of the type known as Chlorendic or HET acid or anhydride. This acid is prepared by the Diels-Alder addition reaction of maleic acid and hexachlorocyclo entadiene or more conveniently by the reaction of maleic anhydride and hexachlorocyclopentadiene to form the corresponding anhydride and then hydrolyzed to form the acid. In place of maleic acid or maleic anhydride, other suitable dicarboxylic acids containing carbon to carbon unsaturation may be employed. Illustrative examples include fumaric acid, itaconic acid, citraconic acid, glutaconic acid, etc. Also, in place of hexachlorocyclopentadiene, other suitable halo-substituted cycloalkadienes may be used. Illustrative examples include 1,2-dichlorocyclopentadiene, 1,5-dichlorocyclopentadiene, 1,2,3-trichlorocyclopentadiene, 1,2,3,4-tetrachlorocyclopentadiene, 1,2,3,4,5-pentachloropentadiene and similar compounds in which all or part of the chlorine is replaced by other halogen and particularly bromine.

A preferred reaction product is the Diels-Alder condensation of 1,3-butadiene with maleic anhydride to form 1,2,3,6-tetrahydrophthalic anhydride, followed by the Diels-Alder condensation with hexachlorocyclopentadiene. The product may be named 5,6,7,8,9,9-hexachloro-1,2,3,4,4a,5,8,8a-octahydro-5,8-methano-2,3-naphthalenedicarboxylic anhydride, hereinafter referred to as A anhydride.

The third reactant is a halogen-free dicarboxylic acid, anhydride or ester. In one embodiment the acid is a saturated dibasic acid as illustrated by oxalic acid, malonic acid, succinic acid, glutaric acid, adipic acid, suberic acid, sebacic acid, etc. In another embodiment the acid is an unsaturated acid including maleic acid, fumaric acid, itaconic acid, citraconic acid, glutaconic acid, etc.

The polyamine, polyhalopolyhydropolycyclicdicarboxylic acid or derivative and halogen-free dicarboxylic acid or derivative are reacted in any suitable manner. These reactants are reacted in proportions of 1 to 2 basic equivalents per 1 to 2 acidic equivalents. The reaction generally is effected at a temperature above 175°F and preferably at a higher temperature which usually will not exceed 500°F, although higher or lower temperatures may be employed under certain conditions depending upon whether a solvent is used, and, when employed, on the particular solvent.

These reaction products can be used as an additive in lubricants and function as a detergent, dispersant, extreme pressure additive, as well as serving as a peroxide decomposer, corrosion inhibitor, rust inhibitor, antioxidant, etc. Other substrates which may be improved by the additive include gasoline, naphtha, kerosene, jet fuel, lubricating oil, diesel fuel, fuel oil, residual oil, drying oil, grease, wax, resin, plastic, rubber, etc.

Example: The product is prepared by reacting 2 mol proportions of N-tallow-1,3-diaminopropane, 1 mol proportion of A anhydride and 1 mol proportion of polyisobutene-succinic anhydride, the polyisobutene moiety having an average molecular weight of about 1,200. The reaction product is prepared by refluxing the above reactants in the presence of xylene solvent for about 6 hours, with the water of reaction being continuously removed. Following completion of the reaction, the product is recovered in the xylene solvent and utilized in this manner as an additive.

Evaluation is made by the Falex Test (page 2) using a mineral oil marketed commercially as Carnes 340 White Oil. The unstabilized mineral oil undergoes seizure at a load of less than 500 pounds. In contrast another sample of the oil containing 2% by weight of the reaction product prepared in the above example will not undergo seizure until a load of above 1,200 pounds is attained. In addition to uses of these products as flame retardants and insecticides, the patent also shows the stabilization of polyester lubricants.

PHOSPHORUS-CONTAINING ANTIOXIDANTS

Amine Salts of Bis(Hydroxyalkyl) Phosphinic Acids or Esters

Two processes are disclosed for stabilizing hydrocarbon oil, grease or synthetic lubricant against oxidative deterioration by incorporating an amine salt of bis(hydroxyalkyl) phosphinic acid or ester thereof.

In the first process, *H.A. Cyba; U.S. Patent 3,542,679; November 24, 1970; assigned to*

Universal Oil Products Company discloses the amine salts of bis(hydroxyalkyl) phosphinic acid illustrated by the following formula:

$$
\begin{array}{c}
\text{O} \\
\parallel \\
\text{HO}-\text{R}-\text{P}-\text{R}_1-\text{OH} \\
\mid \\
\underset{\mid}{\text{O}}\text{H}\cdot\text{R}_2-\text{N}-\text{R}_3 \\
\text{R}_4
\end{array}
$$

where R and R_1 are alkyl, R_2 and R_3 are hydrogen or alkyl and R_4 is alkyl or alkenyl. In a particularly preferred embodiment R and R_1 are alkyl containing 1 to 6 carbons, R_2 and R_3 are hydrogen or alkyl containing 1 to 12 carbons and R_4 is alkyl containing 4 to 50 carbons, preferably from 8 to 40 carbons. The number of carbons in the alkyl groups will be selected with reference to the use of the additive. For example, when the additive is used in organic substrates and particularly hydrocarbon oils, a higher number of carbon atoms is desired to insure ready solubility of the additive in the substrate.

In another embodiment of this process, the additive comprises an amine salt of an ester of bis(hydroxyalkyl) phosphinic acid. The ester may be a monoester, a polyester, or mixture thereof, depending upon whether a monocarboxylic acid or polycarboxylic acid is employed in forming the ester and upon the mol ratios of reactants used.

Any suitable amine is used in preparing the salt and may be a primary, secondary or tertiary amine. In a preferred embodiment the amine is an alkyl amine in which the alkyl group or groups may be of primary, secondary or tertiary configuration. Preferred primary amines include those in which R_2 and R_3 in the above formula are hydrogen and R_4 is an alkyl of 4 to 50 carbons and more particularly 8 to 40 carbons. In some cases, high boiling primary amines are available commercially, generally at a lower cost, as mixtures of amines. For example, one such mixture is marketed as Primene 81-R and is said to comprise a mixture of tertiary alkyl amines containing 12 to 14 carbons in the alkyl group. Another mixture is marketed commercially as Primene JM-T and is said to comprise a mixture of tertiary alkyl amines containing 18 to 22 carbons per molecule.

Example 1: The salt of this example was prepared by mixing and heating bis(hydroxymethyl) phosphinic acid and a mixed amine comprising tertiary alkyl amines containing from 18 to 22 carbons per molecule. The mixed amines used in this example are marketed commercially under the name of Primene JM-T. The salt was prepared by commingling, with stirring, 27.2 grams (0.2 mol) of bis(hydroxymethyl) phosphinic acid and 67 grams (0.2 mol) of the mixed amines. The reaction was exothermic. However, in order to insure completion of the salt formation, the reaction mixture was heated to 110°C. This resulted in a very viscous product. In order to prepare a more fluid solution for easier handling, 94 grams of a commercial lubricating oil was added and the mixture was stirred and heated. This resulted in a homogeneous solution of 50% by weight concentration of active ingredient when heated.

Example 2: The salt of this example is the dimethyl octadecyl salt of an ester of bis(hydroxymethyl) phosphinic acid. The salt was formed by commingling 34 grams (0.25 mol) of bis(hydroxymethyl) phosphinic acid and 73 grams (0.25 mol) of the dimethyl octadecyl amine, the mixture was stirred and heated on a steam bath, resulting in the formation of the salt as a white precipitate.

Xylene was added to the reaction mixture while refluxing. This formed a homogeneous solution, to which 70.5 grams of dodecenyl-succinic anhydride was added. Heating and refluxing of this mixture was continued with the temperature of refluxing ranging from 140° to 210°C. A total of 5.2 cc of water was collected from the reaction. The reaction mixture was heated at 165°C under water pumped vacuum to remove the xylene and to recover the salt as the residue. The salt contained 4.18% by weight of phosphorus.

Example 3: Evaluations were made on the Falex Machine (page 2) using a mineral oil marketed as Carnes 340 White Oil. Typical specifications of this oil are shown on the next page.

Distillation range, °F	740 - 975
Specific gravity at 60°F	0.8836
Viscosity:	
At 100°F	360
At 210°F	52.2
Flash point, CIC, °F	440
Pour point, °F	-20
Refractive index at 68°F	1.4805
Saybolt color	+30

Run No. 3 in the table below is a run using no additive and is the blank or control run. Run No. 4 is a run using the white oil to which has been added 4% by weight of the salt solution prepared as described in Example 1 (2% by weight of active ingredient).

	Temperature, ° F.			Torque, lbs.			Wear, teeth			Seizure conditions		
	250	500	750	250	500	750	250	500	750	Load	Time	Tempera-ture,° F.
Run No.:												
3	172	350–S		5–6	30–S		0	S		425	0.1	275
4	158	244	405	4–5	11–14	17–30	0	0	26	1,500	2	700

NOTE.—S=Seizure.

In the second disclosure, tertiary amine salts are disclosed by *H.A. Cyba; U.S. Patent 3,668,237; June 6, 1972; assigned to Universal Oil Products Company.* Here the salts are a tertiary amine salt of a polycarboxylic acid ester of a bis(hydroxyalkyl) phosphinic acid. The composition may be illustrated by the formula:

$$R_3O[-R-\overset{\overset{O}{\|}}{\underset{\underset{R_6}{|}}{\underset{OH \cdot R_4-N-R_5}{P}}}-R_1-O-\overset{\overset{O}{\|}}{\underset{\underset{R_2}{|}}{C}}-(CH)_n-\overset{\overset{O}{\|}}{C}-O-]_mH$$

where R and R_1 are alkyl of 1 to 18 and preferably 1 to 8 carbons, R_2 is hydrogen, a hydrocarbyl or substituted hydrocarbyl group, R_3 is hydrogen or a polycarboxylic acid residue, R_4 R_5 and R_6 are alkyl, alkylene, cycloalkyl, carbons of a heterocyclic ring, or substituted hydrocarbyl in which the substitution is hydroxyl or nitrogen free of hydrogen, n ranges from 1 to 40 and m ranges from 1 to 50 and preferably from 1 to 5.

Any suitable tertiary amine having 3 to 60 carbons can be used to prepare these salts. Generally, there are available commercially tertiary amines in which two of the alkyl groups contain 1 to 4 and possibly 1 to 12 carbons and the third alkyl group is of longer chain and contains 4 to 50 and more particularly 8 to 40 carbons. Because of the ready availability of such tertiary amines, they advantageously are used in preparing the salt. For example, one such tertiary amine is available commercially as Armeen DMHTD and is dimethyloctadecyl amine.

Example 1: The salt of this example is the dimethyloctadecyl amine salt of an ester of bis(hydroxymethyl) phosphinic acid. The tertiary amine used is dimethyl hydrogenated tallow amine and is marketed commercially as Armeen DMHTD. The salt was prepared by commingling 34 grams (0.25 mol) of bis(hydroxymethyl) phosphinic acid and 73 grams (0.25 mol) of the dimethyloctadecyl amine. The mixture was stirred and heated on a steam bath, resulting in the formation of the salt as a white precipitate. Xylene was added to the reaction mixture while refluxing.

This formed a homogeneous solution, to which 70.5 grams of dodecenyl-succinic anhydride was added. Heating and refluxing of this mixture was continued with the temperature of refluxing ranging from 140° to 210°C. A total of 5.2 cc of water was collected from the reaction. The reaction mixture was heated at 165°C under water pumped vacuum to remove the xylene and to recover the salt as the residue. The salt contained 4.18% by weight of phosphorus.

Example 2: The salt prepared as described in Example 1 was evaluated in mineral oil in the same manner and using the same Carnes 340 White Oil as described in U.S. Patent 3,542,679. Run No. 3 in the following table does not contain an additive and is the blank or control run. Run No. 4 is a run made with the white oil to which has been added 2% by weight of the salt prepared as described in Example 1.

Run Number	Temperature,° F.			Torque, lbs.			Wear, teeth			Seizure conditions		
	250	500	750	250	500	750	250	500	750	Load	Time	Temp., ° F.
3.............	172	350–S		5–6	30–S		0	S		425	0.1	275
4.............	159	284	385	4–5	13–15	17–22	0	0	12	1,500	0.1	500

S = Seizure.

In this patent and in U.S. Patent 3,542,679, additional examples were given showing the stabilization of fuel oil, grease and polyester lubricants with these amine salts.

Esters of Phosphorodithioates

A series of antioxidant derivatives of phosphorodithioates has been disclosed by *M. Braid; U.S. Patents 3,544,465; December 1, 1970; 3,654,155; April 4, 1972; and 3,654,154; April 4, 1972; all assigned to Mobil Oil Corporation.* Broadly, these compounds have the structure:

$$[(RO)_2\overset{S}{\overset{\uparrow}{P}}S-\overset{R''}{\underset{|}{C}}H-\overset{R'}{\underset{|}{C}}H-O]_nX(Y)_m(Z)_b(M)_r$$

where R, R' and R" may each be a hydrocarbyl radical, including alkyl, aralkyl, aryl or alkaryl, and substituted derivatives thereof, containing 1 to 30 carbons, and R' and R" may also be hydrogen or a cyclic hydrocarbon ring or heterocyclic ring containing oxygen, nitrogen or sulfur, or a polymeric chain having over 30 carbons, X may be boron, carbon, nitrogen, silicon, phosphorus or sulfur. Y, Z and M may each be oxygen, sulfur, acyl, alkyl, aralkyl, aryl or alkaryl, alkoxy, aralkoxy, aryloxy and alkaryloxy, and when each contains an organic radical, the radical may contain 1 to 30 carbons; n is an integer of 1 to 3 and the total of m, b and r may range from 0 to (v-n), v being the valence of X. Preferably, at least one of m, b or r is at least 1. When X is phosphorus, one or more of Y, Z or M is an organic group.

These esters are strikingly effective as anticorrosion agents and antioxidants in industrial fluids, especially in lubricating oils and are particularly effective in preventing corrosion of copper surfaces. The intermediate product is prepared by a reaction between a diorganophosphorodithioic acid and an organo-1,2-oxide. The acid is produced by known means, usually by the reaction between an alcohol or a phenol or naphthol with phosphorus pentasulfide. This intermediate, which is also referred to as an O,O-diorgano-S-(2-hydroxyalkyl) phosphorodithioate, is then reacted with the reactive acyl, hydroxyl or halogen compound in a condensation reaction to produce the final product.

In another aspect of this process, R' or R" or both may also contain additional epoxy groups, as in the cases of the diepoxides and polyolefin polyoxides. The resulting intermediate reaction product could contain two or more hydroxy groups and diorganophosphorodithio groups attached through the sulfur atom to the β-carbon relative to the hydroxide, as in the abbreviated structure shown:

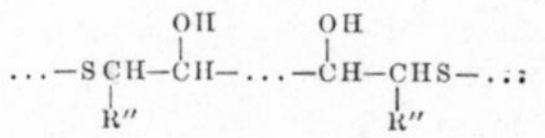

$$...-S\underset{\underset{R''}{|}}{C}H-\overset{OH}{\underset{|}{C}}H-...-\overset{OH}{\underset{|}{C}}H-C\underset{\underset{R''}{|}}{H}S-...; \quad \text{or} \quad ...-S-\overset{OH}{\underset{\underset{R''}{|}}{C}}H-CH-\overset{OH}{C}H-C\underset{\underset{R''}{|}}{H}-S-;;.$$

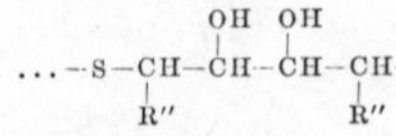

The final products could then have the structure:

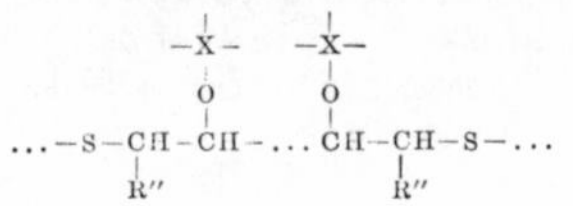

$$...-S-C\underset{\underset{R''}{|}}{H}-\overset{-\overset{|}{X}-}{\overset{|}{\underset{|}{O}}}CH-...CH-\overset{-\overset{|}{X}-}{\overset{|}{\underset{|}{O}}}CH-C\underset{\underset{R''}{|}}{H}-S-... \quad \text{or} \quad ...-S-C\underset{\underset{R''}{|}}{H}-CH....\overset{\diagdown\diagup X\diagdown}{\underset{O\quad O}{}}....CH-C\underset{\underset{R''}{|}}{H}-S-...$$

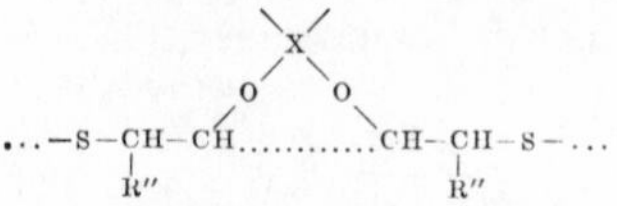

The intermediate is reacted with the active acyl, hydroxyl, or halogen compound, where the nonmetallic atom, X, is attached to 1 to 3 hydroxyl or acyl groups or halogen atoms. Ester formation may take place by condensation with elimination of water, hydrogen halide or acid. As identified above, X may be boron, carbon, nitrogen, silicon, phosphorus or sulfur. When X is boron, suitable reactants include halides, boric, boronic or borinic acids, and partial esters thereof produced by reacting the acid or halide with an alcohol or a phenol.

When X is carbon, such reactants include acyl halides, such as acetyl chloride, propionyl chloride, and the like, acid anhydrides, such as acetic, propionic, butyric anhydride and the like, and acids such as acetic, propionic and the like. When X is silicon, the preferred reactants include mono-organotrihalosilane, diorganodihalosilane, and triorganohalosilane. The groups attached to the silicon atom may also be organo-oxy radicals. Thus Y, Z, and M may include alkyl, aryl, alkaryl and aralkyl and halogen derivatives thereof, as preferred groups.

When X is phosphorus, at least one of Y, Z or M is organic or organo-oxy. Suitable reactants include phosphorus and thiophosphorus acid derivatives, such as mono- or diorganophosphates and phosphonates and their thiophosphorus analogs, pyrophosphates or anhydrides, halophosphites, halophosphates, phosphonyl halides, and their thiophosphorus analogs, and the like. As with the boron compounds, the reactant may be formed in situ by adding a phosphorus or thiophosphorus halide or anhydride to the reaction mixture containing an alcohol or phenol.

When X is sulfur, the reactant is a thionyl or sulfuryl halide, organosulfonyl halide, organosulfonic acid, sulfate ester, bisulfate ester and the like. Thus, Y, Z or M may be an organic or inorganic group or mixtures of the two, or members of one cyclic group, such as a cycloalkyl group or alkylenedioxy or arylenedioxy group. If one substituent attached to X is divalent, a multiple bond linkage may occur as in a carbonyl, sulfoxide or sulfone functional group. The organic radicals may contain from 1 to 30 carbons, and preferably 1 to 20.

Example 1: To a solution of 100 grams (0.32 mol) of O,O-ditolylphosphorodithioate in 100 ml of benzene, 25.2 grams (0.35 mol) of 1,2-butylene oxide is added over a 30 minute period while stirring and maintaining the reaction temperature at about 40°C. The resulting reaction mixture is then heated at 60° to 80°C for 30 minutes, filtered and distilled at reduced pressure to remove solvent and unreacted butylene oxide. There remains 119.4 grams (97% yield) of the reaction product, O,O-ditolyl-S-(2-hydroxybutyl) phosphorodithioate.

Example 2: To the product of Example 1 in 100 ml of benzene there is added 38 grams (0.49 mol) of acetyl chloride while stirring and maintaining the temperature at 50°C. The reaction mixture is then refluxed at 80° to 84°C for 1 additional hour. Solvent and unreacted acetyl chloride is removed by reduced pressure distillation. There remains 139 grams (94% yield) of the esterified product O,O-ditolyl-S-(2-acetoxybutyl) phosphorodithioate.

Example 3: A mixture of 7.3 grams (0.118 mol) of boric acid and 130 grams (0.353 mol) of O,O-ditolyl-S-(2-hydroxypropyl) phosphorodithioate is refluxed in 250 ml of benzene, while the water is distilled off azeotropically and collected in a Dean-Stark tube. When no more water is produced, the reaction mixture is filtered and the solvent is distilled from the filtrate under reduced pressure. The product remaining is the borate ester of the reactant phosphorodithioate, a viscous yellow liquid.

Example 4: To a solution of 80 grams (0.209 mol) of O,O-ditolyl-S-(2-hydroxybutyl) phosphorodithioate, 13.7 grams (0.105 mol) of isooctyl alcohol, and 60 grams (0.6 mol) of triethylamine in 300 ml of benzene there is added over a period of about 30 minutes 14.4 grams (0.105 mol) of phosphorus trichloride while stirring and maintaining the temperature at 25° to 40°C. After addition is completed the reaction mixture is heated for about 1.5 hours at 45° to 52°C and then hydrolyzed. The organic layer is separated, dried and distilled under reduced pressure to remove solvent. There remains 94 grams of the isooctyl phosphite ester of the phosphorodithioate, a clear, slightly viscous liquid.

Example 5: To a solution of 100 grams (0.272 mol) of O,O-ditolyl-S-(2-hydroxypropyl) phosphorodithioate in 100 ml of benzene there is added over a 30 minute period while stirring at 86°C, a solution of 16.2 grams (0.136 mol) of thionyl chloride in 100 ml of benzene. After addition is completed, stirring and heating at 83°C is continued for about 5.5 hours with continuous evolution of hydrogen chloride. Benzene and unreacted thionyl chloride are removed from the reaction mixture by distillation under reduced pressure. The crude sulfite ester of the phosphorodithioate remains as a clear brown viscous liquid.

Example 6: To a solution of 73.7 grams (0.2 mol) of O,O-ditolyl-S-(2-hydroxybutyl) phos- phorodithioate in 200 ml of benzene there is added over a 30 minute period while stirring at 30° to 42°C, 12.9 grams (0.1 mol) of dichlorodimethylsilane. After addition is completed, the reaction mixture is stirred and heated at 81°C for about 4 hours. Solvent is removed from the reaction mixture by distillation under reduced pressure. There remains 78.5 grams of the crude dimethylsilyl ester of the phosphorodithioate, a slightly viscous yellow liquid.

Evaluation of Products: The compounds produced were blended into a refined mineral oil lubricant and tested in an oxidation test. A sample of the test composition is heated to 325°F and air at the rate of about 10 liters per hour is passed through for a period of about 40 hours. Present in the test sample are specimens of iron, copper, aluminum, and lead. The loss in the weight of lead sample is measured, as are the increase in kinematic viscosity measured at 210°F (percent KV change) and the change in the neutralization number (NN change).

It should be noted that the metals are typical metals of engine or machine construction, and they also provide some catalysis for oxidation of organic materials. The compositions are also rated for oxidation stability, the numbers being based on the amount of phosphorus present in the sample required to limit the neutralization number increase to a maximum of 2.0. The results are tabulated in the table below.

Additive of Example	Conc., wt. percent	NN change	Percent KV change	Lead loss, mg.	Stability
None		20.75	271	80	....
2	1	0.22	13	1.1	....
3	0.25	0.92	15	4	....
4	1	7.10	48	0.5	....
	0.5	4.70	47	12.9	....
5	1	0.33	8	0	....
	0.5	1.25	43	1.5	....
6	1.0	−0.19	8	0.9	....
	*0.5	1.17	8	1.4	....

*With 3% by weight of a boron-containing non-metallic detergent.

Phosphorodithioate Ester-Aldehyde Adducts

M. Braid; U.S. Patent 3,644,206; February 22, 1972; assigned to Mobil Oil Corporation has also disclosed a process for production of antioxidants by the reaction between dior- ganophosphorodithioate esters and hindered aldehydes, i.e., those having no alpha-hydrogen atoms. The reaction is one of addition rather than condensation. Broadly, this process has to do with a reaction product of a phosphorodithioate ester, having the structure:

$$\begin{array}{c} RO \\ \diagdown \\ RO \diagup \end{array} P \begin{array}{c} \diagup S \\ \diagdown \\ SH \end{array}$$

where each R is a hydrocarbyl or substituted hydrocarbyl radical having 1 to 35 carbons, with an aldehyde having no alpha-hydrogen atoms.

Preferably the aldehydes have the structures:

$$
\underset{H-\overset{O}{\overset{\|}{C}}-[Cy],}{} \quad
\underset{H-\overset{O}{\overset{\|}{C}}-\underset{\underset{R''}{|}}{\overset{R'}{\overset{|}{C}}}-R''',}{} \quad
\text{or} \quad
\underset{H-\overset{O}{\overset{\|}{C}}-\underset{\underset{R''}{|}}{\overset{R'}{\overset{|}{C}}}=C-R'''}{}
$$

where Cy is a cyclic radical including an aromatic radical, a cyclic alkenyl radical, substituted cyclic alkyl radical or a heterocyclic radical; and the R', R" and R''' are hydrocarbyl groups, such as alkyl, cycloalkyl, aralkyl, aryl, and alkaryl, each having 1 to 20, and preferably 1 to 10, alkyl carbons and these groups may be the same or different. R, R', R" and R''' may also be substituted by halogen, hydroxy, alkoxy, amino, nitro, alkylthio, or cyano groups, and the like. The reaction is believed to occur at the carbonyl group of the aldehyde. Condensation does not occur, since the product no longer contains a carbonyl group, and the formation of water as a side product is not observed.

The aldehydes used in this process are hindered such that the carbon attached to the carbonyl carbon contains no hydrogen atoms. Thus, the 2-carbons may be a member of an aromatic nucleus. Benzaldehyde, naphthoic aldehyde, anthraldehyde, and substituted derivatives thereof are contemplated as suitable. As for the nonaromatic aldehydes, suitable representatives include the 2,2-substituted aldehydes, such as 2,2-dimethylpropionaldehyde, 2,2-dimethylbutyraldehyde, and the like.

The cyclic aldehydes include cycloalkenyl aldehydes having one or more unsaturated bonds, in which the carbonyl group is attached to an unsaturated carbon. Typical of this class are cyclopentyl, cyclohexyl, cyclohexadienyl and the like; the heterocyclic aldehydes, as represented by those containing pyridyl, unsaturated piperidyl and pyrrolidyl, furyl, and thiophenyl; and the alpha-substituted cycloalkyl aldehydes.

The reaction between the aldehyde and the phosphorodithioate ester simply involves the mixing of the two components alone or in the presence of an inert organic solvent, such as benzene, toluene, hexane and the like. The reaction is usually maintained at a moderate temperature, preferably from 20° to 150°C. The reaction appears to involve an equal number of mols of the phosphorodithioate and of the aldehyde. Product analysis shows this 1:1 ratio regardless of whether the phosphorodithioate ester is added to the aldehyde reactant or the reverse additive is employed. The molar ratio of reactants may range from about 0.5 to 2:1 of the phosphorodithioate to the aldehyde, preferably 1:1. The specific structure of the reaction product cannot be determined with certainty, however it is believed to be the carbonyl adduct.

Example 1: To a solution of 62.5 grams (0.5 mol) of 4-cyano-2,2-dimethylbutyraldehyde in 200 ml of benzene there is added while stirring at 68° to 70°C during 1 hour 130 grams (0.5 mol) of crude O,O,di-n-butylphosphorodithioate. After the addition is completed the reaction mixture is stirred at 68° to 70°C for a total of 5 hours. The reaction mixture is then subjected to reduced pressure distillation to remove solvent and remaining reactants. There remains 189 grams of a reddish clear liquid addition product.

Example 2: To a solution of 130 grams (0.5 mol) of crude di-n-butylphosphorodithioate in 200 ml of benzene there is added while stirring during about 1 hour 62.5 grams (0.5 mol) of 4-cyano-2,2-dimethylbutyraldehyde. The temperature is maintained at 38° to 40°C during the addition by ice bath cooling and the reaction mixture is then stirred at 40° to 50°C for an additional 1.75 hours. The reaction mixture is washed with 20% sodium carbonate solution. The organic layer is then washed with water, dried and distilled under reduced pressure to remove solvent and remaining reactants. The addition product remains as a clear amber liquid.

The reaction products may be used in a number of organic fluids and solids to prevent the oxidation deterioration thereof. Primarily, these additives are used in lubricating oils, such as petroleum mineral oils, and synthetic hydrocarbon oils, synthetic polyester lubricants, olefin-derived fluids, and polymers thereof.

Evaluation of Products: The products were evaluated as antioxidants in a mineral oil stock at a number of concentrations. The oil is a solvent refined mineral oil. In the oxidation test, air is passed through an oil sample containing the additive at the rate of 5 liters per hour for 40 hours. The temperature of the sample is held at 325°F. Present in the oil are samples of iron, copper, lead and aluminum. The neutralization number and the kinematic viscosity of the oil sample (at 210°F) are measured before the test and afterward to determine increase in acidity, in thickening and sludge formation caused by oxidation of the oil. The lead sample is weighed before and after the test to measure any weight loss, as a further indication of the effects of oxidation. The following results were obtained:

Additive	Concentration, weight percent	ΔNN	KV Increase, percent	Lead Loss, mg
None	–	17.0	230	39
Product of Example 1	1.0	0.27	17	11
	0.5	3.53	21	23
	0.25	9.71	61	4.0
Product of Example 2	1.0	0.53	12	5.0
	0.5	9.66	78	38.0
	0.25	13.48	93	28.0

1-(O,O-Diorganophosphorodithiato)Alkyl Carboxylates

H. Myers; U.S. Patents 3,646,172; February 29, 1972; and 3,350,348; October 31, 1967; both assigned to Mobil Oil Corporation has produced antioxidants by reacting an O,O-diorganophosphorodithioic acid with a vinyl-type carboxylate. The compounds produced have the structure:

$$\left[(RO)_2 - \overset{\overset{S}{\uparrow}}{P} - S - \underset{\underset{R''}{|}}{C}H - O - \overset{\overset{O}{||}}{C} - R' \right]_n$$

where n is 1 or 2; R is an alkyl, including both primary and secondary alkyl, or cycloalkyl or alkenyl radical containing 1 to 18 carbons, especially alkyl and alkenyl having at least 6 carbons, or an aryl, alkylaryl or alkenylaryl radical having 1 to 5 alkyls attached to the aromatic nucleus, the alkyl containing 1 to 12 carbons and having a total of up to 18 carbons or a hydroxy or halogen derivative of the above-defined alkyl (especially hydroxyalkyl containing at least 6 carbons) or aryl radical; R' is hydrogen or an alkyl or cycloalkyl or alkenyl radical or (when n is 2) an alkenylene or arylene radical having 1 to 11 carbons; or an aryl radical, such as phenyl or naphthyl, or aralkyl or alkaryl or an alkenylaryl radical, the aromatic nucleus being substituted with up to 5 alkyl groups each having 1 to 12 carbons with a total number of up to 18 carbons or the halo derivatives thereof; and R" is alkyl, haloalkyl and aralkyl having similar substituent groups as R' above. Suitable dicarboxylates include oxalates, succinates, maleates, fumarates, phthalates, or cyclohexane dicarboxylates.

The following examples and test results illustrate the typical manner of carrying out and utilizing this process. Parts and percentage in these examples unless otherwise specified are on a weight basis.

Example 1: Into a flask equipped with a stirrer, condenser, dropping funnel and thermometer are added 484.6 grams (2 mols) of the O,O-diisobutylphosphorodithioic acid and thereafter with stirring 258.3 grams (3.0 mols) of vinyl acetate are added dropwise to the acid over a half-hour period. The temperature during this addition is maintained at 78°C. At the end of the addition period, the reaction mixture is heated for 1 hour at a temperature ranging from 85° to 90°C. The reaction mixture is then passed into a rotary film evaporator heated by a boiling water bath and the unreacted vinyl acetate removed under reduced pressure. The yield of 1-(O,O-diisobutylphosphorodithiato)ethyl acetate is 650.9 grams of an amber-colored oil indicating a yield of about 99%.

Example 2: Several products prepared by the method of Example 1 were evaluated by the oxidation stability test and the bearing corrosion test.

Oxidation Stability Test: The product is added to a solvent-refined, mineral lubricating oil, heated to 325°F and dry air at the rate of 10 liters per hour is passed through it in the presence of iron, copper, aluminum and lead. After 40 hours the neutralization number for each composition is obtained using the ASTM D 974-1 method or procedure. The additives are rated in terms of the minimum weight percent of phosphorus required to limit the rise in the neutralization number to 2.0. The additives which are effective at approximately 0.125% or less by weight of phosphorus are deemed to be satisfactory additives.

Bearing Corrosion Test: The minimum amount of the additive to be tested is added to a solvent-refined mineral base oil in the presence or absence of a detergent and the oil composition is used to lubricate a copper-lead bearing in a CRC L-38 test engine run for 40 hours. At the end of the run the test bearing is removed and weighed. If there is a loss of weight of the bearing of over 50 mg, the lubricating oil is deemed to have failed. Selected data obtained in the above tests are given in the table below.

	Phosphorus, percent*	Bearing Weight Loss, mg
1-(O,O-diisobutylphosphorodithiato)ethyl acetate	0.087	4
1-(O,O-dioleylphosphorodithiato)ethyl acetate	0.098	8
1-(O,O-dimethylphosphorodithiato)ethyl acetate	0.112	22
1-(O,O-diisodecylphosphorodithiato)ethyl acetate	0.059	25**
No additive	–	3,669

*In oxidation stability test
**Detergent present

Polymeric Metal Dialkaryldithiophosphates

Monomeric metallic dialkaryldithiophosphates are employed as oxidation and corrosion inhibitors and antiwear extreme pressure additives in petroleum hydrocarbon compounds, such as lubricating oils, fuels, greases, and asphalts. In lubricating compositions, high temperature performance has become more and more critical. Modern, more efficient engines are designed to operate at increasingly higher temperatures and under more severe conditions, and the lubricating oils and greases must withstand these high temperatures with as little deterioration as possible.

T.V. Liston; U.S. Patent 3,654,328; April 4, 1972; assigned to Chevron Research Company has found that the polymeric metal dialkaryldithiophosphates show excellent thermal stability in the thermogravimetric test. These polymeric metal dialkaryldithiophosphate compositions are produced by first polymerizing a bisphenol, or alkylene-di-p-phenol, with phosphorus pentasulfide, followed by reaction of the resulting polymeric dithiophosphate with a Group II metal. The product polymer contains at least two monomer units. The polymeric compositions are predominately of the following recurring monomeric unit:

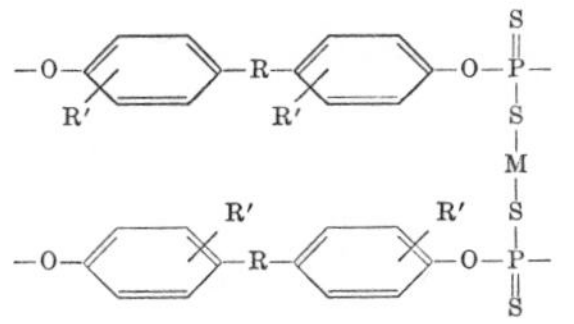

where R is a bivalent alkylene radical of 1 to 50 carbons, preferably 5 to 30 carbons; R' is an alkyl radical of 1 to 15 carbons, with the provision that when R is C_1 to C_3 alkylene, R' will be at least C_6 to impart oil solubility to the molecule; and M is a Group II metal. The R' radical may be attached at any position ortho- or meta- to R. These polymeric compositions include among their properties the ability to withstand degradation, measured by weight loss, at temperatures of about 800°F. This thermal stability is obtained without any adverse effect on the antioxidant and extreme pressure properties of the composition when used as an additive in lubricants. The metal dithiophosphates are used in lubricating oils in amounts sufficient to inhibit oxidation; that is, 0.25 to 20% by weight, preferably from 1.5 to 10% by weight. The following examples will illustrate the preparation and use of these compounds.

Example 1: p-(1-Methyl-1-hydroxy)decylanisole was refluxed for 16 hours in a toluene solution of p-toluenesulfonic acid. After separation of the water of reaction and removal of the solvent, the product dimer was dissolved in alcohol and hydrogenated overnight with 1,350 psig hydrogen at 100° to 300°F in the presence of 5% palladium on carbon. The hydrogenated dimer was then dissolved in acetic acid and reacted with hydrogen iodide by stirring at reflux temperature for about 60 hours in a nitrogen atmosphere. The bisphenol product 10-methyl-10,12-di(4'-hydroxyphenyl)heneicosane was recovered at greater than 98% of theoretical yield.

The bisphenol was dissolved in xylene and, under a nitrogen atmosphere, was heated to 100°C. Phosphorus pentasulfide was added, and the temperature raised to 135°C. The mixture was stirred for about 16 hours. An 87% yield of polymeric O,O'-dialkaryl dithiophosphoric acid was obtained. This material was dissolved in toluene and reacted with zinc carbonate. The final product was filtered and stripped and yielded a polymeric zinc dialkaryl-dithiophosphate having a number average molecular weight of 4,065. With the alkaryl portion of the polymer being derived from the described bisphenol, this number average molecular weight defines a polymer having a number of approximately 3.3 monomer units. This material was labeled Polymer A. A similar reaction produced a polymer (Polymer B) having a number average molecular weight of 3,445, corresponding to a number average of approximately 2.8 monomer units.

Example 2: Polymers A and B were subjected to the Falex Machine Test to determine EP characteristics, (see page 2). The additive was dispersed in a base oil consisting of a neutral oil having a viscosity of 480 SUS at 100°F and a gravity of 29° API and containing 5% by weight of a polyisobutenyl succinimide detergent additive and a small amount of terephthalic acid as a copper-lead corrosion inhibitor. In two tests the base oil containing Polymer A had a Falex failure point of 1,190 and 1,250 pounds, while the oil containing Polymer B had a Falex failure point of 1,060 pounds. The base oil containing only 3.5% by weight of the succinimide failed at 970 pounds.

Bismethylene Amides of Phosphoric or Phosphonic Acids

A process for preparing these bismethylene amides and the use of these compounds in lubricants have been disclosed by *K. Hunger; U.S. Patents 3,725,278; April 3, 1973; and 3,646,134; February 29, 1972; both assigned to Farbwerke Hoechst AG, Germany.* Broadly, these compounds are bismethylene amides of phosphoric or phosphonic acids and their thio-derivatives of Formula 1:

(1)
$$\begin{array}{ccc} R_1 & Z & R_3 \\ \diagdown & \parallel & \diagup \\ C{=}N{-}P{-}N{=}C \\ \diagup & \mid & \diagdown \\ R_2 & X & R_4 \end{array}$$

where R_1, R_2, R_3 and R_4, which may be identical or different, each represent lower alkyl radicals, especially alkyl radicals containing 2 to 6 carbons, the cyclohexyl or phenyl, mono- or di-chloro- or bromophenyl radical or an alkylphenyl radical containing 1 to 4 carbons in the alkyl groups, or R_1 and R_2 as well as R_3 and R_4, respectively, together stand for an alkylene radical containing 4 to 5 carbons as part of a cycloalkyl radical, X represents an alkyl radical containing 1 to 12 carbons, the cyclohexyl, phenyl or an alkylphenyl radical containing 1 to 9 carbons in the alkyl group, which radicals may be bound to the phosphorus atom via oxygen or sulfur, or a morpholino or dialkylamino radical the alkyl groups of which contain 1 to 4 carbons and Z represents oxygen or sulfur.

Compounds of Formula 1 are prepared by reacting a ketimine of Formula 2:

$$(2) \qquad \begin{array}{c} R_1 \\ \diagdown \\ C=NH \\ \diagup \\ R_2 \end{array}$$

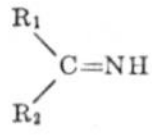

in which R_1 and R_2 have the meanings above, or a mixture of such ketimines in an organic solvent and in the presence of anhydrous bases for binding the hydrogen halide set free, either with a dihalogenophosphorus compound of Formula 3:

$$(3) \qquad \begin{array}{c} Y-P-Y \\ | \\ X \end{array}$$

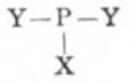

in which X has the meaning given above and Y is chlorine or bromine, and is then exposed to the action of an oxidizing agent or sulfur to form the compounds of Formula 1, or is reacted with a dihalogenophosphorus compound of Formula 4:

$$(4) \qquad \begin{array}{c} Z \\ \| \\ Y-P-Y \\ | \\ Z \end{array}$$

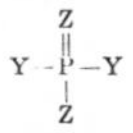

where X, Z and Y have the meanings given above, to form directly the compounds of the Formula 1. The reaction of the ketimines with the dihalogenophosphorus compounds proceeds smoothly at temperatures of from $-30°$ to $+80°C$. Preferably, the reaction is carried out at $0°$ to $+30°C$ in the absence of oxygen, suitably under an inert atmosphere, for example, under nitrogen or carbon dioxide.

As anhydrous bases for binding the hydrogen halide set free during the reaction, there may be used bases that contain tertiary nitrogen atoms, for example, pyridine, triethylamine, picoline, dialkyl-aniline, lutidine or even alkali alcoholates. As organic solvents, there may be used those inert towards the reaction partners which dissolve the starting materials to a sufficient degree. There may be mentioned, for example, dialkyl ethers, aliphatic or aromatic hydrocarbons, halogenated hydrocarbons, nitriles or mixtures of such solvents. If suitable organic bases are selected, these may simultaneously serve as solvents.

Owing to their extraordinary antioxidizing action and to their thermic stabilizing properties, connected with a very low volatility, these bismethylene amides are highly effective as additives to lubricants that are exposed to a high thermic stress in an oxidizing atmosphere, for example, motor oils. The additives may also be used for the stabilization of other aliphatic or aromatic hydrocarbons or of mineral oil products, for example, asphalt, furthermore for the stabilization of synthetic or natural high polymers, for example, rubber or of polyolefins. The following examples illustrate the preparation and use of these compounds.

Example 1: 20.0 grams (0.115 mol) of dichlorophosphorous acid n-butyl ester were added dropwise, while cooling with ice, to a solution of 41.5 grams (0.229 mol) of diphenyl-ketimine and 23.2 grams (0.229 mol) of triethylamine in 300 ml of benzene. After heating to room temperature, 3.7 grams (0.115 mol) of sulfur powder were added and the whole mixture was heated for 2 hours to $50°C$. After cooling to $20°C$, the triethylamine hydrochloride was filtered off with suction, the filtrate was evaporated under reduced pressure and the residue was recrystallized twice from ethanol. There were obtained 44 grams (77% of the theory) of the compound below having a melting point $126°C$.

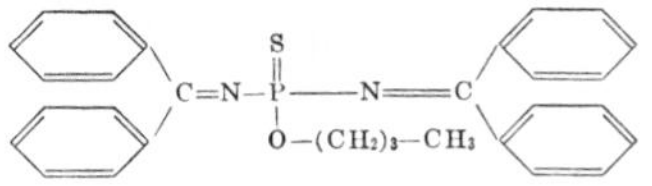

Example 2: Test for Stability to Oxidation — 0.75% by weight of the substance to be tested was dissolved in samples of a mineral oil mixture (500 grams of a mixture of Kirkuk mineral oils of the types HVI 160 B and HVI 65, at a ratio by weight of 1:4) with addition of 15 ppm of iron and 20 ppm of copper in the form of iron and copper stearate as catalysts. The whole was placed into a closed system and then oxygen was pumped through the oil. The time required for the absorption of 25 ml of oxygen was determined. The test was carried out at 160°C. The results of these tests are shown in the following table. For comparison, the known compounds (A) and (B) were also used in the test. Product (A) was 1,1-bis-(3,5-di-tert-butyl-4-hydroxyphenyl)-methane; Product (B) was N,N'-bis-(diphenylamido)-thiophosphoric acid-O-ethyl ester.

Additive		Oxidation, minutes
1	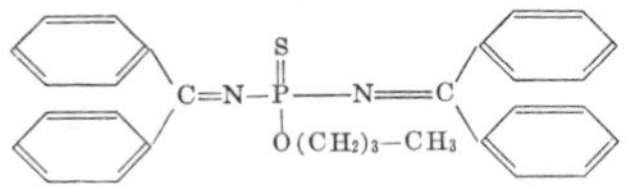	220
2	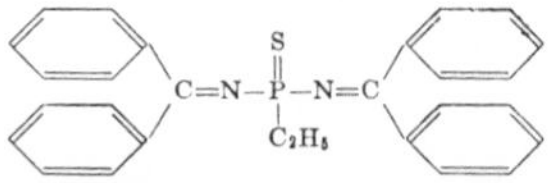	275
3	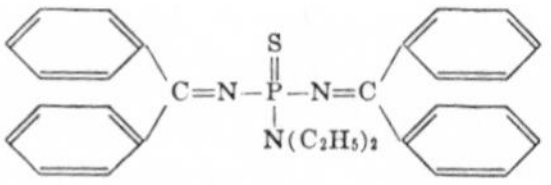	355
No additive		20
A		185
B		100

Amine Derivatives of Dithiophosphonic Acids

Processes for stabilizing lubricating oils and preparing the dithiophosphoric acid derivatives used as antioxidants are disclosed by *K. Pollak; U.S. Patents 3,637,499; January 25, 1972; and 3,546,324; December 8, 1970; both assigned to Esso Research and Engineering Co.* Broadly, the additive is a dithiophosphoric acid neutralized with a monoamine or polyamine. The dithiophosphoric acid is prepared by treating an N-(hydroxy-containing hydrocarbyl) alkenyl-substituted C_3 to C_8 monocarboxylic amide with P_2S_5. The hydrocarbyl referred to is alkyl, cycloalkyl, aryl, or alkylaryl containing 1 to 30 carbons, preferably 1 to 12 carbons. The hydrocarbyl may also include alkoxyalkyl, alkoxyaryl, iminoalkyl and iminoaryl C_1 to C_{30} radicals having the formula $+R-X\}_n R-X-R$ where X represents oxygen or nitrogen, n represents an integer from 0 to 10 and R represents an alkyl and/or aryl group.

A preferred amide is N-(hydroxy-containing C_1 to C_6 alkyl) alkenyl-substituted C_3 to C_8 monocarboxylic amide. Even more preferred is N-di(hydroxy-containing C_1 to C_6 alkyl) alkenyl-substituted C_3 to C_8 monocarboxylic amide. The alkenyl group referred to is C_2 to C_5 olefin polymerized to a molecular weight of 400 to 3,000. The N-(hydroxy-containing hydrocarbyl) alkenyl-substituted C_3 to C_8 monocarboxylic amide is prepared by simple reaction between a hydroxy-containing amine and an alkenyl-substituted C_3 to C_8 monocarboxylic acid under conditions of amide formation. In general, the alkenyl-substituted C_3 to C_8 monocarboxylic acid may be derived from an alpha, beta-unsaturated monocarboxylic acid of 3 to 8 carbons and the C_2 to C_5 monoolefin polymer in accordance with well-known techniques.

Example 1: This illustrates the preparation of a polyisobutenyl propionic acid. A 110-pound portion of polyisobutylene of 780 molecular weight (as determined by osmometry) was heated to 250°F, then a stream of chlorine was passed through the heated polyisobutylene at the 250°F temperature at a rate of 2.5 pounds of chlorine per hour for a total of 4 hours, the total chlorine treated thus being 10 pounds. A sample of the chlorinated product analyzed 4.3% chlorine and had an API gravity of 23.3. To the chlorinated polyisobutylene there was added 10.5 pounds of acrylic acid. Over a period of 2 hours the temperature was raised from 250° to 425°F and the pressure was increased to 20 psig. Heating was continued for 5 hours at 425°F and the reaction vessel was vented to maintain the pressure of 20 psig. The pressure was then released and the mixture was purged with nitrogen for 2 hours to remove unreacted acrylic acid. The polyisobutenyl propionic acid thereby obtained weighed 109.3 pounds and had a total neutralization number (ASTM D-644) of 46.2 mg of KOH per gram. The chlorine content was found to be 0.3% by weight.

Example 2: Into a glass reaction vessel fitted with a mechanical stirrer, heating mantle, thermometer and condenser containing 1,245 grams of polyisobutenyl propionic acid produced in the manner of Example 1 (number average molecular weight 1,245, ASTM Neut. No. 45) in 1,000 grams of a solvent neutral mineral oil (150 SUS viscosity at 100°F) there were charged 105 grams of 2,2'-iminodiethanol. The resulting mixture was then heated at about 300°F for a period of 16 to 18 hours.

The reaction mixture was then cooled to 150°F whereupon 111 grams of P_2S_5 was added over a period of 15 minutes. Upon completion of the P_2S_5 addition, the mixture was heated at 300°F for 4 hours. The mixture was cooled to room temperature and 52.5 grams of diethylene triamine was slowly added over a period of 30 minutes. After stirring for 1 hour, the product was filtered through Dicalite in the cold. The final product recovered totaled 2,322 grams of which 55% by weight was additive product, the remainder being the mineral oil.

Example 3: A number of routine tests were carried out on a typical base oil containing the additive to illustrate the beneficial effects derived therefrom. The following tests were performed.

Oxidation Stability Test: This test was used for a laboratory evaluation of the antioxidant properties of the additive. This test involves heating the compound oil to a temperature of about 340°F in the presence of a copper-lead oxidation catalyst while intimately mixing the compounded oil with air at the rate of 2 cfh. The viscosity increase (SUS, at 100°F) after 23 hours is measured and a determination of the percentage of viscosity increase over that of the original unoxidized oil is made.

Copper-Lead Bearing Weight Loss Test: This test (in milligrams) involving the compounded oil was also conducted. The measure of the change in weight of the Cu-Pb catalyst in the first test, in milligrams is determined.

Oxidation Stability Test

Oil tested	Percent viscosity increase SUS at 100° F., 23 hours	Cu-Pb bearing weight loss, mg.
Base oil alone................................	85	143
Base oil plus 5.0 weight percent of product of Example 2 (55 weight percent active ingredient)........................	8.6	27
Base oil plus 5.5 weight percent of PIBA/TEPA condensate [1]................	110	330
Base oil plus 5.0 weight percent of PIBA/TEPA condensate [1] plus 0.5 weight percent ethyl 728...............	85	223
Base oil plus 3 weight percent of PIBA/TEPA condensate [1] plus 0.5 weight percent ethyl 728 [2] plus 2.0 weight percent of product of Example 2......	7.2	28

[1] Condensation product of 3 parts by weight of polyisobutenyl propionic acid (830 molecular weight) and 1 part by weight of tetraethylenepentamine (50% A.I.).
[2] Bisphenol antioxidant.

THIOORGANOMETALLIC COMPLEXES

A known technique for improving the stability of lubricants and particularly motor oils to oxidation consists of adding zinc dithiophosphates, dithiocarbamates, phenols or amines as antioxidants. These products have the following disadvantages: their antioxidant activity is rather low, particularly in the presence of such metals as iron and copper; they are affected by temperature increases; they produce sludge; and, they are corrosive with respect to certain engine parts, for example, the silver bearings.

C. Blejean and B. Bourdoncle; U.S. Patent 3,764,534; October 9, 1973; assigned to Institut Francais du Petrole, des Carburants et Lubrifiants, France have found that the thioorganometallic complexes defined below have a high antioxidant acitivity, even at high temperature and in the presence of metals at high concentrations. These compounds may be used as well with base oils of petroleum origin as with synthetic base oils. They give good antiwear and extreme pressure properties to the lubricating oils to which they are added. These thioorganic complexes have the formula:

where M may be tin, antimony, lead, bismuth, zinc, cadmium or a transition metal element, for example, chromium, manganese, iron, cobalt, nickel or copper, the element M, at the oxidation degree n, being linked with n coordinates, either identical or different, as defined below.

R_1 and R_2 are each a monovalent radical which may be a hydrocarbon, for example, an aliphatic, alicyclic or aromatic radical, or a halo- or nitro- derivative thereof. They may contain 1 to 3 heteroatoms such as oxygen, sulfur or nitrogen. They usually contain 1 to 20 carbons. Y is a hydrogen atom or a radical R', R'—O—, R'—S— or R'—CO— in which R' is a monovalent hydrocarbon radical of 1 to 20 carbons. Y and R_1 or R_2 may form a divalent hydrocarbon radical of 1 to 20 carbons with 0 to 3 oxygen, sulfur or nitrogen atoms. Each Z may be oxygen or sulfur, provided that at least one Z is sulfur in at least one of the coordinates.

The thioorganic complexes may be manufactured according to known methods in U.S. Patent 3,184,410, pertaining to molybdenum complexes, as well as the *Bulletin of the Chemical Society of Japan,* Volume 40, 2819-2822 (1967). The synethesis of the thioorganic complexes which are used in this process comprises the step of sulfurizing an available or manufactured β-diketone. Hydrogen sulfide may be used, for example, as the sulfurizing agent, either in acidic medium or not, optionally in a solvent. This sulfurization may be carried out in the presence of a salt of the desired metal.

In that case, there is obtained the desired thioorganic complex or a mixture of complexes of the given formula. When the sulfurization is carried out without a metal salt, there is obtained, in some cases, a monothioketone or a dithioketone, or a mixture of both, or a mixture of one or two of them with the starting β-diketone. It is sufficient as a rule, to contact the desired salt of metal with the ketones or their mixtures to obtain a thioorganic complex or a mixture of thioorganic complexes of the given formula. The outstanding antioxidant properties that the thioorganic complexes confer to the lubricating oils appear to result from the hydroperoxides destruction power and the reactivity with free radicals of these complexes.

Examples 1 through 5: The thioorganometallic complexes of the table below have been mixed with the base oils in the given amounts. The resulting mixtures have been subjected to a particularly severe oxidation test in which the sample is vigorously stirred with iron naphthenate (6 ppm) and lead oxide (6 grams per liter) at 160°C in oxygen, and then the amount of oxygen absorbed in 7 hours is noted. The lower this amount, the better the resistance to oxidation of the mixture. By way of comparison a pure base oil of the solvent type, a base oil of the solvent type containing a conventional antioxidant and a pure synthetic oil of the ester type have been subjected to the same test. The results are given in the table below.

Example number	Oil	Additive	Amount, percent b.w.	Absorbed oxygen, moles/liter
	200 neutral solvent (zarzaitine)			14.2
	do	Zincdialkyldithiophosphate (8.7 % b.w. of zinc).	0.25	8.32
1	do	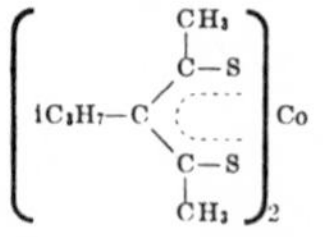 (structure)	0.30	6.54
2	do	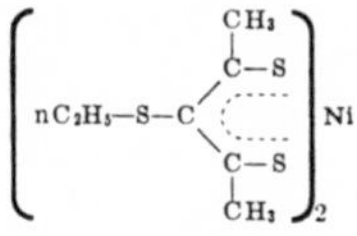 (structure)	0.15	0.11
3	do	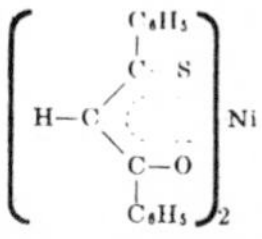 (structure)	0.20	0.16
4	do	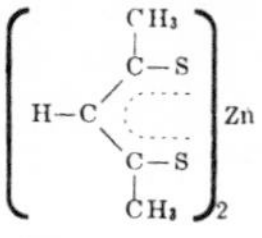 (structure)	0.20	0.09
	2-ethyl hexyl sebacate	None		12.4
5	do	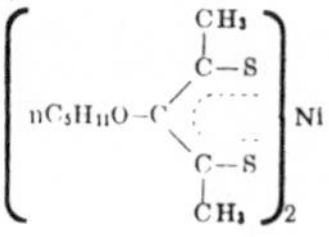 (structure)	0.20	0.28

Example 1 structure:

$$\left[\ iC_3H_7-C\ \begin{matrix} CH_3 \\ | \\ C-S \\ \vdots \\ C-S \\ | \\ CH_3 \end{matrix}\ \right]_2 Co$$

Example 2 structure:

$$\left[\ nC_2H_5-S-C\ \begin{matrix} CH_3 \\ | \\ C-S \\ \vdots \\ C-S \\ | \\ CH_3 \end{matrix}\ \right]_2 Ni$$

Example 3 structure:

$$\left[\ H-C\ \begin{matrix} C_6H_5 \\ | \\ C-S \\ \vdots \\ C-O \\ | \\ C_6H_5 \end{matrix}\ \right]_2 Ni$$

Example 4 structure:

$$\left[\ H-C\ \begin{matrix} CH_3 \\ | \\ C-S \\ \vdots \\ C-S \\ | \\ CH_3 \end{matrix}\ \right]_2 Zn$$

Example 5 structure:

$$\left[\ nC_3H_{11}O-C\ \begin{matrix} CH_3 \\ | \\ C-S \\ \vdots \\ C-S \\ | \\ CH_3 \end{matrix}\ \right]_2 Ni$$

SYNERGISTIC AND OTHER MIXED ANTIOXIDANT SYSTEMS

Mixtures of Metal Dialkyldithiocarbamate and tert-Alkylamines

D. Milsom; U.S. Patent 3,707,498; December 26, 1972; assigned to Cities Service Oil Co. has developed antioxidant additives for hydrocarbon lubricating oils that are effective at low concentrations and for extended periods of time. These additives comprise mixtures of metal dialkyldithiocarbamates and tertiary-alkyl primary amines. Metal dialkyldithio-carbamates and tertiary-alkyl primary amines are known and used individually as antioxidants in lubricating oils. However, when a mixture of a metal dialkyldithiocarbamate and a tertiary-alkyl primary amine is incorporated in a hydrocarbon lubricating oil there is an unexpectedly enhanced resistance of the lubricating oil to oxidative degradation.

The metals usually associated with the dialkyldithiocarbamates are from Groups IIb, IVa, and Va of the Periodic Table. The preferred metals are zinc, cadmium, lead, and antimony. Each of the alkyl groups of the metal dialkyldithiocarbamate will contain 3 to 10 carbons and may be straight chain or branched. The two alkyl groups in any one metal dialkyl-dithiocarbamate molecule may be either the same or different. Examples of suitable metal dialkyldithiocarbamates are zinc di-n-butyldithiocarbamate, zinc diamyldithiocarbamate, lead diamyldithiocarbamate, cadmium dipropyldithiocarbamate, antimony propyloctyldi-thiocarbamate, and the like.

The preferred dialkyldithiocarbamates are cadmium diamyldithiocarbamate and a 50% by weight solution in oil of an antimony dialkyldithiocarbamate having the trade name of

Vanlube 73. The tertiary-alkyl primary amine component of the additive has 8 to 30 carbons and preferably 12 to 22 carbons. The amines are saturated and are, of course, characterized in that they are primary-amines in which the amino nitrogen is attached to a tertiary-carbon of an alkyl group. Examples of suitable amines are tertiary-octylamine, 1-methyl-1-ethyl-n-dodecylamine, etc. The preferred amines are a mixture of C_{12} to C_{14} tertiary-alkyl primary amines, sold under the trade name Primene 81-R, and a mixture of C_{18} to C_{22} tertiary-alkyl primary amines, sold under the trade name Primene JM-T.

The antioxidant additive contains tertiary-alkyl primary amine and metal dialkyldithiocarbamate at a weight ratio of 0.5:1 to 10:1, and preferably 1:1 to 9:1, amine to carbamate. Where the additive is a mixture of Primene JM-T and cadmium diamyldithiocarbamate, a preferred weight ratio is 2:1 to 5:1. Where the additive is a mixture of Primene JM-T and the antimony dialkyldithiocarbamate (Vanlube 73), a preferred weight ratio is 2:1 to 7:1. The hydrocarbon lubricating oil compositions contain 0.5 to 4.5% by weight, and preferably 1.0 to 3.5% by weight, of the antioxidant additive. Where the additive is a mixture of Primene JM-T and cadmium diamyldithiocarbamate, the lubricating oil contains 1.0 to 2.5% by weight of additive. Where the additive is a mixture of Primene JM-T and Vanlube 73 which is 50% by weight of an antimony dialkyldithiocarbamate in oil, the lubricating oil composition contains 1.0 to 3.5% by weight of the active ingredients of the additive.

Example: Several oil compositions are prepared by dissolving antioxidant additives in a major proportion of a hydrocarbon gas engine oil and the oil compositions are subjected to the catalyzed oxidation test. The additives are cadmium diamyldithiocarbamate and Primene JM-T. For comparison, a base gas engine oil containing no antioxidant and gas engine oil compositions containing cadmium diamyldithiocarbamate alone and Primene JM-T along are also subjected to the catalyzed oxidation test. For each oil composition, the end point of the test is the time in hours for the viscosity at 210°F to increase by 2.5 SUS.

The difference in time for each composition relative to the time for the base oil is recorded as △ hours. The table below contains the results of the catalyzed oxidation tests and the amount of each component of the additive. All percents are weight percents of the total oil compositions.

Cadmium diamyl- dithiocarbamate, wt. percent	Primene JM-T, wt. percent	End point, hrs.	△ hours
		53	0
		141	88
	1.0	53	0
0.4	0.5	156	103
0.4	1.0	208	155
0.4	2.0	180	127
0.4	3.0	175	122

Metal Dialkyldithiocarbamate-Metal Sulfonate Mixtures

A second long acting antioxidant mixture has been developed by *D. Milsom; U.S. Patent 3,772,197; November 13, 1973; assigned to Cities Service Oil Company* for lubricating oils. This antioxidant additive comprises a metal dialkyldithiocarbamate and a Group IIa metal sulfonate. The metal dialkyldithiocarbamates in this additive mixture are the same as described in U.S. Patent 3,707,498.

The Group IIa metal sulfonate component of this antioxidant is the oil-soluble Group IIa metal salt of either a synthetic sulfonic acid or a natural sulfonic acid. The synthetic sulfonates are derived from the sulfonation of synthesized alkylated aromatic hydrocarbons and the natural sulfonates are derived from the fuming sulfuric acid treatment of hydrocarbon oils. Chemically, the natural sulfonates are sulfonates of mixtures of alkyl aryl molecular structures of varying molecular weights. The alkyl aryl sulfonic acids from which the Group IIa metal sulfonates are prepared have average molecular weights in the range from 400 to 520. The average molecular weights of the Group IIa metal sulfonates are in the range from 840 to 1,180 and preferably from 940 to 1,030. While Group IIa metal sulfonates in general may be used in this antioxidant additive, barium and calcium sulfonates are preferred. Lubricating oil compositions containing these additives have unexpectedly superior resistance to oxidative degradation as evidenced by their ability to withstand long periods of use without appreciable sludge formation, viscosity increase, and acid number increase. This is of particular utility in sour gas engine operation where the additive increases engine oil life from about 400 hours to greater than about 2,500 hours.

Example: Several oil compositions are prepared by dissolving the antioxidant additives of this process in a major proportion of a hydrocarbon gas engine oil and the oil compositions are subjected to the catalyzed oxidation test. The additives are comprised of cadmium diamyldithiocarbamate and the Group IIa metal sulfonate is the barium sulfonate containing barium carbonate which is marketed under the tradename of Bryton Hybase. For comparison, a base gas engine oil containing no antioxidant and gas engine oil compositions containing cadmium diamyldithiocarbamate alone and Bryton Hybase alone are also subjected to the catalyzed oxidation test.

For each oil composition, the end point of the test is the average time, in hours, based on the above-mentioned parameters of viscosity increase, acid number increase, and capacitance loss. The difference in time to reach the end point for each composition relative to the time for the base oil to reach the end point is recorded as Δ hours. The table below contains the results of the catalyzed oxidation tests and the amount of each component of the additive. All percents are weight percents of the total oil compositions.

Cadmium Diamyl Dithiocarbamate, weight percent	Bryton Hybase, weight percent	Barium Sulfonate, weight percent	End Point, hours	Δ, hours
–	–	–	53	–
0.4	–	–	141	88
–	1.0	0.47	36	-17
0.4	0.5	0.24	181	128
0.4	1.0	0.47	188	135
0.4	2.0	0.94	148	95
0.4	3.0	1.41	146	93
0.4	10.0	4.7	133	80

The data in the above table show that the addition of cadmium diamyldithiocarbamate alone improves resistance to oxidative degradation while the addition of a barium sulfonate alone causes a reduction in resistance to oxidative degradation. Surprisingly, when a mixture of cadmium diamyldithiocarbamate and a barium sulfonate is incorporated in the oil, there is a marked improvement in the resistance to oxidative degradation which clearly illustrates the synergistic interaction of metal dialkyldithiocarbamates and Group IIa metal sulfonates as antioxidants.

Zinc Dialkyldithiophosphate-Zinc Dialkylphenoxyethyldithiophosphate Mixtures

A synergistic antioxidant mixture comprosing zinc dialkyldithiophosphate and zinc dialkylphenoxyethyldithiophosphate is disclosed by *T.O. Brown and J.H. Cupit; U.S. Patent 3,720,613; March 13, 1973; assigned to Texaco Inc.* This mixture provides improved oxidation resistance, nitration inhibition and antiwear properties to a wide variety of organic oil substrates.

These synergistic combinations are useful in any natural and synthetic, hydrocarbon and substituted hydrocarbon oil substrate where oxidative or thermal degradation is a problem. Among such oil substrates are included lubricating oils such as those of the aliphatic ester type; oils of animal and vegetable origin; saturated and unsaturated hydrocarbons such as gasolines, jet fuels, diesel oils, mineral oils, fuel oils, drying oils and greases.

For purposes of convenience and brevity, the zinc dialkyldithiophosphate will be referred to by the designation ZADP and the zinc dialkylphenoxyethyldithiophosphate will be referred to by the designation ZPEP.

Example 1: This example illustrates the synergistic stabilization by the use of these blends. The ZADP used was the zinc salt resulting from the reaction of a mixture of methylisobutyl carbinol and isopropanol with phosphorus pentasulfide in about a 2.7:2.3:1.0 mol ratio and then neutralizing the resulting dithiophosphoric acid with zinc oxide. The ZPEP used was the zinc salt of dinonylphenoxyethyldithiophosphate prepared by reacting p-nonyl phenoxyethyl alcohol with phosphorus pentasulfide and then neutralizing the resulting acid with zinc carbonate.

Example 2: The respective additives were admixed with a paraffinic base oil at a temperature of 130°F with stirring for a period of 30 minutes. The resulting oil sample was then run in a Climax Model V-125 4-cycle natural gas engine for one month. Used crankcase oil samples were withdrawn at seven day intervals and at the end of the test. The samples were then tested for the rate of viscosity increase, the rate of oxidation as determined by measuring the neutralization number of the sample and the rate of oxidation and nitration as measured by the Nitro Oxidation Test.

This test consisted of bubbling an air-NO_2 gas mixture [~0.2 vol % NO_2] through a 150 cc oil sample for 4.5 hours at a gas flow rate of 68 cc/min and an oil temperature of 280°F. Differential infrared analysis was then run on the used oil sample with the degree of oxidation and nitration being determined by measuring the peaks at 5.85 and 6.14 microns, respectively. The results are presented in the following table.

Additives	Percent by Weight	
ZADP (as in Example 1)	0.795	0.88
ZPEP (as in Example 1)	0.265	0
Alkenylsuccinimide (dispersant)	6.0	6.0
Polymethacrylate (pour depressant)	0.12	0.12
Silicone (antifoamant)	150	150
Zinc, in blend (ppm)	0.1	0.1
Test Results		
Viscosity increase rate (SUS at 100°F/100 hrs)	11.7	11.2
Increase in neutralization number after 600 hours service	0.96	1.9
Differential infrared value (abs/cm after 600 hours service)		
5.85 microns (oxidation)	8.75	10.7
6.14 microns (nitration)	7.0	10.0

Five Component Synergistic Additive Blends

A lubricating composition resistant to oxidation at bulk oil temperatures of 300°F and above has been developed by *W.D. Foucher, Jr., W.R. Siegart and H.C. Morris; U.S. Patent 3,732,167; May 8, 1973; assigned to Texaco Inc.* This composition comprises a major proportion of a mineral lubricating oil containing in combination:

(1) 0.1 to 2.5% of an alkylated diphenylamine of the formula:

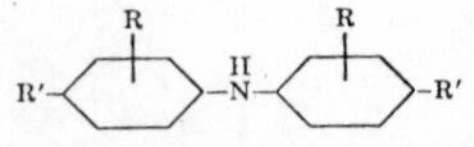

where R is an alkyl radical having 1 to 4 carbons and R' is an alkyl radical having 4 to 16 carbons;

(2) 0.1 to 0.5% of a zinc dithiophosphate of the formula:

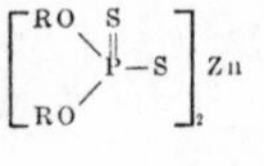

where R is a hydrocarbyl radical or a hydroxy substituted hydrocarbyl having 4 to 12 car bons;

(3) 0.5 to 5.0% of a monohydroxyalkyl hydrocarbyl phosphonate having the formula:

$$R-\overset{\overset{\displaystyle X}{\|}}{\underset{\underset{\displaystyle OH}{|}}{P}}-O-\overset{\overset{\displaystyle R'}{|}}{\underset{\underset{\displaystyle H}{|}}{C}}-\overset{\overset{\displaystyle R''}{|}}{\underset{\underset{\displaystyle H}{|}}{C}}-OH$$

where R is a hydrocarbyl radical having at least 12 carbons, R' and R" are selected from hydrogen and monovalent aliphatic hydrocarbyl radicals containing 1 to 6 carbons and X is sulfur;

(4) 0.5 to 5.0% of an oil-soluble, basic amino nitrogen-containing addition type methacrylate copolymer derived from an alkyl methacrylate copolymer derived from an alkyl methacrylate in which the alkyl radical has 4 to 20 carbons and dialkylaminoalkyl methacrylate in which the alkyl radicals have a total of 4 to 8 carbons, the copolymer containing 0.1 to 3.0% by weight of basic amino nitrogen and having an inherent viscosity of 0.1 to 30; and

(5) 0.25 to 3.5% of a calcium carbonate overbased calcium sulfonate having 5 to 30 mols of dispersed calcium carbonate per mol of calcium sulfonate and having a Total Base Number ranging from 100 to 300.

Examples of typical alkylated diphenylamines include 2,2'-diethyl-4,4'-tert-dioctyldiphenylamine, 2,2'-dimethyl-4,4'-tert-dioctyldiphenylamine, and 2,2'-dipropyl-4,4'-tert-dibutyldiphenylamine. Examples of zinc dithiophosphates include zinc isobutyl 2-ethylhexyl dithiophosphate, zinc di(2-ethylhexyl) dithiophosphate, and zinc di(2,4-diethylphenoxyethyl) dithiophosphate.

The mono-hydroxyalkyl hydrocarbyl thiophosphates used in the mixture can be prepared by reacting alkylene carbonates, such as ethylene carbonate or propylene carbonate, with a hydrocarbyl thiophosphonic acid. The reaction of alkylene carbonate with hydrocarbyl thiophosphonic acid is usually effected in the presence of an alkaline catalyst, such as potassium carbonate. The preferred hydrocarbyl radical is a polybutene radical having a molecular weight between 600 and 5,000.

The copolymers used in the additive mixture are described in detail in U.S. Patent 2,737,496. They should introduce an oil-solubilizing or oleophilic structure to insure that the polymer is soluble to the extent of at least 0.1% by weight in naphthenic or paraffinic lubricating oils. In addition, the presence of basic amino groups, either primary, secondary or tertiary is necessary to impart the unique sludge dispersing properties which characterize these polymers.

The preferred overbased calcium sulfonate used in these additives will have from 10 to 20 mols of dispersed calcium carbonate per mol of calcium sulfonate. The preparation of this component is fully described in U.S. Patent 3,537,996. The motor oil composition was tested in a laboratory engine test designed to simulate extreme service conditions and called an Oxidative Oil Test.

In the laboratory engine test, a 1969 Ford 289-CID V-8 engine was installed on a dynamometer test stand instrumented to control engine operating conditions. The engine was modified by replacing the filter housing with a blank plate and by enclosing the engine oil pan with 1 inch thick fiber glass insulation around the outside. The test stand included an intake air temperature control to maintain a prescribed carburetor inlet air temperature. The automotive radiator was submerged in a water tank with means to control the engine jacket water temperature.

The engine in the laboratory engine test was operated under the following conditions:

Engine speed, rpm	3,200
Load, BHP	105
Jacket outlet, °F	233 ± 2
Intake air, °F	115
Exhaust back pressure, in Hg	5
Oil pressure, psi (min)	30
Spark advance, °BTC	32
Air-fuel ratio	14.0 ± 0.5

Base Oil A, used in preparing the lubricating oils was a blend of mineral oils of lubricating viscosity having the following inspections tests.

Gravity, °API	31.0
Flash, COC °F	410
Viscosity, SUS at:	
0°F (extrap)	7,500
100°F	160
210°F	44

The compositions of a lubricating oil and a comparison oil on a weight percent basis and the terminal increase in viscosity are shown in the table below.

Oxidative Oil Test

Motor oil	A	B	C	D	E
Base oil A	92.56	92.06	92.06	92.06	92.06
Mono (2-hydroxyethyl) polybutene (1,100) average mol wt. thiophos-phonate)	3.00	3.00	3.00	3.00	3.00
Basic amino nitrogen-containing addition type methacrylate copolymer[1]	2.00	2.00	2.00	2.00	2.00
Zinc isopropyl methyl isobutyl carbinyl dithiophosphate	1.09	1.09	1.09	1.09	1.09
Calcium carbonate overbased calcium sulfonate[2]	1.35	1.35	1.35	1.35	1.35
2,2'-diethyl-4,4-tertiary dioctyldiphenylamine[3]		0.5			
Anti-oxidant 450[4]			0.5		
Dimethylaniline				0.5	
Anti-oxidant 237					0.5
Terminal increase in viscosity at 100° F., percent	741	113	543	666	790

[1] Copolymer of butyl, lauryl, stearyl and dimethylaminoethyl methacrylates in 21:53:22:4 weight ratio.
[2] Approximately 15 moles of dispersed calcium carbonate per mole of calcium sulfonate, 300 TBN.
[3] Commercial mixture in which approximately ½ is 2,2'-diethyl-4-tert. octyldiphenylamine.
[4] Commercial anti-oxidants.

Run B in the above table illustrates the outstanding improvement in Motor Oil B as compared to other motor oil compositions including C, D and E which contained a variety of oxidation inhibitors.

Substituted Phenol-Thiobisphenol Mixtures

Highly efficient lubricating oils have been developed by *T. Fujisawa, G. Tsuchihashi, T. Takahashi and Y. Okada; U.S. Patent 3,745,117; July 10, 1973; assigned to Sagami Chemical Research Center and Daiko Oil Co., Ltd., Japan* using a mixture of phenol additives. These additives comprise a 4,4'-thiobisphenol, and a substituted phenol having at least one tertiary butyl group in the ortho position to the hydroxyl group.

The 4,4'-mono-, di- or trithiobis(2,6-di-tert-butylphenols) to be used in the stabilizing mixture are compounds represented by the formula shown on the following page.

$$\text{HO}-\underset{\underset{\overset{|}{\text{H}_3\text{C}-\overset{\overset{\text{CH}_3}{|}}{\underset{|}{\text{C}}}-\text{CH}_3}}{\overset{\overset{\text{CH}_3}{|}}{\underset{|}{\text{H}_3\text{C}-\text{C}-\text{CH}_3}}}}{\bigcirc}-\text{S}_x-\underset{\underset{\overset{|}{\text{H}_3\text{C}-\underset{|}{\text{C}}-\text{CH}_3}}{\overset{\overset{\text{CH}_3}{|}}{\text{H}_3\text{C}-\text{C}-\text{CH}_3}}}{\bigcirc}-\text{OH}$$

In the above formula x is an integer of 1 to 3. The compounds in the additives are substituted phenols having 1 or 2 tertiary-butyl groups in the ortho position to the hydroxyl group, for example, 2,6-di-tert-butyl-p-cresol, 2,6-di-tert-butyl-4-ethylphenol, 4,4'-methylenebis(2-tert-butyl-5-methylphenol) and also 4,4'-bis(2-tert-butyl-5-methylphenol) and the like.

The amount of a thiobisphenol and the substituted phenols to be used in the mixed additives may vary depending on the use of the lubricating oil. The ratio of the thiobisphenols to the substituted phenols in amount may also vary accordingly. Generally, a thiobisphenol is used in an amount of less than 5% by weight based on the weight of total composition, preferably 0.01 to 0.1% by weight, while substituted phenols in an amount of less than 5% by weight, preferably 0.1 to 0.5% by weight, respectively. In other words, about 1 to 50 parts by weight of the substituted phenol is used for each part by weight of the thiobisphenol.

Examples 1 through 20: By using a solvent refined lubricating base oil, a commercially available rust preventative, an antifoamer, 0.50% of 2,6-di-tert-butyl-para-cresol and thiobisphenols illustrated in the table below, 20 turbine oil blends were prepared. An oxidation stability test was conducted on each of these turbine oils on the basis of ASTM D 943. The results are shown in the table below.

Turbine Oil Oxidation Stability Test

Ex. No.	Composition	Time required for the total acid value to reach 1.0 mg. KOH/g. (hr.)
1*	Base oil A [1]	1,120
2*	Base oil A and 0.01% of organic zinc dithiophosphate.	1,310
3	Base oil A and 0.05% S [3]	3,040
4	Base oil A and 0.05% SS [4]	3,690
5*	Base oil A and 0.01% of 4,4'-thiobis (6-t-butyl-o-cresol).	1,260
6	Base oil A and 0.01% S [3]	2,820
7	Base oil A and 0.01% SS [4]	2,960
8	Composition in Example 2 and 0.01% S [3]	2,800
9	Composition in Example 2 and 0.01% SS [4]	2,910
10	Composition in Example 2 and 0.05% SS [4]	3,170
11*	Base oil B [2]	1,220
12	Base oil B and 0.01% of organic zinc dithiophosphate.	1,340
13	Base oil B and 0.01 S [3]	2,750
14	Base oil B and 0.05% S [3]	3,070
15	Base oil B and 0.01% SS [4]	2,860
16	Base oil B and 0.05% SS [4]	3,570
17	Composition in Example 12 and 0.01% S [3]	2,720
18	Composition in Example 12 and 0.05% S [3]	2,980
19	Composition in Example 12 and 0.01% SS [4]	2,690
20	Composition in Example 12 and 0.05% SS [4]	3,110

[1] The lubricating base oil contains 0.50% of 2,6-di-tertiary butyl para-cresol. This base oil used is from the Middle East and is solvent refined. It contains 0.52% of sulfur and has 31.50 centistokes of kinematic viscosity at 37.8° C. and 5.18 centistokes of kinematic viscosity at 98.9° C., respectively.

[2] The lubricating base oil contains 0.50% of 2,6-di-tertiary butyl para-cresol. This base oil used is from the Middle East and is solvent refined. It contains 0.32% of sulfur and has 30.30 centistokes of kinematic viscosity at 37.8° C. and 5.09 centistokes of kinematic viscosity at 98.9° C., respectively.

[3] 4,4'-thiobis (2,6-di-t-butylphenol).

[4] 4,4'-dithiobis (2,6-di-t-butylphenol).

* Reference example.

Mixtures of Dihydrocarbyl Tin Sulfides with Phenolic Antioxidants

Synergistic systems of antioxidants have been developed by *J.D. O'Neill; U.S. Patents 3,442,806; May 6, 1969; 3,530,069; September 22, 1970; 3,692,679; September 19, 1972; all assigned to Ethyl Corporation* containing a dihydrocarbyl tin sulfide plus a phenolic antioxidant. These mixtures are eminently useful for stabilizing lubricants. For example, they improve the stability of mineral oils and greases; silicon-containing oils and greases including the siloxanes, silanes, and silicate esters; fluorocarbon oils and greases; diester oils and greases, aromatic ether oils and greases; phosphate ester oils and greases; polyalkylene glycol oils and greases; synthetic hydrocarbon oils and greases formed from polybutene oils and other low molecular weight polyolefin oils and tetrahydrofuran polymer oils and greases. Broadly, these synergistic stabilizers comprise:

(A) from 1 to 99% by weight of a tin compound having the formula

(1)

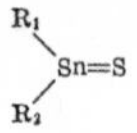

$$\begin{array}{c} R_1 \\ \diagdown \\ \diagup Sn{=}S \\ R_2 \end{array}$$

where R_1 and R_2 are independently selected from alkyl radicals containing 1 to 12 carbons, cycloalkyl radicals containing 6 to 12 carbons, aralkyl radicals containing 7 to 12 carbons and aryl radicals containing 6 to 12 carbons; and

(B) from 1 to 99% by weight of a compound selected from

(1) compounds having the formula

(2)

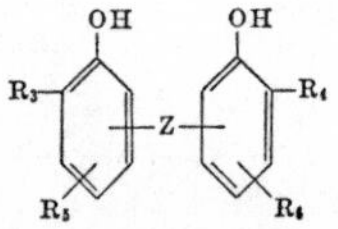

where R_3 and R_4 are alpha-branched alkyl radicals containing 3 to 20 carbons, alpha-branched aralkyl radicals containing 7 to 20 carbons, or cycloalkyl radicals containing 6 to 20 carbons; R_5 and R_6 are hydrogen, alkyl radicals containing 1 to 20 carbons, cycloalkyl radicals containing 6 to 20 carbons, or aralkyl radicals containing 7 to 20 carbons, and Z is a divalent linking radical selected from sulfide radicals having the formula $-S_n-$ where n is an integer from 1 to 3, alkylidene radicals containing 2 to 12 carbons and alkylene radicals containing 1 to 12 carbons;

(2) compounds having the formula

(3)

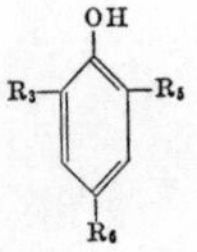

where R_3, R_5 and R_6 are previously defined;

(3) compounds having the formula

(4)

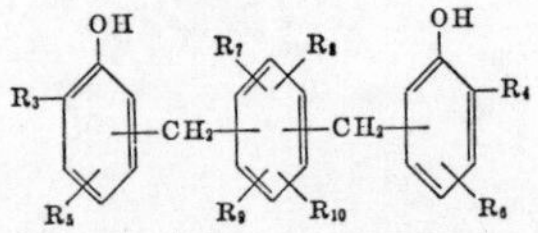

where R_3 R_4, R_5 and R_6 are previously defined and R_7, R_8, R_9 and R_{10} are selected from hydrogen, hydroxyl, alkyl radicals containing 1 to 6 carbons, radicals having the formula $-OR_{11}$ where R_{11} is selected from alkyl radicals containing 1 to 6 carbons, radicals having the formula below;

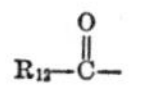

$$R_{12}-\overset{\text{O}}{\underset{}{C}}-$$

where R_{12} is selected from alkyl radicals containing 1 to 6 carbons, aryl radicals containing 6 to 12 carbons, and aralkyl radicals containing 7 to 18 carbons; and radicals having the formula:

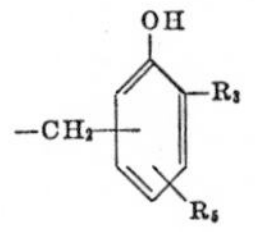

where R_3 and R_5 are previously defined;

(4) compounds having the formula

(5)

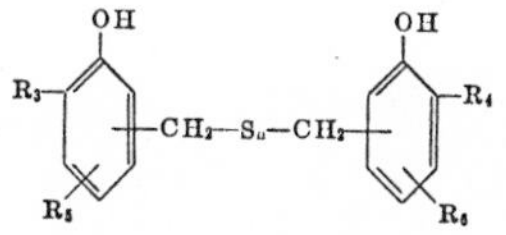

where n is an integer from 1 to 3, and R_3, R_4, R_5 and R_6 are previously defined;

(5) compounds having the formula

(6)

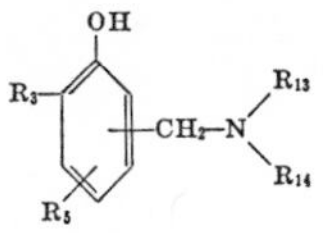

where R_3 and R_5 are previously defined, and R_{13} and R_{14} are selected from alkyl radicals containing 1 to 12 carbons, aryl radicals containing 6 to 18 carbons, aralkyl radicals containing 7 to 18 carbons, and radicals having the formula

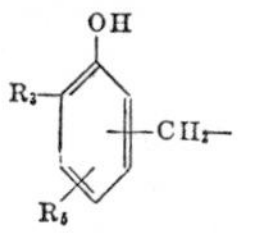

where R_3 and R_5 are previously defined;

(6) compounds having the formula

(7)

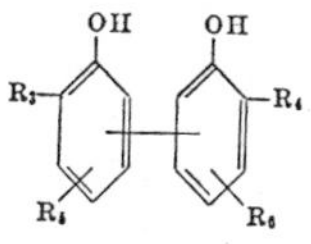

where R_3, R_4, R_5 and R_6 are previously defined; and

(7) compounds having the formula

(8)

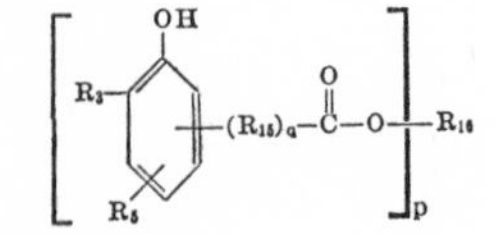

where R_3 and R_5 are previously defined, R_{15} is a divalent hydrocarbon radical containing 1 to 3 carbons, R_{16} is a hydrocarbon radical containing 1 to 20 carbons and having the valence p, p is an integer from 1 to 4, and q is an integer from 0 to 1.

Example 1: Seven one-hundredths parts of 50% dibutyltin sulfide and 50% pentaerythritol-tetrakis[3(3,5-di-tert-butyl-4-hydroxyphenyl)propionate] are blended with 99.93 parts of tricresyl phosphate. Tricresyl phosphate has a viscosity of 25°C of 285 SUS, its flash point is 250°C, its boiling range at 10 mm of mercury is between 275° and 290°C and its autoignition temperature is above 1000°C.

The synergistic stabilizers impart outstanding oxidative and thermal stability to hydrocarbon-derived lubricating oils. To demonstrate this property comparative tests were conducted. The test used was the Panel Coker Test. This test is described in *Aeronautical Standards of the Departments of Navy and Air Force,* Spec. MIL-L 7808C, dated Nov. 2, 1955. In the test, a solvent-refined neutral hydrocarbon lubricating oil is placed in a sump under a metal plate heated to 550°F. The oil is periodically splashed against the heated plate and allowed to drain back into the sump. The oil is splashed for 5 seconds and drained for 55 seconds. This cycle is repeated for 10 hours.

Following this, the metal plate is washed with hexanes and the weight gain determined. Any gain in weight is due to thermal and oxidative breakdown of the oil leaving a carbonaceous deposit. The first series of tests were carried out employing as stabilizers dibutyltin sulfide, 4,4'-methylene bis(2,6-di-tert-butylphenol), and the combination of the two. The deposit weight formed is shown in the following table.

Additive	Conc., %	Deposit wt.
4,4'-methylene bis(2,6-di-tert-butylphenol)	1	143
Di-butyl tin sulfide	0.1	22
Do	0.5	13
4,4'-methylene bis(2,6-di-tert-butylphenol)	1	4
Di-butyl tin sulfide	0.1	

As the above data shows, 0.1% dibutyltin sulfide results in a deposit of 22 mg. On increasing the amount of dibutyltin sulfide five-fold, to 0.5%, the deposit weight only decreases to 13 mg. Surprisingly, the combination of 0.1% of dibutyltin sulfide with 1% of 4,4'-methylene bis(2,6-di-tert-butylphenol) resulted in a deposit weight of only 4 mg. This, despite the fact that 1% of 4,4'-methylene bis(2,6-di-tert-butylphenol) by itself gave 143 mg of deposit.

Further tests were conducted with sulfur-bridged bisphenols. The combination tested was 4,4'-thiobis(2,6-di-tert-butylphenol) and 4,4'-thiobis(2-methyl-6-tert-butylphenol), both in combination with dibutyltin sulfide. The following results were obtained.

Additive	Conc., %	Deposit wt.
4,4'-thiobis(2,6-di-tert-butylphenol)	1	6
4,4'-thiobis(2-methyl-6-tert-butylphenol)	1	16
Di-butyl tin sulfide	0.1	22
4,4'-thiobis(2,6-di-tert-butylphenol)	1	4
Di-butyl tin sulfide	0.1	
4,4'-thiobis(2-methyl-6-tert-butylphenol)	1	8
Di-butyl tin sulfide	0.1	
Do	0.5	37
4,4'-thiobis(2,6-di-tert-butylphenol)	0.5	137
Di-butyl tin sulfide	0.5	4
4,4'-thiobis(2,6-di-tert-butylphenol)	0.5	

Referring to the above table, it is seen that 1% of 4,4'-thiobis(2-methyl-6-tert-butylphenol) resulted in 16 mg of deposit, and 0.1% dibutyltin sulfide yielded 22 mg of deposit. The combination of the two gives a lubricant which formed only 8 mg of deposit.

Even more striking are the results obtained with 4,4'-thiobis(2,6-di-tert-butylphenol). At the 1% level it gives a lubricating oil depositing 6 mg. However, when combined with 0.1% dibutyltin sulfide, which by itself gives a lubricating oil depositing 22 mg, a highly stable oil yielding only 4 mg of deposit is obtained. Even when the amount of 4,4'-thiobis(2,6-di-tert-butylphenol) and dibutyltin sulfide is decreased 50% the oil still retains its unusual stability and yields only a 4 mg deposit. The following example shows the use of an aminophenol as the phenolic compound of the synergistic mixture.

Example 2: Three one-hundredths part of 30% diphenyltin sulfide and 70% 2,6-di-tert-butyl-α-dimethylamino-p-cresol are blended with 99.97 parts of a commercial polybutene oil. The oil has a molecular weight of approximately 330, a viscosity of 114 SUS at 100°F, and a viscosity of 40.6 SUS at 210°F. Its viscosity index is 101, its flash point is 230°F, and its pour point is –65°F.

Other examples in the patent show the addition of these synergistic stabilizers systems to polyethylene, polypropylene, polystyrene, PVC, polyvinyl acetate, polyesters, polymethyl methacrylate, polytetrafluoroethylene, polychlorotrifluoroethylene, various silane and siloxanes, SBR, NBR, natural rubber and lithium greases.

Imide-Amine Phosphate Mixtures

It is known that the reaction products of polyhalopolyhydropolycyclicdicarboxylic acid or derivatives thereof with certain amino compounds possess desirable properties as additives to organic substrates, particularly lubricating oils. It also has been demonstrated that phosphate salts of such reaction products also were extremely effective as additives for such use.

This process by *E.J. Latos and R.H. Rosenwald; U.S. Patent 3,635,823; January 18, 1972; assigned to Universal Oil Products Company* is based on the discovery that mixtures of the reaction products and of certain phosphate salts are very effective additives for use in organic substrates and particularly in lubricating oils.

The synergistic mixture comprises (1) the reaction product of from 1 to 2 mol proportions of amino compound and 1 mol proportion polyhalopolyhydropolycyclicdicarboxylic acid or anhydride and (2) the salt of phosphorus compound and amino compound. In a specific embodiment, the polyhalopolyhydropolycyclicdicarboxylic acid or anhydride is 5,6,7,8,9,9-hexachloro-1,2,3,4,4a,5,8,8a-octahydro-5,8-methano-2,3-naphthylenedicarboxylic acid or anhydride and the amino compound is a long-chain alkyl monoamine containing from 8 to 26 carbons or an N-alkyl-diaminoalkane containing from 8 to 26 carbons in the alkyl and from 1 to 6 carbons in the alkane.

Example 1: The reaction product was prepared by first adding about 4,000 grams of toluene to a reactor and then slowly adding, with stirring, 1,700 grams (4 mols) of 5,6,7,8,9,9-hexachloro-1,2,3,4,4a,5,8,8a-octahydro-5,8-methano-2,3-naphthylenedicarboxylic anhydride, after which 1,070 grams (4 mols) of oleylamine were added with stirring. The mixture was then refluxed and a total of 79 cc of water collected. The reaction mixture was allowed to cool and then treated with potassium carbonate. The resultant imide was recovered as a viscous amber oil.

The mixture of this example was prepared by commingling the reaction product prepared as above with a phosphate salt prepared by the reaction of oleylamine with polyoxyethylenated nonylphenol phosphate containing an average of about 5 oxyethylene groups. The oxyethylenated nonylphenol phosphate is a liquid at room temperature and has a phosphorus content of 4.9% and a specific gravity at 25°C of 1.07. The salt was prepared by mixing at room temperature 108 grams (0.4 equivalents) of oleylamine and 236 grams (0.4 equivalent) of the polyoxyethylenated nonylphenol phosphate, then warming on a steam bath and further mixing. The salt was recovered as a clear, amber, viscous liquid. The reaction product and the salt, prepared as described above, were commingled to form a mixture having a chlorine:phosphorus ratio of 24:1. This mixture is used in different concentrations as an additive in lubricating oils. One example is given below; others are included in the full patent.

Example 2: The mixture prepared as described in Example 1 is used in a concentration of 1% by weight as an additive in grease. The additive is incorporated in a commercial Mid-Continent lubricating oil having an SAE viscosity of 20. Approximately 92% of the lubricating oil then is mixed with approximately 8% by weight of lithium stearate. The mixture is heated to about 450°F, with constant agitation. Subsequently the grease is cooled, while agitating, to approximately 250°F and then the grease is further cooled slowly to room temperature.

The stability of the grease is tested in accordance with ASTM D942 method, in which method a sample of the grease is placed in a bomb and maintained at a temperature of 250°F. Oxygen is charged to the bomb, and the time required for a drop of 5 pounds pressure is taken as the Induction Period. A sample of the grease without additive will reach the Induction Period in about 8 hours. On the other hand, a sample of the grease containing 1% by weight of the additive will not reach the Induction Period for more than 100 hours. Other examples in the full patent show the improved stabilization of lubricating oils by such synergistic mixtures.

Synergistic Mixtures Containing 1-n-Butoxy-1-(1-Naphthoxy)Ethane

1-n-Butoxy-1-(1-naphthoxy)ethane has been prepared and described as an antioxidant in U.S. Patent 3,497,181. *M. Braid; U.S. Patent 3,825,496; July 23, 1974; assigned to Mobil Oil Corporation* has found that a synergistic effect is obtained when this material is mixed with a coantioxidant selected from tert-nonylpolysulfide, phenylthiobenzoquinone and dioctyldiphenylamine.

The mixtures are particularly effective in organic compositions such as lubricating oils, greases, liquid hydrocarbon fuels, plastic materials and other organic materials normally susceptible to oxidative deterioration. The antioxidant 1-n-butoxy-1-(1-naphthoxy)ethane is, in general, prepared as follows.

To a solution of 144.2 grams (1 mol) of 1-naphthol in 200 ml of benzene heated at 85° to 90°C there are added, while stirring, 125 grams (1.25 mols) of n-butyl vinyl ether. The addition is completed in 0.5 hour, and heating is continued for 1 additional hour. The reaction mixture is washed with a 20% aqueous sodium hydroxide solution. The organic part is washed with water, dried and distilled to remove benzene and unreacted ether. The residue, 171 grams (70%), of 1-n-butoxy-1-(1-naphthoxy)ethane is a clear mobile liquid. The coantioxidants, tert-nonylpolysulfide, phenylthiobenzoquinone and dioctyldiphenylamine are commercially available materials.

For most applications, 1-n-butoxy-1-(1-naphthoxy)ethane and coantioxidants tert-nonylpolysulfide, phenylthiobenzoquinone or dioctyldiphenylamine are generally used in a mol ratio from 1:10 to 10:1, preferably from 1:4 to 4:1. In general, the synergistic mixture may be incorporated in the organic composition in any amount which is sufficient to increase oxidation resistance. For most applications, the synergistic mixture is used in an amount from 0.01 to 20%, preferably, from 0.05 to 5%, by weight, of the total weight of the organic composition.

Examples 1 through 8: The data were obtained by means of an antioxidant test, in which the antioxidant, or antioxidant synergistic mixture, is added to a solvent-refined mineral lubricating oil. The oil is then heated to 163°C and dry air at a rate of 10 pounds per hour is passed through it in the presence of iron, copper, aluminum and lead. After 40 hours, the neutralization number (NN) for each oil composition is obtained according to ASTM Method D-741-1. The effectiveness of the antioxidants is revealed by a comparison of the control of acids (change in neutralization number) with the antioxidant-free oil. The oil employed in accordance with the test results shown in the following table comprises a solvent-refined mineral lubricating oil, having a 128/132 SUS viscosity at 100°F and a 390°F minimum flash point. In the data of the table all percentages are expressed in weight percent.

Example	Lubricant formulation	NN Increase
1	Base lubricant	21.5
2	Base lubricant plus 1-b-butoxy-1-1-(naphthoxy) ethane (1%).	1.15
3	Base lubricant plus t-nonylpolysulfide (1%)	1.4
4	Base lubricant plus 1-n-butoxy-1-(1-naphthoxy) ethane (0.5%) and t-nonylpolysulfide (0.5%).	0.58
5	Base lubricant plus phenylthiobenzoquinone (1%).	1.08
6	Base lubricant plus 1-n-butoxy-1-(1-naphthoxy) ethane (0.5%) and phenylthiobenzoquinone (0.5%).	0.49
7	Base lubricant plus dioctyldiphenylamine (1%).	21.05
8	Base lubricant plus 1-n-butoxy-1-(1-naphthoxy) ethane (0.5%) and dioctyldiphenylamine (0.5%).	0.88

ANTIOXIDANTS FOR SYNTHETIC LUBRICANTS AND FUNCTIONAL FLUIDS

A number of synthetic materials have been developed in the past few decades as a substitute for petroleum products. Advanced automotive, aircraft and other industrial and military equipment have required lubricants and functional fluids that can withstand long time operation at very high temperatures. Polyolefins, polyesters, polyglycols, silicones, polyphenyl ethers and phosphates are among the materials that have been used for this purpose. Twenty-three of the twenty-nine patents reviewed here are on antioxidant systems for polyester fluids while the remainder cover antioxidants for phosphate, polysiloxane and polyphenyl ether fluids.

AMINE ANTIOXIDANTS FOR POLYESTERS

Anthranilic Acid Esters

J.F. Coburn and S.J. Metro; U.S. Patent 3,642,632; February 15, 1972 have found that an anthranilic acid derivative having the formula:

(1)

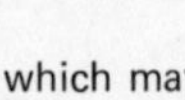

where R is a C_1 to C_{10}, preferably a C_1 to C_8 normal or branched alkyl group and X is selected from hydrogen, a C_1 to C_6 normal or branched alkyl group and an unsubstituted or alkyl substituted phenyl group, is an effective oxidation and corrosion inhibitor in lubricating oils. This compound is especially effective in inhibiting magnesium corrosion. The amount of the ester incorporated into the lubricating oil is usually 0.5 to 4.0 weight percent based on the total amount of the final lubricating composition.

Examples of anthranilic acid derivatives which may be used in the lubricating composition include esters of anthranilic acid such as methyl anthranilate, ethyl anthranilate, propyl anthranilate, 2-ethylhexyl anthranilate, etc. and esters of derivatives of anthranilic acid (i.e., X is other than hydrogen) such as

> methyl-N-methyl anthranilate,
> 2-ethylhexyl-N-methyl anthranilate,
> methyl-N-phenyl anthranilate,
> 2-ethylhexyl-N-phenyl anthranilate,
> isodecyl-N-phenyl anthranilate,
> methyl-N-ethylphenyl anthranilate, etc.

The esters may generally be prepared by reacting an anthranilic anhýdride with an appropriate alcohol. The ester may also be prepared via the acid chloride route which is particularly appropriate, where X of Formula 1 is a phenyl group. The ester additive will generally be used in lubricants which encounter high performance service conditions such as the operation of modern jet type aircraft. Generally, the basestocks of such lubricants are synthetic ester oils. It is in this type of lubricant which the ester dramatically demonstrates its effectiveness. However, the ester additive may be used in mineral oils. The mineral or synthetic oils generally should have a viscosity within the range of 35 to 200 SUS at 210°F and flash points of 350° to 600°F. Lubricating oils having a viscosity index of 100 or higher may be employed.

Example: To 100 grams of a synthetic lubricating base oil was added 1.3 grams of methyl anthranilate and 3.14 grams of a combination of conventional antioxidants, corrosion inhibitors and load carrying agents. This combination was heated and stirred at 210°F until a solution was effected. The conventional additives were used so the finished lubricant would have the qualities more nearly exhibited by a working lubricant. The synthetic lubricating base oil was composed of a mixture of about 25 weight percent of an ester of neopentylglycol and fatty acids having an average chain length of C_8 and about 75 weight percent of an ester of trimethylolpropane and the same fatty acid. The methyl anthranilate was prepared by reacting isatoic anhydride (a commercial product of Maumee Chemical Company) with methyl alcohol at a temperature of about 65°C in the presence of sodium hydroxide.

An Oxidation-Corrosion-Stability Test was carried out on several lubricating compositions containing the anthranilic esters described above. Such test determines the oxidation and corrosion inhibiting effect of the ester additive. The same test was conducted on a lubricant containing di-(octylphenyl)amine, a standard oxidation and corrosion inhibiting additive. The base oil in which the additives were incorporated was the synthetic lubricant as described in the example. Also included in the lubricant compositions which were tested was the combination of conventional additives described in the above example. The lubricant composition contained 100 parts by weight of synthetic oil. The ester additive and the di-(octylphenyl)amine were present in amounts of 13 parts by weight. The conventional auxiliary additives were present in a total amount of 3.14 parts by weight. The results of the tests, an average of several runs, are recorded in the table below.

	425° F., 48 hour O.C.S. test						
	Δmetal weight, mg./cm.³					Δkv./ 100° F.	
Lubricant additive	Cu	Mg	Steel	Al	Ag	cs.	Δtan
Methyl anthranilate	+0.01	−0.03	−0.01	−0.01	−0.04	15.30	3.26
2-Ethylhexyl anthranilate	−0.05	+0.01	+0.01	−0.05	−0.04	14.00	1.41
Methyl-N-phenyl anthranilate	−0.02	−0.07	+0.01	+0.04	+0.04	16.59	7.21
2-ethylhexyl-N-phenyl anthranilate	+0.21	−0.91	+0.09	+0.04	+0.07	15.56	9.84
Isodecyl-N-phenyl Anthranilate	+0.23	−10.43	+0.15	+0.09	+0.14	16.43	11.25
Methyl-N-methyl anthranilate	0.00	+0.02	+0.04	+0.03	−0.01	15.31	3.11
2-ethylhexyl-N-methyl anthranilate	−0.04	+0.01	+0.03	+0.01	−0.03	15.33	3.67
Di-(octylphenyl)amine	−0.25	−13.23	+0.01	+0.01	−0.02	22.07	4.90

The 425°F Oxidation-Corrosion-Stability Test was carried out by blowing air at the rate of 100 volumes per hour through 1 volume of the lubricating composition maintained at a temperature of 425°F, for 48 hours. At the end of the test, the increase in viscosity and the increase in total acid number (tan) were determined. The corrosive characteristic of the lubricant was determined by immersing various weighed metal strips in the oil and measuring weight change at the end of the test. The change in weight signifies either corrosion due to oxidation of the metal or weight gain due to deposits.

Alkylated Diphenylamines

The use of tris-2,4,4'-alkyldiphenylamines is disclosed by *B. Holt; U.S. Patent 3,655,559; April 11, 1972; assigned to Ciba-Geigy Corporation* for stabilizing organic material, especially synthetic lubricating oils against oxidative deterioration. These antioxidants have the following formula.

(1)

$$R'-\bigbenzene-NH-\bigbenzene-R'$$

where R' is a tertiary alkyl having 4 to 12 carbons, R'' is hydrogen or a straight or branched-chain alkyl having 2 to 4 carbons, and R''' is a straight or branched chain alkyl of 2 to 4 carbons. Examples of preferred compounds of Formula 1 include 2,2'-diethyl-4,4'-di-tert-butyl-diphenylamine, 2,2'-diethyl-4,4'-di-tert-octyl-diphenylamine, 2,4,4'-tri-tert-butyl-diphenylamine and particularly 2,2',4,4'-tetra-tert-butyl-diphenylamine. The compounds having the Formula 1 are produced by orthoalkylating in a first stage, diphenylamine with a straight- or branched-chain olefin having 2 to 4 carbons in the presence of a catalyst comprising aluminum, and in a second stage, contacting the orthoalkylated diphenylamine with a secondary olefin having 4 to 12 carbons in the presence of a Friedel-Crafts or Bronsted acid catalyst.

The compounds of Formula 1 are thus conveniently produced by first alkylating diphenylamine in one or both of the ortho- (2 and 2' positions) of the diphenylamine molecule, and subsequently alkylating the orthoalkylated material in both of the para- (4 and 4') positions. The compounds having the formula:

(2)

$$H_9C_4t-\bigbenzene-NH-\bigbenzene-t-C_4H_9$$

where R is hydrogen or a tertiary-butyl group, can be also produced by contacting in a single stage diphenylamine with isobutylene in the presence of a Friedel-Crafts or Bronsted acid catalyst.

Example 1: 69 parts of 2,2'-diethyldiphenylamine and 0.7 part of anhydrous aluminum chloride were charged into a reactor and heated to 130°C, cooled to 100°C. At this temperature 85.9 parts of diisobutylene were added over a period of 2 hours and the mixture heated under reflux conditions until the temperature reached 160°C. After cooling, the reaction mixture was taken up in 500 parts of toluene and washed with aqueous 10% sodium hydroxide and then with water to neutrality. Removal of the toluene under vacuum furnished 110.7 parts of a crude product as an oil. This oil was distilled to give a product which solidified on cooling. Recrystallization of this solid from ethanol gave 2,2'-diethyl-4,4'-di-tert-octyl-diphenylamine having melting point of 63°C.

Example 2: 169 parts of diphenylamine and 4.4 parts of anhydrous aluminum chloride were charged into a reactor and heated to 140°C under an atmosphere of nitrogen to give a liquid melt. Isobutylene was then passed through the melt at a rate of 200 ml per minute until absorption of isobutylene ceased, after a period of 5.5 hours. After cooling, the reaction mixture was taken up in 500 parts of toluene and washed with aqueous 10% sodium hydroxide and then with water to neutrality. Removal of the toluene solvent under vacuum gave a viscous brown oil which slowly solidified. Recrystallization from ethanol gave 2,2',4,4'-tetra-tert-butyl-diphenylamine melting at 161° to 162°C.

Example 3: A synthetic ester-based lubricant was formulated and subjected to the Pratt and Whitney Type II oxidation-corrosion test. The base fluid was a complex ester derived from sebacic acid, caprylic acid and trimethylol propane, the complex ester being described and claimed in British Patent 971,901. Each test was carried out for 48 hours at a temperature of 425°C using dry air at a rate of 5 liters per hour and in the presence of specimens of magnesium alloy, aluminum alloy, copper, silver and steel.

To each lubricant sample there was added, prior to commencing the test, a proportion of the alkylated diphenylamine and a proportion of benzotriazole. For comparison, further tests were carried out using a control containing no antioxidant and also using a lubricant composition diphenylamine or 4,4'-di-tert-octyldiphenylamine and benzotriazole. The results are summarized in the following table.

Additive	Proportion Additive, Weight %	Percent Viscosity Increase, at 100°F	Acid Value Increase, mg KOH/g	Sludge, mg	Weight Change in Specimens (mg/sq cm)				
					Mg	Al	Cu	Ag	Steel
None		113.0	7.3	10,700	–51.27	+0.05	–0.08	+0.07	–0.14
Diphenylamine	2.0	209.0	2.4	280	– 0.02	–0.03	–1.02	+0.01	–0.02
4,4'-di-tert-octyldiphenylamine plus Benzotriazole	4.0 0.5	57.0	2.2	34	– 6.90	–0.04	–0.62	–0.08	–0.02
2,2'-diethyl-4,4'-di-tert-octyldiphenylamine plus Benzotriazole	4.0 0.5	34.46	1.63	2.0	– 0.11	–0.12	–0.20	–0.12	–0.11
2,2',4,4'-tetra-butyldiphenylamine plus Benzotriazole	4.0 0.5	18.93	1.78	0.5	– 0.02	Nil	–0.10	–0.01	+0.02
2,2'-diethyl-4,4'-di-tert-butyl-diphenylamine plus Benzotriazole	4.0 0.5	7.35	3.37	34.7	+ 0.01	+0.04	+0.05	+0.01	+0.01

Examples were also included in the complete patent on the stabilization of polypropylene and SBR with these antioxidants.

Alkoxydiarylamines

M. Braid; U.S. Patent 3,781,206; December 25, 1973; assigned to Mobil Oil Corporation has found that etherified diarylamines are valuable antioxidants for various lubricant compositions. These amines have the formula: $(RO)_m$$\{Ar\}$$NH$$\{Ar'\}$$(OR')_n$ where Ar and Ar' are phenyl, naphthyl, phenanthryl or anthryl, R and R' are alkyls of 1 to 20 carbons, and m and n are 0 to 5, with at least one of them being at least 1.

The method for preparing the above compounds comprises reacting the hydroxy derivative of the above compound (i.e., where R or R' is hydrogen) with an alkyl halide in a dialkyl formamide solvent, or in dimethylsulfoxide or acetonitrile, in the presence of an alkali metal carbonate. This preparative process was not previously known.

The known methods for producing the compounds involved the preparation of the alkali metal derivative of the starting hydroxydiarylamine prior to reaction with the alkyl halide. This is necessary in the known procedures because in the absence of the alkali metal derivative there is a substantial competitive reaction for the alkyl halide with the amine function. By running the reaction in the presence of an alkali metal carbonate and a suitable solvent as disclosed here, there is no need to make, as a separate first step, the alkali metal salt of the aminophenol.

The reaction of the aminophenol with alkali metal carbonate (the alkali metal including sodium, lithium, potassium and cesium) is not merely an in situ reaction. It appears that the dimethyl sulfoxide, acrylonitrile or dialkyl formamides, and especially dimethylformamide, have a selective effect for etherification, yielding up to 97% of etherified product. On the other hand, the same reaction when run in different solvents yields very substantial amounts of N-alkylation rather than etherification.

In running this reaction, good yields can be expected using temperatures of 80° to 200°C, preferably from 130° to 150°C. Usually the reaction can be completed in 2 to 3 hours, but may take several hours, e.g., up to 10 or 12, depending upon the temperature and specific reactants employed. The following Examples 1 and 2 further illustrate the process.

Example 1: A mixture of 19 grams of 4-hydroxydiphenylamine, 16 grams of 1-chloro-octane and 57.6 grams of anhydrous potassium carbonate in 150 ml of N,N-dimethylformamide was refluxed for 6.5 hours. The resulting reaction mixture was cooled below 100°C and was poured into a large excess of cold water. The resulting crystalline solids were collected by filtration. There was thus obtained 29.5 grams (97%) of the 4-n-octoxydiphenyl-amine, melting point 42° to 43°C.

Example 2: A mixture of 50 grams of 2-chlorobenzoic acid, 66.1 grams of anhydrous po-tassium carbonate, 79 grams of 2-methoxyaniline and 300 ml of diethyleneglycol dimethyl ether was heated to 140°C. To this mixture about 1 gram of copper bronze and about 0.1 gram of copper iodide were added and heating at 140° to 145°C while stirring was con-tinued for about 3 hours. The reaction mixture was cooled to about 100°C and poured into water. The aqueous mixture was filtered and the filtrate was acidified with acetic acid, heated to boiling and filtered. There was collected 58 grams (75%) of tan crystalline 2-methoxydiphenylamine-2'-carboxylic acid, MP 171° to 172°C.

171 grams of 2-methoxydiphenylamine-2'-carboxylic acid was heated at 260°C under a nitrogen atmosphere for 5 hours. 2-Methoxydiphenylamine was distilled from the result-ing reaction mixture as a pale yellow oil, boiling point 198° to 204°C at about 6 mm pres-sure.

Example 3: The antioxidants were blended into a synthetic ester oil lubricant (made by reacting pentaerythritol with an equimolar mixture of C_5 and C_9 monocarboxylic acids) and tested in an oxidation test by the following procedure. A sample of the test composi-tion is heated and air at the rate of 5 liters per hour is passed through for a period of 24 hours. Present in the test sample are specimens of iron, copper, aluminum, and lead. The kinematic viscosity is measured at 100°F before and after treating to give the change in viscosity (percent KV change). The change in the neutralization number (NN change) measures the increase in acid content. It should be noted that the metals present in the test are typical metals of engine or machine construction, and they provide some catalysis for the oxidation of organic materials. The results are tabulated in the following table.

Additive, Example	Weight percent additive	Temp., °F.	Initial NN	ΔNN	Initial KV, cs. at 100° F.	ΔKV, percent	Sludge
None		425		5.9		226	Nil.
		450		8.3		585	Trace.
1	2	425	0	1.0	25.72	17	Do.
	1	425	0	1.0	25.72	14	Do.
	2	450	0	7.6	25.72	191	Light.
	1	450	0	7.6	25.72	180	Trace.
2	2	425	0	1.3	25.28	24	Do.
	1	425	0	3.6	25.28	51	Do.
	2	450	0	5.1	25.28	88	Do.
	1	450	0	5.6	25.28	95	Light.

Aminobenzoquinones and Aminonaphthoquinones

It has also been found by *M. Braid and D.A. Law; U.S. Patent 3,445,391; May 20, 1969; and U.S. Patent 3,682,980; August 8, 1972; both assigned to Mobil Oil Corporation* that or-ganic compositions susceptible to deterioration by oxidation have improved stability by the addition of a minor amount of a quinone having at least one amino group attached. These aminoquinones preferably have the following specific structures

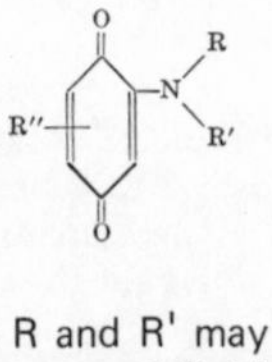

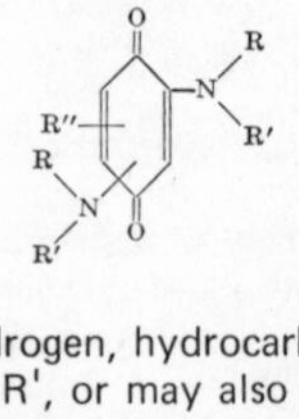

and

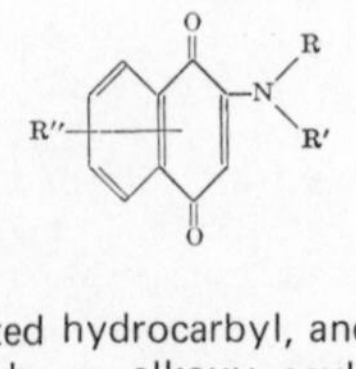

where R and R' may each be hydrogen, hydrocarbyl or substituted hydrocarbyl, and R'' has the same definition as R and R', or may also be halogen, hydroxy, alkoxy, acyloxy, acylamido, carbalkoxy or substituted derivatives of these. The preferred substituents are those organo or substituted organo groups, and especially alkyl or substituted alkyl, having 1 to 40 carbons.

Although the alkyl groups on each nitrogen atom may be different, symmetrical alkyl amines are used to illustrate the essential features of this process. These aminoquinones may be prepared by the reaction between a quinone and a primary or secondary amine; or by the reaction between the amine reactant and a hydroquinone. In the latter reaction, the reactants are dissolved in a suitable solvent and a stream of air or oxygen or other oxygen-containing gas is dispersed therethrough with agitation at or above room temperature. Alternatively, the oxidation step may be performed with an oxidizing agent, such as hydrogen peroxide, potassium permanganate, manganese dioxide, sodium chlorate and the like. The mol ratio of the reactants may be varied to produce the desired product. Approximately a 0.5:1 to 1:1 ratio of amine to quinone may usually be used to produce monoaminobenzoquinones and naphthoquinones; a 2:1 to 10:1 ratio for the diaminobenzoquinone. It is preferred to have an excess of amine present in the reaction mixture. The following examples will illustrate the preparation and testing of these aminoquinone antioxidants.

Example 1: In a suitable reactor, 165 grams (1.5 mols) of hydroquinone was dissolved in 1 liter of methanol, and 230 grams (3.15 mols) of n-butylamine was added at 25°C as the mixture was stirred. The temperature rose to 40°C during which a color change was observed. After 5 minutes of stirring, a slow stream of oxygen was passed through the mixture. The temperature rose to 51°C over a two-hour period. A red crystalline product, 2,5-bis-n-butylamino-p-benzoquinone, commenced to precipitate. The total oxygen treatment lasted for 16 hours. Afterward, the solid was filtered off and washed in methanol, yielding 237 grams (63%) of product; MP 157° to 158°C.

Example 2: The quinones as prepared by this process were tested in a catalytic oxidation test for lubricants, using as the base medium a synthetic ester lubricant. This lubricant is prepared by the esterification of technical grade pentaerythritol with a mixture of commercial valeric and pelargonic acids. The test lubricant composition is subjected to a stream of air which is bubbled through the composition at a rate of 5 liters per hour at 425°F for 24 hours. Present in the composition are metals commonly used as materials of engine construction, namely:

(1) 15.6 sq in of sand-blasted iron wire,
(2) 0.78 sq in of polished copper wire,
(3) 0.87 sq in of polished aluminum wire, and
(4) 0.167 sq in of polished lead surface.

Inhibitors for oil are rated on the basis of prevention of oil deterioration as measured by the increase in acid formation or neutralization number (NN) and kinematic viscosity (KV) occasioned by the oxidation. The results are reported in the table below.

Additive	Conc., Weight Percent	NN Increase	Percent Increase of KV at 100° F.	Sludge	Lead Loss, mg.
None		5 to 9	390	Trace	19.2
2,5-di-t-butyl-p-benzoquinone	1	8.98	415	Nil	3.5
2,5-bis-t-butylamino-p-benzoquinone	1	0.79	8	Trace	6.3
2,5-bis-n-hexylamino-p-benzoquinone	1	1.0	5	Heavy	0.9
2,5-bis-n-octylamino-p-benzoquinone	1	1.7	16	Nil	7.2
2,5-bis-n-dodecylamino-p-benzoquinone	1	1.0	14	Trace	21.7
Product of Example 13	0.5	4.8	128	Nil	2.1
2,5-bis-piperidinyl-p-benzoquinone	2	7.37	106	Heavy	1.0
2,5-bis-2-hydroxyethylamino-p-benzoquinone	<0.75	4.84	404	Nil	6.0

An example of this stabilization of mineral oil lubricant by these compounds was also included in the complete patent.

Alkylphenylalkylnaphthylamines

R.T. Schlobohm; U.S. Patent 3,660,290; May 2, 1972; assigned to Shell Oil Company has found that 4-alkylphenyl-1-alkyl-2-naphthylamines are effective in improving the oxidation resistance, cleanliness and bearing performance properties of polyester lubricating oils. The effectiveness of these compounds is attributed in substantial part to the presence of an alkyl substituent on the naphthyl nucleus which was found to have a remarkable effect on the performance characteristics of the resulting compound. These 4-alkyphenyl-1-alkyl-2-naphthylamines have the formula:

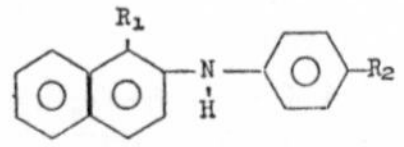

where R_1 and R_2 are alkyl groups having 2 to 80, preferably 2 to 16, carbons. Compounds where R_1 and R_2 have 4 to 12 carbons and have a tertiary alkyl structure are especially advantageous for use as antioxidants, particularly those where R_1 and R_2 are tertiary-butyl or tertiary-octyl groups. These alkylphenyl-alkylnaphthylamines can be used in lubricant compositions either singularly, in mixtures, or in combination with alkylphenyl-2-naphthylamines which have alkyl substituents exclusively on the phenyl nucleus.

Alkylphenyl-2-naphthylamines suitable for use with the additives of this process are those having one or more alkyl substituents on the phenyl ring. The alkyl groups may contain 2 to 16 carbons but preferably have 4 to 12 carbons and a tertiary-alkyl structure. Alkylphenyl-2-naphthylamines having a single tertiary-butyl or tertiary-octyl group in the 4 position of the phenyl have been found to be particularly effective when used in combination with the present additives.

The alkylphenyl-alkylnaphthylamines are generally prepared by reacting phenyl-2-naphthylamine with a 1- or 2-alkene having 2 to 16, or more, carbons at an elevated temperature in the presence of a Friedel-Crafts catalyst, e.g., aluminum chloride. The reaction conditions largely govern the nature of the alkylated products formed. Conditions conductive to naphthyl ring substitution are described in Example 1. Using these conditions it is possible to introduce alkyl substituents into the naphthyl nucleus.

Example 1: 5.36 grams (0.04 mol) of aluminum trichloride was added to 87.6 grams (0.4 mol) of phenyl-2-naphthylamine and heated to 120°C. While stirring and under a nitrogen atmosphere, 89.6 grams (0.8 mol) of diisobutylene was added dropwise to the reaction mixture over a period of one hour. After the addition of the diisobutylene, the reaction was heated to 148°C over a three-hour period and the temperature maintained there for an additional two hours.

The reaction mixture was then allowed to cool, mixed with two volumes of benzene, poured over ice and water, washed with a 10% aqueous NaOH solution and with distilled water until neutral, after which the benzene layer was dried over $CaSO_4$. After filtering and removal of the benzene by distillation, the crude product (146 grams) was vacuum distilled over the range of 210°C/50μ to 260°C/45μ, yielding 139 grams of product. 4-tert-octylphenyl-1-tert-octyl-2-naphthylamine was isolated by means of gas chromatographic preparative techniques and was identified by infrared spectroscopy, nuclear magnetic resonance (NMR) and elemental analysis. This compound constituted 54.99% of the reaction product.

Gas chromatographic analysis also demonstrated the presence of a mixture of two other naphthyl-substituted phenyl-2-naphthylamines constituting 15.79% of the reaction product. This mixture was separated from distilled product and identified by infrared spectroscopy and nuclear magnetic resonance as being 4-tert-octylphenyl-1-tert-butyl-2-naphthylamine and 4-tert-butylphenyl-1-tert-octyl-2-naphthylamine. The compositions used in testing these products as antioxidants are given in the table below.

		Additive, percent weight			
	Base oil	Phenyl-2-naph-thyl amine	4-tert-octyl-phenyl-2-naph-thyl-amine	Addi-tive A	Addi-tive B
Composition:					
I	W	....	[1]1.5	....	....
II	W	....	....	[1]2.02	....
III	W	....	....	....	[1]1.84

[1] Equal molar concentrations equivalent to 1.0% w. phenyl-2-naphthyl amine in base oil.

Additive A is 4-tert-octylphenyl-1-tert-octyl-2-naphthylamine and Additive B is a mixture of 4-tert-octylphenyl-1-tert-octyl-2-naphthylamine, 4-tert-butylphenyl-1-tert-octyl-2-naphthylamine and 4-tert-octylphenyl-1-tert-butyl-2-naphthylamine with 4-tert-octylphenyl-2-naphthylamine; ratio of alkylphenyl-alkylnaphthylamines to 4-tert-octylphenyl-2-naphthylamine is approximately 3 to 1. Base Oil W is mixed C_4–C_{10} acid esters of pentaerythritol and dipentaerythritol containing 0.17% weight of phosphorus extreme pressure agents, 0.1% weight of triazole corrosion inhibitors, 0.25% weight of a copolymeric dispersant, 1.5% weight of an amine antioxidant, 0.02% of a dibasic acid corrosion inhibitor and 10 ppm silicone fluid antifoamant.

Example 2: To evaluate the antioxidation and anticorrosion properties of these compositions, a series of Corrosion and Oxidation Stability Tests were run in accordance with the procedures set forth in Military Specification MIL-L-23699. The results are shown in the following table.

[Corrosion and oxidation stability, 400° F., 72 hours]

	Composition—		
	I	II	III
Weight change of specimens:			
Mg	−0.01	+0.01	+0.01
Al	−0.03	−0.01	−0.01
Cu	−0.13	−0.10	−0.16
Fe	−0.02	+0.01	+0.01
Ag	−0.10	−0.11	−0.09
Viscosity change, 100° F., percent	23.4	37.8	15.2
Acid number change	0.81	1.43	1.54
Sludge, mg./100 ml	19.0	2.0	3.0

It is evident from these results, that Compositions II and III have less tendency to form sludge than Composition I which contains a molar equivalent of an additive not included in the process.

Arylindano Secondary Amines

Antioxidants useful in greases, mineral oils, but particularly in synthetic polyester lubricants are disclosed by *J.W. Schick and R.M. Gemmill, Jr.; U.S. Patent 3,655,561; April 11, 1972; assigned to Mobil Oil Corporation.* These antioxidants have the structure

where Ar is phenyl, naphthyl, alkyl substituted phenyl or alkyl substituted naphthyl; where, when x = 1, y = 0; when x = 0, y = 1; and when x = 1, y = 1. These aryl-indano secondary amines may be prepared, in general, by reacting a halogenated phenyl indan with a metal derivative of an aryl primary amine under conditions effective to produce the corresponding aryl-indano secondary amine. For most purposes, the reaction is carried out at a temperature from 130°C to the boiling point of the aryl primary amine. Preferably, the reaction is carried out at 130° to 200°C. The metal of the metal derivative of the aryl primary amine may comprise any metal, although metals of Group I of the Periodic Table are preferred. The following examples illustrate the preparation and use of these aryl-indano secondary amines.

Example 1: To a stirred, one-liter flask containing 112 grams (1.2 mols) of dry, distilled aniline and 0.4 grams of copper turnings was added 9.2 grams (0.4 mol) of metallic sodium freshly cut into small pieces. This mixture was heated slowly under nitrogen for a total of five hours to a maximum temperature of 130°C. At this point, the sodium was completely dissolved and hydrogen evolution had ceased. Formation of phenyl sodamide was complete.

125 grams (0.4 mol) of monobrominated-1,1,3-trimethyl-3-phenyl indan was then added at room temperature. Upon heating, a strong exothermic reaction occurred, starting at 65°C, which elevated the reaction temperature to 196°C, even with air cooling. The exotherm was of brief duration and the reaction reached completion rapidly. The reaction was allowed to continue for a total of four hours to assure completion. Isomeric phenylamino-1,1,3-trimethyl-3-phenyl indan was produced in a yield of 65% according to gas chromatographic analysis. The molecular weight of the amine was found to be 319 (327 calculated) and the nitrogen content was 4.18% (4.28% calculated). The bromine content was found to be negative and the distilled product was a clear, pale yellow-brown, nearly solid, amorphous material. The phenylamino-1,1,3-trimethyl-3-phenyl indan thus produced, can be depicted as having the structure

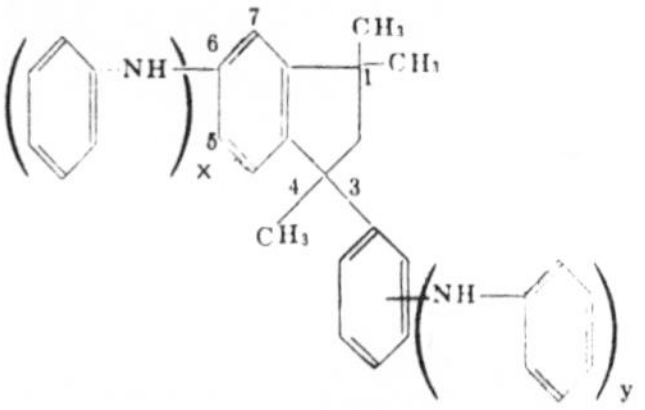

where, when $x = 1$, $y = 0$, and when $x = 0$, $y = 1$.

The aryl-indano secondary amines as produced by this process were evaluated by being subjected to a catalytic oxidation test. This test determines the effectiveness of the additive in preventing oxidation of an oil sample under oxidizing conditions. The oil sample employed comprised an ester of technical grade pentaerythritol and a mixture of C_5 and C_9 monocarboxylic acids.

The test procedure is as follows: in a 200 mm x 25 mm test tube is placed a 25 gram sample of a test oil, having immersed therein (a) 15.6 sq in of sand-blasted iron wire, (b) 0.78 sq in of polished copper wire, and (c) 0.167 sq in of a polished lead specimen. The oil sample is heated to a temperature of 450°F and maintained at this temperature while dry air is placed therethrough at the rate of 5 liters per hour for a period of 24 hours. The change in neutralization number and kinematic viscosity before and after the oxidation are recorded, and the weight loss of the lead specimen is obtained. In the table below are shown the effects of the additives of this process compared with the uninhibited lubricant.

Antioxidant, wt. percent	Percent	Base oil			
		ΔNN	ΔKV100, percent	Sludge	Pb loss, mg.
None		8.25	585	Trace	13.7
Compound 1	8	8.60	99	Nil	3.1
	4	6.40	99	Nil	8.6
	2	8.65	116	Nil	6.1
Compound 2	8	8.34	420	Trace	15.0
	4	6.47	138	Light	13.0
	2	8.03	171	Trace	6.0
Compound 3	8	5.84		Heavy	2.0
	4	5.07	218	Moderate	1.0
	2	7.03	39	Heavy	0.4
Compound 4	8	4.80	111	Heavy	23.7
	4	4.25	35	Trace	15.8
	2	4.27	35	Trace	9.5

In the table Compound 1 is monophenylamino-1,1,3-trimethyl-3-phenyl indan; Compound 2 is mono-(p-n-butyl)phenylamino-1,1,3-trimethyl-3-phenyl indan; Compound 3 is di-phenylamino-1,1,3-trimethyl-3-phenyl indan; and Compound 4 is mono-α-naphthylamino-1,1,3-trimethyl-3-phenyl indan.

Amine Salts or Amides of Fluorocarboxylates

Reaction products of an aromatic amine with fluorinated monobasic acids (or acid chlorides) have been used by *D.S. Bosniack and S.J. Metro; U.S. Patent 3,634,242; January 11, 1972; assigned to Esso Research and Engineering Company* as stabilizers for lubricating oils including synthetic polyester lubricants. The oil-soluble reaction product will be an amide or amine salt depending on whether the acid or acid chloride of the fluorinated compound is used as a reactant. If the fluorinated acid is used, the product will be an amine salt, whereas the acid chloride will produce an amide. The preferred aromatic amine reactant has the formula:

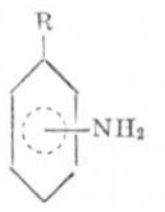

where R is H, C_1 to C_{20} normal or branched alkyl, or $-COOR_1$, where R_1 is a C_1 to C_{16}, preferably C_1 to C_9 normal or branched alkyl group. Specific examples of these aromatic amines include methyl anthranilate, propyl anthranilate, hexyl anthranilate, ethyl p-aminobenzoate, toluidine, octylaniline and aniline. The preferred fluorinated reactant has the formula: $R_3(CF_2)_nCOZ$ where R_3 is hydrogen or fluorine, preferably fluorine, Z is hydroxyl or chloride and n is a number from 1 to 20, preferably 1 to 12. This fluorinated reactant is preferably of a normal structure. Examples of operable acid and acid chlorides include trifluoroacetic acid, heptafluorobutyric acid, pentadecafluorooctanoic acid, and their corresponding acid chlorides.

Example 1: A solution of 60.5 grams (0.4 mol) methyl anthranilate in 300 ml of anhydrous ether was charged to a one-liter 4-neck flask fitted with an air stirrer, condenser, thermometer and dropping funnel. A solution of 165.7 grams (0.4 mol) pentadecafluorooctanoic acid in 300 ml of anhydrous ether was added dropwise with rapid stirring over a period of 30 minutes. The mixture was stirred at reflux for about 2 hours and cooled to 0°C. The product, a white precipitate, was filtered, washed with additional cold ether and dried. The crude o-carboxymethyl anilinium pentadecafluorooctanoate was recrystallized from chloroform to yield 158 grams (70% yield) of white needles having a melting point of 124.5° to 125°C.

Example 2: Methyl anthranilate and heptafluorobutyric acid were reacted according to the procedures of Example 1. The purified o-carboxymethyl anilinium heptafluorobutyrate was a white solid having a melting point of 122.5° to 123.5°C.

Example 3: To 100 parts by weight of a synthetic ester lubricating oil having as components about 70 weight percent of an ester formed from trimethylolpropane and a C_8 average normal carboxylic acid and about 30 weight percent of an ester formed from dipentaerythritol and a C_5 average normal carboxylic acid was added 0.25 part by weight of the above reaction products. Also included in the ester oil was 5.5 parts by weight of a combination of antioxidants, corrosion inhibitors and dispersants. Such commercial additives were included to more fully approximate the properties of an actual working lubricant. This fully formulated lubricant was then tested for oxidation and corrosion stability, the results of such test incorporated into the table below.

| | Oxid.-corr. stability test 425° F./72 hrs. | | | |
| | Cu corr. | Mg corr. | Vis. @100° F., per- cent | tan |
Lubricant composition				
Base oil	−0.11	−10.96	39.66	5.38
Base oil (100 parts by wt.) plus 0.25 parts by wt. of Ex. I amine salt	−0.34	−0.01	38.28	8.03
Base oil (100 parts by wt.) plus 0.25 parts by wt. of Ex. 2 amine salt	−0.59	−0.92	35.55	6.82

The 425°F Oxidation Corrosion Stability Test was carried out by blowing air at the ratio of 5 liters per hour through 100 grams of the lubricating composition at 425°F for 72 hours. At the end of the test, the percentage increase in viscosity and change in total acid number (tan) were determined. The corrosive characteristics were determined by immersing various weighed metal coupons in the oil and measuring weight change at the end of the test. The change in weight signifies either corrosion due to dissolving of the metal or weight gain due to deposits.

AMINE ANTIOXIDANT MIXTURES FOR POLYESTERS

The use of aryl amines as antioxidants for synthetic ester functional fluids is well-known. Thus, the secondary aryl amines such as the phenyl naphthyl amines, the diphenyl amines and the like have been found to decrease the amount of sludge buildup in the fluid. Unfortunately, these materials have proven unsatisfactory in stabilizing the fluids against changes in viscosity and acid number, problems very detrimental to the high temperature performance needed in modern jet engines. Hindered phenolic type compounds, including phenolic amine compounds have been used as antioxidants but these materials tend to be corrosive. Acylating the phenolic amines to give better corrosion characteristics in hydrocarbon oil and dicarboxylate type fluids has also been suggested. None of these materials, however, have adequately solved the problems of acid buildup and viscosity change mentioned above. The following processes using mixtures of antioxidants containing aryl amines have been developed to overcome these problems.

N-Acylated Phenylenediamines with Secondary Arylamines

High temperature antioxidant mixtures for polycarboxylate functional fluids have been developed by *W.F. Gentit; U.S. Patent 3,699,053; October 17, 1972; assigned to Stauffer Chemical Company.* These antioxidants comprise a mixture of an acylated phenylene diamine and a secondary aryl amine. The acylated phenylene diamines used in the present composition have the formula:

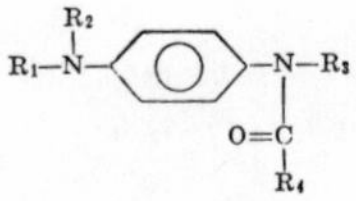

where R_1 and R_3 can each be alkyl, cycloalkyl, aryl, aralkyl or alkaryl; R_2 can be hydrogen, alkyl, cycloalkyl, aryl, aralkyl or alkaryl; and R_4 can be hydrogen, alkyl, phenyl, substituted alkyl or substituted phenyl. In the preferred compounds R_1 and R_3 can each be a C_1–C_{20} alkyl, a C_5–C_{18} cycloalkyl, phenyl, a C_7–C_{26} alkylphenyl, naphthyl or C_{11}–C_{30} alkylnaphthyl; R_2 is hydrogen, and R_4 is C_1–C_{20} alkyl, phenyl, substituted alkyl or substituted phenyl. The terms substituted alkyl and substituted phenyl as used here designate alkyl or phenyl groups having at least one substituent of the type: halogen, cyano, carboxyl, carboxylate, amido, amino, nitro hydroxy or alkoxy. Illustrative of these compounds are the following:

> N-heptanoyl-N,N'-di-sec-butyl-p-phenylene diamine,
> N-benzoyl-N,N'-di-sec-butyl-p-phenylene diamine,
> N-heptanoyl-N,N'-bis(3,5-methylheptyl)-p-phenylene
>   diamine,
> N'-heptanoyl-N-phenyl-N'-(1,3-dimethylbutyl)-p-phenylene
>   diamine; and the like.

The acylated phenylene diamines are normally used in amounts from 0.1 to 10% by weight of the entire fluid. The secondary aryl amines are well-known and as used here are compounds having the formula

$$R_6\text{—}\overset{\displaystyle H}{\underset{\displaystyle |}{N}}\text{—}R_7$$

where R_6 and R_7 are phenyl, naphthyl, C_1–C_{20} alkyl substituted naphthyl. The preferred compounds are: phenyl-α-naphthyl amine, phenyl-β-naphthyl amine, octylphenyl-α-naphthyl amine, octylphenyl-β-naphthyl amine, diphenyl amine and p,p'-dioctyl diphenyl amine. The secondary aryl amines are normally used in amounts from 0.01% to 10% by weight of the entire fluid. They are preferably present in a weight ratio to the acylated phenylene diamine of from 3:1 to 0.3:1. The following examples illustrate the preparation of an acylated phenylene diamine and its use in a functional fluid of the polycarboxylate type containing a secondary arylamine.

Example 1: A two-liter flask, fitted with a reflux condenser to which a water trap is attached, is charged with 200 milliliters of toluene, 110.2 grams of N,N'-di-sec-butyl-p-phenylene diamine and 65.1 grams of heptanoic acid. The flask is heated to reflux and maintained at a pot temperature of 275°C until 9 milliliters of water is formed. The condenser is removed and volatiles are driven off by maintaining the pot temperature at 230°C. The final product weighs 123 grams and is identified by IR spectra, gas chromatography and NMR to be N-heptanoyl-N,N'-di-sec-butyl-p-phenylene diamine.

Example 2: The product of Example 1 is blended with the functional fluid, I(A), to yield the formulation, I(B). The two fluids are tested according to the Alcor Deposition Test, as outlined in the *Proceedings of the United States Air Force Southwest Research Institute— Turbine Engine Lubrication Conference* of September 13 through 15, 1966.

Blend	I(A)	I(B)
Trimethylolpropane triheptanoate	97.85	96.85
Phenyl-α-naphthylamine	1.15	1.15
Dioctyl diphenyl amine	1.00	1.00
N-heptanoyl-N, N'-di-sec-butyl-p-phenylene diamine		1.00
Alcor deposition test:		
Overall demerit rating	91	17.4
Critical temperature, ° F	545	580
Tube deposits, mg	171	5.9
Filter deposits, mg	1.7	3.9
Viscosity change, percent	+25.4	+9.2
Acid number change, mg. KOH/g	+4.08	+0.80

The results contained in the above table demonstrate that the formulation containing the present antioxidants is vastly superior in every category except that of filter deposits where it is comparable and well within normal tolerances.

Mixtures of N-Phenylnaphthylamines with Alkylated Diaminodiphenylmethanes

A mixture of amines suitable as an antioxidant, especially for aviation lubricants has been developed by *G.J. Jervis and R. Robson; U.S. Patent 3,804,762; April 16, 1974; assigned to Esso Research and Engineering Company.* According to this process this antioxidant especially suitable for turbine oils comprises a mixture of (a) an alkylated N-phenylnaphthylamine having at least one alkyl substituent each containing 3 to 14 carbons and (b) an amino compound of the formula:

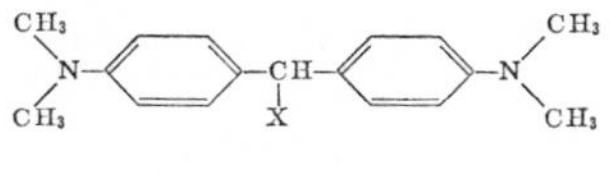

where X is hydrogen, hydrocarbyl containing up to 20 carbons, or the group

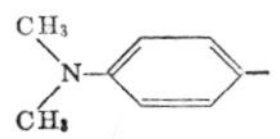

Preferred alkylated N-phenylnaphthylamines are mono- or di-$(C_3$–$C_{14})$alkyl N-phenylnaphthylamines. Thus, one may use isobutyl, hexyl, octyl, decyl, or dodecyl N-phenyl-α-naphthylamine or similarly alkylated N-phenyl-β-naphthylamine; or the dialkyl analogues. The alkyl groups need not be the same for the dialkyl compounds. When there is one alkyl substituent on the phenyl group it is preferably in the para position, although it can be in the ortho- or meta-positions. When there are two alkyl groups the total number of carbon atoms in the two groups is preferably not more than 20. There may be other substituents in any of the aromatic rings, e.g., halogen atoms, nitro groups, etc. The preferred alkylated N-phenylnaphthylamine is N-(tert-octyl phenyl)-β-naphthylamine.

Although preferably it is the phenyl group which is alkylated, one or both of the aromatic rings of the naphthylamine part of the molecule may be alkylated, and the term alkylated N-phenylnaphthylamine covers both possibilities. Suitable alkyl substituents of the naphthylamine part of the molecule include those specifically mentioned above. To avoid corrosion problems it is preferred that component (a) should contain no sulfur atoms as a substituent or part of a substituent group.

The preferred component (b) is N,N'-tetramethyldiaminodiphenylmethane, i.e., when X is hydrogen. It could however be for example 1,1-bis(N,N'-dimethylaminophenyl)heptane, N,N'-tetramethyldiaminotriphenylmethane or N,N',N''-hexamethyltriaminotriphenylmethane. When X is hydrocarbyl, it preferably contains 2 to 12 carbons.

The mol ratio of (a) to (b) must be at least 1:1, and is preferably between 1:1 and 13:1, especially between 1:1 and 10:1. A preferred mol ratio is between 2:1 and 4:1, e.g., about 2.3:1. This antioxidant mixture is suitable for use in a lubricating oil, especially a synthetic polyester aviation turbine oil. When added to a lubricating oil, it should be added in minor proportion, preferably 0.001 to 10.0% by weight, e.g., 0.1 to 5.0% by weight, based on the weight of lubricating oil.

Example: Various antioxidant mixtures were prepared by blending together N-(tert-octyl-phenyl)-β-naphthylamine (abbreviated C$_8$-PBNA) and N,N'-tetramethyldiaminodiphenyl-methane (TMDDPM). Each mixture was separately added to a synthetic ester base oil which also contained 1.0% by weight of tricresyl phosphate. The base oil was a mixture of complete esters obtained by esterification of 90% pentaerythritol and 10% dipentaerythritol with a mixture of (C_6–C_{10}) fatty acids.

The blends of oil plus antioxidant were subjected to the Rolls Royce Oxidation Test (R-R1001) and the results obtained given in the table below. For comparison, tests were carried out using C$_8$-PBNA alone and TMDDPM alone, and a blend where the mol ratio of C$_8$-PBNA to TMDDPM is less than 1:1, i.e., 0.77:1. In Tests (1) and (2) which relate to antioxidants not within the scope of this process, there were vapor phase deposits as a varnish in the test tube, thus indicating that these two antioxidants would be too dirty to be acceptable. In Tests (5) and (6) which also relate to antioxidants not within the scope of this process it is noted that Δkv (increase in kinematic viscosity) and volatility are too high and the induction period too low compared with Tests (7) to (10) on antioxidants of this process.

	Antioxidant and percent. based on weight of oil—		Rolls Royce test (temp†, 215° C., 72 hours duration)					
Test	(a)	(b)	Mole ratio (a):(b)	Percent volatility	Induction period (hrs.)	Δkv. 210° F., percent	Δ tan	Benzene insolubles, percent [1]
(1)		1% TMDDPM		37.5	0			
(2)	1.0% C$_8$-PBNA	1% TMDDPM	0.77:1	28.4	24	125	4.70	0.03
(3)	1.5% C$_8$-PBNA	0.5% TMDDPM	2.31:1	23.4	36	96	5.59	0.03
(4)	2% C$_8$-PBNA			31.6	24	149	4.5	0.01
			Temp. 215° C., duration increased to 192 hrs.					
(5)	2% C$_8$-PBNA			56.6	24	(Solidified after 168 hrs.)		
(6)	3% C$_8$-PBNA			54.7	48	428	4.32	0.03
(7)	3.0% C$_8$-PBNA	1.0% TMDDPM	2.31:1	28.9	~192	64	2.50	0.04
(8)	3.0% C$_8$-PBNA	0.75% TMDDPM	3.07:1	34.7	84	131	4.34	0.04
(9)	3.0% C$_8$-PBNA	0.60% TMDDPM	3.84:1	37.1	82	142	4.22	0.03
(10)	3.0% C$_8$-PBNA	0.50% TMDDPM	4.61:1	40.0	89	118	3.75	0.02

[1] Maximum acceptable value 0.05% by weight.

Mixtures of p,p'-Dioctyldiphenylamine and n-Phenyl-1,2,3,4-Tetrahydro-2-Naphthylamine

The tripropylene glycol diester lubricating base fluid seems to be too unstable for use by itself in the high temperatures of the latest jet engines because of the hydrogen atom attached to a tertiary carbon atom in the tripropylene glycol chain. Accordingly, in order for the tripropylene glycol diester to be used in a jet engine lubricant one must also include an effective antioxidant.

Antioxidant systems have been developed by *R.E. Wann; U.S. Patent 3,681,247; August 1, 1972; assigned to The Procter & Gamble Company* for such lubricant compositions comprising fatty acid diesters of tripropylene glycol where each fatty acid moiety contains from 6 to 10 carbons. The antioxidant system comprises from 0.001 to 5% of a mixture of p,p'-dioctyldiphenylamine and N-phenyl-1,2,3,4-tetrahydro-2-naphthylamine.

The p,p'-dioctyldiphenylamine is a known commercial antioxidant. The other antioxidant, N-phenyl-1,2,3,4-tetrahydro-2-naphthylamine, can be readily prepared by reacting 1,2,3,4-tetrahydro-2-naphthol, a known compound whose preparation is described in Brochet et al, *Bull. Soc. Chim.,* 31, 1280-85 (1922), with aniline according to the general procedure for reacting amines with hydroxyl compounds as described by Guyot et al, *Bull. Soc. Chim.,* 47, 203-10 (1930).

The N-phenyl-1,2,3,4-tetrahydro-2-naphthylamine shall make up from 30 to 80% of the mixture, preferably from 50 to 70%. It is preferred that these two amines be used in a ratio of two parts of p,p'-dioctyldiphenylamine to three parts N-phenyl-1,2,3,4-tetrahydro-2-naphthylamine. A preferred level of the antioxidant is about 1.5% by weight of the lubricant composition and a preferred range is from 0.1 to 2%.

It is believed that the p,p'-dioctyldiphenylamine acts (1) as a free radical inhibitor, (2) as a dispersant, and (3) in a secondary role as a base. It is believed that the N-phenyl-1,2,3,4-tetrahydro-2-naphthylamine acts primarily as a base to neutralize any acid produced either in storage or in use. Other materials serving the same functions can be substituted either wholly, or in part, for the abovementioned components of the antioxidant mixture. The following examples are illustrative of the preparation and use of this antioxidant system.

Example 1: N-phenyl-1,2,3,4-tetrahydro-2-naphthylamine is prepared in the following manner. 75 grams of active nickel catalyst is prepared by reduction of nickel oxide with hydrogen at 300°C. The 75 grams of catalyst is mixed with 1,100 grams (7.5 mols) 1,2,3,4-tetrahydro-β-naphthol and 750 grams (8 mols) of aniline and the mixture is reacted under agitation in an autoclave at 180°C and 20 kg/sq cm pressure for approximately three hours. The reaction mixture is then removed from the autoclave, filtered to remove the nickel catalyst, and acidified with dilute sulfuric acid.

The aqueous solution containing the protonated product and aniline is extracted three times with diethyl ether to remove unreacted 1,2,3,4-tetrahydro-β-naphthol. The aqueous solution is then made basic with dilute NaOH and extracted three times with petroleum ether to give a petroleum ether solution of crude N-phenyl-1,2,3,4-tetrahydro-2-naphthylamine contaminated with small quantities of aniline. The latter is removed by multiple washing of the petroleum ether solution with cold H_2O. The petroleum ether solution is then dried with $MgSO_4$, filtered and cooled to give crystals of the desired product, melting point 121° to 125°C.

Example 2: In this example, pour points are determined according to ASTM D97. The corrosion and oxidation stability tests were a modification of the Federal Standard 791, Method 5308 wherein the tests were run at 347°F. The evaporation test was ASTM D972. The following compares a tripropylene glycol diester where the fatty acids have an approximate distribution C_6, 4%; C_8, 55%; C_{10}, 40%; and C_{12}, 1% and the same tripropylene glycol diester in a lubricant composition containing 1.5% of an antioxidant package which is a 40% p,p'-dioctyldiphenylamine and 60% N-phenyl-1,2,3,4-tetrahydro-2-naphthylamine.

	A. Oxidation-corrosion test (347° F.)							
	(1) Percent volume loss	(2) Total acid number	(3) Corrosivity (weight loss mg./cm.²)					B. Percent evaporation [1]
			Al	Mg	Cu	Steel	Ag	
Tripropylene glycol diester (TPG)	23	24	Too bad to run					57
Tripropylene glycol diester and antioxidant package........	2	0.55	0.000	0.008	0.188	0.015	0.008	15

[1] 6½ hours at 400° F.

Aromatic Amine-Metal Antioxidant Mixtures

R.F. Bridger; U.S. Patent 3,634,238; January 11, 1972; assigned to Mobil Oil Corporation has found that an additive combination consisting essentially of a secondary or tertiary aromatic amine, a bis(diaromatic amine) or an arylene diamine and a metal from Series 3 of the Periodic Table having an atomic number of at least 27, or an acid salt thereof, are excellent antioxidants.

The secondary and tertiary amines are characterized in that each aromatic portion may be a single or a multiple ring system, including fused rings, containing up to 20 carbons each. Thus, the term aromatic will include radicals derived from benzene, naphthene, anthracene, and the like. Also, as used here, the term shall include radicals from the quinones, such as benzo-, naphtho- and anthroquinone. Still further, aromatic amine may have the amino nitrogen as part of a fused ring system containing from 3 (including the one in which the nitrogen appears) to a total of 5 fused rings. The aromatic portion may be substituted with alkyl (C_1–C_{18}), alkoxy (C_1–C_{12}), halo (i.e., Br, Cl, F, I), nitro, alkylthio, alkylamino, arylamino, and carboxyl.

The bis(diaromatic amines) used in the additive are those containing aromatic groups totaling 24 to 40 carbons. In addition, the aromatic portions may be substituted as above. The arylene diamines are the N-alkyl or -aryl-N'-alkyl or -aryl arylene diamines. The alkyl or aryl portions may have 1 to 24 carbons and aryl may be a single or multiple ring system including fused rings. The arylene portion may be a single ring (as phenylene) or a fused ring containing up to 18 carbons, including those derived from naphthalene, anthracene, and, for the purposes of this disclosure, the quinones. Arylene may also be a quinone radical in which one of the double bonded oxygens is replaced by one of the N's, as for example in 2-anilino-1,4-naphthoquinone-4-anil. These aryl and arylene groups may be substituted in the same manner as defined for the other amines.

The metals which may be used are, as already mentioned, those appearing in Series 3 of the Periodic Table and which have an atomic number of at least 27. Examples of such metals are cobalt, nickel, copper and zinc. Cobalt is the preferred metal. In addition to the metals per se, they may be used in the form of their acid salts. By acid is meant a mono- or polycarboxylic acid, the latter preferably containing no more than 2 carboxyls, which contains a saturated or unsaturated hydrocarbyl chain of 2 to 24 carbons. The carboxylic acid may also contain a cyclic structure, either cycloaliphatic or aromatic containing a total of 5 to 15 carbons in the cyclic structure.

Preferably the aliphatic carboxylic acids will contain 4 to 18 carbons, and the most preferred is stearic acid. Among the cycloaliphatic and aromatic acids, those having 6 to 12 carbons are preferred, and the most preferred is one containing 10 carbons, for example, naphthenic acid. The amine may be effectively used over the range of 0.05% to 10% by weight of the stabilized organic compound. The preferred range is 0.1 to 5% by weight, and most preferably 0.1% to 1.0%. When the metal is used in combination with the amine and organic compound, the effective range will be from 1 cm^2 surface area per kg of organic compound to 1,000 cm^2 per kg. The acid salt may be used at a concentration of 0.0005 to 2% by weight of the organic compound, preferably from 0.001 to 1% by weight.

Example: This test is conducted in an oxygen circulation apparatus of the type described by Dornte, *Ind. Eng. Chem.*, 28, 26-30, (1936) modified so the rate of oxygen absorption can be recorded automatically. In general, a tube containing 30 grams of an organic sample and the additive combination is placed in a thermostated heater. After thermal equilibrium is established, the sample tube is connected with the closed oxygen circulation system. Oxygen is circulated through a fritted glass disk near the bottom of the sample tube at the rate of 5 liters per hour. The time required for the adsorption of 1 mol of oxygen per kg of sample is taken as the inhibition period. The longer the inhibition period, the greater is the oxidation resistance of the sample.

The following table shows the results obtained with copper metal and certain amines using a base stock prepared by reacting 1 mol of pentaerythritol with 3 mols of commercial valeric acid and 1 mol of pelargonic acid. The same fluid was used in the other examples unless stated otherwise.

Amine used	Amine, weight percent	Temperature, 0° C.	Inhibition period, hours	
			Without copper	With copper, 100 cm.²/kg.
1,1'-bis-PBN[1]	None	175	2.0	2.0
	...do...	185	1.3	----
	0.218	175	6.0	25.3
	.436	175	15.7	71.0
	.872	185	43.8	64.1
1,1'-bis-DBNA[2]	None	175	2.0	2.0
	.268	175	27.2	49.8

[1] 1,1-bis(N-phenyl-2-naphthylamine)
[2] 1,1-bis[(N-2-naphthyl)-2-naphthylamine]

HETEROCYCLIC ANTIOXIDANTS FOR POLYESTERS

Substituted Benzodiazoboroles

A.K. Sparks; U.S. Patent 3,677,945; July 18, 1972; U.S. Patent 3,481,978; December 2, 1969; and U.S. Patent 3,629,190; December 21, 1971; all assigned to Universal Oil Products Company has prepared a series of 2-hydrocarbyl-1,3-di-sec-alkyl or dicycloalkyl-2H-1,3,2-benzodiazoboroles. These compounds act as stabilizers for lubricants, greases, gasolines, as well as polymeric materials which normally tend to deteriorate in storage, transportation and/or in use due to oxidation, ozonation, ultraviolet light absorption and/or other reactions.

These benzodiazoboroles can be represented by the formula:

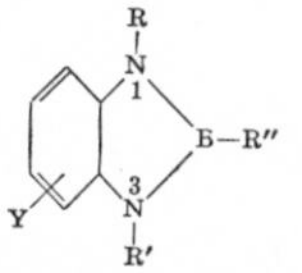

where R and R' are sec-alkyl or cycloalkyl, R'' is hydrocarbyl, and Y is hydrogen, hydrocarbyl, hydrocarbyloxy, halogen or nitro. It is an essential feature of the above compounds that R and R' are secondary alkyl or cycloalkyl. These compounds possess improved potency as additives to organic substrates. The sec-alkyl groups may contain 3 to 20 carbons each and thus will be selected from isopropyl, sec-butyl, sec-pentyl, sec-hexyl, sec-heptyl, sec-octyl and the like. The cycloalkyl groups may contain 3 to 12 carbons each and, in preferred compounds comprise cyclohexyl.

Referring to the above formula, R'' is hydrocarbyl and will be selected from alkyl, alkaryl, aryl, aralkyl or cycloalkyl. The alkyl moiety may be primary, secondary or tertiary and will contain 1 to 20 carbons or more. Where R'' is aryl, it will be selected from phenyl, naphthyl, anthracyl, etc., and may contain alkyl substituents attached to the aryl nucleus. Where R'' is aralkyl, illustrative groups include benzyl, phenylpropyl, phenylbutyl, phenylpentyl, phenylhexyl, phenylheptyl, phenyloctyl, etc., which also may contain one or two alkyls attached to the phenyl nucleus. Where R'' is cycloalkyl, the alkyl contains 3 to 12 carbons in the ring and thus will be selected from cyclopropyl, cyclobutyl, cyclopentyl, cyclohexyl, cycloheptyl, cyclooctyl, cyclononyl, cyclodecyl, cycloundecyl and cyclododecyl. Here again, cyclohexyl is particularly preferred.

Where Y is hydrocarbyl, it may be selected from those described above. Where Y is hydrocarbyloxy, it may comprise alkoxy or phenoxy; the latter also may contain alkyls attached to the phenyl nucleus. The hydrocarbyl moiety of the hydrocarbyloxy group will be selected from the hydrocarbyl groups described above. Where Y is halogen, it will be selected from chlorine, bromine, fluorine or iodine, preferably being chlorine or bromine. Illustrative preferred compounds include:

>2-nonyl-1,3-di-sec-hexyl-2H-1,3,2-benzodiazoborole
>2-nonyl-1,3-di-sec-heptyl-2H-1,3,2-benzodiazoborole
>2-phenyl-1,3-di-sec-hexyl-2H-1,3,2-benzodiazoborole
>2-phenyl-1,3-di-sec-heptyl-2H-1,3,2-benzodiazoborole
>2-phenyl-1,3-di-sec-octyl-2H-1,3,2-benzodiazoborole
>2-phenyl-1,3-di-sec-nonyl-2H-1,3,2-benzodiazoborole

Example 1: 2-Nonyl-1,3-di-sec-octyl-2H-1,3,2-benzodiazoborole was prepared by reacting nonyl boronic acid with N,N'-di-sec-octyl-o-phenylenediamine, the latter being prepared by reductive alkylation of o-phenylenediamine with octyl ketone at about 160°C, 100 atmospheres of hydrogen and in contact with an alumina-platinum catalyst. The reaction was effected by refluxing a mixture of 37 grams of N,N'-di-sec-octyl-o-phenylenediamine, 23 grams of nonyl boronic acid and 250 cc of benzene.

The refluxing was continued for 6 hours, and 2.5 cc of water was recovered from the distillation. Following completion of the reaction, 56 grams of 2-nonyl-1,3-di-sec-octyl-2H-1,3,2-benzodiazoborole was recovered as a reddish liquid. This corresponds to the theoretical yield of 56.9 grams. Analysis of the product found a boron content of 2.35% by weight and basic nitrogen of 1.97 meq/g which equals a molecular weight of 507.6 and corresponds to the theoretical molecular weight of 513.5.

Example 2: This example illustrates the use of 2-nonyl-1,3-di-sec-octyl-2H-1,3,2-benzodiazoborole, prepared as in Example 1, as an additive in lubricating oil. The lubricating oil used is a synthetic lubricating oil marketed under the trade name of Plexol 201 and is dioctyl sebacate. The lubricating oil was evaluated using a standard oxygen stability test in which a 100 cc sample of the lubricating oil is placed in a batch maintained at 204°C, and air is blown therethrough at a rate of 5 liters of air per hour.

The test is continued for 48 hours. The kinematic viscosities at the start of the test, after 24 hours and after 48 hours were determined. In addition, the percent of isooctane insoluble materials was determined. The following table reports the results of an evaluation of the control sample of the lubricating oil (not containing the additive) and a sample of the lubricating oil containing 2% by weight of 2-nonyl-1,3-di-sec-octyl-2H-1,3,2-benzodiazoborole.

	Control sample			Sample with additive		
	Start	24 hr.	48 hr.	Start	24 hr.	48 hr.
Kinematic viscosity	7.958	11.39	16.73	8.106	8.636	8.878
Percent increase		49	100		6	9.5

From the data in the above table it will be seen that the control sample of the lubricating oil (without additive) underwent an increase of approximately 100% in kinematic viscosity. In contrast, the sample containing the additive underwent an increase of less than 10% in kinematic viscosity.

In the control sample, the percent of material insoluble in isooctane was 8.2%. In contrast the percent of isooctane insolubles in the sample containing the additive was 0.1%. This again demonstrates the effectiveness of the compound of the process to retard deleterious reactions in the lubricating oil during evaluation in the above manner.

U.S. Patent 3,677,945 also includes examples of the use of these antioxidants in petroleum based greases and lubricating oil. U.S. Patent 3,481,978 and U.S. Patent 3,629,190 also include the use of these antioxidants in polypropylene, SBR and gasoline.

Alkylated Phenothiazines

Substituted phenothiazines as described below are used by *B. Cook and D.R. Randell; U.S. Patent 3,803,140; April 9, 1974; assigned to Ciba-Geigy Corporation* as antioxidants for organic materials. These antioxidants are particularly effective in the stabilization of synthetic polyester lubricants.

These compounds may be represented by the formula

(1)

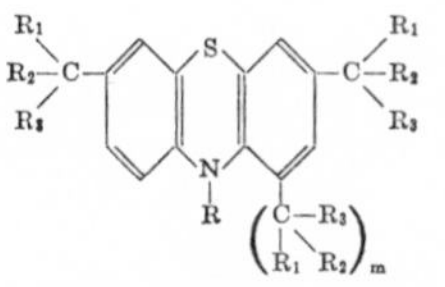

where R is hydrogen; alkyl or alkenyl each having 2 to 12 carbons; cycloalkyl having 5 to 12 carbons; aralkyl having 7 to 9 carbons; cyanoalkyl or hydroxyalkyl each having 2 to 4 carbons; or $YOCH_2-$ where Y is an alkyl radical having 1 to 4 carbons; or a cycloalkyl having 5 to 12 carbons; R_1 is alkyl having 1 to 4 carbons; R_2 is methyl; R_3 is phenyl either substituted or unsubstituted with 1 to 3 alkyl substituents each having 1 to 4 carbons; or R_2 and R_3 together with the carbon to which they are bound form a monocyclic ring having 5 to 12 carbons in the ring which is preferably unsubstituted or has 1 to 3 alkyl substituent groups each having 1 to 4 carbons; m is 0 or 1. Because of their ease of preparation and their high level of stabilizing activity in organic material, compounds of Formula 1 are preferred in which R is hydrogen. Particularly preferred compounds are: 3,7-di(α,α-dimethylbenzyl)phenothiazine, 1,3,7-tri(α,α-dimethylbenzyl)-phenothiazine and 3,7-di(1'-methylcyclohexyl)phenothiazine.

The compounds of Formula 1 are produced by reacting phenothiazine with the corresponding olefin or alcohol, in the presence of an acid catalyst to produce a compound of formula

(2)

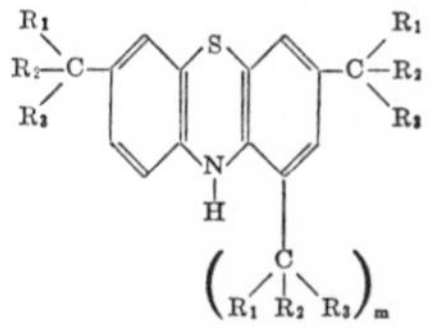

where R_1, R_2, R_3 and m have their previous significance, optionally converting a compound of Formula 2 into the corresponding N-alkali metal salt, and then reacting this salt with the corresponding alkyl, cycloalkyl, alkenyl or aralkyl halide, to produce a compound of Formula 1 in which R is an alkyl, cycloalkyl, alkenyl or aralkyl radical. 3,7-di-substituted phenothiazines are the principle products of these alkylation reactions but they may be accompanied by 1,3,7-tri-substituted phenothiazines or even 3-mono-substituted phenothiazines.

The ring alkylation step of the process is preferably effected by adopting the procedure described in British patent 1,036,696. Suitable olefins or alcohols for use in this stage include α-methylstyrene, α,4-dimethylstyrene, α-methyl-4-isopropylstyrene, 1-methylcyclohexene, or 1-methylcyclodecanol. In the N-substitution reaction stage, a suitable alkyl halide is butyl bromide, allyl bromide is a suitable alkenyl halide and benzyl chloride is a suitable aralkyl halide.

If R in the compound of Formula 1 is a cyanoalkyl group, the compound of Formula 2 may be reacted with the corresponding cyanoolefin, for instance acrylonitrile, preferably in the presence of a basic catalyst, for instance trimethylbenzyl ammonium hydroxide. In order to obtain a compound of Formula 1 in which R is alkoxymethyl, or cycloalkoxymethyl, N-alkoxymethylation or N-cycloalkoxymethylation of the compound of Formula 2 may be effected using a mixture of formaldehyde with the appropriate alcohol, preferably in the presence of sodium dihydrogen phosphate. N-hydroxyalkylation of the compound of Formula 2 may be achieved for example by reaction with the appropriate olefin oxide, for instance ethylene oxide or propylene oxide. The following examples will illustrate the preparative process and the use of these antioxidants.

Example 1: 118 parts by weight of α-methylstyrene were dissolved in 350 parts by volume of petroleum ether (boiling range 100° to 120°C). 80 parts by volume of this solution was added to a mixture of 99.6 parts by weight of phenothiazine and 9.5 parts by weight of p-toluenesulfonic acid. The mixture was heated to reflux in a nitrogen atmosphere and the remainder of the α-methylstyrene solution added over a period of 2 hours at the reflux with stirring, the mixture then being stirred at reflux for a further 4 hours. Without cooling, 100 parts by volume of 10% weight/volume aqueous NaOH solution was added to the mixture. Over a period of 15 minutes the color of the mixture went from deep purple to green and a precipitate was formed.

This solid was dissolved by the addition of 150 parts by volume of petroleum ether (boiling range 100° to 120°C) at 95°C. The aqueous phase was siphoned from the mixture and a further 100 parts by volume of 10% weight/volume aqueous NaOH solution added. The suspension so formed was stirred for 15 minutes at 95°C and the aqueous layer again removed. The petroleum phase was washed with water (6 x 250 parts by volume) until neutral, and the washed solution left to cool with stirring. On standing 116 parts by weight (52% theory yield) of crude 3,7-di(α,α-dimethylbenzyl)phenothiazine was obtained. Recrystallization from petroleum ether (boiling range 100° to 120°C) gave pure material having MP 131.5° to 132.5°C.

Example 2: A synthetic ester-based lubricant was formulated and subjected to a slightly modified Pratt and Whitney Type II oxidation-corrosion test. The base fluid was a complex ester derived from sebacic acid, caprylic acid and trimethylol propane, as described in British Patent 971,901. Each test was carried out for 48 hours at a temperature of 425°F using dry air at a rate of 5 l/hr and in the presence of specimens of titanium, aluminum alloy, copper, silver and steel. To the lubricant sample, there was added, prior to commencing the test, 4.0% by weight of the 3,7-di-(α,α-dimethylbenzyl)phenothiazine and 0.25% by weight of benzotriazol, each amount being based on the total weight of the lubricant. The results observed in the test and in the tests using equivalent amounts of certain known antioxidants are summarized in the following table.

Ex	Additive	Percent additive by wt.	Percent viscosity increase, 100° F.	Acid value increase (mg. KOH/g.)	Sludge mg./100 ml.	Weight changes in specimens, mg./cm.³				
						Ti	Al	Cu	Ag	Steel
	Phenothiazine	2.0	17.9	2.7	1,850	+0.34	+0.28	+0.34	+0.39	+0.31
	Benzotriazole	0.25								
	3,7-di-t-octyl phenothiazine	4.0	26.9	19.9	1.8	−0.03	−0.04	−0.41	−0.07	−0.02
	Benzotriazole	0.25								
2	3,7-di-(α,α-dimethylbenzyl)phenothia-zine.	4.0	28.2	9.2	8.7	+0.01	+0.01	−0.19	−0.02	−0.02
	Benzotriazole	0.25								

Thiooxazolidinedione or Thiazolidinedione Additives

The synthetic lubricating oil composition disclosed by *E.L. Patmore, F.G. Oberender and D.D. Reed; U.S. Patent 3,779,921; December 18, 1973; assigned to Texaco Inc.* comprises a major portion of an aliphatic ester-base oil containing an effective load-carrying amount of a thiooxazolidinedione, thiazolidinedione or corresponding amine salt. The additives are represented by the formulas:

(1)   or   (2)

in which X is sulfur when Y is oxygen, and X is oxygen when Y is sulfur, and R is a hydrocarbyl radical having 4 to 24 carbons. In general, the compounded fluid will also contain an alkylphenyl or alkarylphenyl naphthylamine, a dialkyldiphenylamine, a polyhydroxyanthraquinone and a hydrocarbyl phosphate.

Methods for preparing these thiooxazolidinediones, thiazolidinediones and their corresponding amine salts are well known. The preparation of 2,4-oxazolidinedione is described in *Chemical Abstracts,* 50, 9387 and in *J. Am. Chem. Soc.,* 80 973 (1958). The following examples illustrate the preparation of a representative number of the prescribed compounds which can be employed in the synthetic aircraft turbine oil compositions.

Example 1: Formaldehyde (40 ml of a 37% solution) was added with stirring and cooling (temperature held at 10°C) to a solution of sodium thiocyanate (40.5 grams) and sodium cyanide (27.0 grams) in water (55 ml). Concentrated hydrochloric acid was added while maintaining the temperature at 10°C. The reactants were allowed to warm to room temperature and set overnight. Solids were removed by filtration and the filtrate was heated at reflux for 1.5 hours. Extraction with ether (5 x 100 ml), concentration on the rotary evaporator, and two recrystallizations from water gave 7.1 grams of 2-thiooxazolidinedione, MP 107° to 109°C (lit MP 113°C).

Example 2: A reaction mixture of pseudothiohydantoin (6.4 grams) and hydrochloric acid (50 ml concentrated HCl/150 ml of water) was heated at reflux for 6 hours, concentrated on the rotary evaporator, and treated with 50 ml of methanol. The ammonium chloride was removed by filtration and the filtrate concentrated to give 5.4 grams of crude product. Recrystallization from ethanol gave 4.2 grams of 2,4-thiazolidinedione, MP 124° to 126°C (lit MP 126° to 127°C).

The prescribed compounds are employed in the lubricating oil composition in an amount ranging from 0.01 to 5 weight percent are effective and are preferred for imparting load-carrying and corrosion resistance properties to the lubricant composition. The base fluid component of the lubricant is an ester-base fluid prepared from pentaerythritol or trimethylolpropane and a mixture of hydrocarbyl monocarboxylic acids. Polypentaerythritols, such as dipentaerythritol, tripentaerythritol and tetrapentaerythritol can also be employed in the reaction to prepare the base oil.

The effectiveness of the lubricating oil is enhanced by also adding: one or more antioxidants such as the (1) alkyl or alkarylphenyl naphthylamines, or (2) dialkyldiphenylamines; a metal deactivator such as polyhydroxyanthraquinone; and an antiwear hydrocarbylphosphate ester. Such a composition was tested containing the compounds of Examples 1 and 2.

The lubricating oil composition was tested for its load-carrying properties in the Ryder Gear Test. This test was conducted in accordance with Federal Test Method Standard 791, Test Method 6508. The base fluid blend employed for conducting the tests consisted of a commercial ester base from pentaerythritol and a mixture of C_5 to C_{10} fatty acids containing 0.10 weight percent quinizarin, 1.00 weight percent p,p'-di-tert-octyldiphenylamine, 1.50 weight percent N-(4-tert-octylphenyl)-1-naphthylamine, 2.00 weight percent tricresylphosphate and 50 ppm of a dimethyl silicone fluid. The results of the Ryder Gear Test are given in the table below:

Run	Additive	Load-Carrying Additive, Wt %	Failure Load, ppi
1	Base blend	–	2,689
2	Example 1	0.15	3,325
3	Example 2	0.20	3,560

Substituted 2-Oxazolidones

Lubricating oils and greases are stabilized using substituted 2-oxazolidones in the process disclosed by *A.O.M. Okorodudu; U.S. Patent 3,785,982; January 15, 1974; assigned to*

Mobil Oil Corporation. Broadly, the oxazolidones have the formula

(1)

$$R'-\underset{\underset{CH_2-N}{|}}{\overset{\overset{R}{|}}{C}}\overset{O}{\underset{3}{\overbrace{5\quad1}}}\overset{}{\underset{R''}{\underset{|}{N}}}C=O$$

where R is (1) alkyl of C_7 to C_{20}, (2) members containing 1 to 18 carbons selected from cycloalkyl, aryl, alkaryl and aralkyl or (3) members containing from 2 to 25 carbons selected from alkoxyalkyl and aryloxyalkyl, R' is (a) hydrogen, (b) members containing 1 to 18 carbons selected from alkyl, cycloalkyl, aryl, alkaryl and aralkyl, or (c) members containing 2 to 25 carbons selected from alkoxyalkyl and aryloxyalkyl and R" is R' or NO.

The compounds where R" in Formula 1 is hydrogen are conveniently prepared by the nitrous oxide treatment of the hydrazide of the product of the Reformatsky reaction of a ketone or aldehyde and ethylbromoacetate, followed by heating. The N(3)-substituted 2-oxazolidones, where R" in Formula 1 is other than hydrogen or NO, may be prepared by reacting an organic isocyanate with an epoxide in the presence of a catalytic amount of lithium chloride. The nitroso derivative, where R" is NO, is made by reacting the 2-oxazolidone with sodium nitrite in the presence of HCl or with nitrosyl chloride.

More specific procedures for preparing the above compounds may be found in an article by Martin E. Dyen et al entitled, "2-Oxazolidones," in *Chem. Rev.,* 67, pages 197 to 246 (1967). The 2-oxazolidones are effective as antioxidants when used at concentrations of 0.01 to 10% by weight of the organic composition. They may, for example, be used in natural and synthetic rubbers and in a wide variety of lubricants, such as greases, mineral oils, as well as synthetic oils such as synthetic esters, synthetic hydrocarbons and silicones.

Example 1: Zinc, 65 grams (1 gram atom) and 400 ml of reagent grade benzene were charged into a 1 liter 4-necked flask equipped with a condenser, (carrying a drying tube), mechanical stirrer and an addition funnel. After distilling off 100 ml of benzene to dry the system, the heat was turned off and a mixture of acetophenone, (90 grams, 0.75 mol) and ethylbromoacetate (143 grams, 0.85 mol) was added dropwise to maintain the rapid ebullition. After the addition, the reaction mixture was heated at reflux, with stirring for 35 minutes, cooled and treated with ice cold 2 N HCl. The mixture was extracted with benzene-ether, the organic layer washed with dilute sodium carbonate solution, and then saturated salt solution. After stripping off solvent, distillation afforded 140 grams (90% yield) of ethyl 3-phenyl-3-hydroxybutyrate (A), BP 110°C/0.5 mm.

The ester (A) was treated with a 2 molar equivalent of anhydrous hydrazine and a few cc of ethanol, heated briefly (10 minutes) to reflux and allowed to stand. The solid hydrazide of 3-phenyl-3-hydroxybutyric acid (B) was collected, and washed with petroleum ether, MP 84° to 85°C, yield, 82%. The hydrazide (B) was dissolved in 2 N HCl and treated at 5° to 10°C with a slight excess of $NaNO_2$ dissolved in water. Benzene was then added to the reaction mixture and while stirring vigorously, it was heated slowly to about 70°C. After the rapid gas evolution subsided, the mixture was allowed to stand overnight. The 5-phenyl-5-methyl-2-oxazolidine which precipitated was collected, washed and dried. Yield, about 80%.

Example 2: To illustrate the antioxidant effect of these oxazolidones, certain of them were combined with a lubricating oil prepared from pentaerythritol and an acid mixture containing C_5 and C_9 monocarboxylic acids in approximately equal amounts and tested in the following test.

In this test, a catalytic oxidation test for lubricants, the lubricating composition is subjected to a stream of air which is bubbled through the composition at a rate equivalent to 5 l/hr at 425°F for 24 hours. Present in the composition are metals known to be catalysts for oxidation, e.g., (a) sand-blasted iron wire; (b) polished copper wire; (c) polished aluminum wire; and (d) polished lead. Inhibitors for oil are rated on the basis of their ability to prevent oil deterioration by measuring the increase in acid formation or neutralization number (NN), and kinematic viscosity (KV) occasioned by the oxidation. Following are the results.

Item	Additive	Conc., Wt. percent	Final acidity, NN	ΔNN	Viscosity, KV at 100° F. Final	Viscosity, KV at 100° F. Initial	ΔKV, percent
1	5-phenyl-5-methyl-2-oxazolidone	1	2.8	2.7	47.03		
		0.5	3.8	3.75	61.86		
2	5,5-diphenyl-2-oxazolidone-Ref	Saturated	5.9	5.55	115.9	26.52	338
3	5-(2-ethylpentyl)-2-oxazolidone	4	1.0	−0.6	38.31	27.34	40
		2	2.3	1.38	49.45	26.78	84
		1	3.1	2.64	45.49		69.8
		0.5	3.3	3.1	48.45		81
4	3-p-tolyl-5-phenyl-2-oxazolidone	2	3.3	3.1	47.23	26.90	75
		1	3.7	3.6	56.56		110
5	3-p-tolyl-5-phenoxymethyl-2-oxazolidone	1	6.1	6.0	79.23	26.76	191
		0.5	5.6	5.55	76.65		185
6	3-phenyl-5-phenoxymethyl-2-oxazolidone	1	5.6	5.5	81.20	26.83	201
		0.5	6.8	6.75	91.64		240
7	3,5-diphenyl-2-oxazolidone	2	3.8	3.7	43.81	26.76	63
		1	4.2	4.15	58.74		118
8	3-phenyl-5-decyl-2-oxazolidone	2	5.4	5.3	66.24	26.54	150
		1	4.6	4.55	65.13		112
9	3-nitroso-5,5-diphenyl-2-oxazolidone	4	5.4	4.91	53.04	27.10	95
		2	4.44	4.19	60.81		124
		1	5.16	5.03	78.69		190
10	1-oxa-3-azaspiro[4,5]decan-2-one	4	2.4	2.4	57.3	28.20	102
		2	3.3	3.2	53.9		91
		1	4.6	4.6	61.9		120
11	3-nitroso-1-oxa-3-azaspiro[4,5]decan-2-one	4	4.70	3.99	59.30	28.43	108
		2	4.34	3.98	58.38		102
		1	5.88	5.70	75.38		164
12	3-nitroso-5-phenyl-5-methyl-2-oxazolidone	4	5.7	5.48	59.35	27.00	118
		2	5.43	5.32	54.18		100
		1	4.34	4.28	53.34		98
13	3-p-tolyl-5-phenyl-2-oxazolidone	5	3.8	3.69	44.04	27.79	58
		4	3.8	3.71	54.68		96
		3	4.07	4.01	48.12		73
14	3-phenyl-5-decyl-2-oxazolidone	6	2.7	2.65	46.66	27.04	72
15	3-naphthyl-5-phenoxymethyl-2-oxazolidone	4	3.3	2.2	50.24	28.87	73
16	3-nitroso-5-(2-ethylpentyl)-2-oxazolidone	6	7.3	3.3	76.80	26.79	186
		4	7.05	4.3	70.70		164
		2	5.43	4.1	52.59		96
17	3-naphthyl-5-decyl-2-oxazolidone	6	4.5	4.39	48.89	29.4	66
		4	4.86	3.79	58.71		100
	None		8.0	7.9	142.6	26.14	447

In addition when the 2-oxazolidones are combined with 0.05 to 2.0% by weight of the total composition of phenyl-naphthylamine, especially phenyl-α-naphthylamine, or of dioctyl diphenylamine, the acid number is even more effectively reduced and in many cases so is the increase in viscosity.

POLYMERIC ANTIOXIDANTS FOR POLYESTERS

Epihalohydrin-Amine Condensates with Substituted Di(Aminophenyl)Propanes

Lubricants containing a stabilizing mixture of a di-(sec-alkylamino)-diphenylpropane or di-(cycloalkylamino)-diphenylpropane and polymeric condensation product of epihalohydrin compound and amine are disclosed by H.A. Cyba and R.H. Rosenwald; U.S. Patent 3,755,171; August 28, 1973; assigned to Universal Oil Products Company.

In a specific embodiment of the process the lubricant contains from 0.01 to 10% by weight of a mixture of (1) 25 to 75% by weight of a 4,4'-di-(sec-C_3-C_{50}-alkylamino)-diphenylpropane or 4,4'-di-(cycloalkylamino)-diphenylpropane in which the cycloalkyl moiety contains 4 to 20 carbons in the ring and (2) from 75 to 25% by weight of the polymeric condensation product of epihalohydrin compound or a mono- or polyamine containing 4 to 50 carbons. Any suitably substituted diaminodiphenylpropane is used as one component of the additive mixture. In a preferred embodiment, this is a 4,4'-di-(sec-alkylamino)-diphenylpropane in which the sec-alkyl moiety contains 3 to 50 carbons.

In another embodiment, this component of the mixture comprises a 4,4'-di-(cycloalkyl-amino)-diphenylpropane in which the cycloalkyl moiety contains 4 to 20 carbons in the ring. A particularly preferred compound is 4,4'-di-(cyclohexylamino)-diphenylpropane. Another component of the additive mixture comprises a polymeric condensation product of an epihalohydrin and a mono- or polyamine containing at least 4 carbons and more particularly from 4 to 50 carbons. A preferred epihalohydrin compound is epichlorohydrin. In one embodiment the amine reacted with the epihalohydrin compound is an alkyl monoamine. Illustrative examples of preferred amines include butylamine, hexylamine, nonylamine, and more particularly longer chain primary alkylamines. Conveniently the long chain amines are prepared from mixtures of fatty acids formed as products or by-products. Such mixtures are available commercially, generally at lower prices, and the mixtures may be used without the necessity of separating individual amines in pure state.

An example of such a mixture is hydrogenated tallow amine which is available under various trade names including Alamine H26D and Armeen HTD. These products comprise mixtures predominating in alkylamines containing 16 to 18 carbons per alkyl group, although they contain a small amount of alkyl groups having 14 carbons. Illustrative examples of secondary amines, which may be reacted with the epihalohydrin compound, include di-(dodecyl)amine, di-(tridecyl)amine, di-(tetradecyl)amine, di-(pentadecyl)amine, and the like. Here again, mixtures of secondary amines are available commercially, e.g., Armeen 2HT which consists primarily of dioctadecylamine and dihexadecylamine.

In another embodiment the amine to be reacted with the epihalohydrin compound is a polyamine. A preferred amine is a N-alkyl-1,3-diaminopropane in which the alkyl group contains 6 to 50 carbons. Here again, mixtures are available commercially, e.g., Duomeen T which is N-tallow-1,3-diaminopropane and predominates in alkyl groups containing 16 to 18 carbons each.

Example 1: This example describes an additive mixture of 4,4'-di-(sec-butylamino)-diphenylpropane and the polymeric condensation product of epichlorohydrin and hydrogenated tallow amine. The 4,4'-di-(sec-butylamino)-diphenylpropane was prepared by the reactive alkylation of 4,4'-diaminodiphenylpropane with methyl ethyl ketone in the presence of a platinum–containing catalyst and hydrogen. The hydrogenated tallow amine used is marketed commercially as Armeen HTD and is a mixture of primary amines predominating in 16 to 18 carbons per alkyl group. The condensation is effected by first forming a solution of 2 mols of epichlorohydrin in 600 cc of a solvent mixture comprising 400 cc of xylene and 200 cc of 2-propanol.

A separate solution of 2 mols of Armeen HTD is prepared in an equal volume of xylene. One mol of the latter solution is added gradually to the epichlorohydrin solution, with stirring and heating at 130° to 140°F for a period of 2.5 hours. Then another mol of Armeen HTD is added gradually to the reaction mixture, stirred and reacted at 175°F for 2.5 hours. 1 mol of sodium hydroxide then is added with stirring and heating at 185° to 195°F for 3.5 hours, after which another mol of sodium hydroxide is added and the mixture stirred and reacted at 185° to 195°F for 1 hour. Following completion of the reaction, the mixture is cooled, filtered, and the filtrate then is distilled under vacuum to remove the alcohol and xylene. The resultant product is a hard, waxy, brittle solid of light amber color containing 3.11 meq/g of basic nitrogen. The 4,4'-di-(sec-butylamino)-diphenylpropane and the polymeric condensation product are mixed together in approximately equal weight concentrations.

Example 2: This example illustrates the use of the additive mixture of Example 1 in a synthetic lubricant. This synthetic lubricant is pentaerythritol ester available commercially as Hercoflex 600 and is stated to be monomeric pentaerythritol ester having an acid number of 0.10 maximum, a saponification number of 410, a refractive index at 20°C of 1.453 and a specific gravity at 25/25°C of 0.997.

The evaluation was made in accordance with an Oxygen Stability Test, in which a 100 cc sample of the synthetic lubricating oil is placed in a bath maintained at 260°C and air is blown therethrough at a rate of 5 liters of air per hour. The sample of synthetic lubricating oil is examined periodically and the time to reach an acid number of 5 is reported. It is apparent that the longer the time required to reach an acid number of 5, the more stable is the sample of the lubricating oil. In other words, it takes longer for the more stable oil to deteriorate. In addition to determining the acid number of 5, the number at 22 hours and the percent viscosity change were also determined. The results of these evaluations, along with the evaluation of a sample of the lubricating oil without additive, are reported in the following table.

Run Number	Additive	Hours to Acid Number of 5	Acid Number at 22 Hours	% Viscosity Change at 26 Hours
1	None	6	13.9	111
2	1% by weight of 4,4'-di-(sec-butylamino)-diphenylpropane	12	8.5	75
3	1% by weight of 4,4'-di-(sec-butylamino)-diphenylpropane plus 1% by weight of the polymeric condensation product of Example 1	26	3.9	68.4

Another example in the patent shows the incorporation of similar antioxidant mixtures in grease. No quantitative stabilization data is given.

Polymeric Imides of Maleic Anhydride Copolymers

G. Frangatos; U.S. Patent 3,714,045; January 30, 1973; assigned to Mobil Oil Corporation has developed a reaction product from a primary arylamine and a alpha-olefin-maleic anhydride heteropolymer as a stabilizer for lubricants such as lubricating oils and greases including the mineral oils and synthetic polyester oils.

These polymeric imides are made by reacting a heteropolymer of maleic anhydride and an α-olefin with an aromatic amine. With reference to the heteropolymer, there are free anhydride groups along the polymeric chain and the number of these is proportional to the amounts of maleic anhydride and olefin which are coreacted, e.g., when equimolar amounts of maleic anhydride and olefin are copolymerized, the olefin and anhydrode portions alternate in the copolymer chain. The heteropolymer is made up of recurring units of

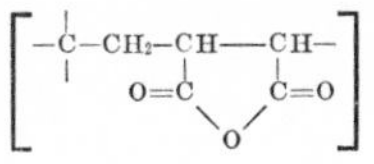

$$\left[\begin{array}{c} -\overset{|}{C}-CH_2-CH-CH- \\ \underset{O=C}{|} \quad \underset{C=O}{|} \\ \diagdown O \diagup \end{array} \right]$$

The aromatic amine reacts with the anhydride portion of the heteropolymer as follows:

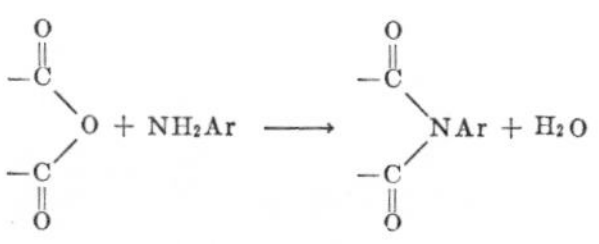

$$\begin{array}{c} O \\ \| \\ -C \\ \diagdown O + NH_2Ar \longrightarrow \\ -C \\ \| \\ O \end{array} \quad \begin{array}{c} O \\ \| \\ -C \\ \diagdown NAr + H_2O \\ -C \\ \| \\ O \end{array}$$

In its preferred form, the heteropolymer is reacted with sufficient amine to form an imide with each anhydride unit along the polymer chain.

Example 1: Into 300 ml of xylene were placed 40 grams (0.5 mol) maleic anhydride, 126 grams (0.5 mol) 1-octadecene and 5 grams di-tert-butyl peroxide. The mixture was refluxed and stirred under nitrogen for 5 hours. Yield: 68% based on maleic anhydride. A mixture of 35 g (0.1 mol) of this heteropolymer, 14.3 g (0.1 mol) of α-naphthylamine and 250 ml of xylene were placed in a flask. The reaction mass was brought to reflux. After recovery of about 0.8 ml of water, gradual removal of the xylene was begun. As the xylene was removed, the temperature of the reaction medium was gradually increased, and such increase was continued until a temperature of 205°C was reached. 49.2 g of the polyimide was recovered.

Example 2: The polyimides were blended into a synthetic ester oil lubricant (made by reacting pentaerythritol with an equimolar mixture of C_5 and C_9 monocarboxylic acids) and tested in an oxidation test in accordance with the following procedure. A sample of the test composition is heated and air at the rate of about 5 l/hr is passed through for about 24 hours. Present in the test sample are specimens of iron, copper, aluminum, and lead. It should be noted that the metals are typical metals of engine or machine construction, and they also provide some catalysts for the oxidation of organic materials. The neutralization number (NN) measures the amount of acidity in the oil. The percent change in viscosity (ΔKV, percent) occurring as a result of the test conditions is determined from the initial and final measurements at 100°F. The results, tabulated in the following table, concern the product of Example 1.

Base	Additive, percent	Temperature, °F.	Initial NN	final NN	ΔNN	Initial KV	final KV	ΔKV, percent
PE 1 ‑‑‑‑		425	0.1	9.5	9.4	26.69	98.97	270.81
		450	0.1	10.7	10.6	26.69	206.0	671.82
PE 2 ‑‑‑‑		450	0.1	8.6	8.5	27.86	57.21	105.35
PE 1 ‑‑‑‑	3	425	0.66	1.40	0.74	30.13	56.26	86.72
	3	450	0.66	1.40	0.74	30.13	43.43	44.14
PE 2 ‑‑‑	3	450	0.81	3.10	2.29	31.34	43.04	37.33

[1] This is the pentaerythritol ester described in the procedure.
[2] This is the same pentaerythritol ester having therein about 4% of a mixture of an arylamine antioxidant, an antiforming agent, an antiwear agent and a metal scavenger.

Cetyl Vinyl Ether Telomers with N-Vinylpyrrolidone

The properties of lubricating oils are also found by *G. Frangatos; U.S. Patent 3,663,439; May 16, 1972; assigned to Mobil Oil Corporation* to be improved by adding a telomer prepared from cetyl vinyl ether and N-vinylpyrrolidone in the presence of a trihydrocarbyl phosphite. The trihydrocarbyl phosphite acts as a telogen in the copolymerization of the two vinyl monomer.

The telomer may be made using molar ratios of cetyl vinyl ether and N-vinylpyrrolidone of from 1:1 to about 1:20 to 20:1. Preferably such ratio will be 1:1. The trihydrocarbyl phosphite is used in an amount equal to or larger than the molar concentration of the monomer present in the higher concentration. If the trialkyl phosphite is in excess, this excess will generally range from about 10 to 30%. Preferably, however, such excess should not exceed 20%.

The product is made up of recurring units of copolymerized vinyl monomers, terminated with a phosphorus moiety linked to such copolymer through direct linkage with the phosphorus atom. More precisely, it is believed that the structure of the telomer will conform to the following

where n may vary from 2 to 200 and R is a hydrocarbyl group as defined below. In general, the process contemplates the use of from about 0.005 to 15% of the telomer in lubricating oils. Preferably, the concentration of additive in such oil will be from about 0.01 to 10% by weight thereof, more preferably from about 1.0 to 5.0%.

The trihydrocarbyl phosphites include those where each hydrocarbyl portion contains 1 to 20 carbons. Preferably among these are those phosphites having lower alkyl groups, i.e., those of 1 to 6 carbons. Specifically, there may be mentioned the trimethyl, triethyl, tributyl, and trihexyl phosphites and the alkyl portions thereof may be straight or branched chain. The hydrocarbyl group of the phosphite may also be an aryl, such as phenyl or naphthyl, an alkaryl, such as tolyl or ethylphenyl, or an aralkyl such as benzyl or phenethyl.

Example 1: Into a reaction vessel equipped with a condenser, stirrer and thermometer was placed a mixture of 83.1 grams (0.5 mol) of triethyl phosphite and 200 ml of chlorobenzene and the temperature brought up to reflux (about 130°C). 44.4 grams (0.4 mol) of N-vinylpyrrolidone, 107.2 grams (0.4 mol) of cetyl vinyl ether and 10 grams of di-tert-butyl peroxide were placed in 200 ml of chlorobenzene, and this mixture was added to the refluxing chlorobenzene over a period of 1½ hours with stirring, under a nitrogen atmosphere. Heating at 125° to 130°C was continued for 10 hours. An additional 5 grams of di-tert-butyl peroxide was added and heating at 125° to 130°C was continued for another 4 hours. The solvent and unreacted monomers were distilled off under reduced pressure and finally at 0.6 mm of Hg at 240°C. The product, 128 grams, was a clear viscous fluid. An analysis of this product showed it to contain 0.88% of phosphorus and to have a molecular weight of 1,232.

Example 2: Oxidation tests in synthetic ester lubricants are carried out as follows. The telomers were blended into a synthetic ester oil lubricant and tested in an oxidation test in accordance with the procedure of U.S. Patent 3,714,045. The results, tabulated in the following table, concern the product of Example 1.

Oil	Percent additive	Initial NN	Final NN	ΔNN	Initial KV	Final KV	ΔKV percent
A[1]	0	0.10	10.70	10.60	26.69	206.0	671.82
B[2]	0	0.30	6.90	6.60	27.37	50.5	84.44
A	3	0.05	7.00	6.95	30.87	102.2	231.07
B	1	0.27	2.10	1.83	28.89	39.84	37.90

[1] Synthetic ester made from pentaerythritol and an equimolar mixture of C_8 and C_9 monocarboxylic acids.
[2] Same as oil A, except it contains about 5% of an additive package comprising a major amount of a neutral phosphate ester and lesser amounts of an amine mixture and metal suppressor, as well as about 0.3% of bis(nonylphenyl)phosphonate.

Aryliminodialkanol-Phosphate Condensates

G. Frangatos; U.S. Patent 3,654,157; April 4, 1972; assigned to Mobil Oil Corporation has also developed a third antioxidant for lubricants comprising a copolymer of a dialkyl hydrocarbylphosphonate and an aryliminodialkanol.

The copolymer is produced by a condensation reaction, so it is important that a 1:1 molar ratio of phosphonate to dialkanol be maintained. The reaction produces a copolymer believed to be made up of the following unit recurring along the polymer chain

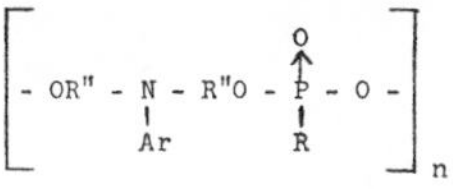

$$\left[- OR'' - N - R''O - \overset{\overset{O}{\uparrow}}{\underset{R}{P}} - O - \right]_n$$
$$\quad\quad\quad\;\; Ar$$

where n is a number from 2 to about 200 and R, R' and Ar are as defined in connection with the starting materials.

The dialkyl hydrocarbylphosphonates contemplated as starting materials are those having the formula

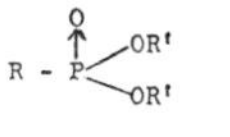

$$R - \overset{\overset{O}{\uparrow}}{P}\overset{OR'}{\underset{OR'}{\diagdown}}$$

where R may be alkyl, aryl, aralkyl and cycloalkyl of 1 to 200 carbons, preferably 1 to 50 carbons and R' may be individually selected from alkyl groups having 1 to 10 carbons. Since the reaction involves transesterification with consequent removal of an alkanol, it is preferred that R' be kept from 1 to 6 carbons, and more preferably from 1 to 3 carbons. Included among the phosphonates which may be used are dimethyl methylphosphonate, dimethyl ethylphosphonate and the like.

The aryliminodialkanols contemplated as starting materials are those having the formula $ArN(R"OH)_2$ where Ar is an aryl group having 6 to 30 carbons in the ring or condensed ring portion and which may have substituted thereon an alkyl group of 1 to 50 carbons, a nitro, halo (preferably chloro, iodo or fluoro) or cyano group, and R" is an alkylene having 1 to 50 carbons.

Among those aryliminodialkanols which can be used are: phenyliminodiethanol, naphthyliminodiethanol, chlorophenyliminodimethanol, nitrophenyliminodimethanol and the corresponding diethanol, dipropanol and similar derivatives.

The lubricants which may be improved by the addition of the copolymer are mineral oils, both paraffinic and naphthenic, and synthetic oils. The synthetic oils include polyolefin fluids, polyglycols, polyacetals, the siloxanes and the like.

Example 1: Xylene (250 ml) was charged to a reaction flask. To this were added 1.1 grams of metallic sodium, 36.1 grams (0.1 mol) of dimethyl octadecylphosphonate and 18.1 grams (0.1 mol) of 2,2'-phenyliminodiethanol while maintaining an atmosphere of nitrogen over the reaction medium.

Thereafter, the reaction mixture was heated to 140°C and maintained at this temperature for 6 hours. The solvent was slowly distilled under atmospheric pressure. It contained the theoretical amount of methanol (6.4 grams, 0.2 mol) determined by gas liquid chromatography (GLC). The remaining traces of solvent were removed in vacuo at 200°C and 0.65 mm of Hg. 45.3 grams of product was obtained. The stoichiometry of the reaction, the quantity of the methanol recovered and the yield of final product indicated that a condensation copolymer was obtained.

The dimethyl octadecylphosphonate used in this example was prepared by reacting 1-octadecene and dimethylphosphonate at a 1:3 molar ratio in the presence of di-tert-butyl peroxide. Specifically the phosphonate and 1-octadecene were mixed, heated to 150°C and the peroxide was added dropwise over a period of 30 minutes. Following addition of the peroxide, the reaction was completed by heating the reaction mixture for 60 minutes at 150°C.

The compounds produced in accordance with this process were blended into a synthetic ester oil lubricant (made by reacting pentaerythritol with an equimolar mixture of C_5 and C_9 monocarboxylic acids) and tested in an oxidation test in accordance with the procedure given in U.S. Patent 3,714,045. The results, tabulated in the following table, concern the product of Example 1.

Percent Additive	Temp., °F.	Initial NN	Final NN	Δ NN	Initial KV	Final KV	ΔKV, percent
0	425	0.10	9.50	9.40	26.69	98.97	270.81
0	450	0.10	10.70	10.60	26.69	206.00	671.82
3	425	0.15	5.70	5.55	27.06	90.21	233.37
3	450	0.15	15.60	15.45	27.06	104.00	284.33

Complex Phosphorus Esters

Additives which impart superior oxidation resistance to synthetic ester base functional fluids but do not adversely affect the load-bearing properties of the lubricants are disclosed by *Q.E. Thompson, S.L. Reid and R.W. Weiss; U.S. Patent 3,684,711; August 15, 1972; assigned to Monsanto Company.*

The synthetic ester base lubricants and particularly the lubricants derived from pentaerythritol and polypentaerythritol are stabilized against oxidation at elevated temperatures by incorporating in the ester an inhibiting amount of a complex alkali metal organophosphorus compound prepared by esterifying a polyhydric alcohol free of beta hydrogen with an acylating agent which is a carboxylic acid or acid derivative and a polybasic acid of phosphorus or equivalent derivative to produce a mixed acid ester of the polyol having both carboxylic acid and phosphorus acid residues, and contacting the acid ester with an alkali metal base to yield a complex alkali metal organophosphorus salt inhibitor.

The inhibitors can be prepared separately and added to the ester base stock lubricant, or where the lubricant base stock is an ester derived from a polyhydric alcohol free of beta hydrogen, the inhibitors can be prepared in situ by causing the phosphorus acid or acid derivative to react with the base stock itself to form the complex mixed organophosphorus ester, and then contacting the ester with an alkali metal base.

Useful carboxylic acids are the mono- and polycarboxylic acids generally, and include those having straight, branched or cyclic hydrocarbon structures. The acids may be saturated and may contain 4 to 22 carbons while the polycarboxylic acids may contain up to 50 or more carbons. The preferred acids are the monocarboxylic acids or mixtures of mono- and dicarboxylic acids represented by the structure RCOOH where R is an alkyl, aryl, alkaryl, or alicyclic hydrocarbon.

The more preferred monocarboxylic acids, however, are the acyclic acids having from 4 to 12 carbons and including specifically the fatty acids and the common branched chain acids such as isovaleric, 2-ethyl hexanoic, isodecanoic, and 2-propylheptanoic acid.

The size and structure of the organic groups in the carboxylic acids affects the solubility of the material, and the optimum size of this group is determined largely by the nature of the polyol to be esterified and the type of base stock to be inhibited. For example, in the esterification of dipentaerythritol with a mixture of phosphorus acid and monocarboxylic acids, the monocarboxylic acids can contain up to 18 carbons while in the esterification of tripentaerythritol it is generally advantageous to use lower molecular weight acids of 4 to 8 carbons.

Illustrative of the polyols useful in the preparation of the inhibitors are polyhydric alcohols free of beta hydrogen such as neopentyl glycol, trimethylolethane, trimethylolpropane, pentaerythritol, dipentaerythritol, tripentaerythritol, 2-butyl-2-ethyl-1,3-propane diol, and the like.

The phosphorus compounds useful in the esterification of the polyol include the free acids of phosphorus such as phosphorous, phosphoric and the lower alkyl phosphonic acids and derivatives of such acids which are capable of esterifying the polyol. Examples of such useful derivatives of these acids include the various acid anhydrides, phosphites, phosphonates, halophosphates, halophosphites, halophosphonates, phosphorous amides and phosphonous amides. In general, the free acids of phosphorus provide good results and are the preferred reactants, while the acid derivatives are useful as permissible alternatives.

Example 1: Preparation of Inhibitor Composition — To a 5 liter reactor equipped with a stirrer, reflux condenser and water separator were charged 3 mols of dipentaerythritol, 3 mols of crystalline phosphorous acid, 15.3 mols octanoic acid, and 200 ml toluene. The reactants were brought to vigorous reflux at an initial temperature of 120° to 130°C and water released during the esterification was separated as formed. Reactor temperature was gradually increased over a 2 hour period to 160°C, and finally increased to 170°C and held for 30 minutes to complete the reaction.

When the esterification was complete as indicated by the lack of water of reaction, the reactor pressure was decreased to 10 mm to remove water, toluene and other volatile materials. A light yellow complex organophosphorous acid ester was decanted from heavier insoluble materials such as polyphosphorous acids.

The complex acid ester was treated at 140°C with 1.9 mols of anhydrous potassium carbonate (2 equivalents per equivalent of acid) added in small increments with vigorous agitation. After addition and reaction was complete, the potassium organophosphorus compound was separated from excess carbonate as a clear yellow filtrate. The atomic ratio of potassium to phosphorus in the inhibitor product was determined to be about 1.3.

Example 2: The complex organophosphorous compound prepared in Example 1 was added to a synthetic ester base stock comprised of a mixture of PE and diPE esters of C_5 to C_9 aliphatic acids containing approximately 2% arylamine antioxidant, 0.1% of a corrosion inhibitor, and 15 ppm silicon oil defoamer.

The inhibitor was added to the base stock at four levels of concentration, and the inhibited fluid evaluated for oxidation and corrosion stability. The results obtained are compared in the table below with the results obtained without the inhibitor, and for the base stock inhibited with potassium octanoate (KC_6) and potassium neodecanoate (KC_{10}).

	Inhibitor, meq. alkali metal/20 g. base stock	Lead corrosion, mg./in.[2]	Appearance	O & C Test			
Run				Percent viscosity increase	Mg loss	Cu loss	Ryder Test [1]
1	Control	0	Clear	([2])	−7.8	−0.5	100
2	0.02 KC₈	−57.2	Suspension	71	−0.43	−0.16	96
3	0.02 KC₁₀	−74.4	Clear	162	−3.7	−0.23	87
4	0.005	−1.8	do	([2])	−10.4	−0.54	
5	0.01	−1.0	do	173	−4.3	−0.30	
6	0.02	−3.2	do	54	−0.08	−0.21	104
7	0.045	−4.8	do	58	−0.04	−0.26	

[1] Test results reported as percent of control.
[2] Too viscous to measure.

Comparison of Run 5, a preferred embodiment of this process, with the control (Run 1) and the prior art (Runs 2 and 3) clearly shows the generally superior results obtained with the inhibitor of Example 1. Particular improvement over the control is noted in percent viscosity increase and Mg corrosion, while improvement over the prior art is noted in Pb corrosion, appearance, and Ryder Test.

PHOSPHATE ESTER BASED FLUIDS

Phosphate ester based fluid compositions are widely used as the operating fluid in aircraft hydraulic systems where the fluids are exposed to elevated temperatures in the order of 300°F. It is essential to the successful operation of such hydraulic systems that the fluid used be resistant to oxidation at the operating conditions.

Many hydraulic systems employ magnesium and copper and their alloys in pumps, seals, etc. contacted by the hydraulic fluid. Phosphate ester based hydraulic fluids which are not effectively stabilized against oxidation form corrosive decomposition products which are particularly aggressive toward magnesium and copper. In order to prevent corrosive damage to mechanical components of such hydraulic systems, it is essential that the hydraulic fluid be suitably stabilized.

2,6-Diaminopyridines

A stabilized phosphate ester base stock has been developed by *J.F. Herbert; U.S. Patent 3,783,132; January 1, 1974; assigned to Monsanto Company*. This comprises a major amount of a phosphate ester base stock and an oxidation inhibiting amount of a 2,6-diaminopyridine compound represented by the structure

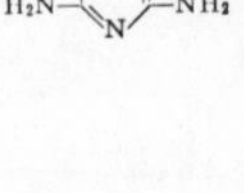

In this formula each R is individually an alkyl of 1 to 8 carbons, a phenyl or a methyl substituted phenyl, and n is an integer of 0 to 2. The composition may also contain minor amounts of other conventional base stock and/or additives such as viscosity index improvers.

Specifically these comprise a major amount of one or more phosphate esters represented by the formula

$$R-O-\overset{\overset{\displaystyle O}{\|}}{\underset{\underset{\displaystyle R}{|}}{P}}-O-R$$

where each R is individually an alkyl or alkoxyalkyl group containing 2 to 12 carbons, a phenyl group, or a substituted phenyl group containing up to 16 carbons, where the substituents are alkyl, phenyl, or phenylalkyl and the alkyl has 1 to 10 carbons.

The compositions preferably comprise at least 65% by weight of the phosphate ester and at least 0.001% by weight of the phosphate ester of 2,6-diaminopyridine inhibitor. Any remainder of the composition may be selected from other base stock constituents such as, for example, polyesters, polyphenyl ethers, polyphenyl thioethers, polyamides, silicate esters, and the like which may be present in amounts of up to 35% by weight of the composition and from conventional functional fluid additives.

An amount of the 2,6-diaminopyridine inhibitor sufficient to improve the oxidative stability of the fluid composition is employed. This amount may be from as little as 0.001 to as much as about 5% by weight of the phosphate ester in the composition.

The oxidative stability of the stabilized compositions were determined according to the basic procedure set forth in Federal Test Method Standard 791-5308 under specific test conditions as follows: sample size, 100 cc; airflow, 5 l/hr of dry air; temperature 300°F; exposure time, 168 hours; and metals present, Mg, Al, Cd, Fe, Cu.

The effect of incorporating 0.1% of 2,6-diaminopyridine in one base stock consisting of dibutyl phenyl phosphate and in a second base stock consisting of a mixture of tributyl phosphate and tricresyl phosphate is illustrated by the Oxidation and Corrosion Test results given in the table below. It is evident from these data that in both instances the addition of the inhibitor effectively inhibited the corrosion rate experienced during the test, particularly with respect to magnesium and copper. There was also significant improvement in reducing the amount by which viscosity and acidity increased during the test.

| Fluid composition | Corrosion rate, mg./cm.² | | | | | Coking | Sludge | 100° F. viscosity, percent increase | Acidity, TAN | |
	Mg	Al	Cd	Fe	Cu				Initial	Final
A. Dibutyl phenyl phosphate	−60.85	−0.04	−82.09	−2.75	−187.94	Light	Heavy	514	0.02	60.6
B. (A) plus 0.1% 2,6-diaminopyridine	−0.23	−0.06	−0.03	+0.06	−12.52	Heavy	do	−4.0	0.02	12.1
C. 88.5% tributyl phosphate; 11.5% tricresyl phosphate	−0.14	0.00	−6.89	+0.04	−51.04	None	None	5.7	0.02	10.1
D. (C) plus 0.1% 2,6-diaminopyridine	−0.06	−0.03	−0.05	+0.06	+0.04	Heavy	do	0	0.02	1.8

Nitrogen Antioxidant-Nitrogen Heterocycle Mixtures for Phosphoroamidates

Functional fluid compositions comprising a phosphoroamidate base stock, a known nitrogen-containing antioxidant and a nitrogen-containing heterocyclic compound, are disclosed by *J.F. Herbert; U.S. Patent 3,778,376; December 11, 1973; assigned to Monsanto Co.* These compositions have the ability to inhibit and control corrosion damage to mechanical members in contact with the functional fluid.

More specifically, the corrosion of metal in contact with a phosphoroamidate can be inhibited and controlled by the incorporation into the functional fluid of a unique combination of a nitrogen-containing antioxidant and a nitrogen-containing heterocyclic compound selected from:

(A) A compound of the structure

$$(R_1)_c-X_1 \overline{\qquad} X_1-(R)_a$$
$$R_2-C \underset{\displaystyle N}{\overset{\displaystyle \|}{\diagdown}} \diagup X_1-(R)_b$$
$$\underset{H}{\overset{|}{N}}$$

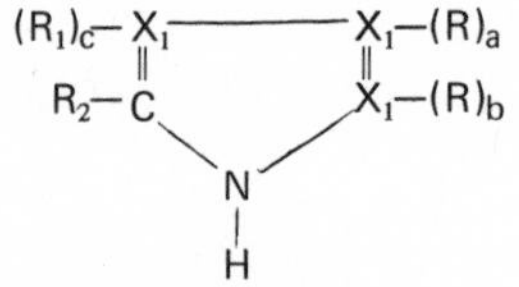

where each R is selected from hydrogen, alkyl, amino, substituted amino, hydroxyl and cyano amino; R_1 and R_2 are each selected from hydrogen, amino, substituted amino, alkyl, substituted alkyl, cycloalkyl, aryl and substituted aryl and R_1 and R_2 together can form a cyclic or a substituted cyclic ring, selected from carbon- and nitrogen-containing heterocyclic rings having 4 to 10 atoms optionally interrupted by 1 to 4 nitrogens, and a carbocyclic ring containing 4 to 10 carbons; a, b and c are each 0 or 1; each X_1 is carbon or nitrogen provided that when each X_1 is nitrogen a, b and c, respectively, are 0 and provided that at least one X_1 is nitrogen; and mixtures thereof;

(B) A compound of the structure

$$(R_3)_c$$
$$\underset{X_2}{\overset{|}{}}$$
$$R_4-C \diagup\qquad\diagdown X_2-(R_3)_d$$
$$R_5-C \qquad X_2-(R_3)_e$$
$$\underset{(R_3)_b}{\overset{|}{X_2}}$$

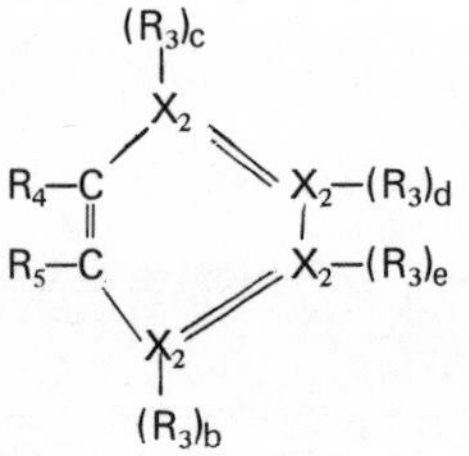

where each R_3 is selected from hydrogen, alkyl, amino, substituted amino, hydroxyl and cyano amino; R_4 and R_5 are each selected from hydrogen, amino, substituted amino, alkyl, substituted alkyl, cycloalkyl, aryl and substituted aryl and R_4 and R_5 together can form a cyclic or a substituted cyclic ring selected from heterocyclic ring having 4 to 10 atoms optionally interrupted by 1 to 4 nitrogens and carbocyclic rings containing 4 to 10 carbons; c, d, e and f are each 0 or 1; each X_2 is nitrogen or carbon provided that when X_2 is nitrogen, c, d, e and f are 0 and provided that there is present within the compound (a) at least one nitrogen atom represented by X_2 or (b) at least one nitrogen atom represented by X_2-R_3 where X_2 is carbon and R_3 is selected from NH_2, monoalkylamino, dialkylamino and cyanoamino, and mixtures thereof;

(C) A compound of the structure:

$$R_7-N \overline{\qquad} X_3-(R_6)_g$$
$$R_8-C \underset{\displaystyle N}{\overset{\displaystyle \|}{\diagdown}} \diagup X_3-(R_6)_h$$

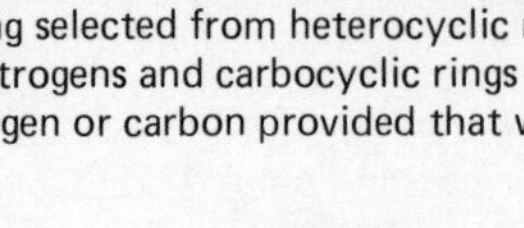

where R_6 is selected from hydrogen, alkyl, amino, substituted amino, hydroxyl and cyano amino; R_7 and R_8 are each selected from hydrogen, amino, substituted amino, alkyl, substituted alkyl, cycloalkyl, aryl and substituted aryl and R_7 and R_8 together can form a cyclic or a substituted cyclic ring selected from heterocyclic rings having 4 to 10 atoms optionally interrupted by 1 to 4 nitrogens and carbocyclic rings containing 4 to 10 carbons; g and h are each 0 or 1; X_3 is nitrogen or carbon provided that when X_3 is nitrogen, g and h are 0, and mixtures thereof; and

(D) Mixtures of any combination of (A), (B) and (C).

Typical examples of compounds represented by (A) are imidazoles, imidazolines, indazoles, triazoles, and indoles. Typical examples of nitrogen-containing heterocyclic compounds represented by (B) are pyrimidines, pyridines, quinolines, pteridines, and naphthylimides. Typical examples of heterocyclic compounds represented by (C) are triazines and indolizines.

Typical examples of nitrogen-containing antioxidants which can be utilized in this composition are the naphthylamines, the carbazoles, the diphenylamines, the aminophenols, aminodiphenyl ethers, aminodiphenyl thioethers, the aryl-substituted alkylenediamines, the aminobiphenyls, the reaction products of an aldehyde or ketone with an amine, and the like.

Typical examples of phosphoroamidate base stocks used in the composition are the amides of an acid of phosphorus which have the structure

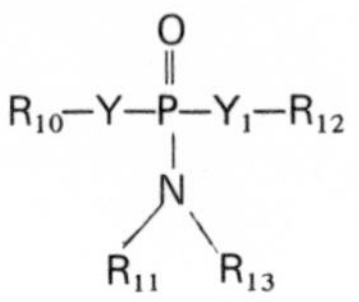

$$R_{10}-Y-\underset{\underset{\underset{R_{11}}{N}}{|}}{\overset{\overset{O}{||}}{P}}-Y_1-R_{12}$$

where Y is oxygen, sulfur or

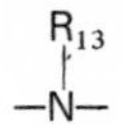

$$-\underset{}{\overset{R_{13}}{N}}-$$

and Y_1 is oxygen, sulfur or

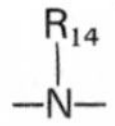

$$-\underset{}{\overset{R_{14}}{N}}-$$

R_{10}, R_{11}, R_{12}, R_{13} and R_{14} are each selected from alkyl, aryl, cycloalkyl, substituted aryl, substituted alkyl and a monovalent heterocyclic and substituted heterocyclic ring having 4 to 10 atoms optionally interrupted by 1 to 4 hetero atoms in the ring and where R_{10}, R_{11}, R_{12}, R_{13} and R_{14} can be identical or different with respect to any other radical and mixtures thereof.

It is also within the scope of this composition that the phosphoroamidates can be blended with minor amounts, i.e., up to 10 weight percent of ester compounds, such as di- and triester compounds, polyester compounds, complex ester compounds and mixtures thereof.

Various compositions were tested according to the procedure of Modified Federal Test Method 791, Method Number 5308. The metal specimens used were steel, copper, cadmium, magnesium and aluminum. The results are recorded in the table below.

Example Number	Nitrogen-Containing Antioxidant	Heterocyclic Compound	Base Stock	Copper	Cadmium	Magnesium	Total Acid	Sludge
1	1% p,p'-dioctyl diphenylamine, 1% N-phenyl-α-naphthylamine	None	A	−29.70	−4.44	−0.39	14.0	Slight
2	None	0.1% 3,5-diamino-1,2,4-triazole	A	−20.56	−36.12	−14.95	24.8	Heavy
3	1% p,p'-dioctyl diphenylamine, 1% N-phenyl-α-naphthylamine	0.1% 3,5-diamino-1,2,4-triazole	A	−0.16	−0.11	−0.01	3.10	None
4*	None	0.1% 5-amino indazole	A	−7.43	−2.53	−0.30	–	–
5	1% p,p'-dioctyl diphenylamine, 1% N-phenyl-α-naphthylamine	0.05% 5-amino indazole	A	−2.16	−0.17	0.17	–	Slight
6	1% p,p'-dioctyl-diphenylamine, 1% N-phenyl-α-naphthylamine	0.1% 4,5-diamino pyrimidene	A	−0.30	−0.60	−0.06	17.0	Slight
7	1% p,p'-dioctyl diphenylamine, 1% N-phenyl-α-naphthylamine	0.1% 7-amino indazole	A	−1.33	−2.15	−0.47	14.0	Slight
8	2% p,p'-dioctyl diphenylamine	None	A	−30.13	−4.21	−3.77	21.9	Heavy
9	2% p,p'-dioctyl diphenylamine	0.1% 3,5-diamino-1,2,4-triazole	A	−2.19	−0.37	−0.39	7.2	Slight
10	2% p,p'-dioctyl diphenylamine	0.10% 5-amino indazole	A	−0.48	−0.32	+0.22	5.0	None

The corrosivity to metals was determined by weighing the metal specimens before and after the test. The weight difference in mg/cm^2 of metal surface exposed to the fluid is reported. A minus sign (-) indicates that the metal specimen had a net weight loss after the test. In the table the asterisk (*) indicates that the oxidation and corrosion test as described above was run at a temperature of 260°F.

In all other examples, the temperature of the oxidation and corrosion test was at a temperature of 300°F and the flow rate of dry air at both temperatures was 5 l/hr. The designation A refers to a diamidate base stock which in N-methyl-N-butyl-N'-methyl-N'-butyl-phenylphosphorodiamidate. The duration of the oxidation and corrosion test was 168 hours.

POLYSILOXANE FLUIDS

Silylorganometallocene Antioxidants

Recently, automobiles have been manufactured with a variable speed fan. The fan is connected to the crankshaft of the motor by means of a fluid clutch. In order to operate such a clutch, it is necessary to utilize a fluid that is capable of withstanding high torsional forces at high temperatures without breaking down by oxidizing and gelling.

For such an application dimethylpolysiloxane fluid has been found especially suitable. However, this fluid oxidizes at high temperatures above 200°C after continued use in such fluid clutch for 50 hours or more. Various antioxidants were added to the polysiloxane fluid to prevent its oxidation and gelling.

Examples of such antioxidants are iron oxide, iron octoate, and manganese oxide. However, with all such antioxidants the compound either precipitated out of the fan clutch fluid or did not sufficiently protect the polysiloxane fluid and, in particular, dimethyl-polysiloxane, from oxidizing and gelling.

E.D. Brown, Jr. and A. Berger; U.S. Patents 3,745,129; July 10, 1973; and 3,649,660; March 14, 1972 have found that a class of silylorganometallocenes can stabilize and prevent polysiloxane fluids from oxidation.

These silylorganometallocenes are selected from the class of compounds consisting of:

(a) Polymers having structural units of the formula

$$(1) \qquad S{-}W{-}R''{-}\overset{\displaystyle (R)_a}{\underset{\displaystyle }{Si}}O_{\frac{3-a}{2}}$$

(b) Copolymers composed of structural units of the formula

$$(2) \qquad \overset{\displaystyle (R)_b}{\underset{\displaystyle }{Si}}O_{\frac{(4-b)}{2}}$$

and at least one unit of (a);
(c) Disiloxanes of the formula

$$(3) \qquad [S{-}W{-}R''{-}(R)_2Si]_2O$$

where R is selected from monovalent hydrocarbon radicals, halogenated monovalent hydrocarbon radicals, cyano radicals and fluoroalkyl radicals; S is an organometallocene radical having the formula

$$(4) \qquad -[C_5Q_4]M[C_5Q_5]$$

where W is a carbamyl radical; R" is selected from an arylene radical and an alkylene radical; Q is chemically bonded to a cyclopentadienyl radical and is a member selected from hydrogen, a monovalent electron donating organic radical and a monovalent electron withdrawing organic radical; and M is a transition metal bonded to cyclopentadienyl radicals. In the above formula, a is a whole number from 0 to 2, and b is a whole number from 0 to 3.

The organopolysiloxanes are produced by hydrolyzing metallocenyl halides of the formula

$$(5) \qquad S-W-R''\overset{(R)_a}{\underset{|}{Si}}X_{3-a}$$

where S, W, R", R and a are as defined above and X is a halogen radical. The copolymeric organopolysiloxanes are produced by cohydrolyzing the metallocenyl halide of Formula 5 with halosilanes of the formula

$$(6) \qquad \overset{(R)_b}{\underset{|}{Si}}X_{4-b}$$

where R, b, and X are as defined above.

The disiloxane of Formula 3 is produced by hydrolyzing a metallocenyl halide of the formula

$$(7) \qquad S-W-R''-\overset{(R)_2}{\underset{|}{Si}}X$$

where S, W, R", R and X are as defined above.

The metallocenyl halides of Formulas 5 and 7 are prepared by reacting a metallocene having the formula

$$(8) \qquad [(Q'')_e(R')_d(H)_cC_5]_2M$$

with a silyl isocyanate halide of the formulas

$$(9) \qquad X_{3-a}-\overset{(R)_a}{\underset{|}{Si}}R''NCO \qquad\qquad (10) \qquad X-\overset{R_2}{\underset{|}{Si}}R''NCO$$

where M, R, R", X and a are as defined previously, Q' is an electron donating radical, Q" is an electron withdrawing radical, c is an integer equal to from 1 to 5, d is a whole number equal to from 0 to 4 and e is a whole number equal to from 0 to 1, while the sum of c, d and e is equal to 5. The reaction is a modified Friedel Crafts reaction carried out in the presence of a Lewis acid such as boron trifluoride, phosphoric acid, hydrogen fluoride, zinc chloride, stannic chloride and aluminum chloride, which is preferred.

Molar amounts of the reactants are used to carry out the reaction under preferred conditions. The reaction is preferably carried out in a chlorinated hydrocarbon solvent such as chloroform, dichloromethane, dichloroethane, etc. Other suitable solvents are benzene, nitrobenzene and carbon disulfide. The temperature at which the reaction can be carried out varies widely, for instance a temperature range of –25° to 100°C has been found operable, while a range of 0° to 25°C is preferred.

Example 1: Into a 3 necked flask equipped with a magnetic agitator, thermometer, condenser and maintained under a nitrogen atmosphere there was added 9.4 parts (0.05 mol) of ferrocene and 100 ml of dry ethylene chloride. After agitation had begun, there was added immediately 8.8 parts (0.05 mol) of chlorodimethylsilylpropylisocyanate.

The reaction mixture was then heated at a temperature in the range of 15° to 90°C and there was added over a two hour period 6.7 parts (0.05 mol) of anhydrous aluminum chloride. A blood red complex was formed. The reaction was kept at reflux for 48 hours.

At the end of that period the flask was cooled and the contents poured over ice. The deep blue aqueous phase was separated from the red organic phase, then the aqueous phase was washed with methylene chloride and the washings combined with the organic phase. The organic phase was dried, stripped of solvent and then chromatographed. The resulting product was eluted with ethanol and purified by crystallization from ether-benzene. The product was obtained in 82% yield as yellow solid with MP of 156° to 158°C and having the structure:

$$O\left(\underset{\underset{CH_3}{|}}{\overset{\overset{CH_3}{|}}{Si}}-CH_2CH_2CH_2-\underset{\overset{|}{H}}{N}-\overset{\overset{O}{\|}}{C}C_5H_4FeC_5H_5\right)_2$$

Example 2: The silylorganoferrocene of Example 1, which is 1,3-bis(ferrocenoylaminopropyl)tetramethyldisiloxane, was dispersed at different concentrations in various samples of dimethylpolysiloxane fluids of 1,000 and 5,000 centistokes viscosity. The silylorganometallocene was insoluble and when heated to 140°C a clear yellow solution was formed.

On cooling the fluid became cloudy and microscopic examination showed it to be full of ribbon-like crystals. These crystals remained suspended in the fluid during freeze-thaw cycles and did not settle out. The samples of the mixtures were tested by placing 40 parts of the samples in a 150 ml beaker and placing the beaker in an oven maintained at 290°C. The time for gelation as well as the iron concentration and the silylorganometallocene concentrations in the fluid is set forth in the table below.

Fluid viscosity of dimethylpolysiloxane, cs.	Concentration of iron, percent by weight	Concentration of silylorganometallocene, percent by weight	Time to gelation at 290° C., hours
1,000	0.004		168
1,000	0.0085		692
1,000	0.017		>1,384
1,000	0	0	>24
5,000	0.017		692

All of the samples which exceeded a gelation time of 200 hours were placed in a fluid clutch which was operated continuously for 200 hours. All these fluid materials passed the test satisfactorily.

Phenolic Thin Film Antioxidants

Hydraulic systems containing poly(alkoxy)siloxane fluids as the power transmission medium are often used in aircraft hydraulic systems. Experience with these fluids has shown that they suffer from a serious bulk oxidation problem. This problem has been kept within reasonable limitations by including small amounts of a bulk oxidation inhibitor in commercial siloxane fluids.

It has also been found that in the hydraulic systems of high speed aircraft, a second type of oxidation of the fluid is encountered. This is referred to as thin film oxidation, and is manifested by the formation of crystals on portions of the hydraulic apparatus where the fluid is drawn out into a thin film and heated by the frictional resistance of the passing air. The crystals prevent smooth operation of the jacks and can seriously affect control of the aircraft. The conventional bulk oxidation inhibitors are not capable of controlling this crystallization.

M.L. Burrous and N.W. Furby; U.S. Patent 3,732,169; May 8, 1973; assigned to Chevron Research Company have developed a crystallization inhibitor or thin film antioxidant for these polysiloxane fluids. These crystallization inhibitors have the following formula:

(1)

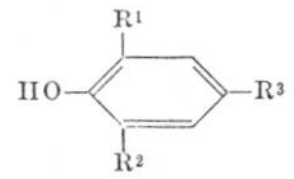

$$HO-\langle\ \rangle-R^3$$

with R^1 top and R^2 bottom of the ring.

where R^1 is a secondary or tert-alkyl group having 4 to 8 carbons; R^2 and R^3 are each a hydrocarbon group or a group containing carbon, hydrogen, and oxygen, and together have a total of 22 to 40 carbons and 0 to 5 oxygens.

When these phenols are used in the transmission fluid, the fluid has good oxidative stability at temperatures in the range of 300° to 400°F. The fluid comprises 55 to 99.8 weight percent poly(alkoxy)siloxane, the alkoxy radical containing 3 to 8 carbons and the siloxane polymer having a number average molecular weight of between 1,000 and 1,600 and consisting predominantly of polymer chains containing at least 4 monomer units; a bulk oxidation inhibitor; and a crystallization inhibitor as defined above.

The crystallization inhibitor should be present in amounts of approximately 0.1 to 5.0 weight percent and, more preferably, 0.5 to 3.0 weight percent of the total fluid. The fluid must also contain 0.1 to 3.0 weight percent of a bulk oxidation inhibitor. Several of these are described in the art. A typical, and widely used inhibitor is di-tert-butyl-p-cresol.

Effectiveness of the crystallization inhibitors is illustrated in Table 2 below. In each experiment the additive to be tested (described in Table 1) was put into a base fluid which consisted of 84 weight percent of poly(2-ethylbutoxy)siloxane and 15 weight percent of di(2-ethylhexyl)sebacate. The additive was present as an additional 1 weight percent in the fluid during the test. The fluid was then heated as a thin film in the presence of air at 392°F. Visual examination of the fluid was made at the stated intervals.

TABLE 1

Additive	Compound	R^2		R^3				R^2+R^3	
		C	O	C	O	N	S	C	O
A	di-t-Butyl-p-cresol	4	0	1	0	0	0	5	0
B	bis (3,5-di-t-butyl-4-hydroxyphenyl)methane.	4	0	15	1	0	0	19	1
C	Octadecyl 3-(3′,5′-di-t-butyl-4′-hydroxyphenyl)propionate.	4	0	21	2	0	0	25	2
D	2,4-di-(3′,5′-di-t-butyl-4′-hydroxyphenoxy)-6-octylthio-1,3,5-triazine.	4	0	25	3	3	1	29	3

TABLE 2

	Fluid appearance after—				
Additive	1 hr.	4 hrs.	7 hrs.	16 hrs.	23 hrs.
None	Clear liquid	Opaque and crystalline			
A	do	do			
B	Liquid	Slight crystallization	Complete crystallization		
C (Exp-1)	Clear liquid	Clear liquid	Clear liquid	Liquid	Light yellow liquid; slight crystallization.
C (Exp. 2)	do	do	do	Clear liquid	Clear liquid.
D	do	Yellow liquid	Dark yellow liquid		Brown liquid

It is apparent from these data that those compounds which contain less than 22 total carbons in the R^2 and R^3 groups have little effect on the crystallization of the base fluid. These compounds extend the life of the fluid by no more than a factor of two. The compounds of Formula 1, however, extend the fluid life by a factor six or more.

POLYPHENYL ETHERS

Lipid Extracts of Yeast Cultures

It is possible to grow microorganisms by the cultivation of microorganisms on a hydrocarbon substrate in the presence of nutrient media and oxygen. The recovered microorganisms may be purified by solvent extraction are then available as food-stuff.

E.S. Forbes and A.D. Forbes; U.S. Patent 3,658,702; April 25, 1972; assigned to The British Petroleum Company Limited, England have found that some of the waste products from the purification stage, referred to as lipid extracts, when added to a lubricating base oil possess lubricating load-carrying properties, antioxidant and anticorrosion properties.

In order to separate the lipid extract from the microorganisms, a solvent system consisting of a polar and nonpolar solvent may be used. Preferably the polar solvent contains a hydroxyl group. Suitable solvent systems are ethanol/diethyl-ether, methanol/chloroform, and isopropanol/n-hexane. Especially useful solvent systems are azeotropic mixtures of alcohols and hydrocarbons. Solvent systems consisting of alcohol/water mixtures are also useful, and the preferred solvent system is an azeotropic isopropanol/water system. The extraction may be carried out at room temperature.

Diethyl-ether may be used as a sole extractant but careful temperature control is required for efficient separation. After the initial extraction of the lipid extract the solvents used can be evaporated off. When water is present in the solvent system an aqueous mixture is left which is then distilled to remove the water.

Various yeast culture, molds and bacterial cultures may be used in the growth process and are listed in the complete specification. The preferred yeast culture for use in this process is *Candida lipolytica.* The following examples will illustrate the process.

Example 1: A yeast of the family *Candida tropicalis* was grown in a gas oil of boiling range 300° to 400°C in the presence of a nutrient medium containing nitrogen and phosphorus. During the growth period air was blown through the liquid mixture as described in U.K. Patent 914,568.

When the growth had reached the desired stage as measured by the cellular density of the yeast the mixture was centrifuged. A pasty phase containing yeast cells impregnated with hydrocarbons and aqueous medium was thus separated. This pasty phase was washed with water to remove the bulk of the gas oil, and the product obtained heated to 80° to 90°C in a rapid current of air and ground to a powder.

The powder was treated by solvent extraction using a mixture of isopropanol, n-hexane and water. The solids not removed by the extracting liquids are the purified food-yeasts and the extracting liquids contain the yeast lipids extract. The extracting liquids can then be treated in two ways. If they are allowed to settle, two phases are formed, an upper phase containing isopropyl alcohol, n-hexane, any residual gas oil and some of the yeast lipids extract and a lower phase consisting of mainly, isopropyl alcohol, water and the remainder of the yeast lipids extract.

The solvents can be evaporated off from both these phases to yield two yeast lipids fractions. Alternately the extracting liquids can be subjected to distillation and all the solvent removed, prior to settling, to give a total yeast lipids extract, TL 9.

Example 2: The total yeast lipid extract TL 9 prepared as in Example 1 was subjected to the following separation stages to isolate various fractions having enhanced anticorrosion properties. Crude lipids extract TL 9 was dissolved in n-heptane to yield TL 9.31 freed from residual yeast and mineral salts.

Example 3: Lipid extract TL 9.31 prepared as above was tested as antioxidant in inhibiting the oxidation of a phenylene oxide. Compositions with and without TL 9.31 were shaken in a flask immersed in a silicone oil bath at 200°C with air passing through the flask at constant mass flow. The decrease in oxygen content of the air from the test flask was measured. The induction period, maximum rate of oxidation and the total oxygen uptake were determined. The results are shown below.

Sample	Induction Period (minutes)	Maximum Rate of Oxidation (mol O_2 mol^{-1} sec^{-1})	Total Oxygen Uptake (mol O_2/mol Squalane)
A*	0	0.55	2.3
B**	16	0.47	1.8

*0.8 gram squalane plus 2.3 grams polyphenylene oxide
**0.8 gram squalane plus 2.3 grams polyphenylene oxide plus 0.0147 gram TL 9.31, i.e., 1.8 weight percent

The temperature was 200°C, the air flow rate was 65 ml/min with a duration of 2 hours. The results show the antioxidant properties of the lipid extract.

Further fractionation of the lipid extracts could be done by dialysis over a 24 hour period using a rubber membrane and n-hexane as solvent. The fractions obtained gave improved antiwear properties in liquid paraffin lubricants.

ANTIOXIDANTS FOR ELASTOMERS

ANTIOZONANTS

Unsaturated polymers, whether natural or synthetic vulcanized or unvulcanized, are normally susceptible to degradation by ozone. By and large this occurs as a result of prolonged exposure to ozone contained in the atmosphere. Ozone degradation can manifest itself in rubber by the scission of polymer chains, resulting in a decrease in tensile strength, flexibility and other desirable properties. Therefore it is often necessary to provide compounds which will, by incorporation into the polymers, protect the polymers against ozone degradation.

Tetrahydroquinoxaline-Aldehyde Condensates

It was found by *F.H. Wilson, Jr.; U.S. Patent 3,706,742; December 19, 1972 and U.S. Patent 3,580,884; May 25, 1971; both assigned to The Goodyear Tire & Rubber Company* that polymers may be protected against the deleterious effects of ozone by incorporating a product prepared by reacting aldehydes with tetrahydroquinoxalines. The aldehydes that may be used in preparing the products are compounds of the structural formula:

$$\overset{\displaystyle O}{\underset{\displaystyle \|}{R-C-H}}$$

where R is selected from hydrogen, alkyl radicals having 1 to 20 carbons, cycloalkyl radicals having 5 to 10 carbons, heterocyclic radicals having 4 to 10 carbons, and 1 to 4 additional atoms selected from sulfur, nitrogen and oxygen, aryl radicals having 6 to 8 carbons and aralkyl radicals having 7 to 12 carbons. Among the preferred aldehydes are formaldehyde, acetaldehyde, propionaldehyde, benzaldehyde, furfural, tetrahydrofurfural and butyraldehyde. The most preferred aldehyde is formaldehyde.

The tetrahydroquinoxalines that are to be used in preparing the reaction products are compounds having the structural formula:

222

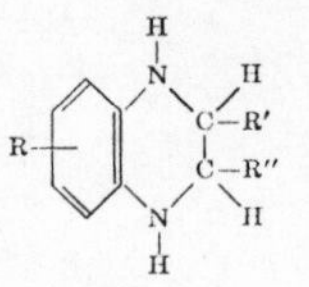

where R is selected from hydrogen, alkyl radicals having 1 to 12 carbons, alkoxy radicals having 1 to 12 carbons, cycloalkyl radicals having 5 to 12 carbons, cycloalkoxy radicals having 5 to 12 carbons, aryl radicals having 6 to 10 carbons, aralkyl radicals having 7 to 12 carbons, alkaryl radicals having 7 to 12 carbons, aryloxy radicals having 6 to 10 carbons and heterocyclic radicals having 4 to 10 carbons and 1 to 4 additional atoms selected from sulfur, nitrogen and oxygen, and where R' and R" are selected from hydrogen, alkyl radicals having 1 to 12 carbons, aryl radicals having 6 to 10 carbons, cycloalkyl radicals having 5 to 10 carbons and radicals where the R' and R" are joined together to form a carbocyclic ring having 5 to 10 carbons.

Within this definition the preferred tetrahydroquinoxalines includes 1,2,3,4-tetrahydro-quinoxaline; and 2,3-dimethyl-1,2,3,4-tetrahydroquinoxaline. The products are prepared by reacting the tetrahydroquinoxalines with an aldehyde in an aqueous solution and in the presence of an acidic catalyst.

A preferred combination comprises approximately two mols of the tetrahydroquinoxaline and one mol of the aldehyde. The combination is permitted to react for an extended period of time at a temperature of –20° to 200°C. A preferred temperature range is 0° to 120°C. The reaction mixture is then cooled and the acidic catalyst neutralized by pouring it into an aqueous alkaline solution where it is vigorously agitated. The desired product is then separated by filtration and thoroughly washed with water and subsequently dried. The desired reaction products have melting points between 65° and 150°C. Yields in the range of 90% of theoretical are routinely obtained.

Example: Into a reaction flask equipped with stirrer, thermometer, dropping funnel and reflux condenser were charged 20 grams of 2,3-dimethyl-1,2,3,4-tetrahydroquinoxaline, 26 grams of concentrated sulfuric acid and 85 ml of water. The mixture was heated to 55°C with stirring to obtain solution and then cooled to 7.5°C. To this cooled reaction mixture was gradually introduced 5.5 grams of formalin added over an interval of 15 minutes. The reactants were stirred for one hour at a temperature between 11° to 22°C and then gradually heated to reflux and stirred for an additional 24 hours.

The reaction mixture was then cooled to 70°C and poured into an aqueous alkaline solution containing 24 grams of sodium hydroxide. The slurry was vigorously stirred for approximately 30 minutes. The solid reaction product was then filtered and washed several times with water and dried. The resulting reaction product weighed 18 grams, representing a yield of 85%. The melting point of the resulting reaction product was 65° to 105°C.

The effectiveness of the stabilizers is demonstrated by subjecting rubber samples containing them to accelerated aging in an ozone chamber and comparing the relative deterioration of the sample compared to the deterioration shown in a similar sample containing a commercially available stabilizer. The polymer in which these tests were conducted was a SBR rubber conventionally referred to as 1502 black stock prepared by a cold polymerization procedure and containing approximately 75% bound butadiene and 25% bound styrene. This rubber stock was formulated and cured as sheets in a conventional manner.

Ingredients	Proportion
Cold SBR (1502)	100.00
High abrasion furnace black	50.00
Stearic acid	2.00
Hydrocarbon processing oil	5.00
Zinc oxide	3.00
Benzothiazole disulfide	1.00
Sulfur	1.75
Diphenyl guanidine	0.2

Sheets of the above rubber formulation were cured. Dumbbells of 2" x 0.075" x 0.075" with ¼" square ends were cut from the sheets. These dumbbells were immersed in benzene solutions containing an antiozonant concentration sufficient to give 4 phr of antiozonant in the dumbbell when it was completely swollen. The dumbells were removed from solution, allowed to dry 3 hours in a hood and then were dried for 3 hours in a vacuum oven at 26" mercury vacuum at 46° to 48°C. Samples of each antiozonant were tested three ways: First, without prior stretching (unaged); second, aged at 20% elongation for 24 hours at room temperature; and third, aged at 20% elongation for one hour at 100°C.

These dumbbells were tested at 20% elongation in an ozone chamber continuously charged with air containing 50 pphm O_3. The temperature was maintained at 100°F. The time, in hours, required for the first visible crack to develop in the test samples is summarized in the following table.

Stabilizer	Hours to first cracking: Unaged	Aged 24 hours at room temp.	Aged one hour at 100° C.
Control (a commercially available mixture of diaryl-p-phenylenediamine)	7	24	7
Product of Example	336	412	216

N-Substituted Dimethylpyrroles

Nondiscoloring antiozonants or those having limited discoloring properties have been developed by *E.A. Fike; U.S. Patents 3,580,885; May 25, 1971 and 3,702,331; November 7, 1972; both assigned to Security Chemicals, Inc.*

It has been found that rubber compositions sensitive to oxygen or ozone can be prevented from the degrading action of oxygen or ozone, or the effects can be greatly retarded if a slight amount of N-substituted dimethylpyrroles are added. These compounds correspond to the following formula:

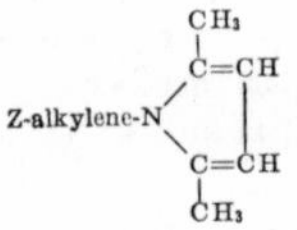

Where Z is a substituted amino group from the following:

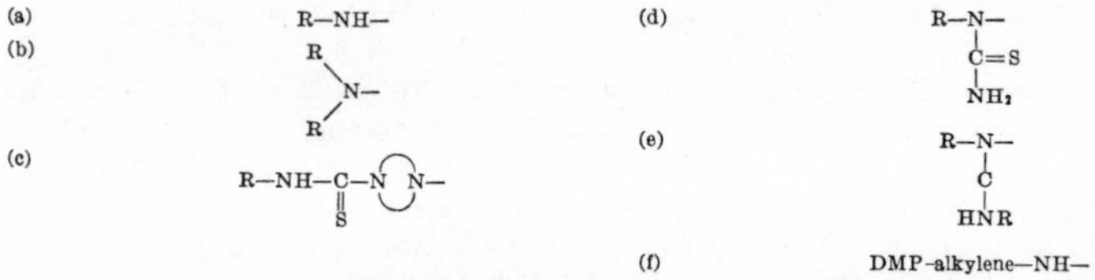

in which R is alkyl containing 1 to 18 carbons. Among the many examples coming within the scope of the formula are the following where DMP is dimethylpyrrole:

(1) DMP-$(CH_2)_3$—NH—$(CH_2)_3$-DMP

(2) $(C_2H_5)_2$—N—$(CH_2)_3$-DMP

(3) $(CH_3)_2$—N—$(CH_2)_2$-DMP

(4) $C_{12}H_{25}$—NH—$(CH_2)_3$-DMP

(5) CH_3—NH—$(CH_2)_3$—DMP

(6) C_2H_5—NH—$(CH_2)_3$-DMP

(7)
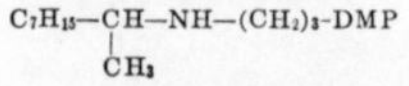

(8)
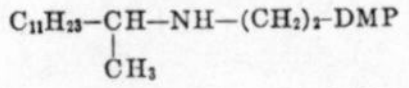

(9)
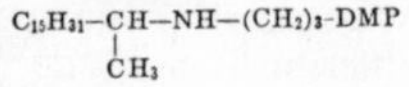

(10)
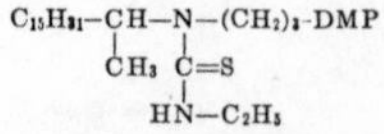

(11)
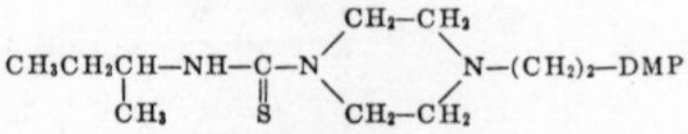

(12)
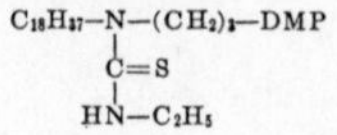

(13)
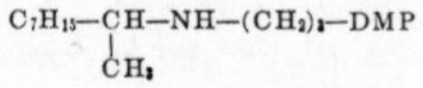

In the above formula the alkylene group may be ethylene, propylene or butylene, may be a straight or branched chain and may contain hydroxy substituents. The alkyl groups R may be branched or straight chains. In general, the above compounds may be prepared by refluxing a solution of an amino compound, e.g., a primary or β-amine and a carbonyl compound in a suitable solvent, such as ethanol, methanol, or water. Specifically, as an example, DMP—(CH$_2$)$_3$—NH(CH$_2$)$_3$—DMP was prepared by charging 2 mols (262 g) of imino bispropylamine into a flask with an agitator, feeding through a funnel into the flask 4.4 mols (500 g) of 2,5-hexanedione at 90° to 100°C, and thereafter the contents heated to reflux to remove water. After about four hours 142 cc of water were removed.

The product was distilled under vacuum and after a first cut of 21 grams, the main fraction of product consisted of 475 grams which distilled at a vapor temperature of 250° to 254°C at a vacuum of 20 mm. The 475 grams represented an 83% yield and had a crystallization point of 45°C.

In the table below are given data showing the effectiveness of certain of the compounds in preventing degradation of rubber vulcanizates. The compounds are identified from the above listing by number and Compound A is a commercially available antioxidant which is a substituted phenylenediamine. The control is a test strip containing no additive.

Compound	Black stock 8 hrs. (ozone)	White stock 8 hrs. (ozone)	Color
(1)	2	1	4
(2)	2	1	4
(3)	3	1	2
(4)	2	1	5
(5)	1	1	6
(6)	1	1	6
(7)	2	5	5
(8)	3	4	3
(9)	3	4	3
(10)	3	4	3
(11)	3	1	2
(12)	4	2	4
(13)	1	3	3
Control	6	6	1
A	3	1	6

The test procedure involved preparing a 5% solution of the compound to be tested in xylene. Rubber strips (2" x 2" of commercial GRS stock ⅛" thick) were immerse ½ into the solution for thirty seconds and then allowed to dry. The rubber strips were bent to give stress and exposed to ozone of approximately 50 parts per 100 million for eight hours. The condition of the strip was determined by visual observation and given a 1 to 6 rating for both ozone attack and color change, with a 1 for best rating and a 6 for the poorest rating in each case. The above tests establish the effectiveness of the compounds to give ozone protection and prevent degradation.

Ternary Mixtures of Substituted p-Phenylenediamines

Antiozonant mixtures which are homogeneous, compatible, nonscorching and nonblooming have been disclosed by *A.E. Hoffman; U.S. Patent 3,663,505; May 16, 1972; assigned to Universal Oil Products Company*. This antiozonant composition comprises from about 20% to about 50% by weight of an N,N'-di-sec-alkyl-p-phenylenediamine in which each alkyl contains 6 to 10 carbons, N-phenyl-N'-sec-alkyl-p-phenylenediamine in which the alkyl contains 3 to 6 carbons and N-phenyl-N'-sec-alkyl-p-phenylenediamine in which alkyl contains 7 to 10 carbons.

The first component is an N,N'-di-sec-alkyl-p-phenylenediamine in which each alkyl contains 6 to 10 carbons. A preferred component is N,N'-di-sec-octyl-p-phenylenediamine, particularly, N,N'-di-(1-methylheptyl)-p-phenylenediamine. Other derivatives for use as this component include N,N'-di-sec-hexyl-p-phenylenediamines, N,N'-di-sec-heptyl-p-phenylenediamines, other N,N'-di-sec-octyl-p-phenylenediamines, N,N'-di-sec-nonyl-p-phenylenediamines and N,N'-di-sec-decyl-p-phenylenediamines. The second component is N-phenyl-N'-sec-alkyl-p-phenylenediamine in which the alkyl contains 3 to 6 carbons. A preferred derivative is N-phenyl-N'-(1,3-dimethylbutyl)-p-phenylenediamine. Other derivatives for this component include N-phenyl-N'-isopropyl-p-phenylenediamine, N-phenyl-N'-(1-methylpropyl)-p-phenylenediamine, N-phenyl-N'-(sec-pentyl)-p-phenylenediamines, and other N-phenyl-N'-(sec-hexyl)-p-phenylenediamine. The third component is an N-phenyl-N'-sec-alkyl-p-phenylenediamine in which the alkyl contains 7 to 10 carbons. A preferred component is N-phenyl-N'-(1-methylheptyl)-p-phenylenedimaine. Other derivatives comprise N-phenyl-N'-(sec-heptyl)-p-phenylenediamines, other N-phenyl-N'-(sec-octyl)-p-phenylenediamines, N-phenyl-N'-(sec-nonyl)-p-phenylenediamines, and N-phenyl-N'-(sec-decyl)-p-phenylenediamines.

The three components of the composition are used in a proportion of from about 20 to about 50% by weight of each of the components. These proportions are essential in order to obtain the improved benefits. The composition is used in rubber in a concentration sufficient to effect the desired stabilization. The concentration may range from 1.5 to 6% and more particularly from 2 to 4% by weight of the rubber.

These concentrations are based on the rubber hydrocarbon exclusive of the other components of the rubber composition. When desired, the composition may be used along with an additional antioxidant and also is used along with other additives incorporated in rubber for specific purposes including accelerators, softeners, extenders, wax reinforcing agents, etc.

Example 1: The 3-component mixture was prepared of equal parts by weight of N,N'-di-(1-methylheptyl)-p-phenylenediamine, N-phenyl-N'-(1,3-dimethylbutyl)-p-phenylenediamine and N-phenyl-N'-(1-methylheptyl)-p-phenylenediamine.

Example 2: The 3-component mixture described in Example 1 was utilized as an antiozonant in a commercial polyisoprene base rubber stock. The uninhibited rubber stock was milled with 3.5 phr of the 3-component composition of Example 1 and cured for 25 minutes at 300°F.

In one evaluation, the rubber sample was evaluated in a dynamic antiozonant activity test in which a sample of the rubber is cured onto a belt and the belt is flexed at 72°F in an atmosphere of 40 pphm of ozone. The time to first crack is noted. When evaluated in this manner, the rubber sample containing the antiozonant composition did not undergo cracking for more than 168 hours, at which time the test was terminated. In contrast to the above, three other samples of the same rubber containing different commercial antiozonants all underwent cracking in less than 72 hours when evaluated in the same manner.

For comparative purposes another sample of the uninhibited rubber was prepared to contain 3.5 phr of a 2-component mixture comprising equal parts by weight of N,N'-di-(1-methylheptyl)-p-phenylenediamine and N-phenyl-N'-(1-methylheptyl)-p-phenylenediamine. The rubber stock was cured and evaluated in the same manner as described above. This sample underwent cracking in less than 120 hours. Thus it is seen that the 3-component mixture was more effective than the 2-component mixture in retarding cracking of the rubber.

Cyclohexen-3-ylidenemethyl Ethers for Polychloroprene Rubbers

A series of ether or thioether antiozonants having a cyclohexen-3-ylidenemethyl or corresponding 2,5-endomethylene derivatives have been developed by *R. Nast, K. Ley and T. Kempermann; U.S. Patent 3,639,485; February 1, 1972; assigned to Farbenfabriken Bayer AG, Germany.* These are useful for elastomer compositions containing at least 20% by weight of polychloroprene. These antiozonants corresponding to the formulas:

in which R_1 represents a hydrocarbon radical containing 3 to 18 carbons which may optionally contain oxygen or sulfur moieties, X represents oxygen or sulfur, R_2 and R_3 each represent hydrogen or a methyl radical. One particularly significant technological advantage of the compounds is that they do not discolor. The enolethers may be prepared by conventional methods, for example, by reacting aldehydes with alcohols or mercaptans in the presence of acid catalysts to form the corresponding acetals or thioacetals. The compounds formed in the first stage are converted in a second reaction stage into the corresponding enol- or thioenolethers by heat with the elimination of alchohol or mercaptan. Thioenolethers may also be directly formed from mercaptans and aldehydes provided the reaction is carried out with a molar ratio of 1:1.

As a rule, the water formed during the acetal formation is azeotropically distilled off from a mixture of 1 mol of the aldehyde and at least 2 mols of an alcohol in the presence of catalytic quantities of a strong acid such as p-toluenesulfonic acid, for example, by means of an organic solvent which is immiscible with water such as, for example, chloroform, benzene, xylene or washing spirit or, optionally, by means of an excess of the alcohol used. After the water has been removed, the reaction mixture is fractionated through a column at reduced pressure to split up the acetal formed in the first stage into alcohol and enol ether.

Example: The following mixtures were prepared on mixing rolls:

	Parts by Weight
Polychloroprene	100.0
Magnesium oxide	4.0
Stearic acid	0.5
Precipitated silica (BET-surface 180 m^2/g)	20.0
Soft kaolin	170.0
Titanium dioxide	5.0
Antimony oxide	5.0
Chloroparaffin	10.0
Naphthenic mineral oil plasticizer	20.0
Paraffin	4.0
Zinc oxide	5.0
Ethylene thiourea	1.0
Antiozonant (as listed on the following page)	1.0

Tests specimens measuring 0.4 x 4.5 x 4.5 cm were prepared from these mixtures and vulcanized (press vulcanization: 30 minutes at 151°C). Groups of four of the test specimens were then clamped in a plastics frame in such a way that elongations of 10%, 20%, 35% and 60% were developed over their surfaces. The test specimens were then treated with a stream of air containing 1,000 parts of ozone to 100 million parts of air, at room temperature. Crack formation was then assessed at regular intervals as specified in the table on the following page by counting the total number of cracks formed that were visible with the naked eye, and also by measuring their average length in accordance with the following system.

Number of Cracks

No cracks	0
1 to 2 cracks	1
3 to 9 cracks	2
19 to 24 cracks	3
25 to 79 cracks	4
80 to 249 cracks	5
More than 250 cracks	6

Average Length of the Cracks

No crack formation	0
Just visible	1
1 to 3 mm	2
3 to 8 mm	3
More than 8 mm	4

In the following table, the results obtained are separated by a vertical line with the number

of cracks indicated first in each case. In the tables, the symbol + means that the test specimen broke.

Hours	2	10	33	66	168
No anti-ozonant present					
Elongation, percent:					
10	0/0	0/0	3/2	3/2	3/4
20	0/0	5/1	5/2	5/2	4/4
35	0/0	5/1	5/2	5/2	+
60	5/1	5/2	4/4	+	+
[cyclohexen-(3)-ylidene-methyl]-n-butylether					
Elongation, percent:					
10	0/0	0/0	0/0	0/0	0/0
20	0/0	0/0	0/0	0/0	0/0
35	0/0	0/0	0/0	0/0	0/0
60	0/0	0/0	0/0	1/3	1/4
[3- (or -4)-methylcyclohexen-(3)ylidene-methyl]-n-butylether					
Elongation, percent:					
10	0/0	0/0	0/0	0/0	0/0
20	0/0	0/0	0/0	0/0	0/0
35	0/0	0/0	1/2	1/4	1/4
60	0/0	4/2	4/4	+	+
[2,5-endomethylene-cyclohexen-(3)-ylidene-methyl]-n-hexylether					
Elongation, percent:					
10	0/0	0/0	0/0	0/0	0/0
20	0/0	0/0	0/0	0/0	0/0
35	0/0	0/0	0/0	0/0	0/0
60	0/0	2/1	3/3	+	+

Free-Flowing Diaryl-p-Phenylenediamines for Polychloroprene

*F.P. Hytrek; U.S. Patent 3,674,705; July 4, 1972; assigned to E.I. du Pont de Nemours
and Company* has prepared a free-flowing, nonmassing antiozonant composition by mixing
about 100 parts by weight of a molten diaryl-p-phenylenediamine with about 2 to 20 parts
by weight of a finely divided inert inorganic solid. The mass is solidified by cooling and
then crushed and ground to the desired particle size.

The inorganic solids used to improve the form of the diaryl-p-phenylenediamines can be
any inert inorganic material having a surface area of 40 to 200 m^2/g, with a high capacity
for absorbing oil, i.e., 200 to 600% of oil based on the weight of the inorganic solid. By
inert is meant that the inorganic solid will not react with the diaryl-p-phenylenediamine
or interfere with its antiozonant properties. Suitable inorganic solids include clays (such
as the kaolin clays), precipitated calcium carbonates, carbon blacks, colloidal silicas and
synthetic colloidal silicates.

The preferred solids are the synthetic hydrous calcium silicates that are commonly used
in compounding rubbers, paints, printing inks, and the like. Representative of such synthetic hydrous calcium silicates are a class of materials containing 49 to 55% by weight
silica (SiO_2), 22 to 28% by weight lime (CaO), 14 to 19% by weight water and the remainder is small quantities of alumina (Al_2O_3), iron oxide (Fe_2O_3), magnesia (MgO) and
alkalies ($Na_2O + K_2O$) in varying amounts. These preferred inorganic materials are sold
commercially under the trade name Micro-Cel. They are prepared by the hydrothermal
reaction of crude diatomaceous silica (diatomite), hydrated lime and water.

These antiozonant mixtures once reduced to a granular or pulverulent form have excellent
resistance to massing or agglomeration. They can be readily handled and incorporated into
a chloroprene polymer rubber stock during compounding. Surprisingly, intimate physical
mixing of solid diaryl-p-phenylenediamines of the types described here with finely divided
absorbent organic solids is relatively ineffective in preventing massing of the product under
storage conditions.

Example: A diaryl-p-phenylenediamine composition is prepared as follows. A one-liter
electrically heated flask equipped with an agitator and an offset vapor take-off line leading
to a water-cooled condenser is used. The condensed vapors are collected in a decanter,
from which the water layer is intermittently removed and the organic phase is continuously
returned to the reactor. Prior to heating, 73 grams of phenylamine composition, 290 grams
of o-toluidine, 165 grams of hydroquinone, 7 grams of aluminum chloride and 2 grams of
ferric chloride are charged to the reactor. The phenylamine composition used is a technical
grade product sold as Xylidines Mixed o-m-p Technical (Du Pont). The purity of the
phenylamine composition as determined by the sodium nitrite test is 99% minimum. The
mixture is heated until reflux (212°C). Heating is continued and the temperature slowly

rises to 252°C. The total heating time is 12 hours. When no more water appears in the condensate, vacuum is applied at 252°C to remove any low-boiling materials. The product is cast in an aluminum pan and allowed to cool and crystallize overnight. It is solid melting at 100° to 110°C.

To about 45 parts by weight of diaryl-p-phenylenediamine prepared as above is added about 4.9 parts by weight of a hydrous calcium silicate (Micro-Cel E) having a surface area of 95 m²/g and an oil absorption capacity of 490 weight percent. Micro-Cel E has the following typical chemical analysis in percent by weight: SiO_2, 54.3; CaO, 25.1; alumina, 3.6; iron oxide, 1.2; magnesia, 3.0; alkalies, 1.3 and ignition loss, 14.0. It is prepared by the hydrothermal reaction of crude diatomaceous silica (diatomite), hydrated lime and water. The mixture is heated to 120° at which temperature the diamine mixture is completely molten and the resulting mixture is stirred until the calcium silicate is completely dispersed.

The mixture is poured into an aluminum pan and allowed to solidify after which it is broken into small chunks, ground in a mortar and sieved so that all product passes a 20-mesh screen. A sample of this product is placed in a cylindrical glass container, and the sample is compressed by a slightly smaller, weighted glass cylinder such that a pressure of about 0.65 lb/in² is applied, simulating loading conditions expected in normal storage. The entire assembly is held in a circulating air oven for extended periods to simulate temperatures that are experienced in summer warehouse storage. For comparison, samples of the particulate diaryl-p-phenylenediamines (Samples 2 and 3) that are mechanically mixed with the hydrous calcium silicate without melting are similarly tested. Results are as follows:

Sample No.	Calcium Silicate (Calculated)	Oven Temp ° C	Time in Oven, Days	Massing Behavior
1	10%	45	25	Free flowing
2	5%*	35	22	Heavy caking
3	10%*	45	22	Heavy caking

*Control

Antiozonant-Antioxidant Mixtures

For certain uses it is desirable to have an antiozonant-antioxidant that is readily dispersible in elastomeric polymers at low temperatures, without loss of the beneficial properties associated with polymers compounded with the type antiozonant referred to hereinabove. For example, in the preparation of covered wire by the extrusion of the compounded polymer over the wire, rapid curing must follow. This requires a fast-acting accelerator system and, therefore, the compounding step, that is, the mixing of the polymer with the compounding ingredients, must be carried out at relatively low temperatures in order to prevent premature vulcanization.

J. Kalil; U.S. Patent 3,785,995; January 15, 1974; assigned to E.I. du Pont de Nemours and Company has developed an antiozonant-antioxidant composition that is crystalline, and readily dispersible in elastomeric polymers 70° to 85°C, and can be handled with ease in rubber processing procedures.

This comprises a composition containing (1) 94 to 86%, by weight, based on the weight of the total composition, of a secondary amine, the amine containing (a) 30 to 65%, by weight, of a diaryl-p-phenylenediamine prepared by condensing hydroquinone with an amine mixture comprising 75 to 90%, by weight, o-toluidine and 25 to 10%, by weight, mixed xylidines, and (b) 70 to 35%, by weight, N-phenyl-2-naphthylamine, and (2) 6 to 14%, by weight, of hydrous calcium silicate. The antiozonant-antioxidant prepared by mixing the secondary amines in the molten state and calcium silicate so as to uniformly incorporate hydrous calcium silicate into the molten amines. The composition functions as an effective combined antiozonant and antioxidant when incorporated in elastomers, especially chloroprene and butadiene-styrene elastomers.

Any hydrous calcium silicate can be used in the composition. Representative hydrous calcium silicates include those containing 49 to 65%, by weight, silica (SiO_2), 19 to 28%, by weight, lime (CaO), and the remainder being water and small quantities of alumina (Al_2O_3), iron oxide (Fe_2O_3), magnesia (MgO), and alkalies ($Na_2O + K_2O$) in varying amounts. The preferred calcium silicates are available commercially under the trade names Micro-Cel manufactured by Johns-Manville and Silene manufactured by PPG Industries, Inc. Generally, the surface area of the silicates is about 80 to 200 m^2/g.

Example: The process is carried out in a steam-jacketed steel kettle equipped with agitator and bottom outlet. The steam pressure in the jacket is about 60 psig. To the kettle are charged 1,419 lb (44%) of the diaryl-p-phenylenediamine prepared by reacting 20% mixed xylidines and 80% o-toluidine with hydroquinone in the presence of aluminum chloride, and 1,419 lb (44%) of N-phenyl-2-naphthylamine while maintaining an atmosphere of nitrogen in the vessel. The mixture is heated to about 135°C until entirely molten. Agitation is begun as soon as the charge has melted enough to allow agitation without splashing.

When the charge is completely molten, 387 lb (12%) of hydrated calcium silicate having an average particle size of 2.1 microns and a surface area of 95 m^2/g, and identified as Micro-Cel E, are added gradually. After stirring for one hour to ensure a uniform blending, the mixture is fed by nitrogen pressure through steam-jacketed transfer lines maintained at 120° to 130°C to a Thermascrew apparatus containing a seed of already solidified material.

The Thermascrew apparatus used is a double-screw device (operating essentially as described in Figures 6 and 7 of U.S. Patent 2,610,033). The hollow screw and jacketed trough are brine-cooled. The seed bed is maintained at 20° to 50°C. The product issuing from the Thermascrew is screened to remove all particles above about 0.5 inch in size. The product is in the form of brownish-to-grey pellets. The melting point is 80° to 85°C.

As a test to determine crystallization time, the following procedure is carried out. A total of 9 to 10 grams of a mixture of the composition is prepared by adding the solid ingredients to a test tube and heating to about 120°C. The molten contents are then stirred and allowed to cool. When the temperature reaches about 90°C the material in the test tube is poured into an aluminum cup, Mixing is continued until the mixture solidifies. The time from pouring until the composition becomes a nontacky solid is the crystallization time. Crystallization time of the sample should be one minute or less if the mixture is to solidify rapidly enough so that it can be recrystallized in an apparatus such as the herein-described Thermascrew apparatus. The table shows the crystallization time for various mixtures. The following abbreviations are used: DAPD, diaryl-p-phenylenediamine (same as above); NPNA, N-phenyl-2-naphthylamine and Silicate, same calcium silicate used above.

	Grams			Percent silicate	Crystallization time, seconds
Expt.	DAPD	NPNA	Silicate		
A	4.37	4.37	1.25	12.5	21
B	4.50	4.50	1.0	10	34
C	4.62	4.62	0.75	7.5	47

PHOSPHORUS-CONTAINING ANTIOXIDANTS

Tetrakis (Hindered Phenolic) Phosphonium Halides

The preparation and use of these phosphonium halides are disclosed by *C.J. Worrel; U.S. Patents 3,483,260; December 9, 1969 and 3,642,691; February 15, 1972; both assigned to Ethyl Corporation.* These tetrakis-hydroxybenzyl phosphonium halides are made by reacting a hydroxybenzyl halide with one of the following: (1) tetrakis-hydroxyalkyl phosphonium halide, (2) tris-hydroxyalkyl phosphine oxide, or (3) tris-hydroxyalkyl phosphine. The compounds are antioxidants either alone or in combination with a dialkylthiodialkanoate synergist. Broadly, these compounds have the formula shown in the following page.

(1)

$$\left[\begin{array}{c} OH \\ \underset{R_1}{\overset{}{\bigcirc}} \underset{R_2}{} CH_2 \overline{} P - X \end{array} \right]_4$$

R_1 and R_2 are independently selected from hydrogen, C_{1-12} alkyl radicals, C_{6-12} aryl radicals, C_{6-12} cycloalkyl radicals, C_{7-12} aralkyl radicals, and X is a halogen having an atomic number from 17 to 53. In a highly preferred embodiment of these compounds the hydroxyl radical is located para to the benzyl group and both positions ortho to the hydroxyl radical are substituted. In this embodiment, the compounds have the formula:

(2)

$$\left[HO - \underset{R_5}{\overset{R_4}{\bigcirc}} CH_2 \overline{} P - X \right]_4$$

where X is the same as in Formula 1; R_4 is selected from alpha-branched C_{3-12} alkyl radicals, alpha-branched C_{8-12} aralkyl radicals and C_{6-12} cycloalkyl radicals, and R_5 is selected from C_{1-12} alkyl radicals, C_{6-12} cycloalkyl radicals anc C_{6-12} aralkyl radicals. The preferred compound is tetrakis(3,5-di-tert-butyl-4-hydroxybenzyl)phosphonium chloride. The new compounds can be made by several methods. The first method is the reaction of a hydroxybenzyl halide with a tetrakis-hydroxyalkyl phosphonium halide. For example, useful hydroxybenzyl halides are described in *J. Am. Chem. Soc.,* 77, 1783—5 (1955), and in U.S. Patent 3,257,321. The tetrakis-hydroxyalkyl phosphonium halides are described by E.L.Gefter, *Organo Phosphorus Monomers and Polymers,* 102—3, Associated Technical Services, Inc., Glenridge, N.J. (1962), and by G.M. Kosolopoff, *Organo Phosphorus Compounds,* 81—7, John Wiley and Sons, N.Y. (1950).

It is generally preferred to conduct the reaction in a solvent. Useful solvents are those that are substantially inert to the reactants and have some solvent effect. These include hydrocarbons, chlorinated hydrocarbons, ethers, and the like. Examples of aliphatic hydrocarbons are hexane, heptane, isooctane, n-nonane, and the like. Typical aromatic solvents are benzene, toluene, xylene, and the like. A second method of preparing the tetrakis-hydroxybenzyl phosphonium halides is by the reaction of a hydroxybenzyl halide with a tris(hydroxyalkyl)phosphine oxide. In a third method of making the new compound a hydroxybenzyl halide is reacted with a tris-hydroxyalkyl phosphine.

Example 1: In a reaction vessel equipped with stirrer, thermometer, heating and cooling means and provided with a nitrogen atmosphere place 2,000 parts of dioxane, 1,016 parts of 3,5-di-tert-butyl-4-hydroxybenzyl chloride, 142 parts of tetrakis(hydroxymethyl)phosphonium chloride and 400 parts of triethylamine.

Stir for 30 minutes and then warm the mixture to 50°C. Stir at 50° to 75°C for 2 hours. Cool to 20°C and filter off the precipitate. Wash the precipitate once with diethyl ether and then extract the product from the filter cake with hot chloroform. Evaporate the chloroform from the filtrate, leaving the solid product. Recrystallize the product from methanol, yielding tetrakis(3,5-di-tert-butyl-4-hydroxybenzyl) phosphonium chloride. In the above example other hydroxybenzyl halides may be substituted to obtain the corresponding product. The following table lists various hydroxybenzyl halides and the product which would result from its substitution in the above example.

Hydroxybenzyl Halide	Product
2-methyl-5-tert-butyl-4-hydroxybenzyl chloride	Tetrakis(2-methyl-5-tert-butyl-4-hydroxybenzyl)phosphonium chloride
3,5-dicyclohexyl-4-hydroxybenzyl chloride	Tetrakis(3,5-dicyclohexyl-4-hydroxybenzyl)phosphonium chloride
3-tert-butyl-2-hydroxybenzyl chloride	Tetrakis(3-tert-butyl-2-hydroxybenzyl) phosphonium chloride

(continued)

Hydroxybenzyl Halide	Product
3-sec-dodecyl-5-methyl-2-hydroxybenzyl chloride	Tetrakis(3-dodecyl-5-methyl-2-hydroxybenzyl)phosphonium chloride
3,5-di-sec-butyl-4-hydroxybenzyl chloride	Tetrakis(3,5-di-sec-butyl-4-hydroxybenzyl)phosphonium chloride

The additives of this process are effective in stabilizing rubber against degradation caused by oxygen or ozone.

Example 2: A rubber stock is prepared containing the following components:

Components	Parts
Pale crepe rubber	100.00
Zinc oxide filler	50.00
Titanium dioxide	25.00
Stearic acid	2.00
Ultramarine blue	0.12
Sulfur	3.00
Mercaptobenzothiazole	1.00

To the above base formula is added one part by weight of tetrakis(3-tert-butyl-5-methyl-2-hydroxybenzyl)phosphonium bromide and, following this, individual samples are cured for 20, 30, 45, and 60 minutes, respectively, at 274°C. After cure, all of these samples remain white in color and possess excellent tensile strength. Furthermore, they are resistant to degradation caused by oxygen or ozone on aging.

EP terpolymer, cis-polybutadiene SBR and NBR rubbers are also stabilized in examples in the patents. These phosphonium halides are also useful antioxidants for polyolefins and examples are also included on the stabilization of polypropylene and polyethylene. Additional examples also include the stabilization of ABS, lubricating oils (including the synthetic polyester oil), gasoline, diesel fuel, lard and coconut oil.

O,O-Dialkylhydroxybenzyl Dithiophosphates

An improved preparation process has been developed by *K.H. Shin and E.F. Zaweski; U.S. Patent 3,745,148; July 10, 1973; assigned to Ethyl Corporation* for the preparation of these antioxidants. The process comprises: reacting from 1 to 10 mols of a monohydric alkanol containing from 1 to about 50 carbons with a mol of P_2S_5 at a temperature of from 75° to about 125°C to form a dithiophosphate reaction mixture; neutralizing the dithiophosphate reaction mixture with aqueous ammonia; and adding from about 1 to 3 mols of a hydroxybenzyl chloride to the neutralized reaction mixture and reacting at a temperature of from 50° to 150°C.

A particularly preferred alkanol reactant is a mixture of aliphatic monohydric alcohols containing from about 20 to 50 carbons. Minor amounts of lower alcohols (e.g., C_{18} alcohols) can be present. The major amount of alcohols are primary. The preferred proportion of alcohols in the mixture of alcohols containing from about 20 to 50 carbons is as follows:

Alcohol	%
C_{20}	14 – 29
C_{22}	14 – 29
C_{24}	7 – 21
C_{26}	7 – 21
C_{28}	7 – 21
C_{30-50}	7 – 21

The above percent composition is based upon the alcohol content and does not take into account any diluent or other material which might be present. As stated previously, small amounts, up to about 3%, of C_{18} alcohols can also be present in the preferred alcohol mixtures. The above alcohol mixtures are readily available from an aluminum alkyl chain growth alcohol process such as is shown in U.S. Patents 3,384,651, 3,415,861 and 3,475,501, the disclosure of which is incorporated hereby by reference.

An essential feature of the present process is the use of aqueous ammonia to neutralize the reaction mixture. If other neutralizing agents such as sodium bicarbonate, sodium carbonate, sodium hydroxide, and the like, are used the final product is cloudy and extremely difficult to clarify by filtration due to the presence of a slime-like material. Furthermore, unless the neutralization is carried out in the manner described herein, the final product will tend to discolor the substrate to which it is added by turning it yellow. Although the discoloration does not lessen the effectiveness of the additive in preventing oxidative degradation, it is quite important because in some applications it is necessary that a nondiscoloring antioxidant be used.

The preferred method of conducting the neutralization is to add sufficient aqueous ammonia to the reaction mixture following the alkanol-P_2S_5 reaction to substantially neutralize the reaction mixture. Preferably, the neutralization at this stage is such that the pH is raised to about 5.5 to 7.0. Following this the hydroxybenzyl chloride reactant is added and then additional aqueous ammonia is added at a controlled rate during the course of the reaction of the hydroxybenzyl chloride such that the pH during this reaction remains below about 6 preferably in the range of about 5 to 6. It has been found that if the aqueous ammonia is added too rapidly, such that the reaction mixture becomes alkaline, the course of the reaction is altered in some manner such that the resultant reaction product, although an effective antioxidant, will cause the substrate to which it is added to become yellow.

The hydroxybenzyl chloride used in the process is a benzyl chloride having a hydroxy group substituted in the benzene ring. Other substituents that do not interfere with the reaction can also be substituted on the benzene ring, such as chlorine, bromine, iodine, fluorine, nitro, alkoxy, hydroxyl, alkyl, aralkyl, and the like. The 3,5-dialkyl-4-hydroxybenzyl chlorides are more preferred. These compounds have the formula:

in which R_1 and R_2 are alkyl groups. The most preferred hydroxybenzyl chloride is 3,5-di-tert-butyl-4-hydroxybenzyl chloride. In the following examples, all parts are by weight unless otherwise indicated.

Example 1: In a glass-lined reaction vessel was placed 94 parts of a mixture of aliphatic monohydric alcohols containing from about 18 to 50 carbons (predominantly in the C_{20}-C_{50} range) and containing 35 weight percent hydrocarbons (predominantly C_{20}-C_{50} paraffins). Analysis showed the alcohol mixture to have a bromine number of 10.5 and to contain 2.76 weight percent hydroxyl. Average molecular weight based on hydroxyl analysis was 618. To this mixture was added 94 parts of toluene and 12.44 parts of P_2S_5. While stirring, the mixture was heated to 90°C (Note: Vent evolved H_2S to caustic scrubber.) The mixture was stirred at 90°C for an hour and then cooled to 70°C. The mixture was neutralized to pH 5.5 by adding 4.05 parts of 24.5 weight percent aqueous ammonia. The temperature rose to 76°C during neutralization.

Then, 35.27 parts of 3,5-di-tert-butyl-4-hydroxybenzyl chloride were added at 70°C, causing the pH to drop sharply. While stirring, additional aqueous ammonia was added at a controlled rate such that the pH remained below 6. This reaction stage required 4 hours, during which time a total of 3.56 parts or 24.5 weight percent aqueous ammonia were added. The water phase was then removed and the product was filtered. Toluene solvent was distilled out. A product having the texture of soft wax at room temperature and a liquid when warmed to about 50°C was obtained. This reaction product was an excellent antioxidant which did not cause discoloration of organic sustrates. The additives are incorporated into the organic substrate in a small but effective amount so as to provide the required antioxidant protection. A useful range is from about 0.01 to about 5 weight percent, and a preferred range is from about 0.1 to 3 weight percent.

Example 2: To a synthetic rubber master batch comprising 100 parts to SBR rubber having an average molecular weight of 60,000, 50 parts of mixed zinc propionate stearate, 50 parts carbon black, 5 parts road tar, 2 parts sulfur and 1.5 parts of mercapto benzothiazole is added 1.5 parts of the reaction product of Example 1. After mastication, the resultant master batch is cured for 60 minutes using 45 psi steam pressure, resulting in a stabilized SBR vulcanizate.

Other examples included in the patent cover the quantitative stabilization of butyl rubber, NBR and cis-polybutadiene. Also the stabilization of polypropylene, polyethylene, mineral oil, silicone and polyester lubricants, gasoline, diesel fuel, paraffin, lard and corn oil were covered by examples.

Hindered Phenolic Phosphorodithioates for SBR

A stabilizer for SBR has been disclosed by *B.R. Meltsner; U.S. Patents 3,662,033; May 9, 1972 and 3,801,543; April 2, 1974; both assigned to Ethyl Corporation.* This stabilizer may be used in unvulcanized SBR rubber to inhibit chain scission and cross-linking during storage and prevent a resultant change in Mooney viscosity. This stabilizer has the formula:

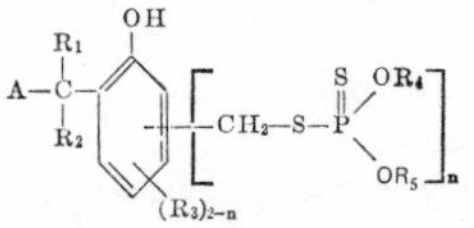

where A is an aryl radical containing 6 to 18 carbons, R_1 is a lower alkyl radical containing 1 to 3 carbons, R_2 is selected from hydrogen and lower alkyl radicals containing 1 to 3 carbons, R_3 is selected from alkyl radicals containing 1 to 20 carbons, cycloalkyl radicals containing 6 to 20 carbons and radicals having the formula:

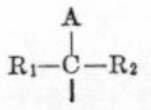

where A, R_1 and R_2 are the same as above, R_4 and R_5 are independently selected from alkyl radicals containing 1 to 50 carbons and aryl radicals containing 6 to 20 carbons and n is 1 or 2. Because of the unusually high degree of stability against Mooney change and concurrent nondiscoloration from UV light provided to unvulcanized styrene-butadiene rubber, a most preferred stabilizer is that having the formula:

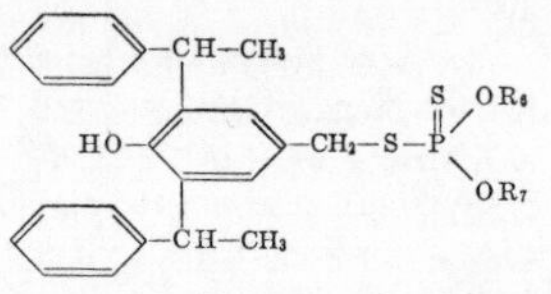

where R_6 and R_7 are primary aliphatic hydrocarbon radicals containing from 20 to 50 carbons. An excellent process for making these compounds is to first react the appropriate alcohol or aromatic hydroxy compound with phosphorus pentasulfide to form the corresponding dihydrocarbyl dithiophosphoric acid and then to react this with the appropriate benzyl halide.

The first reaction is carried out by mixing the phosphorus pentasulfide with the alcohol or aromatic hydroxy compound and heating the mixture to reaction temperature while stirring. Means for conducting this reaction are shown in U.S. Patents 2,386,207, 3,190,833 and

3,293,181. The temperature for the first part of the process should be high enough to promote a reasonable reaction rate, but not so high as to cause reactant or product decomposition. A useful temperature range is from 50° to 200°C. A preferred temperature range is from 75° to 150°C.

The stoichiometry of the reaction requires four equivalents of alcohol or aromatic hydroxy compound for each mol of phosphorus pentasulfide. Generally an excess of phosphorus pentasulfide is employed and the unreacted material filtered off after the reaction. A useful range is from 3 to 4 equivalents of alcohol or aromatic hydroxy compound per mol of phosphorus pentasulfide, and a more preferred range is from 3.5 to 4 equivalents of alcohol or aromatic hydroxy compound per mol of phosphorus pentasulfide.

Example 1: Step A — In a reaction vessel fitted with stirrer, thermometer, reflux condenser and gas inlet tube was placed 163 parts of a mixture of 81 weight percent 2,6-di(α-methylbenzyl)phenol, 12.2 weight percent 2,4,6-tri(α-methylbenzyl)phenol, and 4.8 weight percent 2-(α-methylbenzyl)phenol made by the process shown in U.S. Patent 2,831,898. Following this, 250 parts of concentrated aqueous hydrochloric acid and 60 parts of paraformaldehyde were added.

The mixture was heated to 60°C while stirring, and dry hydrogen chloride was injected into the liquid phase while stirring at this temperature until a vapor phase chromatograph of the reaction mixture showed that all of the 2,6-di(α-methylbenzyl)phenol and 2-(α-methylbenzyl)-phenol had reacted. Following this, the mixture was cooled to room temperature and the aqueous acid phase removed. Then 280 parts of toluene were added and the solution washed three times with water. Toluene was distilled from the mixture under vacuum until no further water came over with the toluene. This left 290 parts of a toluene solution containing 186.5 parts of a mixture of 3,5-di(α-methylbenzyl)-4-hydroxybenzyl chloride, 2-(α-methylbenzyl)-3,5-dichloromethylphenol and 2,4,6-tri(α-methylbenzyl)phenol.

Step B — In a second reaction vessel equipped with stirrer, thermometer, condenser and provided with a nitrogen atmosphere was placed 215 parts of toluene, 54.6 parts of a mixture of primary aliphatic alcohols having the following composition:

	Weight Percent
C_{20} alcohol	16
C_{22} alcohol	15
C_{24} alcohol	12
C_{26} alcohol	10
C_{28} alcohol	6
C_{32} alcohol	1
C_{20-50} paraffinic hydrocarbon	35

Following this, 6.64 parts of phosphorus pentasulfide was added. This mixture was stirred and refluxed for 2.5 hours. It was then cooled to 70°C and 5 parts of sodium bicarbonate added. Following this, 29 parts of the toluene solution prepared in step A was added over a 20 minute period while maintaining the reaction mixture at reflux. Following this, 45 parts of toluene were added and the mixture refluxed for 30 minutes. It was cooled to room temperature and 60 parts of water added. Additional sodium carbonate was supplied to render the mixture alkaline following which the mixture was filtered.

The toluene and other volatiles were then distilled out under vacuum, leaving 59.2 parts of a wax-like solid. This was identified by infrared to consist essentially of S-[3,5-di-(α-methylbenzyl)-4-hydroxybenzyl] O,O-di-(C_{20-50} primary alkyl) phosphorodithioate and a small amount of 2,4,6-tri(α-methylbenzyl)phenol and O,O-di-(C_{20-50} primary alkyl) phosphorodithioate, S,S-diester with α^2,α^4-dimercapto-6-(α-methylbenzyl)-2,4-xylenol.

These additives are eminently useful as stabilizers and antioxidants for SBR rubber compositions. The amount of additives used in the rubber is not critical as long as an amount sufficient to provide the desired protection is present. This amount varies from as little as 0.001 weight percent up to about 5 weight percent. Generally, excellent results are obtained when from about 0.1 to about 3 weight percent of the additive, based on the weight of the SBR rubber, is included in the composition. The following example serves to illustrate the use of the stabilizers of the process in stabilizing both unvulcanized and vulcanized SBR rubber.

Example 2: A styrene-butadiene copolymer containing 30% styrene units and 70% butadiene units is prepared in aqueous emulsion using sodium oleate as emulsifying agent and potassium persulfate/lauryl mercaptan as the polymerization catalyst. The final emulsion contains 20 weight percent solids. To this is added a sodium oleate stabilized aqueous emulsion of S-(3,5-di-tert-butyl-4-hydroxybenzyl) O,O-di(C_{20-50} primary alkyl) phosphorodithioate. The emulsion made by adding a toluene solution of the phosphorodithioate to water containing a sodium oleate emulsifying agent. The amount of phosphorodithioate in the emulsion is equal to one weight percent of the styrene-butadiene copolymer solids.

The fianl emulsion is then vigorously stirred, following which it is added to an aqueous solution containing 3.5 weight percent sodium chloride and 0.25 weight percent sulfuric acid, causing the unvulcanized rubber to coagulate in the form of crumb containing one weight percent of S-(3,5-di-tert-butyl-4-hydroxybenzyl) O,O-di(C_{20-50} primary alkyl) phosphorodithioate. This SBR crumb is extremely resistant to change in its Mooney viscosity during the storage period prior to final compounding and vulcanization.

PHENOLIC ANTIOXIDANTS

Hydroxybenzylphenyl Carbonates and Carboxylates

Antioxidants useful for polyolefins, elastomers and petroleum products have been developed by *B.R. Meltsner; U.S. Patents 3,579,561; May 18, 1971 and 3,644,281; February 22, 1972; both assigned to Ethyl Corporation.* These antioxidants have the formula:

(1)

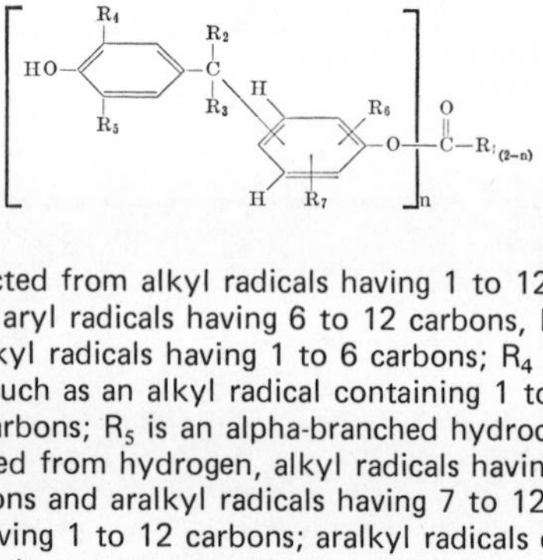

where n is 1 or 2, R_1 is selected from alkyl radicals having 1 to 12 carbons, aralkyl radicals having 7 to 12 carbons, and aryl radicals having 6 to 12 carbons, R_2 and R_3 are selected from hydrogen and lower alkyl radicals having 1 to 6 carbons; R_4 is a hydrocarbon radical containing 1 to 18 carbons such as an alkyl radical containing 1 to 18 carbons or an aralkyl radical containing 8 to 18 carbons; R_5 is an alpha-branched hydrocarbon radical containing 3 to 18 carbons; R_6 is selected from hydrogen, alkyl radicals having 1 to 12 carbons, aryl radicals having 6 to 12 carbons and aralkyl radicals having 7 to 12 carbons; and R_7 is selected from alkyl radicals having 1 to 12 carbons; aralkyl radicals containing 7 to 18 carbons and radicals having the formula:

(2)

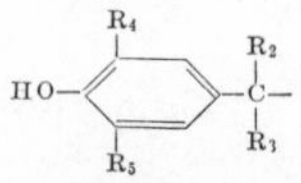

where R_2, R_3, R_4 and R_5 are the same as above. In Formula 1, R_6 and R_7 are bonded to positions ortho or para to the position bearing the

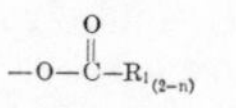

substitution. Some examples of these compounds are shown on the following page.

(3)

2-tert-butyl-4-methyl-6-(3,5-di-tert-butyl-4-
hydroxybenzyl)phenyl acetate

(4)

bis[2-tert-butyl-6-methyl-4-(3,5-di-tert-butyl-4-
hydroxybenzyl)phenyl]carbonate

Another embodiment of this process is a stabilizing composition comprising 10 to 90 weight percent of a compound previously described by Formula 1 and about 10 to 90 weight percent of a sulfur compound having the formula:

(5)
$$R_8O-\overset{O}{\overset{\|}{C}}-R_9-S-R_{10}-\overset{O}{\overset{\|}{C}}-OR_{11}$$

wherein R_9 and R_{10} are divalent hydrocarbon radicals selected from the group consisting of alkylene radicals containing about 1 to 6 carbons and arylene radicals containing about 6 to 12 carbons, and R_8 and R_{11} are alkyl radicals containing about 6 to 20 carbons.

Example 1: In a reaction vessel equipped with stirrer, reflux condenser, thermometer and heating means was placed 13 parts of 3,5-di-tert-butyl-4-hydroxybenzyl chloride, 20 parts hexane, 3.7 parts p-tert-butylphenol and one part anhydrous stannic chloride. The reaction vessel was then flushed with nitrogen and a nitrogen atmosphere retained over the reactants during the remainder of the experiment. While stirring, the reaction mixture was heated to 65° to 70°C and maintained at this temperature for 1.5 hours.

The reaction mixture was then cooled to room temperature, during which period white crystals began to form. About 50 parts of diethyl ether were added, causing the crystals to go back into solution. Following this, the reaction solution was washed with water and then dried over anhydrous sodium sulfate. Following this, the reaction solution was evaporated to dryness, leaving 13 parts of a solid product identified as 4-tert-butyl-2,6-bis(3,5-di-tert-butylbenzyl)phenol by its infrared spectra and carbon-hydrogen analysis.

In a second reaction vessel was placed 1.0 part of the derivative prepared above together with 5 parts of acetic anhydride. This reaction vessel was equipped the same as above. This reaction mixture was refluxed for 3 hours, during which period the solids slowly went into solution. After this period, the reaction mixture was cooled to room temperature and all volatile material removed by evaporation at reduced pressure over a 60° to 70°C hot water bath. The product remaining was identified by its infrared spectra to be 4-tert-butyl-2,6-bis(3,5-di-tert-butyl-4-hydroxybenzyl)phenyl acetate.

Example 2: To a reaction vessel equipped as in Example 1 is added one mol of 3,5-di-tert-butyl-4-hydroxybenzyl chloride and 1,000 parts of hexane. To this is added 0.5 mol of o-tert-butylphenol and 5.0 parts of anhydrous stannic chloride, following which the reaction is refluxed for 4 hours. This results in the formation of 2-tert-butyl-4,6-bis-(3,5-di-tert-butyl-4-hydroxybenzyl)phenol.

Following this, phosgene is passed into the liquid phase of the mixture until a pressure of about 5 psig of phosgene builds up. Stirring is continued for an additional 8 hours, while maintaining the reaction temperature at 30° to 40°C and the phosgene pressure at about 5 psig. A small amount of the gas phase is continually withdrawn and replaced with additional phosgene in order to provide a means of removing by-product HCl. Following this, the reaction is washed with water and dried over anhydrous sodium sulfate. Then the solvent is removed by evaporation at reduced pressure, yielding bis[2-tert-butyl-4,6-bis(3,5-di-tert-butyl-4-hydroxybenzyl)phenyl]carbonate. Qualitative examples are given in the patent on the use of these stabilizers in SBR, butyl rubber, NBR and natural rubber. Stabilizer mixtures such as 50% 2-tert-butyl-4-methyl-6-(3,5-di-tert-butyl-4-hydroxybenzyl) phenyl acetate and 50% dilaurylthiodipropionate are used in qualitative examples for the stabilization of polyethylene, polypropylene, polyisobutylene and ethylene/propylene terpolymer. Petroleum products, e.g. oils, gasoline, and synthetic polyester lubricants as well as lard and olive oil were also stabilized with the compounds of formula 1, optionally mixed with the compounds of formula 5 in additional qualitative examples.

Alkylidenedithiobisphenols

Sulfur containing bisphenols have been prepared by *M.B. Neuworth; U.S. Patent 3,704,327; November 28, 1972; assigned to Continental Oil Company.* They are useful in natural and synthetic rubbers which have high olefinic unsaturation. These compounds have the following formula:

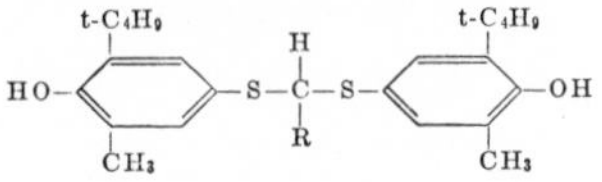

where R is selected from hydrogen and methyl groups. The compounds are prepared as follows. The appropriate 4-mercaptophenol is reacted with the appropriate carbonyl compound in the presence of a strong acid catalyst. The mercaptophenol and the appropriate carbonyl compound are preferably dissolved in an inert organic solvent to provide a homogeneous reaction mixture. At least a stoichiometric amount of the carbonyl compound is used. The catalyst is a strong acid catalyst, for example hydrochloric acid, sulfuric acid, perchloric acid, and strong acid cationic exchange resins. The reaction is mildly exothermic initially; external heating is then required to maintain the reaction temperature, generally between 50° and 100°C. Reaction times of 0.8 to 6 hours are generally required.

Example: 4-mercapto-6-tert-butyl-o-cresol (39.3 grams, 0.2 mol) was dissolved in 50 ml of methanol at room temperature, and 1 ml of concentrated HCl was added. Then, 37% formaldehyde (8.1 grams, 0.1 mol) in aqueous solution was added over five minutes with a resultant temperature rise from 29° to 35°C. Stirring of the homogeneous solution was continued for 40 minutes, at which time, 9.5 ml of 10% $NaHCO_3$ solution was added to neutralize the HCl. The mixture was then extracted with 200 ml of ethyl ether.

The ether extract was extracted with three 30-ml portions of 10% NaOH in aqueous solution to remove unreacted mercaptophenols. The caustic extract was discarded. The ether layer was water washed to pH 7, dried, filtered and evaporated to a dry tan powder which was recrystallized from hexane. Nearly colorless crystalline bis (3-tert-butyl-5-methyl-4-hydroxy phenylmercapto) methane was obtained which had a melting point of 121° to 123.5°C. When recrystallized from isopropyl alcohol and dried in vacuo at 110°C, the product had a melting point of 125.5° to 126.5°C.

The table below tabulates the results obtained by the direct use of these compounds as antioxidants for rubber. In addition, the results obtained on a blank and a commercial rubber antioxidant are included for comparison. In each case, a sample of the compound was incorporated in a natural rubber of the following composition:

Components	Parts by Weight
Pale crepe rubber	100.00
Zinc oxide	50.00
Titanium oxide	25.00
Stearic acid	2.00
Ultramarine blue	1.00
Mercaptobenzothiazole	1.00
Sulfur	3.00

One part by weight of the selected compound was added to the above mixture to provide a batch. A series of samples containing the selected antioxidant was prepared from the batch. A second series of samples was also prepared which contained no antioxidant, to serve as blanks. All the samples were first cured, their tensile strength determined, and then they were subjected to oxygen bomb (ASTM D-572-53). Their tensile strength after the aging treatment was measured. The results obtained are shown in the following table.

Composition	Oxygen bomb aging	
	Aged tensile	Percent of original tensile
Blank	1,640	53.0
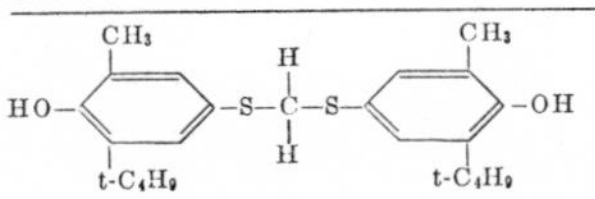 $HO-\underset{t\text{-}C_4H_9}{\overset{CH_3}{\bigcirc}}-S-\overset{H}{\underset{H}{C}}-S-\underset{t\text{-}C_4H_9}{\overset{CH_3}{\bigcirc}}-OH$	2,120	71.3
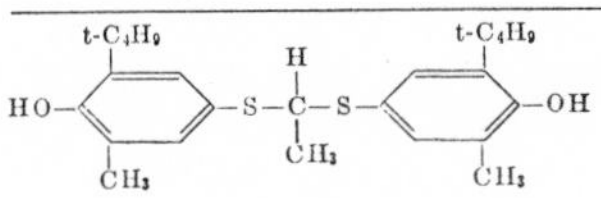 $HO-\underset{CH_3}{\overset{t\text{-}C_4H_9}{\bigcirc}}-S-\overset{H}{\underset{CH_3}{C}}-S-\underset{CH_3}{\overset{t\text{-}C_4H_9}{\bigcirc}}-OH$	2,195	74.0
$HO-\underset{t\text{-}C_4H_9}{\overset{CH_3}{\bigcirc}}-\overset{H}{\underset{(CH_2)_2}{\underset{CH_3}{C}}}-\underset{t\text{-}C_4H_9}{\overset{CH_3}{\bigcirc}}-OH$	2,265	78.5

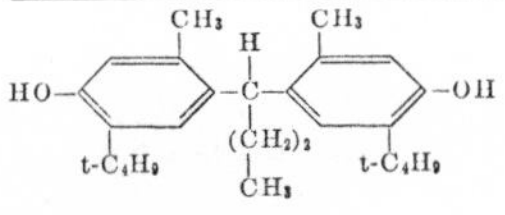

(Commercial antioxidant)

OTHER RUBBER ANTIOXIDANTS

Mixtures of N,N'-Substituted Phenylenediamines for Polyisoprenes

Solution polymerized polyisoprene having high resistance to thermal and mechanical stresses which is equivalent to that of natural rubber has been produced by *B. Berg and K.-H. Nordsiek; U.S. Patent 3,770,694; November 6, 1973; assigned to Chemische Werke Huels AG, Germany.* This improvement is obtained by adding to the polyisoprene polymerization solution, optionally after the addition of a conventional shortstop agent of a stabilizing amount: (1) 0.0005 to 0.05 part by weight per 100 parts by weight of the polyisoprene, of a difunctional, secondary aryl amine of Formula 1

$$(1) \qquad R_2-NH-\bigcirc-NH-R_1$$

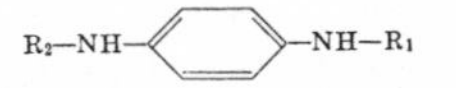

where R_1 and R_2 which can be identical or different, are alkyl of 1 to 20 carbons, cycloalkyl of 5 to 12 carbons, or mono- or dicyclic carbocyclic aryl; and (2) 0.01 to 1.0 part by weight per 100 parts by weight of polyisoprene, of an aliphatic amine of Formula 2

$$(2) \qquad R_n(NH)_{n-1}(NH_2)_x$$

where n and x are 1 and R is C_{2-20} alkyl or n is 1 to 10, x is 2 and R is C_{2-10} alkylene bridging adjacent amino groups. Precipitation of the polyisoprene from solution produces stabilized new unvulcanized solid polyisoprene of the difunctional secondary aryl amines of Formula 1 employed in the process, preferred are (a) those wherein at least one of R_1 and R_2 is alkyl, particularly those wherein alkyl is of 3 to 8 carbons; and (b) those wherein one of R_1 and R_2 is aryl, preferably phenyl, especially those wherein the other of R_1 and R_2 is alkyl as defined in (a). Especially suitable difunctional secondary aromatic amines are N-isopropyl-N'-phenyl-p-phenylenediamine, N-(1,3-dimethylbutyl)-N'-phenyl-p-phenylenediamine, N,N'-di-1,4-dimethylpentyl-p-phenylenediamine and N,N'-dioctyl-p-phenylenediamine.

Preferred compounds of Formula 2 are those wherein: (a) n is 2 and x is 2, and (b) R is alkylene of 2 to 6 carbons, preferably ethylene, propylene respectively trimethylene or tetramethylene etc., especially those of (a). Examples of such amines are propylamine, isopropylamine, butylamine, cyclohexylamine, stearylamine, laurylamine, ethylenediamine, hexylenediamine (hexamethylenediamine), diethylenetriamine, dipropylenetriamine, tetra-ethylenepentamine. The stabilization of the polyisoprene is conveniently effected in the solution phase of the polymerization charge after the polymerization has been terminated. Three different modes of operation are possible:

(1) If the polymerization catalyst is inactivated conventionally, e.g., by addition of an alcohol or water, a solution of the above-described mixture of amines (0.005 to 0.05 part by weight, per 100 parts by weight of polyisoprene, of the aromatic amine of Formula 1 and 0.01 to 1.0 part by weight, per 100 parts by weight of polyisoprene, of the aliphatic amine of Formula 2 is stirred into the shortstopped and optionally water-scrubbed, polymer solution.

(2) An improvement in the stability behavior of polyisoprene can be attained by short-stopping with an amine of Formula 2. Desirably, the polymerization catalyst is deactivated with the same aliphatic amine of Formula 2 employed in the stabilizer composition of this process. The amount of amine required for shortstopping is dependent on the amount of $TiCl_4$ in the mixed catalyst. This amount, in case of ethylenediamine, is about 2.2 mol/mol $TiCl_4$.

Without impairing the thus-obtained superior stability properties, it is impossible to conduct, after shortstopping the polymerization charge with the aliphatic amine of Formula 2 of this process and without any further addition of the aliphatic amine, a sole post stabilization with 0.005 to 0.05 part by weight, based on 100 parts by weight of polyisoprene, of the aromatic amine of Formula 1. Quite surprisingly, the amount of aliphatic amine according to Formula 2 employed as the shortstopping agent also acts as an activator for the small amount of the p-phenylenediamine of Formula 1 employed.

(3) The mixtures of amines of this process of Formula 1 and Formula 2 is employed as the shortstop agent for the polymerization. In such a case, additional stabilization is not necessary. This embodiment is particularly advantageous from the viewpoint of processing technology.

Results of Experiments and Tests — In these experiments a rolling mill is employed having an operating width of 450 mm and a roll diameter of 250 mm. The rotary speed of the front roll is 24 rpm that of the rear roll is 29 rpm (friction 1:1.2). The roll nip is adjusted to a width of 0.7 mm. After heating to 150°C, 300 grams of the sample of raw unvulcanized polyisoprene is exposed for periods of up to 15 minutes to the shear stress produced under these conditions with rotating rolls. The subsequent determination of the ML-4 values is effected according to the DIN [German Industrial Standard] 53,523. The following is a definition of the abbreviation of the chemical compounds and the trade names utilized in the table below:

> DPTA: dipropylenetriamine
> BKF: 2,2'-methylenebis(6-tert-butyl-p-cresol)
> 4010 Na: N-isopropyl-N'-phenyl-p-phenylenediamine
> (commercial product of Farbenfabriken Bayer AG)
> pbw: parts by weight per 100 parts by weight of poly-
> isoprene

The following table shows the properties of polyisoprenes (methanol shortstop agent) stabilized by a conventional nondiscoloring phenolic type stabilizer (Product No. I) and a discoloring arylamine type stabilizer (Product No. II), with usual dosages. The effect of an aliphatic amine (Product No. III) is also shown. The effect of the combination of an aliphatic amine with an aromatic amine is clearly shown by the jump-like increase in stabilization achieved with Product No. IV. The usual discoloration occurs in the range of the concentration selected for this example.

Product number	Stabilizers		Polyiso- prene color	ML–4 after rolling test at 150° C.				
	Type	P.b.w.		0′	2½′	5′	10′	15′
I	BKF	0.4	Light	87	49	40	23	15
II	4010 Na	0.4	Dark	86	50	42	25	19
III	DPTA	0.4	Light	86	46	39	20	12
IV	{4010 Na {DPTA	0.4 0.4	}Dark	87	73	65	48	43

Acyl Derivatives of Aromatic Nitroso Compounds

p-Nitrosoanilines are of value as antioxidants for rubbers, especially since they are resistant to extraction from the rubber by solvents. The acyl derivatives used in this process developed by *B.T. Ashworth, K. Crawford, and P.M. Quan; U.S. Patent 3,826,779; July 30, 1974; assigned to Imperial Chemical Industries Limited, England* have advantages over nitroso anilines in that they are less prone to stain and irritate the skin, they disperse more easily in the rubber and have less effect on the processing safety of the rubber. Broadly, the rubber compositions contain in a stabilizing amount, an acyl derivative of a nitroso compound of the formula

$$X-\langle\bigcirc\rangle-NO$$

where X is a hydroxyl group or a group NHR or N(OH)R in which R is an alkyl, alkenyl, cycloalkyl or aryl group or substituted derivative thereof and where the benzene ring may optionally be further substituted.

The rubber may be natural rubber or a synthetic rubber for example a polymer or copolymer derived from a conjugated diene such as cis-polybutadiene, cis-polyisoprene, other polymers of butadiene or isoprene, polymers of 2-chlorobutadiene or copolymers of any of the foregoing with each other or with isobutene, styrene, acrylonitrile, methyl methacrylate, or other well-known polymerizable compounds used in the manufacture of synthetic rubbers. The acyl compound which may be incorporated into the rubber by any conventional method is of particular value for the stabilization of vulcanized rubber compositions.

The amount of acyl compound to be used is conveniently from 0.1 to 4.0%, and preferably from 0.25 to 2.0%, of the weight of rubber. The acyl compounds are derived from the quinone oxime or quinone imine oxime tautomers of the nitroso compounds and have compositions of the formulas

$$O=\langle\bigcirc\rangle=N.O.Ac \qquad RN=\langle\bigcirc\rangle=N.O.Ac \qquad \overset{O}{\underset{\uparrow}{R\overset{|}{N}}}=\langle\bigcirc\rangle=N.O.Ac$$

where R has the meaning given above and Ac is an acyl group. The preferred carboxylic acids from which the acyl groups may be derived are alkane carboxylic acids containing a total of four to eighteen carbons, especially lauric and stearic acids, carbonic acid alkyl, e.g., ethyl hydrogen carbonic acid, α,ω-alkanedioic acids containing from six to twelve carbons, especially adipic, azelaic and sebacic acids, and aryl carboxylic acids. for example benzoic acid and readily available substituted derivatives thereof such as alkyl, alkoxy or chloro substituted benzoic acids.

The acyl compounds may be prepared by treating the appropriate nitroso compound of Formula 1 with preferably an acid chloride but other conventional reactive derivatives of an acid which will give rise to an acyl group, for example an acid anhydride may be used. The reaction is desirably carried out in presence of an acid binding agent, preferably a weakly basic metal compound binding agent, preferably a weakly basic metal compound such as calcium carbonate, calcium hydroxide, sodium bicarbonate and especially sodium carbonate. Other acid binding means can be used, for example caustic alkalies or organic tertiary amines, or the nitroso compounds can be used as preformed metal salts but the former afford less pure products and the latter procedure is inconvenient.

Example 1: 10 parts of 4-nitrosodiphenylamine are dissolved in 125 parts of acetone; 12.5 parts of anhydrous sodium carbonate are added. The mixture is stirred, and 5.1 parts of acetic anhydride are added. After a reaction period of 17 hours the mixture is filtered and the filter cake is washed with 100 parts of acetone. The filtrate and washings are poured into 600 parts of water when 11 parts of the required acetyl compound are precipitated. The precipitate is collected and after drying at 50°C under reduced pressure it melts at 87° to 88°C.

Example 2: Rubber mixes of the following composition are prepared by mixing on a two roll mill:

	Parts by Weight
Pale crepe natural rubber	100
Zinc oxide	10
Stearic acid	1
Barium sulfate	75
Sulfur	2.5
Cyclohexylbenzothiazolyl sulfenamide	0.5
Antioxidant	As indicated

The mixes are vulcanized for 20 minutes at 153°C and the vlucanizates, in sheet form of 0.8 mm thickness are examined for antioxidant activity by determining the time taken in hours for an absorption of 2% of their weight of oxygen at 100°C.

The results below show that the antioxidants of this process lose little of their antioxidant activity after extraction.

Antioxidant	None	Lauric acid deriva- tive of 4-nitroso- diphenyl- amine	Isobutyric acid deriva- tive of 4-nitroso- diphenyl- amine	n-Hexa- noic acid deriva- tive of 4-nitroso- diphenyl- amine	n-Butyric acid deriva- tive of 4-nitroso- diphenyl- amine
Percent on rubber hydrocarbon		2	2	2	2
Time (in hours) for absorption of 2% oxygen:					
Unextracted vulcanisate	18	36	39	38	41
Extracted vulcanisate	<8	33	36	34	40

The acyl derivatives used above are prepared by reacting 4-nitrosodiphenylamine with lauryl chloride and isobutyric chloride respectively, and with n-hexanoic anhydride and n-butyric anhydride respectively by the procedure of Example 1.

POLYOLEFIN ANTIOXIDANT SYSTEMS

HINDERED PHENOL DERIVATIVES

Four series of hindered phenol compounds have been developed as antioxidants by the Ethyl Corporation. As disclosed in the following eight patents, they are used in a broad range of organic materials, but their main value appears to be in the polyolefins. Workers at Argus have also produced complex phosphates having hindered phenol groups useful in PVC and polyolefins.

Hindered Hydroxybenzyl-Substituted Thiodicarboxylates

Esters of (3,5-dihydrocarbyl-4-hydroxybenzyl)thiodicarboxylic acids are shown by *P.D. Beirne; U.S. Patents 3,637,585; January 25, 1972; and 3,465,029; September 2, 1969; both assigned to Ethyl Corporation* to be effective stabilizers for organic material. For example, dilauryl-[(3,5-di-tert-butyl-4-hydroxybenzyl)thio]succinate prolongs the life of polypropylene. Effectiveness is synergistically increased by inclusion of an ester of a thiodialkanoic acid such as dilaurylthiodipropionate.

These esters have the formula:

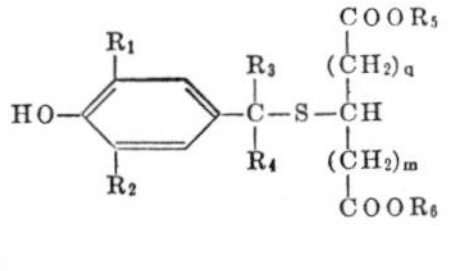

where m is an integer from 0 to 12, q is an integer from 0 to 1, R_1 is selected from alkyl radicals containing 1 to 20 carbons, aryl radicals containing 6 to 20 carbons, aralkyl radicals containing 7 to 20 carbons and cycloalkyl radicals containing 6 to 20 carbons. R_2 is selected from alpha-branched alkyl radicals containing 3 to 20 carbons, alpha-branched aralkyl radicals containing 8 to 20 carbons and cycloalkyl radicals containing 6 to 20 carbons. R_3 and R_4 are selected from hydrogen, alkyl radicals containing 1 to 6 carbons, aryl radicals containing 6 to 12 carbons and aralkyl radicals containing 7 to 12 carbons. R_5 and R_6 are selected from alkyl radicals containing 1 to 20 carbons, aralkyl radicals containing 7 to 20 carbons, and aryl radicals containing 6 to 20 carbons.

In a preferred embodiment of the formula, R_1 and R_2 are both alpha-branched alkyl radicals containing 3 to 20 carbons or alpha-branched aralkyl radicals containing 8 to 20 carbons; R_3 and R_4 are hydrogen; R_5 and R_6 are alkyl radicals containing 6 to 20 carbons; m is 1 and q is 0. Some examples of these compounds are:

Di-n-hexyl-[(3,5-di-tert-butyl-4-hydroxybenzyl)thio]succinate
Didecyl[(3,5-diisopropyl-4-hydroxybenzyl)thio]succinate
Dieicosyl[(3,5-di-sec-butyl-4-hydroxybenzyl)thio]succinate
Dilauryl[(3-tert-eicosyl-4-sec-octyl-4-hydroxybenzyl)thio]succinate
Dicetyl⟨[3-(α-methylbenzyl)-4-hydroxy-5-tert-nonylbenzyl]thio⟩succinate

The most preferred antioxidant is dilauryl[(3,5-di-tert-butyl-4-hydroxybenzyl)thio]succinate. The antioxidant compounds of the formula can be prepared by reacting the appropriate benzyl halide with the proper mercapto derivative of a diester of a dibasic acid. For example, dilauryl[(3,5-di-tert-butyl-4-hydroxybenzyl)thio]succinate is formed by the reaction of 3,5-di-tert-butyl-4-hydroxybenzyl chloride with dilauryl mercaptosuccinate. The following example illustrates the preparation of a typical antioxidant compound. All parts are parts by weight unless otherwise stated.

Example: To a reaction vessel equipped with stirrer and thermometer were added 440 parts of benzene, 12.74 parts (0.05 mol) of 3,5-di-tert-butyl-4-hydroxybenzyl chloride and 24.14 parts (0.05 mol) of dilauryl mercaptosuccinate. Following this, there were added, while stirring, at room temperature, 10.12 parts (0.1 mol) triethylamine. A precipitate of triethylamine hydrochloride formed immediately. The mixture was stirred an additional 2 hours at room temperature and then the precipitate was filtered off. Benzene was distilled from the filtrate, leaving a yellow viscous oil.

This material was eluted with benzene through an alumina column and all of the fractions having the same infrared spectrum were combined. The benzene was distilled from this material, leaving 21.4 parts of a yellow viscous liquid. Analysis showed it to be in good agreement with the theoretical analysis for dilauryl[(3,5-di-tert-butyl-4-hydroxybenzyl)thio]succinate.

In one series of tests, the additive compounds were incorporated into polypropylene samples and compared not only with the unstabilized polypropylene, but with polypropylene stabilized with an equal amount of other recognized antioxidants. Duplicate runs were made on the test stabilizer of this process in order to provide increased confidence in the results. The results obtained in these tests are shown in the following table.

No.	Additive	Concentration (weight percent)	Hours to failure
1	None		2.5
2	2,6-di-tert-butyl-4-methylphenol	0.3	16.0
3	2,2'-methylenebis-(4-methyl-6-tert-butylphenol)	0.3	112.0
4	4,4'-thiobis(2 tert-butyl-5-methylphenol)	0.3	96.0
5	Dilauryl(3,5-di-tert-butyl-4-hydroxybenzyl)thio]succinate	0.3	1,224
6	do	0.3	1,144
7	do	0.3	1,000

These additive compounds (Tests 5-7) provide a 500-fold increase in polypropylene life over the unprotected polypropylene and a 10-fold increase over the protection afforded by some prior art antioxidant compounds. Further Oven Aging Tests showed the effect of the synergistic compounds on these antioxidant compounds; duplicate runs were made to increase the reliability of the results shown below.

No.	Additive	Concentration (weight percent)	Hours to failure
1	Dilaurylthiodipropionate	0.3	288
2	Dilauryl(3,5-di-tert-butyl-4-hydroxybenzyl)thio]succinate	0.1	208
3	do	0.1	280
4	Dilauryl(3,5-di-tert-butyl-4-hydroxybenzyl)thio]succinate dilaurylthiodipropionate	0.1 } 0.2 }	840
5	do	0.1 } 0.2 }	808

As the above results show, although the addition of 0.1 weight percent dilauryl[(3,5-di-tert-butyl-4-hydroxybenzyl)thio] succinate stabilized the polypropylene for 208 hours (Test 2) and 0.3 weight percent dilaurylthiodipropionate stabilized the polypropylene for only 288 hours (Test 1), the combination of 0.1 weight percent dilauryl[3,5-di-tert-butyl-4-hydroxybenzyl)thio] succinate and only 0.2 weight percent dilaurylthiodipropionate (the preferred synergist) stabilized the polypropylene on the order of twice the sum of the stability expected from the two components (Tests 4 and 5).

Examples are included in the complete patents on the addition of these ester antioxidants to lubricating oils, polyester lubricants, transmission fluids, gasolines, NR, SBR, NBR, and polyethylene. No quantitative stabilization results were given in these examples.

Hindered Hydroxyphenoxysilanes

Silanes having a hindered phenol moiety have been prepared by *E.F. Zaweski and B.R. Meltsner; U.S. Patents 3,647,749; March 7, 1972; and 3,491,137; January 20, 1970; both assigned to Ethyl Corporation.* The effectiveness of these antioxidants is also improved by mixing with a dihydrocarbylthiodialkanoate such as dilaruylthiodipropionate, or a phosphonate such as tri-p-nonylphenylphosphite.

These silane antioxidants have the formula:

(1)

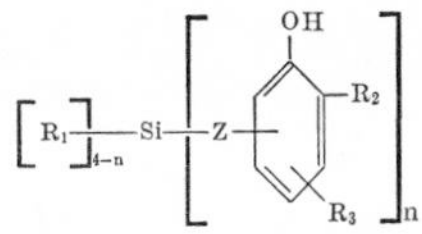

$$\left[R_1 \right]_{4-n} - Si - \left[Z - \left\langle \begin{array}{c} OH \\ \\ \end{array} \right\rangle \begin{array}{c} R_2 \\ \\ R_3 \end{array} \right]_n$$

where n is 1 to 4, R_1 is a hydrocarbon radical containing 1 to 20 carbons, Z is oxygen, sulfur or an imino radical, R_2 is selected from alpha-branched alkyl radicals containing 3 to 20 carbons, alpha-branched aralkyl radicals containing 8 to 20 carbons, aryl radicals containing 6 to 20 carbons, and cycloalkyl radicals containing 6 to 20 carbons, and R_3 is selected from hydrogen, alkyl radicals containing 1 to 20 carbons, arylradicals containing 6 to 20 carbons, aralkyl radicals containing 7 to 20 carbons, cycloalkyl radicals containing 6 to 20 carbons, halogen and alkoxy radicals containing 1 to 12 carbons.

In a preferred antioxidant, the Z in the above formula is oxygen and is bonded to the position para to the phenolic hydroxyl radical. In a most preferred embodiment R_3 is bonded to the carbon atom ortho to the phenolic hydroxyl group. These compounds have the formula:

(2)

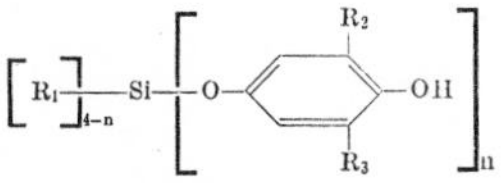

$$\left[R_1 \right]_{4-n} - Si - \left[O - \left\langle \begin{array}{c} R_2 \\ \\ R_3 \end{array} \right\rangle OH \right]_n$$

where n, R_1 and R_2 are the same as defined for Formula (1) and R_3 is selected from the group previously defined excepting hydrogen. Some examples of these highly preferred compounds are:

Diphenyl bis(3,5-di-isopropyl-4-hydroxyphenoxy)silane
Diphenyl bis(3,5-di-tert-butyl-4-hydroxyphenoxy)silane
Diphenyl bis[3,5-di(α-methylbenzyl)-4-hydroxyphenoxy] silane

The following example will serve to illustrate the process of making the silicon-containing antioxidant compounds. All parts are parts by weight unless otherwise specified.

Example: In a reaction vessel equipped with a stirrer, thermometer, heating means and provided with a nitrogen atmosphere were placed 120 parts of toluene, 25 parts of 2,6-di-tert-butyl-p-hydroquinone and 11.4 parts of triethylamine. Following this, 10.5 parts of diphenyl dichloro silane were added and an immediate exothermic reaction occurred. The temperature was maintained at 60° to 65°C for 4 hours and then cooled to about 30°C. The reaction mixture was washed 3 times with 150 parts of water in each.

The toluene was then distilled off under vacuum and the glass-like residue was recrystallized from isopropyl alcohol, yielding a white crystalline product having a MP 171° to 172°C. Infrared analysis confirmed the structure of the product as diphenyl bis(3,5-di-tert-butyl-4-hydroxyphenoxy)silane. Quantitative Oven Aging Tests were conducted with polypropylene.

Test specimens are prepared by mixing the test stabilizers with polypropylene powder for 3 minutes in a Waring Blendor. The mixture is then molded into a 6" x 6" sheet with a thickness of either 0.025" or 0.0625". This is accomplished in a molding press at 400°F under 5,000 psi pressure. Each sheet is then cut into ½" x 1" test specimens in order to obtain the five replicate samples. These samples are then subjected to the Oven Aging Tests.

In order to compare these silane antioxidants, tests were carried out employing several commercially accepted stabilizers with the preferred stabilizer of the process. The results obtained are shown in the following table.

	Additive	Concentration, weight percent	Sample thickness, mil	Hours to failure
1	None		25	2.5
2	2,6-di-tert-butyl-4-methylphenol	0.3	25	19
3	2,2'-methylenebis(4-methyl-6-tert-butylphenol)	0.3	25	112
4	4,4'-thiobis(2-tert-butyl-5-methylphenol)	0.3	25	96
5	Diphenyl-bis(3,5-di-tert-butyl-4-hydroxyphenoxy)silane	0.3	25	480

The effect of synergistic action with dilaurylthiodipropionate (DLTDP) is given in the following table.

	Additive	Concentration, weight percent	Sample thickness, mil	Hours to failure
1	Dilaurylthiodipropionate	0.3	25	288
2	Diphenyl-bis(2,6-di-tert-butylphenoxy)silane	0.3	25	480
3	{Diphenyl-bis(2,6-di-tert-butylphenoxy)silane / Dilaurylthiodipropionate	0.1 / 0.2	25	>528

Other examples in these patents show the addition of these silanes to NR, SBR, NBR, EPT, polyethylene, gasoline, antiknock fluids, diesel fuel, and petroleum and polyester lubricating oils. No quantitative results were given for these formulations.

3,5-Dihydrocarbyl-4-Hydroxybenzylphenyl Alkyl Ethers

Mono- and di-(3,5-dihydrocarbyl-4-hydroxybenzyl)phenyl alkyl ethers are disclosed by *B.R. Meltsner; U.S. Patents 3,637,586; January 25, 1972; 3,476,814; November 4, 1969; both assigned to Ethyl Corporation.* These compounds are useful either alone or in synergistic combination with a dialkyl thiodialkanoate as antioxidants for a broad range of organic material. These antioxidants have the formula:

(1)

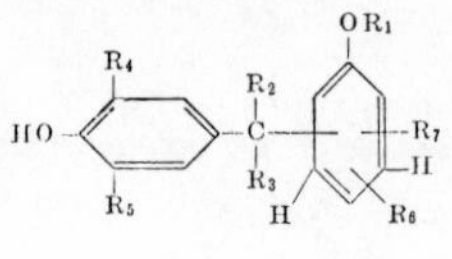

where R_1 is selected from alkyl radicals having 1 to 12 carbons, aralkyl radicals having 7 to 12 carbons, and aryl radicals having 6 to 12 carbons, R_2 and R_3 are selected from hydrogen and lower alkyl radicals having 1 to 6 carbons; R_4 is a hydrocarbon radical containing 1 to 18 carbons; R_5 is an alpha-branched hydrocarbon radical containing 3 to 18 carbons. R_6 is selected from hydrogen, alkyl radicals having 1 to 12 carbons, aryl radicals having 6 to 12 carbons and aralkyl radicals having 7 to 12 carbons; and R_7 is selected from alkyl radicals having 1 to 12 carbons, aralkyl radicals containing 7 to 18 carbons and radicals having the formula:

(2)

where R_2, R_3, R_4 and R_5 are the same as above.

In a highly preferred embodiment, R_7 in Formula (1) is a radical of Formula (2) and is substituted on the benzene ring in a position ortho to the position bearing the OR_1 substitution and R_6 is substituted on the position para to the position bearing the OR_1 substitution. Some examples of these compounds are:

> α,α'-(2-methoxy-5-ethyl-m-phenylene)-bis-(2-methyl-6-tert-butyl-p-cresol)
> α,α'-(2-methoxy-5-tert-butyl-m-phenylene)-bis-(2,6-di-sec-butyl-p-cresol)
> α,α'-(2-methoxy-5-methyl-m-phenylene)-bis-[2,6-di-α-methylbenzyl)-p-cresol]

The most preferred antioxidant has R_7 in Formula (1) equal to Formula (2) and located ortho to the OR_1 substitution, R_6 located para to the OR_1 substitution, and R_4 and R_5 both alpha-branched hydrocarbon radicals containing 3 to 18 carbon atoms, e.g., α,α'-(2-methoxy-5-tert-butyl-m-phenylene)-bis-(2,6-di-tert-butyl-p-cresol). The preparation of such compounds is shown by the following example.

Example: To a reaction vessel equipped with a stirrer, thermometer, reflux condenser and maintained under a nitrogen atmosphere were added 100 parts water and 4 parts sodium hydroxide. When the sodium hydroxide had dissolved, 15 parts of p-tert-butylphenol were added. Following this, 15.8 parts of methanol were added, causing all the p-tert-butylphenol to dissolve.

After this, 12.6 parts of dimethyl sulfate were added. The temperature rose to 40°C and an oil came out of solution. The reaction was stirred for an hour and the oil layer which had formed was separated and washed with water. Following this, the oil was dried over anhydrous sodium sulfate, yielding 10 parts of a material which was identified by infrared analysis as p-tert-butyl anisole.

In a second reaction vessel equipped with stirrer, thermometer, reflux condenser and maintained under nitrogen were placed 20 parts of hexane, 8.8 parts of 3,5-di-tert-butyl-4-hydroxybenzyl chloride, 2.83 parts of the p-tert-butyl anisole prepared above and 0.2 part of anhydrous stannic chloride. It was refluxed for two hours, during which period HCl was evolved. It was then cooled to room temperature, washed with water and then dried over anhydrous sodium sulfate. The hexane solvent was then evaporated, leaving a residue which was crystallized from petroleum ether, yielding 4 parts of white crystals having a melting point of 149° to 151°C. These crystals were identified as α,α'-(2-methoxy-5-tert-butyl-m-phenylene)-bis-(2,6-di-tert-butyl-p-cresol) by carbon and hydrogen analyses.

The following tests were conducted to show the superior properties of these antioxidants. The stabilizing compositions were incorporated into polypropylene and the polymer milled on rollers exposed to the atmosphere and maintained at 425°F, until signs of polymer degradation became discernible. These test conditions simulate the temperature and air exposure encountered during the processing of plastic materials. The procedure followed was to first bring the rollers to operating temperature and then to pour the polypropylene poly-mer, in granular form, together with the stabilizing compositions onto the hot rollers, where-upon the polypropylene melted and became thoroughly mixed with the stabilizing composi-tion. Hot milling was continued until the polymer showed signs of breakdown by discolo-ration or a decrease in viscosity, evidenced by polymer flow, indicating a decrease in mo-lecular weight. The test criterion was the time lapse before polymer degradation was noted for stabilizing composition (A) compared with known phenolic compositions (B) and (C). Results obtained when 0.4 weight percent of each stabilizer composition was added to poly-propylene and the polypropylene then subjected to the foregoing test follow. In each mix-ture 50% dilaurylthiodipropionate was combined with 50% of the ingredient listed.

Stabilizer	Minutes to Failure
(A) α,α'-(2-methoxy-5-tert-butyl-m-phenylene)bis(2,6-di-tert-butyl-p-cresol)	102*
(B) α,α'-(2-hydroxy-5-tert-butyl-m-phenylene)bis(2,6-di-tert-butyl-p-cresol)	30**
(C) 1,3,5-trimethyl-2,4,6-tri-(3,5-di-tert-butyl-4-hydroxybenzyl)benzene	75*

*Polymer breakdown.   **Turned yellow.

The complete patents also included examples of the addition of these antioxidants or their synergistic mixtures with a dialkylthiodialkanoate to a wide variety of substrates. Included are: SBR, NBR, EPT, butyl and natural rubbers; polyester and petroleum lubricants; diesel, gasoline and antiknock fuels; lard and olive oil; and polyethylene and polyisobutylene. No quantitative stabilization data were given in these examples.

Phenolic Phosphates and Phosphites

Mono- or di(dihydrocarbylhydroxyphenyl) alkyl phosphates, phosphites, thiophosphates or thiophosphites, such as 3,5-di-tert-butyl-4-hydroxyphenyl di-n-octadecyl phosphate are disclosed by *J.C. Wollensak and E.F. Zaweski; U.S. Patents 3,755,250; August 28, 1973; and 3,683,054; August 8, 1972; assigned to Ethyl Corporation.* The antioxidant ability of these compounds is synergistically improved by inclusion of a dialkyl thiodialkanoate such as dilaurylthiodipropionate. Broadly, these compounds have the formula:

(1)

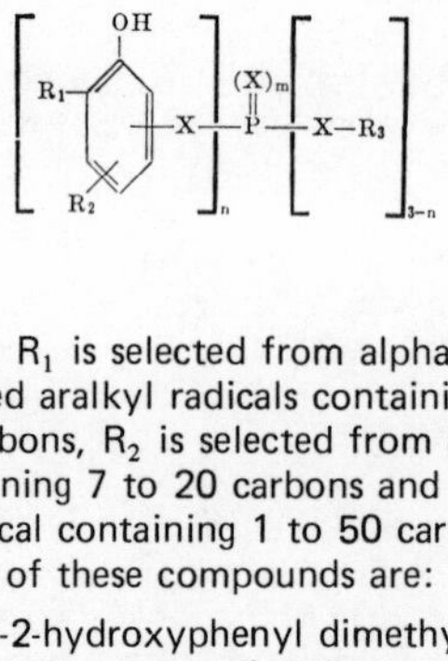

where m is 0 or 1, n is 1 or 2, R_1 is selected from alpha-branched alkyl radicals containing 3 to 20 carbons, alpha-branched aralkyl radicals containing 8 to 20 carbons, and cycloalkyl radicals containing 6 to 20 carbons, R_2 is selected from alkyl radicals containing 1 to 20 carbons, aralkyl radicals containing 7 to 20 carbons and cycloalkyl radicals containing 6 to 20 carbons, R_3 is an alkyl radical containing 1 to 50 carbons, and X is independently oxy-gen or sulfur. Some examples of these compounds are:

3-tert-butyl-5-methyl-2-hydroxyphenyl dimethyl phosphate
S-(3,5-diisopropyl-4-hydroxyphenyl) O,O-di-n-dodecyl thiolothionophosphate
2-methyl-5-(α-methylbenzyl-4-hydroxyphenyl) di-n-hexadecyl phosphite
di-(3,5-dicyclohexyl-4-hydroxyphenyl) methyl phosphite

The above compounds, in which R_3 is an alkyl having 12 to 50 carbons, is preferred. This class is apparently more compatible with a broader range of organic material. More pre-ferred are those in which the phenolic hydroxy radical is in the 4 position.

A most preferred antioxidant is represented by the phosphates, especially those in which both positions ortho to the phenolic hydroxyl radical are tert-butyl groups. This class of compounds has the formula shown on the following page, where n and R_3 are the same as defined in Formula (1).

(2)

$$\left[HO-\underset{\underset{C(CH_3)_3}{\overset{C(CH_3)_3}{\bigcirc}}}{}-O-\overset{O}{\underset{P}{\parallel}}-\left[OR_3\right]_{3-n}\right]_n$$

Examples of these 3,5-di-tert-butyl-4-hydroxyphenyl dialkyl phosphates are the dimethyl, diisobutyl, di(2-ethylhexyl), di-n-dodecyl, di-sec-eicosyl, etc. esters.

These antioxidants are readily prepared by reacting the appropriate hydroquinone or mercaptophenol with the appropriate phosphorus trihalide, phosphorus oxyhalide or phosphorus thiohalide and then reacting the intermediate with the appropriate alcohol or alkyl mercaptan. The reaction is preferably carried out in a solvent such as toluene or xylene and in the presence of a hydrogen halide acceptor such as the tertiary amines, for example, pyridine or triethylamine. The following example serves to illustrate the methods of preparing these antioxidants. All parts are parts by weight unless otherwise specified.

Example: In a reaction vessel equipped with stirrer, condenser, thermometer, heating means and provided with a nitrogen atmosphere were placed 129 parts of toluene and 38.8 parts of phosphorus oxychloride. To this solution was added a solution of 50.6 parts of triethylamine, 20 parts of toluene and 111.3 parts of 2,6-di-tert-butyl hydroquinone. The temperature rose from 10° to 40°C during this addition. The mixture was stirred at room temperature for 2 days. The mixture was then filtered to remove the triethylamine hydrochloride.

One-half of the filtrate was placed in a second reaction vessel and 13.1 parts of triethylamine added. Then a solution of 33.8 parts of 1-octadecanol in 175 parts of toluene was added. The mixture was stirred and heated to 55°C and stirred at this temperature for 23 hours. The mixture was cooled and filtered. The filtrate was washed with water and the solvent distilled out, leaving 88 parts of residue. This was identified by elemental analysis and nuclear magnetic resonance as bis(3,5-di-tert-butyl-4-hydroxyphenyl) n-octadecyl phosphate.

The addition of these antioxidants to mineral lubricating oils, polyester lubricating oils, functional fluids and gasoline is shown in numerous examples in the complete patents. Other examples included the addition of these stabilizers to NR, SBR and NBR elastomers and to polyethylene. No quantitative test results were given for these compositions. However quantitative data were given for the stabilization of polypropylene.

In one series of Oven Aging Tests, these antioxidants were incorporated into polypropylene samples and compared not only with the unstabilized polypropylene, but with polypropylene stabilized with an equal amount of other recognized antioxidants. The results obtained in these tests are shown in the following table.

Number	Additive	Conc. Weight %	Hours to Failure
1	None	- -	2.5
2	2,6-di-tert-butyl-4-methylphenol	0.3	16.0
3	2,2'-methylenebis-(4-methyl-6-tert-butylphenol)	0.3	112.0
4	4,4'-thiobis(2-tert-butyl-5-methyl-phenol)	0.3	96.0
5	bis(3,5-di-tert-butyl-4-hydroxy-phenyl) n-octadecyl phosphate	0.3	1408.0

As the above results show, the additive compounds of this process (Test 5) provide about a 500-fold increase in polypropylene life over the unprotected polypropylene and a 12.5-fold increase over the protection afforded by some known antioxidant compounds.

The effectiveness of these antioxidants is also synergistically increased by using them in combination with a dialkylthiodialkanoate.

Polycarbocyclic Phenolic Phosphites

O.S. Kauder, W.E. Leistner and A.C. Hecker; U.S. Patents 3,655,832; April 11, 1972; and 3,476,699; November 4, 1969; both assigned to Argus Chemical Corporation have developed organic phosphites which are useful as stabilizers in polyolefins and polyvinyl chloride. These phosphites have in the molecule at least one polycarbocyclic phenolic group

$$(Ar)_p - Y - Ar$$
$$(OH)_m$$

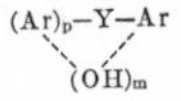

for each phosphite group, the polycarbocyclic phenolic group having one to thirty carbons per phenolic hydroxyl group, and at least one aliphatic or cycloaliphatic group, the phosphite having the formula:

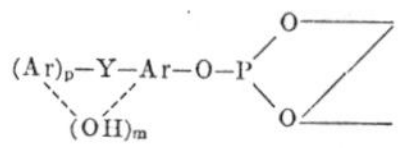

$$(Ar)_p - Y - Ar - O - P$$

where Ar is a carbocyclic aromatic nucleus and at least one Ar nucleus has a phenolic hydroxyl group (OH); m is 1 to 2; p is 2 to 4; and Z is taken in sufficient number to satisfy the valences of the two phosphite oxygen atoms and is hydrogen; monovalent or bivalent saturated aliphatic, aromatic or saturated cycloaliphatic hydrocarbon radicals having 1 to 30 carbons; or monovalent or bivalent phenolic groups having 1 to 30 carbons per phenolic hydroxy group, or the group consisting of $(HO)_m - Ar-$ or

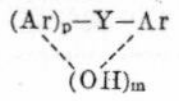

$$(Ar)_p - Y - Ar$$
$$(OH)_m$$

which in polymeric phosphites are linked to additional phosphite groups, such polymeric phosphites containing at least one aliphatic or cycloaliphatic group having 1 to 30 carbons for each one to ten phosphite groups; and Y is a linking group selected from trivalent, tetravalent and pentavalent aliphatic, and aliphatic aromatic hydrocarbon groups, attached to each Ar group through a carbon atom not a member of an aromatic ring, and such aliphatic radicals including carboxylic acid ester groups, having 1 to 33 carbons.

These compounds are more effective as stabilizers than phosphites and phenols in combination, but as separate compounds, in the same relative amounts as the phosphite and phenol moieties of the phosphites of this process. Apparently, the association of the groups in the same molecule has an enhancing effect. Furthermore, the presence of at least one aliphatic or cycloaliphatic group attached to a phosphite group in the molecule also substantially enhances the stabilizing effectiveness of the phosphite.

Usually, in a molecule containing several phosphite groups there should be at least one aliphatic or cycloaliphatic group attached to phosphorus through oxygen for every ten phosphite groups, and preferably at least one for every eight phosphite groups. The compounds having two phosphite groups as a minimum per molecule are generally more effective stabilizers than compounds having one phosphite group and the same relative proportion of phenolic groups.

This formula encompasses a large number of compounds which can be obtained by the classical method of reacting the desired polyphenols and alcohols with PCl_3 in the presence of basic HCl acceptors such as tertiary amines, or alternatively, by first reacting the polyphenols with PCl_3 without basic catalyst to form the aryl chlorophosphites and then reacting the aryl chlorophosphites with alcohol in the presence of tertiary amines. The phosphite ester compounds are also obtained quite readily by transesterifying an aliphatic and/or cycloaliphatic phosphite having the desired aliphatic and/or cycloaliphatic groups with a polycyclic polyhydric phenol, or alternatively, by transesterifying an aryl phosphite with a polycyclic polyhydric phenol and an aliphatic and/or cycloaliphatic alcohol. One can also transesterify a mixture of phenolic phosphates and aliphatic and/or cycloaliphatic phosphites to obtain a final product with the desired proportion of aliphatic and/or cycloaliphatic radicals in the molecule. Exemplary polycyclic phenols used in preparing phosphites of the process are:

> 4,4'-methylenebis(2-tert-butyl-6-methylphenol)
> 2,2'-bis(4-hydroxyphenyl)propane
> methylenebis(p-cresol)
> 4,4'-oxobis(3-methylphenol)
> 2,2'-oxobis(4-dodecylphenol)
> 4,4'-n-butylidenebis(2-tert-butyl-5-methylphenol)
> 2,2'-methylenebis[4-methyl-6-(1'-methylcyclohexyl)phenol]

Example 1: 55 grams of 4,4'-n-butylidenebis(2-tert-butyl-5-methylphenol), 30 grams of triisooctyl phosphite and 0.48 grams of sodium hydroxide were heated at 120° to 125°C for 3 hours, forming a clear brown homogeneous liquid. This was then heated at 140°C under reduced pressure, and the isooctanol which was distilled off was recovered. The weight of isooctanol recovered showed that the reaction product was di-(4,4'-n-butylidene-bis(2-tert-butyl-5-methylphenol) isooctyl phosphite.

Example 2: One mol of triphenyl phosphite, 0.5 mol of 4,4'-n-butylidenebis(2-tert-butyl-5-methylphenol) and two mols of tridecyl alcohol were reacted in two stages. The triphenyl phosphite was first transesterified with the biphenol in the presence of 0.5 gram of sodium hydroxide, reacting the ingredients at 110° to 120°C for 3 hours, and vacuum stripping the mixture to 170°C on the water pump.

Next, the tridecyl alcohol was added, and the mixture again heated to 110° to 120°C for 3 hours, and then vacuum stripped to 170°C at the water pump. The combined distillate gave 89% of the calculated quantity of phenol at the first stage, and 98% at the second stage. The reaction product was tetra-tridecyl(4,4'-n-butylidenebis(2-tert-butyl-5-methyl-phenyl)diphosphite. $D_{25} = 0.931$, $n_D^{25} = 1.4910$, 4.48% trivalent phosphorus. In addition to the stabilization of PVC resins, these phosphates are useful in polyolefins as shown below.

Example 3: A stabilized polypropylene composition was prepared using as the stabilizer the phosphite of Example 2, together with a metal salt, zinc 2-ethyl hexoate. The phosphite, phenol and metal salt were blended together to yield a stabilizer composed of 375 parts by weight tetra-tridecyl-4,4'-n-butylidenebis(2-tert-butyl-5-methylphenyl)diphosphite and 125 parts by weight zinc 2-ethylhexoate.

The stabilizer blend was dispersed by hand-stirring in powdered, previously unstabilized polypropylene (Profax 6501, reduced specific viscosity (RSV) 3.0, melt index 0.4, ASTM D 1238-57T at 190°C) in an amount of 0.5% stabilizer by weight of the resin. The mixture was placed on a 2 roll mill and fluxed for 5 minutes at 170°±2°C. Pieces cut from the milled sheet were used in the standard test described below. The standard sample used in testing was 200 grams, except for the Brabender Plastograph, which was 35 grams. The stabilizers were incorporated as described in the working example and milled to a sheet.

Small squares cut from a milled sheet are exposed in a forced-draft air oven at 205°C lying flat on aluminum foil. Samples are removed at 15 minute intervals and examined for loss of shape, flow-out, or melting, which constitute failure. The time to failure was 2 hours and the sample became light gray in color.

HINDERED PHENOLIC ESTERS FROM UNSATURATED QUINONE ESTERS

Kleiner of Ciba-Geigy laboratories has a series of patents disclosing the use of hindered phenolic esters as antioxidants for synthetic polymers. Although designated as primarily for use in polyolefins such as polyethylene and polypropylene they are also stated to be useful in polystyrene, polyvinyl chloride, nylon and other polyamides, polyesters, cellulosics, poly-acetals, polyurethanes, petroleum and wood resins, mineral oils, animal and vegetable fats, waxes, rubbers such as styrene-butadiene rubber (SBR), acrylonitrile-butadiene-styrene rubber (ABS), olefin-copolymers, ethylene-vinyl-acetate copolymers, polycarbonates, polyacrylonitrile, poly(4-methylpentene-1) polymers, polyoxymethylenes, and the like.

The tests conducted on the materials listed in the following table were conducted in a tubular oven with an airflow of 400' per minute at an oven temperature of 150°C. The oven ageing is set out in hours. In preparing the sample for testing, unstabilized polypropylene powder is blended with the indicated antioxidant, and then milled on a two-roller mill at 182°C for six minutes after which the stabilized polypropylene is sheeted from the mill and allowed to cool. The milled sheet is then cut into small pieces and pressed for 7 minutes on a hydraulic press at 218°C and 174 psi pressure. The resultant sheet of 25 mil thickness is then tested for re-sistance to accelerated ageing in the above described tubular oven.

Esters of Thiosuccinic Acids

In the first process, *E.K. Kleiner; U.S. Patents 3,743,623; July 3, 1973; and 3,637,809; January 25, 1972; both assigned to Ciba-Geigy Corporation* has disclosed the compounds of the following formulas:

$$(1) \quad S\!\!\begin{bmatrix} R_1 & R_3 \\ | & | \\ C-CH \\ | & | \\ R_2 & COOR \end{bmatrix}_2 \qquad (2) \quad R_4-S-\begin{matrix} R_1 & R_3 \\ | & | \\ C-CH \\ | & | \\ R_2 & COOR \end{matrix} \qquad (3) \quad \begin{matrix} R_3 & R_1 \\ | & | \\ CH-C-S-R_5-S- \\ | & | \\ COOR & R_2 \end{matrix}\begin{matrix} R_1' & R_3' \\ | & | \\ C-CH \\ | & | \\ R_2' & COOR \end{matrix}$$

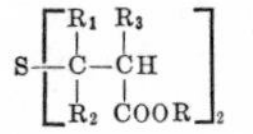

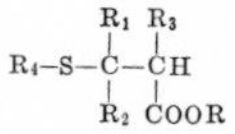

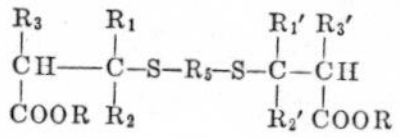

where R is

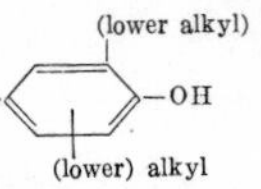

R_1, R_2, R_3, R_1', R_2', R_3' are each —H, lower alkyl, phenyl, aralkyl or —$C_m H_{2m}$COOR, where m is 0 to 6 (preferably 0 or 1) R_4 is —$C_n H_{2n+1}$ where n is 1 to 24 (preferably 8 to 18 or mix-tures thereof), cyclohexyl, phenyl, aralkyl, or —$(CH_2)_y$—COO-alkyl, -phenyl or -aralkyl, where y is 1 or 2. R_5 is —$C_n H_{2n}$— where n is 2 to 12, —$CH_2 CH_2 OCH_2 CH_2$—, —$CH_2 CH_2$—S—$CH_2 CH_2$—

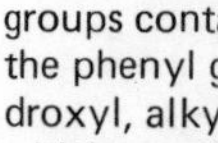

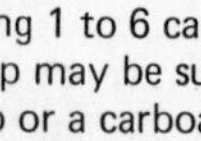

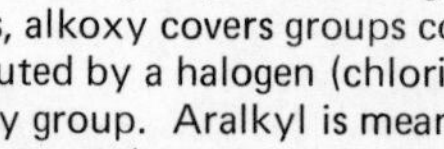

or

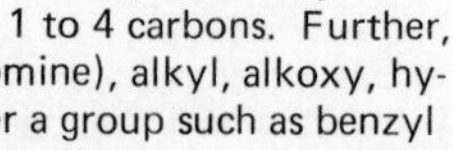

with the proviso that in compounds of Formulas (1) and (2), at least one R_1, R_2 or R_3 must be —$C_m H_{2m}$COOR and in compounds of Formula (3), at least one R_1, R_2, R_3, R_1', R_2' or R_3' must be —$C_m H_{2m}$COOR, where R_1, R_2, R_3, R_1', R_2', R_3', R and m are as defined above.

As used herein, alkyl is meant to cover groups containing 1 to 24 carbons; lower alkyl covers groups containing 1 to 6 carbons, alkoxy covers groups containing 1 to 4 carbons. Further, the phenyl group may be substituted by a halogen (chlorine or bromine), alkyl, alkoxy, hy-droxyl, alkythio or a carboalkoxy group. Aralkyl is meant to cover a group such as benzyl which may be substituted by a halogen (chlorine or bromine), alkyl, alkoxy, hydroxy, alkyl-thio or a carboalkoxy group. These antioxidants are addition products of (a) and α,β-unsat-urated ester of a hindered hydroquinone of the formula:

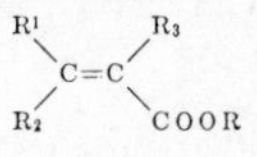

and (b) hydrogen sulfide or a mercaptan of the formula R_4—SH or HS—R_5—SH, where R, R_1, R_2, R_3, R_4, and R_5 are as described above.

The addition of hydrogen sulfide or a mercaptan with the α,β-unsaturated ester is effected in the presence of catalytic amounts (0.01 to 2%) of a base at temperatures varying from room temperature up to an elevated temperature. The preferred bases are alkoxides such as sodium or potassium methoxide or sodium or potassium ethoxide, piperidine, pyridine or benzyltrimethylammonium hydroxide. It is also possible to catalyze the addition by use of a free-radical initiator such as an azo compound, an azonitrile compound or an aliphatic peroxide.

One procedure which is used in preparing antioxidants represented by Formulas (2) and (3) (symmetrical only), method (a), involves dissolving equimolar amounts of the α,β-unsaturated ester and mercaptan in a solvent such as benzene or chloroform together with 1% by weight (based on the ester and mercaptan) of a 35% (by weight) solution of benzyltrimethylammonium hydroxide in methanol. The reaction is exothermic and cooling may be necessary.

After standing several hours at room temperature (or heating to a temperature between 60° and 80°C for 20 to 60 minutes), the base is neutralized with an equivalent of acetic acid. After evaporation of the solvent, the product is either distilled or crystallized. The yields in all cases are excellent that is, in excess of 90%.

A second procedure which can be used to prepare unsymmetrical antioxidants represented by Formula (3) involves adding, to a solution of 5 to 10 mols of a dimercaptan of the formula HS—R_5—SH, in chloroform and 1% benzyltrimethylammonium hydroxide (in a 35% solution in methanol) a solution of 1 mol of the α,β-unsaturated ester of a hindered hydroquinone in chloroform. After standing for several hours at room temperature, the base is neutralized with acetic acid. The solvent and excess dimercaptan are distilled off and the crude intermediate is recrystallized. The addition of the second α,β-unsaturated ester of a hindered hydroquinone is carried out as described under method (a).

The methods (a) and (b) are preferred for synthesizing the antioxidants. However, it is also possible to add first the mercaptan or hydrogen sulfide to the α,β-unsaturated acid followed by esterifying the intermediate with the hindered hydroquinone. This procedure is preferred for preparing antioxidants of the formula:

$$R_4-S-\underset{\underset{R_2}{|}}{\overset{\overset{R^1}{|}}{C}}-\underset{\underset{COOR}{|}}{\overset{\overset{R_3}{|}}{CH}}$$

where R_4 is —$(CH_2)_y$—COOR, y is 1 or 2 and R, R_1, R_2 and R_3 are as defined above. The products which can be prepared by these methods and test results are illustrated in the following tables where R_O = 3,5-di-tert-butyl-4-hydroxyphenyl.

Product	Structural formula	Name of product
A	$C_8H_{17}SCHCOOR_0$ $\quad\mid$ CH_2COOR_0	Bis(3,5-di-tert-butyl-4-hydroxyphenyl)-2-(n-octylthio) succinate.
B	$C_8H_{17}SCH_2CHCOOR_0$ $\quad\mid$ CH_2COOR_0	Bis(3,5-di-tert-butyl-4-hydroxyphenyl)-2-(n-octylthio-methyl)succinate.
C	$C_6H_5(CH_2)_3SCH_2CHCOOR_0$ $\quad\mid$ CH_2COOR_0	Bis(3,5-di-tert-butyl-4-hydroxyphenyl)-2-(3-phenyl-n-propylthiomethyl)succinate.
D	$C_{12}H_{25}SCHCOOR_0$ $\quad\mid$ CH_2COOR_0	Bis(3,5-di-tert-butyl-4-hydroxyphenyl)-2-(n-dodecylthio) succinate.
E	$C_{18}H_{37}SCHCOOR_0$ $\quad\mid$ CH_2COOR_0	Bis(3,5-di-tert-butyl-4-hydroxyphenyl)-2-n-octadecylthio) succinate.
F	$R_0OCOCH_2CH_2SCH_2CH_2SCHCOOR_0$ $\quad\mid$ CH_2COOR_0	Bis(3,5-di-tert-butyl-4-hydroxyphenyl)-2-(3,5-di-tert-butyl-4-hydroxyphenoxycarbonylethylthioethylthio)succinate.

(continued)

Product	Structural formula	Name of product
G.........	$R_9OCOCH_2CH_2SCH_2CH_2SCH_2CHCOOR_9$ $\quad\quad\quad\quad\quad\quad\quad\quad\quad\quad CH_2COOR_9$	Bis(3,5-di-tert-butyl-4-hydroxyphenyl)-2-(3,5-ditert-butyl-4-hydroxyphenoxycarbonylethylthioethylthiomethyl) succinate.
H.........	$\begin{bmatrix} R_9OCOCHCH_2SCH_2 \\ R_9OCOCH_2 \end{bmatrix}_2$	Tetrakis(3,5-di-tert-butyl-4-hydroxyphenyl)-2,2'-(ethylenebisthio disuccinate.
I.........	$\begin{bmatrix} R_9OCOCHCH_2SCH_2CH_2 \\ R_9OCOCH_2 \end{bmatrix}_2$	Tetrakis(3,5-di-tert-butyl-4-hydroxyphenyl)-2,2'-[tetramethylene-bis(thiomethyl)]disuccinate.
J.........	$\begin{bmatrix} R_9OCOCHS(CH_2)_4 \\ R_9OCOCH_2 \end{bmatrix}_2$	Tetrakis(3,5-di-tert-butyl-4-hydroxyphenyl)-2,2'-(octamethylenebisthio)disuccinate.
K.........	$\begin{bmatrix} R_9OCOCHCH_2S(CH_2)_4 \\ R_9OCOCH_2 \end{bmatrix}_2$	Tetrakis(3,5-di-tert-butyl-4-hydroxyphenyl)-2,2'-[octamethylenebis(thiomethyl)]disuccinate.
L.........	$\begin{bmatrix} R_9OCOCHSCH_2CH_2 \\ R_9OCOCH_2 \end{bmatrix}_2 O$	Tetrakis(3,5-di-tert-butyl-4-hydroxyphenyl)-2,2'-[oxybis(ethylthio)]disuccinate.
M.........	$\begin{bmatrix} R_9OCOCHSCH_2CH_2 \\ R_9OCOCH_2 \end{bmatrix}_2 S$	Tetrakis(3,5-di-tert-butyl-4-hydroxyphenyl)-2,2'-[thiobis(ethylthio)]disuccinate.
N.........	$\begin{bmatrix} R_9OCOCHCH_2SCH_2 \\ R_9OCOCH_2 \end{bmatrix}_2 S$	Tetrakis(3,5-di-tert-butyl-4-hydroxyphenyl)-2,2'-[thiobis(ethylthiomethyl)]disuccinate.

Evaluation Antioxidants in Polypropylene (25 mil), Tubular Oven, 150°C

	Hours to fail	
Product	0.25% anti-oxidant	0.1% anti-oxidant plus 0.3% DSTDP*
A..................	1,100	1,370
B..................	1,125	1,315
C..................	945	1,070
D..................	1,430	1,770
E..................	1,820	2,100
F..................	1,000	1,500
G..................	820	1,480
H..................	660	1,340
I..................	430	1,000
J..................	840	1,460
K..................	520	1,000
L..................	780	1,590
M..................	780	1,590
N..................	820	1,440

*DSTDP is distearylthiodipropionate
(a synergist for antioxidants)

Besides activity in the Oven Aging Test, these antioxidants are characterized by excellent color values (no discoloration during the Oven Aging Test) and good gas fading properties.

Esters of Cyclic Aminocarboxylic Acids

E. Kleiner; U.S. Patent 3,681,358; August 1, 1972; assigned to Ciba-Geigy Corporation has also developed the following esters of heterocyclic aminocarboxylates.

$$(1) \quad A{>}N{-}\underset{\underset{R_2}{|}}{\overset{\overset{R_1}{|}}{C}}{-}\underset{\underset{COOR}{|}}{\overset{\overset{R_3}{|}}{CH}} \quad \text{and} \quad (2) \quad \underset{\underset{COOR}{|}}{\overset{\overset{R_3}{|}}{CH}}{-}\underset{\underset{R_2}{|}}{\overset{\overset{R_1}{|}}{C}}{-}N{<}B{>}N{-}\underset{\underset{R_2}{|}}{\overset{\overset{R_1}{|}}{C}}{-}\underset{\underset{COOR}{|}}{\overset{\overset{R_3}{|}}{CH}}$$

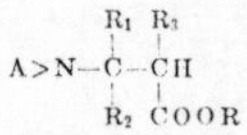

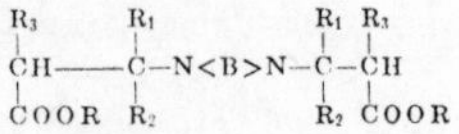

where R is

(lower) alkyl
—⟨benzene ring⟩—OH
(lower) alkyl

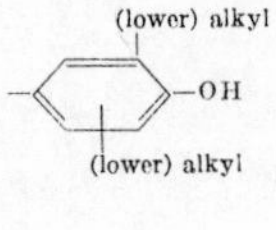

R_1, R_2 and R_3 are each —H, lower alkyl, phenyl, aralkyl or —C_mH_{2m}COOR, where m is 0 to 6 and preferably 0 to 1 and aralkyl has up to 24 carbons and preferably up to twelve carbons.

A>N— is a radical derived from a heterocyclic amine having one replaceable amine hydrogen selected from ethyleneimine, trimethyleneimine, pyrrolidines, piperidines, morpholines, thiomorpholines, 1,2,3,4-tetrahydroquinolines, indolines, isoindolines, carbazoles, N-alkylpiperazines, N-arylpiperazines and N-aralkylpiperazines, the alkyl, aryl and aralkyl groups having up to 12 carbons.

—N<B>N— is a radical derived from a heterocyclic amine having two replaceable amine hydrogens selected from piperazines and 4,4'-polymethylenedipiperidines.

The heterocyclic secondary amines may be substituted by a halogen, alkyl, aryl, aralkyl, alkoxy, hydroxyl, alkylthio or carboalkoxy group or be part of an aliphatic or aromatic ring system. From the above it should be apparent that any heterocyclic secondary amine may be used in preparing these antioxidants. The substituents on the heterocyclic rings are of no substantial consequence as long as they do not interfere with the reaction. The presence of tertiary amines either in the ring or outside similarly do not affect the reaction.

These antioxidants are addition products of (a) an α,β-unsaturated ester of a hindered hydroquinone of the formula:

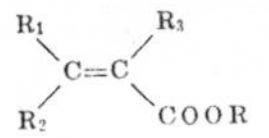

$$R_1\diagdown \quad \diagup R_3$$
$$C=C$$
$$R_2\diagup \quad \diagdown COOR$$

and (b) heterocyclic secondary amines of the formula A>NH and HN<B>NH, where R, R_1, R_2, R_3 and A<N— and —N<B>N— are as defined above. These antioxidants were prepared by the following general procedure.

Equimolar amounts of the α,β-unsaturated ester and the amine were dissolved in five times the amount of chloroform, sealed in an ampule under nitrogen and heated for 8 hours in an oil bath at 80°C. The reaction mixture was then filtered through five times the amount of neutral aluminum oxide and the crude reaction product was purified by crystallization as indicated in Table 1. Yields are generally high, i.e., above 75%.

Nonheterocyclic primary and secondary amines can also be added to the α,β-unsaturated esters to provide antioxidants. However, heterocyclic secondary amines are preferred because higher yields are obtained and amide formation is less favored. Antioxidants prepared by this process and their test results in polypropylene are shown in the following tables, where R_0 is

$$C(CH_3)_3$$
—OH
$$C(CH_3)_3$$

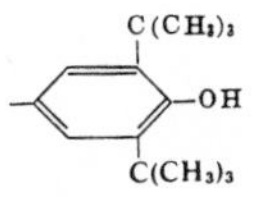

TABLE 1: ANTIOXIDANTS

Product
A .... 3,5-di-tert-butyl-4-hydroxyphenyl 3-[2-(1,2,3,4-tetrahydroisoquinolyl]propionate.

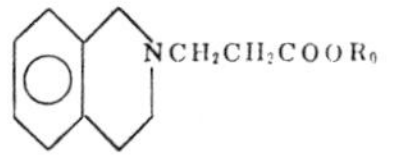

NCH₂CH₂COOR₀

(continued)

TABLE 1: (continued)

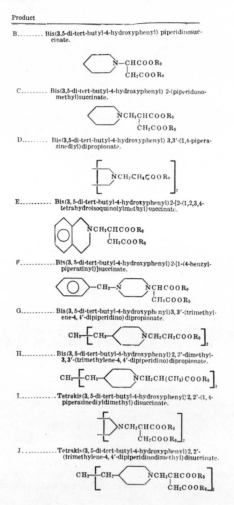

Product

B......... Bis(3,5-di-tert-butyl-4-hydroxyphenyl) piperidinosuc-
cinate.

C......... Bis(3,5-di-tert-butyl-4-hydroxyphenyl) 2-(piperidono-
methyl)succinate.

D......... Bis(3,5-di-tert-butyl-4-hydroxyphenyl) 3,3'-(1,4-pipera-
zinediyl)dipropionate.

E.......... Bis(3,5-di-tert-butyl-4-hydroxyphenyl) 2-[2-(1,2,3,4-
tetrahydroisoquinolylmethyl)succinate.

F.......... Bis(3,5-di-tert-butyl-4-hydroxyphenyl) 2-[1-(4-benzyl-
piperazinyl)]succinate.

G.......... Bis(3,5-di-tert-butyl-4-hydroxyphenyl)3,3'-(trimethyl-
ene-4,4'-dipiperidino)dipropionate.

H.......... Bis(3,5-di-tert-butyl-4-hydroxyphenyl)2,2'-dimethyl-
3,3'-(trimethylene-4,4'-dipiperidino)dipropionate.

I.......... Tetrakis(3,5-di-tert-butyl-4-hydroxyphenyl)2,2'-(1,4-
piperazinediyldimethyl)disuccinate.

J.......... Tetrakis(3,5-di-tert-butyl-4-hydroxyphenyl)2,2'-
(trimethylene-4,4'-dipiperidinodimethyl)disuccinate.

TABLE 2: EVALUATION OF ANTIOXIDANTS IN POLYPROPYLENE (25 MIL), TUBULAR OVEN, 150°C

	Hours to Fail	
Product	0.25% Antioxidant 0.5% UV−2*	0.1% Antioxidant 0.5% UV−2* 0.3% DSTDP**
A	< 20	70
B	160	540
C	40	150
D	60	260
E	140	520
F	300	600
I	70	350
J	80	300

*UV−2: An ultraviolet absorber, 2-(3',5'-di-tert-
butyl-2'hydroxyphenyl)-5-chlorobenzotriazole
**DSTDP: Distearylthiodipropionate

Esters of Thiocarboxylic Acids

A third series of antioxidants disclosed by *E.K. Kleiner; U.S. Patent 3,636,033; January 18, 1972; assigned to Geigy Chemical Corporation* are obtained by reacting (a) an α,β-unsaturated ester of a hindered hydroquinone and (b) a thio acid. These antioxidants are represented by the following formulas:

$$(1) \quad R^4 COS-\underset{\underset{R^2}{|}}{\overset{\overset{R^1}{|}}{C}}-\underset{\underset{COOR}{|}}{\overset{\overset{R^3}{|}}{CH}} \qquad\qquad (2) \quad R^5\left[-COS-\underset{\underset{R^2}{|}}{\overset{\overset{R^1}{|}}{C}}-\underset{\underset{COOR}{|}}{\overset{\overset{R^3}{|}}{CH}}\right]_2$$

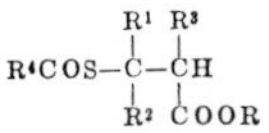

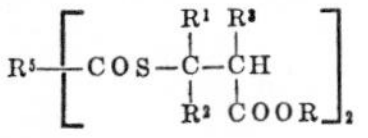

where —R is

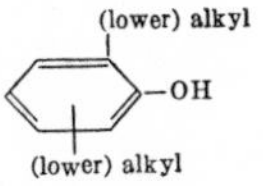

$-R^1$, $-R^2$, $-R^3$ are each hydrogen, lower alkyl, aryl, aralkyl or $-C_m H_{2m}COOR$, where m is 0 to 6, $-R^4$ is straight or branched alkyl, aryl, aralkyl or R and $-R^5$ is $-C_n H_{2n}$ where n is 0 to 12 or $-C_6H_4-$(ortho, meta or para phenylene).

As used here, alkyl covers straight, branched and cyclic alkyl groups having from 1 to 24 carbons and preferably to 12 carbons; lower alkyl covers groups containing from 1 to 6 carbons. These antioxidants were prepared by using the following procedure.

Equimolar amounts of the α,β-unsaturated ester of the hindered hydroquinone and the thio acid were dissolved in three times the amount of chloroform and sealed in a reaction vessel under nitrogen. The vessel is kept from 12 to 24 hours at 80°C depending on the degree of conversion which was checked by thin layer chromatography. After completion of the reaction, the solvent is evaporated and the crude product is purified by recrystallization from hexane, heptane or benzene, and identified by infrared spectroscopy, nuclear magnetic resonance and elemental analysis. Yields are high, that is, higher than 75%.

A thio acid of the formula R^4COSH or $HSCO-R^5-COSH$, where R, R^1, R^2, R^3, R^4 and R^5 are as described above is used in the process. Instead of the free thio acids, their salts, such as the sodium or potassium salts can also be used.

In Tables 2 and 3 are reported the results of the Oven Aging Tests in which the antioxidants (Table 1) of this process were added to polypropylene together with the indicated ultraviolet light absorber and the synergist. R_o is as defined on page 255.

TABLE 1: ANTIOXIDANTS

Product	
3,5-di-tert-butyl-4-hydroxyphenyl 3-(acetylthio)propionate. $R_6OCOCH_2CH_2SCOCH_3$	(A)
3,5-di-tert-butyl-4-hydroxyphenyl 3-(diphenylacetylthio)propionate. $R_6OCOCH_2CH_2SCOCH(C_6H_5)_2$	(B)
Bis(3,5-di-tert-butyl-4-hydroxyphenyl) 2-(acetylthio)succinate. $R_6OCOCHSCOCH_3$ R_6OCOCH_2	(C)
Bis(3,5-di-tert-butyl-4-hydroxyphenyl) 2-(propionylthio)succinate. $R_6OCOCHSCOCH_2CH_3$ R_6OCOCH_2	(D)

(continued)

TABLE 1: (continued)

Product	
Bis(3,5-di-tert-butyl-4-hydroxyphenyl) 2-(propionylthiomethyl)succinate. $R_6OCOCHCH_2SCOCH_2CH_3$ | R_6OCOCH_2	(E)
Bis(3,5-di-tert-butyl-4-hydroxyphenyl) 2-(benzoylthio)succinate. $R_6OCOCHSCOC_6H_5$ | R_6OCOCH_2	(F)
Bis(3,5-di-tert-butyl-4-hydroxphenyl) 2-(benzoylthiomethyl)succinate. $R_6OCOCHCH_2SCOC_6H_5$ | R_6OCOCH_2	(G)
Bis(3,5-di-tert-butyl-4-hydroxyphenyl) 3,3'-(terephthaloylthio)dipropionate. 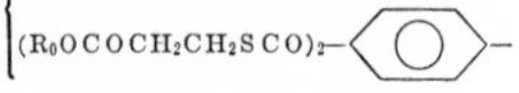	(H)
Bis(3,5-di-tert-butyl-4-hydroxyphenyl) 2-(diphenylacetylthio)succinate. $R_6OCOCHSCOCH(C_6H_5)_2$ | R_6OCOCH_2	(I)
Tetrakis(3,5-di-tert-butyl-4-hydroxyphenyl) 2,2'-(terephthaloylthio)-disuccinate. 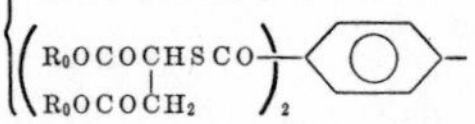	(J)
Tetrakis(3,5-di-tert-butyl-4-hydroxyphenyl) 2,2'-(terephthaloylthiomethyl)-disuccinate. 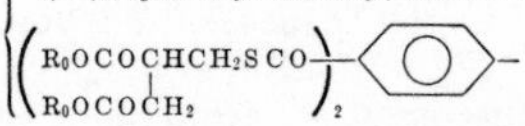	(K)

TABLE 2: EVALUATION OF ANTIOXIDANTS IN POLYPROPYLENE (25 MIL), TUBULAR OVEN, 150°C

	Hours to fail	
Product	0.25% antioxidant plus 0.5% UV-2	0.1% antioxidant plus 0.5% UV-2 [1] plus 0.3% DSTDP [2]
E	160	430
F	380	720

[1] UV-2, an ultraviolet absorber, 2-(3',5'-di-tert-butyl-2'-hydroxyphenyl)-5-chlorobenzotriazole.
[2] DSTDP=distearylthiodipropionate, commercial synergist for antioxidants.
NOTE.—Unstabilized 3 hours.

TABLE 3: EVALUATION OF ANTIOXIDANTS IN POLYPROPYLENE (25 MIL), ROTARY OVEN, 150°C

	Hours to fail	
Product	0.25% antioxidant plus 0.5% UV-2	0.1% antioxidant plus 0.5% UV-2 plus 0.3% DSTDP
A	10	10
B	55	210
C	160	390
D	190	540
G	290	1,450
H	305	1,350
I	550	1,640
J	480	1,030
K	470	1,030

NOTE.—Unstabilized 2 hours.

Esters of Phosphinodithioic Acids and O,O-Diesters of Phosphorothiolothionic Acids

In the fourth series of compounds prepared by *E.K. Kleiner; U.S. Patent 3,639,538; February 1, 1972; assigned to Ciba-Geigy Corporation* an alpha, beta-unsaturated ester of a hindered hydroquinone is reacted with a phosphinodithioic acid or an O,O-diester of phosphorothiolothionic acid. Compounds are obtained which have the formula:

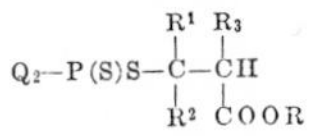

$$Q_2-P(S)S-\underset{\underset{R^3}{|}}{\overset{\overset{R^1}{|}}{C}}-\underset{\underset{COOR}{|}}{\overset{\overset{R_3}{|}}{CH}}$$

where $-Q$ is $-R^4$ or OR^4, $-R$ is

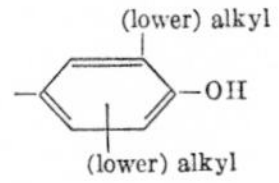

where the (lower)alkyl has from 1 to 6 carbons; $-R^1$, $-R^2$, $-R^3$ are each hydrogen, lower alkyl from 1 to 6 carbons, phenyl, benzyl or $-C_mH_{2m}COOR$, where m is 0 to 6; $-R^4$ is alkyl from 1 to 24 carbons, cycloalkyl from 1 to 6 carbons, phenyl and benzyl and when Q is $-OR^4$ and two $-R^4$ groups can be $-(CH_2)_n-$, where n is 2 or 3, forming a cyclic O,O-diester of phosphorothiolothionic acid.

The antioxidants were prepared by using the following general procedure. Equimolar amounts of the α,β-unsaturated ester and the phosphinodithioic acid or O,O-diester of a phosphorothiolothionic acid are dissolved in 2 to 3 times the amount of chloroform or benzene and sealed under nitrogen. The reaction vessel is kept at about 80°C for 12 to 20 hours until the conversion is complete as checked by thin layer chromatography. The reaction mixture is then washed with a saturated sodium bicarbonate solution and water, and then dried over sodium sulfate. Then the solvent is evaporated and the crude product purified either by distillation or by crystallization or by filtering the solution through neutral aluminum oxide. Yields are high, that is, generally over 80%.

In the reactions, one can use a phosphinodithioic acid or a O,O-diester of a phosphorothiolothionic acid of the formulas: $(R^4O)_2P(S)SH$ and $(R^4)_2P(S)SH$ respectively, where $-R$, $-R^1$, $-R^2$, $-R^3$, $-R^4$ are as defined above.

In Tables 2 and 3 are reported the results of the Oven Aging Tests in which antioxidants (Table 1) prepared by this process were added to polypropylene together with the indicated ultraviolet light absorber and the synergist. R_0 is as defined on page 255.

TABLE 1: ANTIOXIDANTS

	Product
(A)...	3,5-di-t-butyl-4-hydroxyphenyl 3-(diphenylphosphinothioyl-thio)propionate
	$R_9OCOCH_2CH_2S(S)P(C_6H_5)_2$
(B)...	Bis(3,5-di-t-butyl-4-hydroxyphenyl) 2-(diphenylphosphino-thioylthio)succinate
	$R_9OCOCHS(S)P(C_6H_5)_2$
	$\quad\;\;\vert$
	R_9OCOCH_2
(C)...	Bis(3,5-di-t-butyl-4-hydroxyphenyl) 2-(diphenylphosphino-thioylthiomethyl)succinate
	$R_9OCOCHCH_2S(S)P(C_6H_5)_2$
	$\quad\;\;\vert$
	R_9OCOCH_2
(D)...	3,5-di-t-butyl-4-hydroxyphenyl 2-methyl-3-(diethoxyphos-phinothioylthio)propionate
	$R_9OCOCH(CH_3)CH_2S(S)P(OC_2H_5)_2$

(continued)

TABLE 1: (continued)

Product
(E)... Bis(3,5-di-t-butyl-4-hydroxyphenyl) 2-(diethoxyphosphino-thioylthio)succinate

$$R_9OCOCHS(S)P(OC_2H_5)_2$$
$$|$$
$$R_9OCOCH_2$$

| (F)... Bis(3,5-di-t-butyl-4-hydroxyphenyl) 2-(diethoxyphosphino-thioylthiomethyl)succinate |

$$R_9OCOCHCH_2S(S)P(OC_2H_5)_2$$
$$|$$
$$R_9OCOCH_2$$

TABLE 2: EVALUATION OF ANTIOXIDANTS IN POLYPROPYLENE (25 MIL), ROTARY OVEN, 150°C

	Hours to fail	
	0.25% anti-oxidant plus 0.5% UV-2 [1]	0.1% anti-oxidant plus 0.5% UV-2 plus 0.3/ DSTDP [2]
Product:		
A	235	470
B	530	980
C	610	1,130

[1] UV-2, an ultraviolet absorber, 2-(3',5'-di-tert-butyl-2'-hydroxy-phenyl)-5-chlorobenzotriazole.
[2] DSTDP=Distearylthiodipropionate, commercial synergist for anti-oxidants.

TABLE 3: EVALUATION OF ANTIOXIDANTS IN POLYPROPYLENE (25 MIL), TUBULAR OVEN, 150°C

	Hours to fail	
	0.25% anti-oxidant plus 0.5% UV-2	0.1% anti-oxidant plus 0.5% UV-2 plus 0.3%/ DSTDP
Product:		
D	20	20
E	320	380
F	270	270

MIXED OR SYNERGISTIC STABILIZING SYSTEMS

Amineborates with Ketone- or Aldehydephenols

Synergistic stabilizer mixtures of (1) a borate of N,N-dihydrocarbyl-alkanolamine or borate of polyalkyl- or polycycloalkylpolyhydroxyalkyl-alkylenepolyamine and (2) a reaction product of a phenol and ketone or aldehyde are disclosed by *A.K. Sparks and J.J. Louvar; U.S. Patent 3,694,374; September 26, 1972.*

The borate may be illustrated as a borate of an alkanolamine of the following formula:

$$R-N-(R'-N-)_m(R'-N-)_nR''-O-H$$
$$|\qquad |\qquad |$$
$$X\qquad Y\qquad Z$$

where R is hydrocarbyl, R' is alkylene, R" is alkylene, X is hydrocarbyl when m and n are zero or hydroxyalkyl when m is one or more and/or n is one, Y is hydrocarbyl when m is one and n is zero or hydroxyalkyl when m is more than one and n is one, Z is hydrocarbyl, m is an integer of zero to four and n is zero or one.

In a preferred embodiment the alkyl groups attached to the terminal nitrogen atoms are secondary alkyl groups. In another embodiment, these groups may be cycloalkyl groups and particularly cyclohexyl, alkylcyclohexyl, dialkylcyclohexyl, etc., although they may comprise cyclobutyl, cyclopentyl, cycloheptyl, cyclooctyl, etc., and alkyl derivatives thereof. The cycloalkyl groups may be considered as corresponding to secondary alkyl groups. The secondary alkyl configuration is definitely preferred although, when desired, the alkyl groups attached to the terminal nitrogen atoms may be normal alkyl groups but not necessarily with equivalent results.

The borate for use in this process is prepared in any suitable manner and generally by reacting the alkanolamine or polyalkylpolyhydroxyalkylalkylenepolyamine with a suitable borylating agent including boric acid, boric anhydride, mono-, di- or trialkylborate, phenyl or cycloalkyl borate, etc., in the presence of a solvent at a temperature of from 60° to 100°C or up to about 200°C.

The second component of the synergistic mixture is the reaction product of a phenol and ketone or aldehyde. While phenol may be used as the reactant in a preferred embodiment an alkylphenol is used. Nonylphenol is particularly preferred. Other alkylphenols contain from 1 to 30 and preferably 3 to 15 carbons in the alkyl group. In still another embodiment a dialkylphenol is used as a reactant and each alkyl group may contain from 1 to 30 carbons.

The reaction of the phenol and ketone or aldehyde is effected in any suitable manner. In one method, the reaction is effected in the presence of a strong acid such as hydrochloric acid or dry HCl gas. This reaction is well-known and need not be described here in detail.

The reaction products generally comprise a mixture of products including alkylidene-bis-(alkylphenols) and hydroxyphenyl chromans. The hydroxyphenyl chromans generally will be either the 2-(2'-hydroxyphenyl) chromans or the 4-(2'-hydroxyphenyl) chromans, and will contain whatever alkyl substituents are originally attached to the phenol reactant.

Example 1: The synergistic mixture of this example comprises approximately 72% by wt. of the borate of N,N-dicyclohexyl-ethanolamine and 23% by weight of the reaction product of nonylphenol and acetone. The borate of N,N-dicyclohexyl-ethanolamine was prepared by the reaction of 3 mol proportions of N,N-dicyclohexyl-ethanolamine and one mol proportion of boric acid. In a specific preparation, 68.4 grams (0.3 mol) of N,N-dicyclohexyl-ethanolamine and 6.18 grams (0.1 mol) of boric acid are refluxed in the presence of 100 grams of benzene at 85°C. Heating and refluxing are continued until about 5 cc of water is collected.

Following completion of the reaction, the benzene is removed by vacuum distillation at a temperature of about 170°C at 0.4 mm/Hg. The borate is recovered as a liquid having a basic nitrogen content of 4.29 meq/g, an acid value of 0.008 meq/g and a boron content of 1.42% by weight. This corresponds to the theoretical boron content of 1.58% by weight for the compound tris-(N,N-dicyclohexyl-ethoxy) borate.

The reaction product of alkylphenol and acetone is prepared by the general steps of condensing a technical nonylphenol with acetone by saturating the mixture with anhydrous hydrogen chloride at 60°C and holding at this temperature for 70 hours. Technical nonylphenol comprises a mixture of alkylphenols containing approximately 18% octyl, 67% nonyl, 13% decyl and small amounts of other alkylphenols in which the alkyl radical contains more than 10 carbons. The alkyl substituents are primarily in the para position and comprise straight and branched chain alkyl groups. Following completion of the reaction the reaction mixture is distilled. The distilled reaction product contains 34% of 2,2'-isopropylidene-bis-(4-nonylphenol) and about 23% of 2-(2'-hydroxyphenyl)-2,4,4-trimethyl-5',6-dinonyl-chroman.

Example 2: This example reports the results of evaluations made in a commercial solid polypropylene which was free of inhibitors. Samples of the polypropylene, with and without additive, were pressed into sheets, and dumbbell specimens were cut from the sheets.

The specimens were thin tensiles of 5 to 7 mil thickness. As is well-known, these thin tensiles are more difficult to stabilize than the thicker tensiles used in other evaluations. The dumbbell specimens were mounted on boards and exposed to carbon arc rays at about 52°C in a Fade-O-Meter. The specimens were withdrawn periodically, removed from the board and the yield strength determined in an Instron Universal Tester. In the Instron Universal Tester the specimen is gripped firmly at the top and bottom. A constant pull of 2 inches per minute is exerted downwardly and the point at which the sample loses its resistance to permanent deformation is defined as the yield strength. In most cases, the yield strength is equivalent to the tensile strength which is the pounds per square inch force at which rupture occurs.

A control sample of the polypropylene (not containing the additive) had an initial yield strength of 4,480 psi which dropped to 1,260 psi after 72 hours and was brittle after 96 hours of exposure in the Fade-O-Meter. Another sample of the polypropylene was prepared to contain 0.35% by weight of the borate prepared as described in Example 1. This sample had an initial yield value of 5,056 psi and became brittle after 384 hours of exposure in the Fade-O-Meter.

Another sample of the polypropylene was prepared to contain 0.25% by weight of the borate prepared as described in Example 1 and 0.10% by weight of the reaction product of nonylphenol and acetone prepared as described in Example 1. It will be noted that the total concentration of additive is the same as used in the evaluations made with each component individually as described above. However, the sample containing the mixture of additives had an initial yield value of 4,582 psi but did not become brittle until 480 hours of exposure in the Fade-O-Meter. Examples were also included in the patent on the use of such mixtures in the stabilization of polyethylene, polystyrene and polyvinyl chloride.

Mixtures with Thioalkylcarboxylic Acid Compounds

Synergistic antioxidant mixtures have been developed by *I. Yamane, M. Nagayama and M. Takai; U.S. Patent 3,741,909; June 26, 1973; assigned to Lion Fat & Oil Co., Ltd., Japan* containing a compound expressed by formula:

$$\left(R-S-X-\overset{\overset{\displaystyle O}{\|}}{C}-O \right)_{a} \cdot M$$

where R represents hydrocarbon radical having 6 to 22 carbons, X represents a lower alkylene redical having 1 to 5 carbons, M represents nonalkali metal and n represents an integer ranging from 1 to 5.

The maximum efficiency of this antioxidant system can be displayed when the compound expressed by the foregoing general formula is combined with a phenol-type or amine-type antioxidant at the ratio of 15 to 85% (by weight) of the latter. This compound is synthesized through the following process. R is as defined above.

$$RCH{=\!=}CH_2 + HSCH_2COOH \xrightarrow[\text{50° to 70°C–1.5 hr}]{\text{irradiation of ultraviolet ray}} R-CH_2CH_2SCH_2COOH \longrightarrow$$

$$R-CH_2CH_2SCH_2COONa \longrightarrow (R-CH_2CH_2SCH_2COO)_2Ca$$

Typical compounds applicable as the phenol-type antioxidant include:

> p-hydroxyphenyl cyclohexane
> 2,6-di-tert-butyl-4-methylphenol
> 2,4,6-tri-tert-butylphenol
> 1,1'-methylene-bis-(4-hydroxy-2,5-tert-butylphenol)
> 2,2'-methylene-bis-(4-methyl-6-tert-butylphenol)
> 2,6'-(2-tert-butyl-4-methyl-6-methylphenol)-p-cresol
> 2,2'-thio-bis-(4-methyl-6-tert-butylphenol)

4,4'-thio-bis-(3-methyl-6-tert-butylphenol)
4,4'-butylidene-bis-(6-tert-butyl-3-methylphenol)
styrenated phenol
di-p-hydroxyphenyl cyclohexane
dicresyl propane

Typical amine-type antioxidants applicable include:

phenyl-α-naphthylamine
phenyl-β-naphthylamine
diphenylamine
N,N'-diphenyl-p-phenylene diamine
N,N'-di-β-naphthyl-p-phenylene diamine
N,N'-phenyl cyclohexyl-p-phenylene diamine
p-hydroxy diphenylamine
p-hydroxyphenyl-β-naphthylamine
2,2',4-trimethyl dihydroquinoline

Example 1: Polypropylene pellets not containing any other antioxidant and the respective antioxidant shown in the following table were simultaneously extruded by an extruding machine to thereby knead them with each other so as to obtain pellets having overall concentration of 0.5% in terms of antioxidant, and then these pellets were subjected to injection molding to form into 2 mm thick plate.

This plate was placed on a glass plate put in a thermostat having a temperature of 120°±3°C and left standing for 150 hours. Subsequently, the plate was pelletized again by cutting with a cutting machine, and the melt index was measured of the resulting pellets in accordance with ASTM.

Besides, the surface condition and the degree of coloring of the pellets were also judged through observation with the naked eye. The composition under this process proved stable against heat. The results were as shown in the following table.

Antioxidant Under this Process (A)	Known antioxidant (B)	Ratio of A/B	After heating at 120° C. for 150 hrs.		
			Melt index	Surface condition	Coloring.
$(C_{16}H_{33}SCH_2COO)_2Mg$	2,6-di-t-butyl-p-cresol.	100/0	3.62	Satisfactory	Almost none.
		75/25	4.11	____do	None.
		50/50	4.01	____do	Do.
		25/75	3.96	____do	Do.
		0/100	1.16	Luster was slightly lost.	Light yellow.
Comparative examples wherein the known antioxidants were employed					
$CH_2CH_2COOC_{12}H_{25}$ / S \ $CH_2CH_2COOC_{12}H_{25}$	2,6-di-t-butyl-p-cresol.	25/75	2.88	Luster was slightly lost.	Almost none.
$CH_2CH_2COOC_{12}H_{25}$ / S \ $CH_2CH_2COOC_{12}H_{25}$			1.00	Luster was lost.	Light yellow.

NOTE.—Antioxidant: overall concentration=0.5%.

Example 2: One kilogram of ABS resin and 10 grams each of various antioxidants were blended (simultaneously) with each other by means of Henshell mixer for 10 minutes, and the thus blended mixture was pelletized through kneading by an extruding machine. The pellets thus prepared were further subjected to extrusion molding at 220°C to form into 1 mm thick plate.

Upon heating this plate at 120°C to expedite deterioration thereof, the resulting fragility was measured to observe the effect of the stabilizer. Besides, the degree of coloring and the surface condition of the respective plate subsequent to heating 120°C for 150 hours were also judged through observation with the naked eye. The antioxidant of this process displayed satisfactory performances. Examples are also included in the complete patent on the stabilization of polyethylene, and lubricating oil.

Cycloaliphatic Sulfide Synergists

It is customary to stabilize polyolefins, particularly polypropylene, against oxidative degradation by incorporating in the polyolefins a small amount of a phenolic primary antioxidant and a sulfur-containing secondary antioxidant or synergist. The sulfide synergists now used almost exclusively are dilauryl thiodipropionate (DLTDP) or distearyl thiodipropionate (DSTDP). These DLTDP and DSTDP suffer from the fact that they are gradually leached out of polyolefins by hot water, particularly hot water containing soap or detergents. This gradual loss of stabilizer results in premature deterioration (embrittlement and cracking) of polyolefins when they are used for hot water pipe and tubing applications and as components in automatic laundry and dish washers, vaporizers and other hot water equipment.

B. Buchholz; U.S. Patent 3,652,680; March 28, 1972; assigned to Pennwalt Corporation has found that cycloalkanebis(alkyl sulfide) compounds of structure

(1) 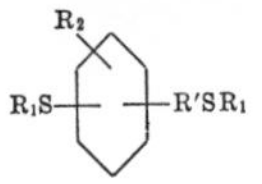 R_1S—⬡—$R'SR_1$ (with R_2 substituent)   and   (2) 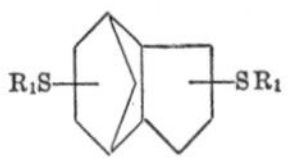 R_1S—⬡—SR_1

where R_1 is higher alkyl, R_2 is H or lower alkyl and R' is lower alkylene, exhibit high activity as antioxidant synergists. They are superior to the thiodipropionates in resistance to hot water leaching and have excellent compatibility with polyolefins. These sulfides are readily prepared from commercially available cyclic diolefins, H_2S and higher molecular weight monoolefins as illustrated by the following three equations:

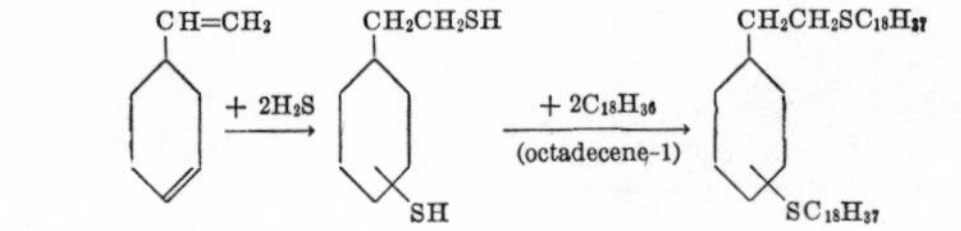

(vinylcyclohexene) + 2H_2S → SH derivative + 2$C_{18}H_{36}$ (octadecene-1) → 1-[β-(octadecylthio)ethyl]-3 (or 4)-(octadecylthio)cyclohexane

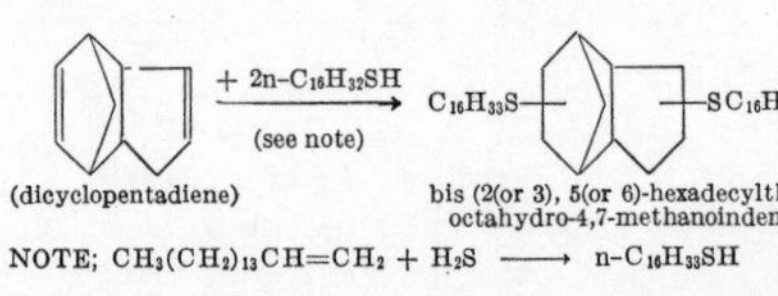

(dipentene or d-limonene) + 2n-$C_{16}H_{33}$SH (see note) → 2,9-bis(hexadecylthio)-p-menthane

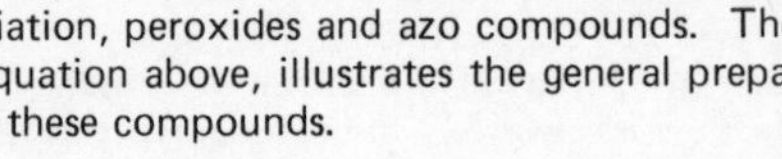

(dicyclopentadiene) + 2n-$C_{16}H_{33}$SH (see note) → bis (2(or 3), 5(or 6)-hexadecylthio)-octahydro-4,7-methanoindene

NOTE; $CH_3(CH_2)_{13}CH=CH_2 + H_2S \longrightarrow$ n-$C_{16}H_{33}$SH

All the above reactions occur in the presence of conventional free radical catalysts such as ultraviolet light, gamma radiation, peroxides and azo compounds. The following example, corresponding to the first equation above, illustrates the general preparative procedure which can be used to make these compounds.

Example 1: The liquid phase reaction of 4-vinylcyclohexene-1 is carried out with excess

H_2S in the presence of ultraviolet light from 15 watt germicidal lamps to produce vinyl-cyclohexane dimercaptan (β-mercaptoethyl-3 (or 4)-mercaptocyclohexane), 97° to 99°C per 1.25 mm in high yield. A solution containing 13 g (0.073 mol) of vinylcyclohexane di-mercaptan and 37 g (0.146 mol) of octadecene-1 in 300 cc of methyl propyl ketone is maintained at about 5°C while irradiating at 47.5 watts with a Nester/Faust ultraviolet lamp for 5 hr. Filtration of the precipitated solid gives 25 g (50%) of the desired product, MP 67° to 69.5°C. Recrystallization from methyl ethyl ketone gives a soft waxy white crystalline product, MP 71° to 72°C.

Example 2: The compounds were evaluated as antioxidant synergists in polypropylene. The polypropylene test samples were prepared by dry blending 0.1% by weight of a com-mercial phenolic primary antioxidant and 0.1 or 0.25% by weight of the synergist into un-stabilized polypropylene (Hercules' Profax 6501 flake), extruding into ⅛" rods, pelletizing, and hot pressing at 200° to 225°C into 10 mil thick sheets. Unless otherwise specified, all alkyl groups corresponding to R_1 are straight chain alkyl. The synergists were compared with control samples containing DSTDP in standard Oven Aging Tests, i.e., the average hours to embrittlement of 10 mil samples in a 140°C air-circulating oven were determined.

Primary antioxidant: 0.1% Irganox 1010

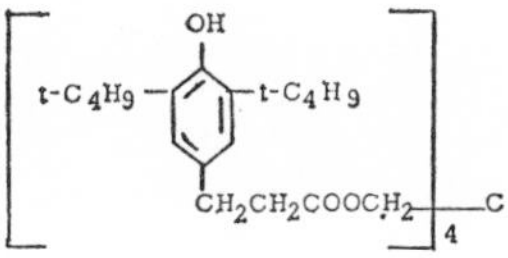

Synergist: 0.1%

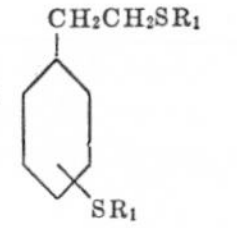

R_1	Average hours stabilization at 140° C.	Percent hours of DSTDP
n-$C_{16}H_{33}$	1,064	109
n-$C_{18}H_{37}$	1,139	117
n-$C_{20}H_{41}$	1,091	112
DSTDP (Control).....	976	....

Alkylated Phenol-Sulfur Compound Mixtures

P.R. Dean II; U.S. Patent 3,652,495; March 28, 1972; assigned to The Goodyear Tire & Rubber Company has disclosed a process for producing relatively saturated polymers pos-sessing resistance to oxidative degradation. These can be polyolefins and polystyrene con-taining very low amounts of a relatively nondiscoloring phenolic stabilizer and possessing adequate resistance to oxidative degradation.

These polymers are effectively stabilized by incorporating an alkylated reaction product where the product is formed by first reacting dicyclopentadiene with a phenol selected from phenol, p-cresol, o-cresol, mixed m,p-cresol and p-ethylphenol to form a phenolic compound, and then alkylating the phenolic compound with a tertiary olefin selected from isobutylene, tert-amylenes and tert-hexylenes, in combination with a sulfur-containing compound conforming to the formula:

$$R(S)_n\overset{\displaystyle R''}{\underset{\displaystyle |}{C}}HCH_2\overset{\displaystyle O}{\overset{\displaystyle \|}{C}}{-}R'$$

where R is selected from hydrogen, alkyl radicals containing 1 to 20 carbons, cycloalkyl radicals containing 5 to 8 carbons, aryl radicals containing 6 to 24 carbons, and a radical of the formula:

$$\begin{array}{cc} R'''' & O \\ | & \| \\ -CHCH_2C-R''' \end{array}$$

where R" and R"" are selected from hydrogen, alkyl radicals containing 1 to 20 carbons, cycloalkyl radicals containing 5 to 8 carbons, aryl radicals containing 6 to 24 carbons, R' and R''' are selected from hydrogen, alkyl radicals containing 1 to 20 carbons, cyclo-alkyl radicals containing 5 to 8 carbons, aryl radicals containing 6 to 24 carbons, alkoxy radicals containing 1 to 20 carbons, cycloalkoxy radicals containing 5 to 8 carbons and aryloxy radicals containing 6 to 24 carbons and where n is a whole number less than 3.

The reaction between dicyclopentadiene and the phenolic compounds is effectively catalyzed by a Friedel-Crafts type catalyst, and in particular the more potent Friedel-Craft catalysts such as aluminum chloride, zinc chloride, ferrous and ferric chloride and boron trifluoride, as well as complexes based on boron trifluoride. Boron trifluoride and complexes based on boron trifluoride are preferred catalysts for the first step of the disclosed process.

The second step of the above described two-step reaction process, wherein the product obtained by reacting dicyclopentadiene and a phenolic compound is further alkylated with a tertiary olefin, is effectively catalyzed by employing one or more of the customary acidic alkylation catalysts such as sulfuric acid, benzenesulfonic acid, toluenesulfonic acid, acid activated clays, boron trifluoride, zinc chloride, ferrous and ferric halides, aluminum halides and the stannous and stannic halides.

Sulfuric acid, benzenesulfonic acid, toluenesulfonic acid and acid activated clay are preferred catalysts for the second step of the disclosed process. The catalysts employed in both the first and second stages of the disclosed process are employed in the customary catalytic amounts, which will normally vary from 0.1 to 5.0% of catalyst based on the total weight of the reactants in the reaction which is to be catalyzed.

In making the alkylated reaction products of this process preferred phenolic materials are p-cresol and mixed m,p-cresol. The preferred olefin is isobutylene. Representative examples of sulfur-containing compounds which may be used are:

> 1-(butylthio)heptanone-3
> 1-(cyclohexylthio)hexanone-3
> 1-(3-methylphenylthio)octanone-3
> 3-(phenylthio)propanal
> 3-(hexylthio)propanal
> octadecyl 3-(cyclohexylthio)propanoate
> dodecyl 3-(phenyldithio)propanoate

Preferred sulfur-containing compounds are esters of thiodipropionic acid of the following formula:

$$\begin{array}{ccc} O & & O \\ \| & & \| \\ X-O-C-CH_2-CH_2-S-CH_2-CH_2-C-O-Y \end{array}$$

where X and Y are alkyl radicals containing 1 to 20 carbons. Most preferred are those containing from 8 to 18 carbons. Details of the reaction conditions are illustrated in the following examples.

Example 1: 330 g of p-cresol and 9.0 g of a phenol BF$_3$ complex containing 26% BF$_3$ were heated to 100°C and then 132 g of dicyclopentadiene were added over a period of 3½ hr. The excess p-cresol was removed by heating to a column temperature of 150°C at 4 mm, this procedure also removed the BF_3 catalyst. A residue of 316 g was obtained. 236 g of this product were dissolved in an equal weight of toluene and 4.0 g of H_2SO_4 added. The solution was heated to 80°C and 168 g of isobutene added over a period of 1¾ hr. The mixture was heated one hour longer then the catalyst was destroyed with a Na_2CO_3 solution. Volatiles and unreacted materials were removed by heating to 175°C at 30 mm. Catalyst residues were removed by filtration. Weight of the product was 313 g.

Examples 2 through 4: The polypropylene samples were prepared in the following manner. The phenolic compound was either dissolved in a suitable solvent such as hexane or acetone in a concentration of 1 to 5% and added to the polypropylene (Pro-Fax 6501) by dispersing the stabilizer solution in the powdered polypropylene using a Henschel blender and agitating at 2,800 rpm or by adding the phenolic compound directly to the polypropylene in the Henschel blender. The sulfur-containing compound was added to the polypropylene in the blender either directly or in solution.

After 15 min the typical batch temperature approached 180°F and a reasonable dispersion of the stabilizers was obtained. After 10 min only traces of the solvent remained where the stabilizers were added in solution. The stabilized polypropylene was then injection molded to produce tensile bars conforming to ASTM-D-638-64 T. The tensile bars were aged at 140°C in a forced air oven. The stress-strain properties of the original and aged samples were measured by an Instron. A 4½" jaw was used, the jaw separation rate being 1"/min. Melt index determinations were made on the aged and unaged tensile bars which had been cut up into small pieces. The melt index test was run according to ASTM-D-1238-62 T, Condition L.

Examples 2 and 3 are based on polypropylene polymer containing the individual components of the system used in Example 4. The samples were prepared, aged and tested as described above. Yield tensile and melt index data are listed in the table below.

Stabilization system	Example					
	2		3		4	
Butylated reaction product[1] of p-cresol and dicyclopentadiene (parts)	0.05		------		0.05	
Dilaurylthiodipropionate (parts)			0.25		0.25	
	A	B	A	B	A	B
Aging time, days:						
0	5,540	1.58	5,540	2.61	5,610	1.52
1	5,140	2.04	5,100	2.64	5,120	1.45
3	4,970	2.45	4,110	3.30	4,990	1.58
5	5,090	2.63	(2)	(2)	5,130	1.81
7	2,910	(2)	------		5,150	2.12
9	610				5,050	2.16

[1] Prepared by a method according to Example 1.
[2] Failed.
NOTE.—A = Yield Tensile (p.s.i.); B = Melt Index, expressed as grams of polymer extruded per 10 minutes.

Four Component Stabilizer System

W.O. Drake and K.R. Mills; U.S. Patent 3,636,031; January 18, 1972; assigned to Phillips Petroleum Company have developed a stabilizer system for poly-1-olefins comprising an organic phosphite ester, a thioester, 2,6-di-tert-butyl-4-methylphenol, and 4,6-di(4-hydroxy-3,5-di-tert-butylphenoxy)-2-octylthio-1,3,5-triazine. This system not only improves the resistance of the polymer to discoloration but also improves the resistance of the polymer to embrittlement upon exposure to air and light at normal atmospheric and at elevated temperatures, particularly over long periods of time. The phosphite ester in the system is characterized by the formula:

$$RO-P\begin{matrix} OR' \\ OR'' \end{matrix}$$

where R is a hydrocarbon radical selected from alkyl, aryl, cycloalkyl, and combinations thereof such as alkaryl and aralkyl, having 1 to 20 carbons, and R' and R" are selected from R and hydrogen. The thioester characterized by the formula:

$$C_nH_{2n}-COOR'''$$
$$|$$
$$S$$
$$|$$
$$C_mH_{2m}-COOR''''$$

where R''' and R'''' are alkyl groups containing 6 to 24 carbons, and n and m are integers from 1 to 6, preferably 2.

Exemplary organic phosphite esters are: trimethyl phosphite, di-2-ethylhexyl phosphite, dibutyl phosphite, diisooctyl tolyl phosphite, tri-2-ethylhexyl phosphite, triphenyl phosphite, isobutyl phosphite, tricresyl phosphite, tri(2,3-dimethylphenyl) phosphite, phenyl phosphite, dioctyl phosphite (DOPI), triisooctyl phosphite, etc.

Exemplary thioester compounds are: laurylhexylthiodipropionate, dilaurylthiodipropionate (DLTDP), butylstearylthiodipropionate, 2-ethylhexylthiodipropionate, diisodecylthiodipropionate, isodecyltetradecylthiodiheptanoate, laurylstearylthiodipropionate, distearylthiodipropionate, etc.

Example: Polypropylene prepared by mass polymerization of propylene (in the presence of a catalyst system comprising diethylaluminum chloride and the reaction product formed on mixing titanium tetrachloride and aluminum, the product having the approximate formula $TiCl_3 \cdot \frac{1}{3}AlCl_3$) was treated with the four component stabilizer system of this process. All additives were introduced as 1% acetone solutions. After evaporation of the solvent accompanied by occasional stirring, the mixtures were blended in the plastograph for 10 minutes under nitrogen at 190°C and 60 rpm.

After blending, the formulations were molded into 20 mil sheets of 217°C. Sheets were then cut into 0.25 x 1.75" strips and five specimens of each sample were placed in the 150°C forced air oven. Any crazing, spotting or crumbling of the specimens was classified as a failure. The oven embrittlement resistance was based on the average time in days for the second, third and fourth specimens to fail.

The amount of the A compound to the B compound was from 0.3:0.1 to 0.1:0.3. All samples in the example contained 0.3 php dilaurylthiodipropionate and 0.1 php of dioctyl phosphite. It can be readily seen from the table below that a synergistic improvement in oven life is obtained using a combination of the substituted triazine and the 2,6-di-tert-butyl-4-methylphenol.

| | Php.[1] | | Oven life, days | |
	A[2]	B[3]	Found	Expected
Sample Number:				
1	0.4	0.0	<1	----------
2	0.3	0.1	33	<13.25
3	0.2	0.2	47	<25.5
4	0.1	0.3	43	<37.75
5	0.0	0.4	49	----------

[1] Parts by weight per 100 parts polymer.
[2] 2,6-di-tert-butyl-4-methylphenol.
[3] 4,6-di(4-hydroxy-3,5-di-tert-butylphenoxy)-2-octylthio-1,3,5-triazine.

Stabilizer Mixtures Containing Nickel Phosphate

A process for improving the thermal and ultraviolet stability of polymer prepared from alpha-monoolefins is disclosed by *K.R. Mills; U.S. Patent 3,642,690; February 15, 1972; assigned to Phillips Petroleum Company.* This process uses nickel phosphate in combination with 2-hydroxybenzophenone and its derivatives and at least one antioxidant to provide a thermal and ultraviolet stabilized polymer prepared from alpha-monoolefins.

Nickel phosphate either as the ortho- or pyrophosphate is suitable for use in this mixture. The nickel phosphate is used in an amount to provide from about 0.05 to 5, preferably 0.2 to 2 parts by weight of nickel phosphate per 100 parts by weight of polymer (php). The 2-hydroxybenzophenone, and its derivatives, with which the nickel phosphate is used to enhance its effectiveness as an ultraviolet stabilizer can be represented by the formula

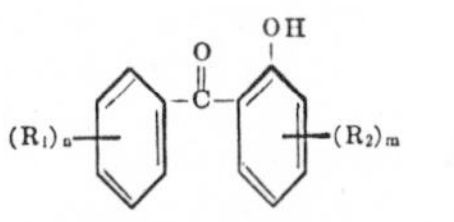

where n is an integer from 0 to 5 and m is an integer from 0 to 4 and the (R_1 and R_2) radicals can be the same or different and are selected from hydroxy ($-OH$), sulfo ($-SO_3H$), halogen (such as fluorine, chlorine, bromine, and iodine), or organic radicals selected from aliphatic, alicyclic, or heterocyclic groups containing 1 to 30 carbons.

The 2-hydroxybenzophenone and derivatives thereof are employed in an amount sufficient to provide from about 0.05 to 10, preferably 0.1 to 3 parts by weight per 100 parts by weight of monoolefin polymer to be stabilized. Any conventional antioxidant can be used with the nickel phosphate and 2-hydroxybenzophenone, or derivatives thereof, to complete the stabilizer combinations.

Examples of conventional antioxidants are disclosed in *Modern Plastics, Encyclopedia,* vol 45, No. 14A, October 1968, pp 505 to 507 (McGraw Hill Publications, N.Y.). At least one of the conventional antioxidants and preferably two or more are employed according to this process. It is preferred that at least one antioxidant is selected from phenols, organic phosphites, thiodipropionates, or triazines and used in an amount to provide from about 0.005 to 5, preferably 0.1 to 2 parts by weight per 100 parts by weight of alpha-monoolefin polymer to be stabilized.

Example: Testing samples of powdered polypropylene having a nominal melt flow of 3 were prepared. A mixture of the additives in acetone were mixed with the base polymer and the solvent evaporated. The mixture was then blended in a Brabender Plastograph for 10 min in a nitrogen atmosphere at 185°C. The prepared samples had the following composition by weight.

Sample Number	I	II	III
Polypropylene, parts	100	100	100
DLTDP [1] (php.) [2]	.1	.1	.1
Irganox 858 [3] (php.)	.1	.1	.1
DOPI [4] (php.)	.01	.01	.01
Cyasorb UV-531 [5] (php.)	.07	1.57	.07
Ferro AM-101 [6] (php.)	1.5		
Nickel Phosphate (php.)			1.5

[1] Antioxidant, dilauryl-3,3'-thiodipropionate. Evans Chemetics, Inc.
[2] Parts by weight of additive per 100 parts by weight of polymer.
[3] Antioxidant, 2,4-bis-(4-hydroxy-3,5-di-tert-butylphenoxy)-6-(n-octylthio)-1,3,5-triazine, Geigy Chemical Company.
[4] Antioxidant, dioctyl phosphite, Hooker Chemical Corp.
[5] Ultraviolet absorber, 2-hydroxy-4-n-octoxybenzophenone, American Cyanamide Co.
[6] Ultraviolet absorber, bis[2,2'-thiobis[4-(1,1,3,3-tetramethylbutyl)]]-nickel (II), Ferro Corp.

Compression molded film 10 mils in thickness were made from each of the three samples shown above. Speciments 1½" long and ⅜" wide were tested for long term thermal stability (oven life) by placing the specimens in glass test tubes with a 0.125" diameter hole in the bottom thereof. The tubes containing the test specimens were placed in a forced air oven at 150°C. Failure of the sample is indicated by deterioration of one exposed edge. The above samples were also tested for melt flow stability at an elevated temperature using the general procedure of ASTM-1238-65T at 290°C and employing a 2,160 g weight. The lower the melt flow the less the polymer sample has been thermally degraded. The results of these tests are reported in the following table.

Sample No.	Oven Life (days)	Melt Flow
1 (control)	13	90
2 (control)	20	56
3 (process)	28	23

The above results demonstrate that the thermal stability of polypropylene is enhanced by employing nickel phosphate in combination with a 2-hydroxybenzophenone derivative. Comparison of Sample 2 (control) and Sample 3 (process) demonstrate that the addition of nickel phosphate for an equal amount of the 2-hydroxybenzophenone derivative vastly improves the stability of a polypropylene polymer. Comparison of Sample 1 (control) and Sample 3 (process) demonstrate the stabilizing superiority of nickel phosphate in combination with 2-hydroxybenzophenone derivatives over an organic nickel compound.

Mixed Esters of a Thiodicarboxylic Acid plus a Hindered Phenol

A stabilizer system which protects polypropylene not only against deterioration of melt viscosity, but also against embrittlement and discoloration has been developed by *C.R. Bresson; U.S. Patent 3,644,282; February 22, 1972; assigned to Phillips Petroleum Co.* This stabilizer comprises mixtures of diesters of thiodicarboxylic acids. In another example, the stabilizer further comprises at least one hindered mono- or polyphenolic compound.

The diesters of thiodicarboxylic acids are produced by reacting a mixture of alcohols characterized by the formulas ROH and R'OH where R and R' are the same or different and are hydrocarbon radicals selected from alkyl or cycloalkyl substituted alkyl in the range of from 10 to 20 carbons per R and R' group with at least one thiodicarboxylic acid of the formula $S-(C_nH_{2n}COOH)_2$ where n is an integer from 1 to 6.

In a preferred example, the alcohol mixture is produced by the Oxo process. Olefin containing feedstock to the Oxo process is reacted with hydrogen and carbon monoxide in the presence of usually a cobalt-containing catalyst to produce an aldehyde-containing product, the aldehydes containing 1 carbon atom per molecule more than their olefin precursors. The crude aldehyde is then generally reduced with hydrogen in the presence of a catalyst, typically a copper catalyst, to form a corresponding alcohol which is then fractionated to remove components which have boiling points outside the desired boiling range.

It is believed that the Oxo alcohol contains predominantly branched constituents since it is well-known that by the nature of the Oxo process even if the starting material contains only linear unbranched olefins, the Oxo product will contain approximately 40 to 60% branched material. It is also well-known that the Oxo process produces only primary alcohols. The great bulk of the esters produced from these alcohols can then be called isoalkyl thiodicarboxylic acid esters or cycloalkylmethyl thiodicarboxylic acid esters.

Diesters of thiodicarboxylic acids are prepared by reacting a thiodicarboxylic acid and the mixture of Oxo alcohols as described above in the presence of sulfuric or a sulfonic acid. In general, temperatures of from 30° to 150°C are employed, preferably from 50° to 100°C. Preferably, the esterification reaction is carried out in a diluent which is capable of azeotroping water. Suitable diluents include toluene, benzene, xylene, carbon tetrachloride, di-n-butyl ether, diethyl ether, chloroform, and the like. In general, conventional esterification conditions can be employed.

Example 1: The thiodipropionate esters were prepared according to the following general procedure. A mixture of one mol thiodipropionic acid, 2.2 mols Oxo alcohol, [a heart cut having a boiling point range of 600° to 650°F (1 atm)], 1 g of methanesulfonic acid and 100 ml of toluene was heated to reflux temperature under a nitrogen atmosphere and water of esterification removed via a Dean-Stark trap. The mixture was cooled to 85°C, washed with 100 ml 5% sodium hydroxide solution, 2 x 100 ml water and 100 ml saturated salt solution. Excess alcohol was removed under vacuum on a 45 cm Vigreux column. The bottoms product was heated with 3 g Nuchar activated charcoal and 0.5 g sodium borohydride for 3 hr on a steam bath. The mixture was filtered through Celite to give a nearly quantitative yield of odorless thiodipropionate ester in each run.

Example 2: Polypropylene prepared by mass polymerization of propylene in the presence of catalyst systems comprising diethyl aluminum chloride and the reaction product of titanium tetrachloride and aluminum having the approximate formula $TiCl_3 \cdot {}^1/_3 AlCl_3$ was treated with exemplary stabilizer systems of the instant process. The stabilized samples were prepared by mixing polypropylene powder with acetone or benzene solutions of the antioxidants. All phenolic compounds were introduced as 1% acetone solutions, and the diesters of thiodipropionic acid were added as 1% benzene solutions. The solvent was evaporated and the polypropylene was compressed and molded in films 20 mils thick.

| | Embrittlement time, days (C) | | Melt flow, grams/10 min. (D) Residence time, minutes | | | | | |
| | | | A | | | B | | |
Secondary antioxidant (0.2 php.)	A	B	5	10	20	5	10	20
C_{13}-C_{15} isoalkyl TDP	24	44	10	15	24	9.1	13	14
C_{16}-C_{18} isoalkyl TDP	33	59	10	14	24	8.8	9.8	12
C_{19}-C_{21} isoalkyl TDP	32	54	12	16	30	8.0	11	18
DLTDP	17	34	10	14	24	8.0	10	14
DSTDP	36	65	10	14	24	8.2	9.9	17
DBTDP	36	64	10	12	19	9.0	11	16
LSTDP	32	57	9.5	16	24	8.1	9.7	15
None	3							

(A) In polypropylene containing 0.1 php. 1,1,3-tris(2-methyl-4-hydroxy-5-tert-butyl-phenyl)butane and 0.1 php. 2,6-di-tert-butyl-4-methylphenol.
(B) In polypropylene containing 0.1 php. tetrakis[3-(3,5-di-tert-butyl-4-hydroxyphenyl) propionyloxymethyl]methane and 0.1 php. 2,6-di-tert-butyl-4-methylphenol.
(C) Five specimens were cut from a compression-molded film 20 mils thick and were aged in an air circulating oven at 150° C. These specimens were checked periodically for failure as indicated by the appearance of spot granulation, usually accompanied by discoloration. The average failure time for the five samples was reported as the embrittlement time.
(D) The change in melt flow was determined by adding 7.5 grams of the stabilized polymer to a melt indexer and the melt flow (grams/10 min.) at 550° F. was determined after dwell times of 5, 10, and 20 minutes.

POLYMER BONDING OF ANTIOXIDANTS

Unfortunately, the antioxidants commonly used are limited in their efficacy by physical loss which is attributed to diffusion with subsequent evaporation or extraction. In order to minimize or eliminate such losses, workers have suggested the use of increasingly larger antioxidants, so tending to immobilize the molecule in the polymer network and prevent diffusive losses, or the chemical bonding of the antioxidant to the polymer chain.

Carbene Bonding of Phenolic Antioxidants

In this disclosure by *M.L. Kaplan and P.G. Kelleher; U.S. Patent 3,723,405; March 27, 1973; assigned to Bell Telephone Laboratories, Incorporated*, the prior limitations are obviated by a procedure for chemically bonding an antioxidant to the olefinic polymer chain. Briefly, the technique involves diazotizing 2,6-di-tert-butylaminophenol to yield 3,5-di-tert-butylbenzene-1,4-diazooxide, adding the resultant diazooxide in solution to the polymer and, after removing the solvent, effecting the decomposition of the diazooxide by thermal or photochemical means.

The decomposition results in the formation of a carbene which chemically bonds with the polymer. During this bonding process, an electronic rearrangement occurs with the formation of a hindered phenol bonded chemically to the polymer. Studies have indicated that the resultant composition has superior stability with respect to oxidative degradation as compared with both unstabilized materials and those stabilized with conventional antioxidants when all the compositions have undergone an aqueous extraction procedure.

Polymers amenable to stabilization against oxidative degradation in accordance with this process are derived from alpha-olefins such as ethylene. Typical polymers in this class are linear and branched (i.e., high and low density) polyethylene, polypropylene, polybutene as well as copolymers of these monomers. The critical reactant in this technique is 3,5-di-tert-butylbenzene-1,4-diazooxide. This compound may be obtained by the diazotization by conventional techniques of the corresponding aminophenol. The aminophenol may be prepared by the catalytic reduction of either 4-nitro-2,6-di-tert-butylphenol or 4-nitroso-2,6-di-tert-butylphenol. Typical procedures would involve reduction at 100°C in the presence of tin and hydrochloric acid or the use of platinum oxide and several atmospheres of hydrogen. The diazooxide may then be prepared by diazotization of the aminophenol by conventional techniques, as for example, with nitrous acid.

The next step involves adding the diazooxide to the polymer to be stabilized. This may be attained by initially forming a solution of the diazooxide. Materials suitable as solvents are the aromatic and aliphatic hydrocarbons, aliphatic ethers and halogenated aliphatics. Preferred compounds are methylene chloride, diethyl ether, hexane and benzene. In the formation of the solution, the ratio of solvent to solute is dictated by practical considerations. Details of this step are shown in the following example.

Example: A solution comprising 0.005 g of 3,5-di-tert-butyl-1,4-diazooxide (DTBDO) in 10 ml of methylene chloride was prepared, the diazooxide having been obtained by diazotization of 4-amino-2,6-di-tert-butylbenzene. The resultant solution was added to 1 g of low density branched polyethylene powder (0.92 g/cm^3). The solvent was next removed at a pressure of the order of 30 torr and 0.010" films were molded at 140°C for 1 min during which carbene insertion occurred.

For comparative purposes, 1 g of polyethylene of the type described was added to 0.5% by weight of 2,6-di-tert-butylphenol (DTBP) and a third sample of polyethylene (1 g) was maintained as a control. The three polymer films, unstabilized, DTBP and DTBDO stabilized were then extracted in a Soxhlet apparatus with water for 30 hr. After drying in vacuo, the films were subjected to oxygen uptake studies at 140°C. The results are set forth in the table.

Stabilizer	Hours to Failure (1% Oxygen Incorporation)
None	3
DTBP	5
DTBDO	14

Silane Bonding of Aromatic Amine Antioxidants

R.V. Albarino and H. Schonhorn; U.S. Patent 3,823,114; July 9, 1974; assigned to Bell Telephone Laboratories, Incorporated have found that the migration of antioxidants from polymeric hydrocarbons may also be retarded by bonding the antioxidant with a silane coupling agent. Briefly, this involves reacting a silane compound of the formula

$$(RO)_x-Si-[(CH_2)_n R']_{4-x}$$

where R is selected from methyl and ethyl radicals, R' is selected from

$$-NH_2, -Cl, -Br, -OH, \quad \diagdown C=C \diagup \quad \text{and} \quad -C-C-$$

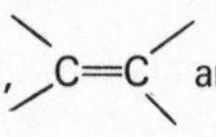

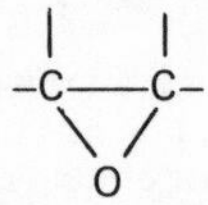

radicals, x is an integer from 1 to 4 and n is an integer from 1 to 10, with a conventional arylamine antioxidant resulting in a compound of the formula

(a) $(RO)_x-Si-[(CH_2)_n A]_{4-x}$ or   (b) $(RO)_x-Si-[(CH_2)_n A]_{4-x}$

where A represents a conventional arylamine antioxidant radical originally having an additional substituent (Y) on the aromatic portion capable of reacting with the silane R' groups, R, x and n are as represented above and R" is selected from —NH— and —O— radicals.

The resultant silane antioxidants are found to be far more compatible with alpha-olefin polymers than the antioxidant alone and upon prolonged exposure to the atmosphere evidence less migration or physical loss than the antioxidant alone.

As indicated, the silane antioxidants may be prepared by reacting an alkoxysilane (of the type described) with an arylamine antioxidant having a substituent Y on the aromatic portion capable of reacting with the R' group in the silane compound. The Y group may conveniently be selected from $-NH_2$, $-OH$, $-Cl$, $-Br$, and $-COOH$ radicals. A typical product is obtained by reacting the following compounds:

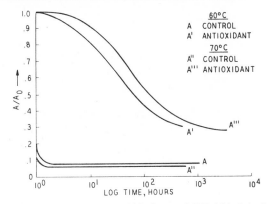

The antioxidants of this process are most effective in the range of 0.005 to 2% by weight, based upon the weight of the polymer. Thus, for example, in a typical case of the antioxidant in which bridging to the silicon is effected through an oxygen atom, 3 mols of 3-hydroxydiphenylamine may be reacted with 1 mol of γ-aminopropyltriethoxysilane while heating to a temperature of 100°C for several minutes to yield the desired silane.

100 g of hydrocarbon polymer pellets were worked up to a melt on a 6"x 12" two-roll mill and various concentrations of antioxidant, ranging up to 1.0%, by weight, based on the weight of the polymer were incorporated into the polymer. Milling was then effected for approximately 5 min at 130°C. The polymer used was a high molecular weight polyethylene high pressure polymer obtained from commercial sources. The samples were obtained by molding the mill massed compositions against 5 mil polished sheet aluminum at 150°C under pressure and then cooled rapidly.

Following molding, the samples were stored in water at room temperature for 64 hr. After storage, the resultant films were cut and placed in a holder suitable for spectral analysis. In order to remove exuded antioxidant from the surfaces of the film prior to insertion in the holder, cleansing was done in water and containing a commercially available detergent followed by a water rinse. Oven aging was done at 60° and 70°C for various time periods and spectral analysis was made to determine the amoung of retained antioxidant. With reference to Figure 11.1, there is shown a graphical representation on coordinates of time in hours against antioxidant concentration as derived from ultraviolet spectra for 60° to 70°C aging temperatures for polyethylene containing 0.8% by weight of aminopropyltri-(diphenylamino)oxysilane.

FIGURE 11.1: TIME/ANTIOXIDANT CONCENTRATION CURVE

Source: R.V. Albarino and H. Schonhorn; U.S. Patent 3,823,114; July 9, 1974

As a control, the procedure was repeated using polyethylene containing 0.1% by weight of 3-hydroxydiphenylamine. Analysis of the figure reveals that the control, the 3-hydroxydiphenylamine exuded far more rapidly from the polyethylene than the silane.

STABILIZATION OF COPPER-POLYOLEFIN SYSTEMS

A wide range of antioxidants have been used in olefinic polymers with various degrees of effectiveness. The stabilizing problem becomes particularly acute when the polymer is used in contact with copper such as in electrical insulation for copper wire. Although many stabilizers provide adequate protection for the polymer under normal use, it has been found that when used in contact with copper the polymer fails prematurely, tending to crack and lose its electrical insulation properties. In fact, some types of oxidative deterioration have been reported to be more severe when a typical antioxidant is used than when none is used (Hansen et al, *J Poly. Sci., Part A,* 2, 587-609, 1964).

Phenolic Antioxidant-Gallic Acid Ester Mixtures

An improved antioxidant system for polyolefins in contact with copper has been disclosed by *K.G. Ihrman and R.E. Malec; U.S. Patent 3,792,014; February 12, 1974; assigned to Ethyl Corporation.* This comprises a hydrocarbyl ester of gallic acid (e.g., propyl gallate) together with a phenolic antioxidant. A wide range of phenolic antioxidants can be used and an extensive list of them is given in the patent.

Superior results are obtained when the antioxidant compound is a tris(3,5-dialkyl-4-hydroxybenzyl)benzene as described in U.S. Patent 3,026,264. Of this class, the most preferred additive is 1,3,5-trimethyl-2,4,6-tris(3,5-di-tert-butyl-4-hydroxybenzyl)benzene. The amount of antioxidant used need only be a small antioxidant amount. A useful concentration is from about 0.05 to 1 weight percent. In general, good results are obtained using about 0.05 to 0.5 weight percent.

Preferred gallates are the alkyl gallates in which the alkyl group contains from 1 to 20 carbons such as methyl gallate, propyl gallate, decyl gallate, dodecyl gallate, and eicosyl gallate. The amount of hydrocarbyl gallate should be a promoter amount. By this is meant an amount sufficient to at least reduce the detrimental effect of copper on the polymer containing the antioxidant. A useful promoter range is from 0.005 to 1 weight percent. A preferred range is from 0.05 to 0.5 weight percent.

Light stabilizers for olefin polymers can also be added, for example, 2-hydroxybenzophenones, o-hydroxyphenylbenzotriazoles, 1-dioxides of α,β-benzoisothiazolones and 1,3,5-triazines and nickel organophosphites (see U.S. Patent 3,395,112). Known synergists for phenolic antioxidant can be included in the polymer in addition to combinations of gallate ester and phenolic antioxidant, e.g., synergists are dialkyl thiodialkanoates such as dilauryl thiodipropionate.

Tests have been carried out to demonstrate the effectiveness of hydrocarbyl gallates in reducing the detrimental effect of copper on phenolic antioxidant stabilized olefinic polymers. In these tests, low density polyethylene was compounded to contain typical phenolic antioxidants widely used in olefinic polymers, alone and in combination with the gallate promoter.

The polyethylene was pressed into 10 mil sheets and placed on a clean copper surface in an air circulating oven at 105°C. Criteria of effectiveness was the hours to polymer failure as evidenced by tearing of the polymer sheet when moderately stretched. The olefinic polymer phenolic antioxidants included in the test were:

    (A) pentaerythritol tetrakis[3-(3,5-di-tert-butyl-4-hydroxyphenyl)propionate]
    (B) 1,3,5-trimethyl-2,4,6-tris(3,5-di-tert-butyl-4-hydroxybenzyl)benzene
    (C) 1,1,3-tris(2-methyl-5-tert-butyl-4-hydroxyphenyl)butane
    (D) 4,4'-thiobis(3-methyl-6-tert-butylphenol)

The following table shows the test results.

Test No.	Additive	Conc. (wt. percent)	Hours to failure Without copper	With copper
1	None		120	72
2	Propyl gallate	0.1		168
3		0.2		168
4	Dodecyl gallate	0.1		336
5		0.2		360
6	"A"	0.1	2,952	456
7	"A" plus Propyl gallate	0.1 0.1		1,200
8	"B"	0.1	2,784	408
9	"B" plus Propyl gallate	0.1 0.1		1,416
10	"B" plus Decyl dodecyl gallate	0.1 0.1		1,536
11	"C" plus Propyl gallate	0.1 0.1		1,128
12	"C" plus Decyl dodecyl gallate	0.1 0.1		1,248
13	"D"	0.1	1,104	456
14	"D" plus Propyl gallate	0.1 0.1		600
15	"D" plus Decyl dodecyl gallate	0.1 0.1		696

Heterocyclic Amines and Amides

Heterocyclic amines or amides are provided by *M. Minagawa, K. Nakagawa and M. Goto; U.S. Patent 3,673,152; June 27, 1972; assigned to Argus Chemical Corporation* which are useful in the enhancement of the resistance of olefin polymers to copper catalyzed oxidative deterioration. Stabilizer compositions are also provided consisting essentially of at least one known olefin polymer stabilizer and heterocyclic amines or amides. This class of stabilizers embrace a wide variety of compounds having the broad general formula

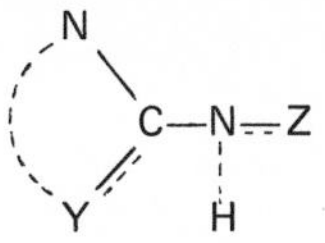

where the dotted lines represent bonds necessary to satisfy the valences of the atoms to which they are connected,

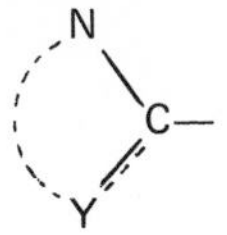

represents a heterocyclic nitrogen-containing ring structure including at least one five or six membered ring and at least two nitrogen atoms; Y is selected from nitrogen, carbon or sulfur, and Z is selected from

$$(1) \qquad -C-(CH_2)_a-(S)_b-(R_oS)_c-R_1 \quad (X)$$

where X is oxygen or sulfur. R_o is methylene, alkyl-substituted methylene, aryl-substituted methylene or arylene, and c is 0 or 1. R_1 is selected from hydrogen, alkyl having 1 to 18 carbons,

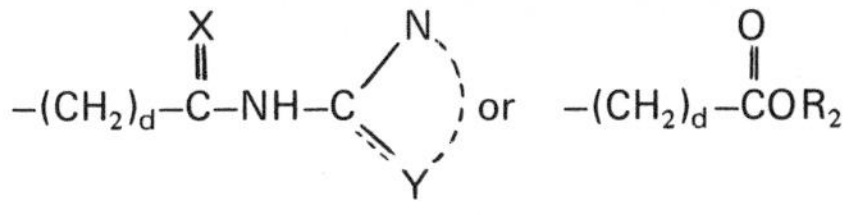

In the above formula R_2 is hydrogen, alkyl having 1 to 10 carbons or benzyl; a is 0, 1 or 2; b is 1 or 2; and d is 0, 1 or 2;

(2)
$$-\overset{\overset{\displaystyle A}{\|}}{C}-R_3$$

where A is oxygen, sulfur or two hydrogen atoms, and R_3 is

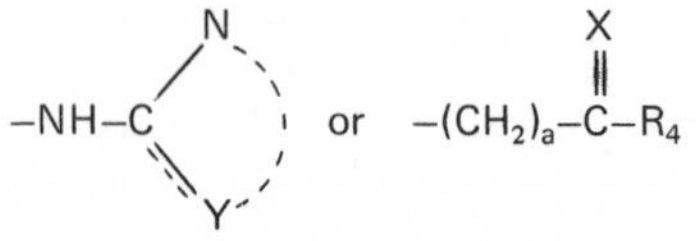

$$-NH-C\underset{\diagdown Y}{\overset{\diagup N}{\Big\langle}}\quad \text{or} \quad -(CH_2)_a-\overset{\overset{\displaystyle X}{\|}}{C}-R_4$$

where R_4 is aryl, o-hydroxyaryl, benzyl, or alkyl having 1 to 18 carbons and X,

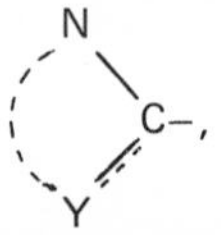

$$\underset{\diagdown Y}{\overset{\diagup N}{\Big\langle}}C-, \text{ and a are as defined above;}$$

(3)   two radicals, $-R_5$ and $-R_6$

where R_5 is hydrogen, methylol or ethylol and R_6 is methylol, ethylol or

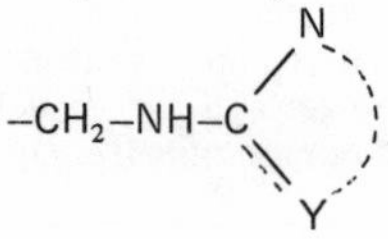

$$-CH_2-NH-C\underset{\diagdown Y}{\overset{\diagup N}{\Big\langle}}$$

(4)
$$-CH_2-\overset{\overset{\displaystyle X}{\|}}{C}-NHNHR_7$$

where X is as defined before and R_7 is hydrogen, alkyl having 1 to 18 carbons, benzyl or aryl;

(5) $-CH\!=\!R_8$

where R_8 is selected from the group consisting of R_4 and

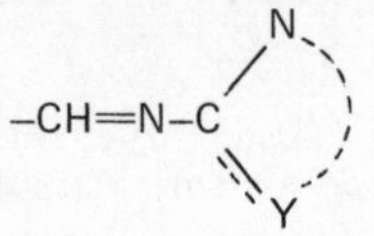

$$-CH=N-C\underset{\diagdown Y}{\overset{\diagup N}{\Big\langle}}$$

and

(6)
$$-\overset{\overset{\displaystyle X}{\|}}{C}-R_9-\overset{\overset{\displaystyle X}{\|}}{C}-NH-C\underset{\diagdown Y}{\overset{\diagup N}{\Big\langle}}$$

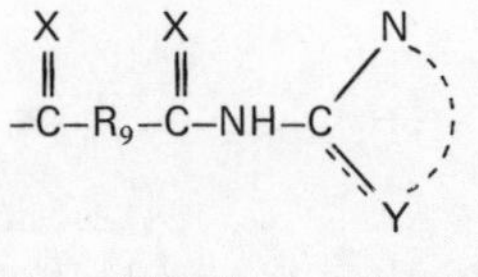

where R_9 is phenyl, $-(CH_2)_e-$, $-\underset{OH}{\overset{|}{C}H}-$, $-\underset{OH}{\overset{|}{C}H}-\underset{OH}{\overset{|}{C}H}-$, $-CH_2-\underset{OH}{\overset{|}{C}H}-$, and $-CH\!=\!CH-$

where e is an integer from 0 to 6, and the known stabilizer is selected from the group consisting of organic phosphites, alkyl substituted phenols, and polynuclear phenols, thio-dipropionic acid esters, polyvalent metal salts of organic acids, hydrocarbon sulfides and polysulfides and alpha-monoolefin polymer light stabilizers. The heterocyclic amine or amide is used in combination with one known and preferably two or more such stabilizers.

Examples 1 through 5: Polypropylene compositions were prepared, stabilized by combina-tions of compounds of the process and known polypropylene stabilizers, and were evaluated for their resistance to oxidative degradation in the presence of copper. An accelerated oxi-dation test was employed, to determine the effective useful life of the polypropylene. The time required for a polypropylene sample to absorb 10 cc of oxygen per gram of sample, when heated at $150°C$ in a closed system was determined. This time is the induction time. The base olefin polymer composition tested was as follows.

	Parts by Weight
Polypropylene (Profax 6501)	100
1,1,3-tris(2'-methyl-4'-hydroxy-5'-tert-butylphenyl)butane	0.05
Distearyl thiodipropionate	0.15
Trinonylphenyl phosphite	0.1
Copper powder	1.0

The components listed were mixed on a two roll mill and sheeted off to form 0.5 mm sheets. To each sample there was also added 0.5 part of the compound listed in the table. As Control A, the base composition was tested, without copper. As Control B, the base com-position was tested with copper. As Control C, the base composition containing added oxanilide also was tested. The table below sets out the results of the test for each com-pound tested.

Example Number	Compound	Induction time (hours)
Control A (no copper)	None	[1] 1,200
Control B (with copper).	do	<20
Control C	Oxanilide	300
1	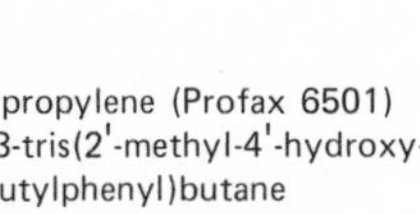	1,430
2	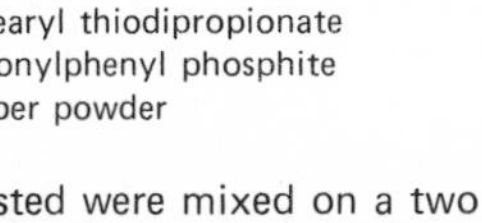	1,450
3	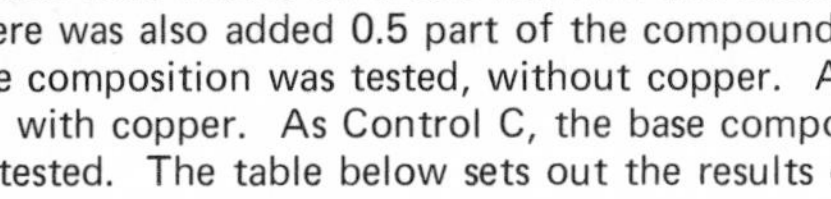	1,150
4		1,650
5	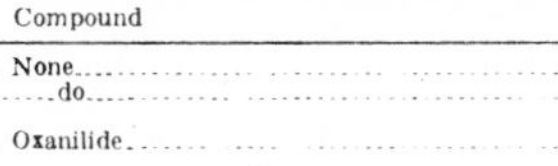	1,600

[1] Absent copper powder.

The preparation of these heterocyclic stabilizers is illustrated by the following examples.

Example 6: Thiodipropionyl aminotriazole was prepared by direct fusion of thiodipropionic acid with 3-aminotriazole as follows. 44.5 g (0.25 mol) of thiodipropionic acid, 42 g (0.5 mol) 3-aminotriazole and 0.44 g p-toluenesulfonic acid were charged into a 300 ml 3-necked flask equipped for downward vacuum distillation and the flask was immersed in an oil bath. The oil bath temperature was brought to 160°C thereby causing the contents of the flask to melt. The contents of the flask were maintained at 160°C for 2.5 hr. Water (8 cc) was removed at reduced pressure. After 2 hr at 160°C, the contents of the flask started to solidify and after 2.5 hr, the flask contents were completely solid. The solid was found to be thiodipropionyl aminotriazole.

Example 7: A mixture of 21 g of 3-amino-1,2,4-triazole and 21.4 g of 25% formaldehyde aqueous solution in 20 g of water was allowed to stand for half an hour. A small amount of sodium hydroxide was added to the mixture and the mixture was maintained at 70°C for an hour. A solid product was separated from the mixture, washed with water and dried in a vacuum oven. The solid material weighed 21.9 g, melted at 231° to 242°C and had an IR spectra corresponding to a heterocyclic amine of the structure

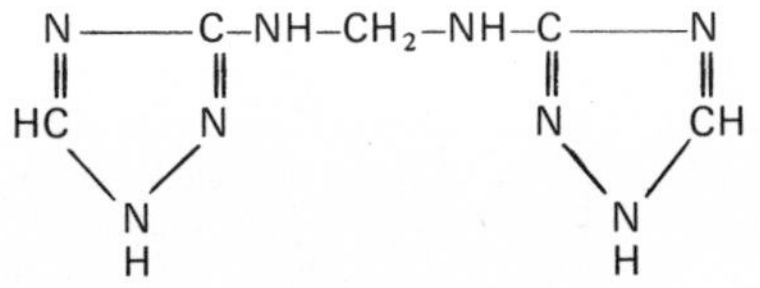

$$
\begin{array}{ccc}
\text{N——C–NH–CH}_2\text{–NH–C——N} \\
\parallel \quad \parallel \qquad\qquad \parallel \quad \parallel \\
\text{HC} \quad \text{N} \qquad\qquad \text{N} \quad \text{CH} \\
\diagdown \;\; \diagup \qquad\qquad \diagdown \;\; \diagup \\
\text{N} \qquad\qquad\qquad \text{N} \\
\text{H} \qquad\qquad\qquad \text{H}
\end{array}
$$

MISCELLANEOUS POLYOLEFIN ANTIOXIDANTS

Phenolic Isocyanurates

Mixed esters of isocyanuric acid have been prepared by *J.C. Gilles; U.S. Patent 3,644,277; February 22, 1972; assigned to The B.F. Goodrich Company.* These bis(hydroxyphenyl-alkylene)alkyl isocyanurates provide excellent stabilization for organic materials, such as polyolefins, against oxidative, thermal and photochemical degradation. These compounds are represented by the formula

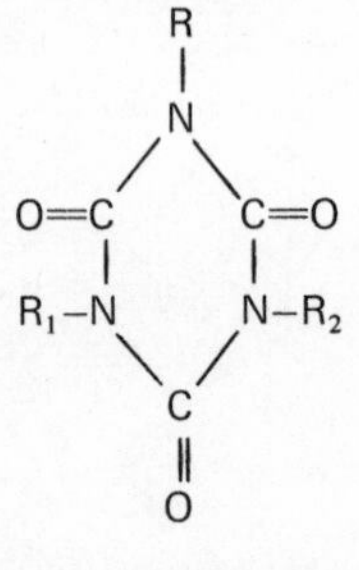

$$
\begin{array}{c}
\text{R} \\
| \\
\text{N} \\
\diagup \;\;\;\; \diagdown \\
\text{O=C} \qquad \text{C=O} \\
| \qquad\qquad | \\
\text{R}_1\text{–N} \qquad \text{N–R}_2 \\
\diagdown \;\;\;\; \diagup \\
\text{C} \\
\parallel \\
\text{O}
\end{array}
$$

where R is a branched or straight chain aliphatic hydrocarbon radical containing 1 to 18 carbons and R_1 and R_2 are hydroxyphenylalkylene radicals having the formula

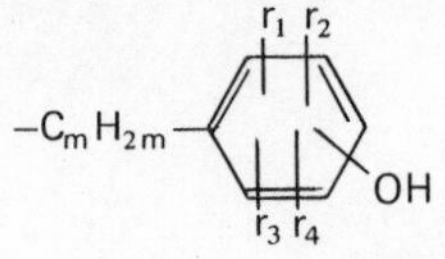

$$
-C_m H_{2m} - \underset{r_3 \; r_4}{\overset{r_1 \; r_2}{\bighexagon}} OH
$$

where m is an integer from 1 to 4, r_1 is an alkyl group, aliphatic or cycloaliphatic, containing 1 to 18 carbons and positioned immediately adjacent to the hydroxyl group on the ring, and r_2, r_3 and r_4 are hydrogen or aliphatic or cycloaliphatic groups containing 1 to 18 carbons. Especially useful isocyanuric acid mixed esters are those compounds where R is an alkyl group containing 6 to 20 carbons, r_1 is a tertiary alkyl group containing 4 to 12 carbons, r_2 is an alkyl group containing 1 to 12 carbons, r_3 and r_4 are hydrogen and m is 1. Preferred hydroxybenzyl radicals include the 3,5-di-tert-butyl-4-hydroxybenzyl radical, the 3-methyl-5-tert-butyl-4-hydroxybenzyl radical, the 2-methyl-5-tert-butyl-4-hydroxybenzyl radical, the 3-tert-butyl-5-methyl-2-hydroxybenzyl radical or like radicals.

The bis(hydroxybenzyl)alkyl isocyanurates are obtained by reacting the monoalkyl substituted isocyanurate with the appropriate phenolic substituent in accordance with any one of a number of procedures. For example, the monoalkyl isocyanurate can be reacted with an alkali metal cyanate and a hydroxybenzyl halide in an aprotic solvent, such as dimethyl sulfoxide or N,N-dimethylformamide, at an elevated temperature.

A process such as that described in U.S. Patent 3,075,979 may also be employed to prepare the bis(hydroxybenzyl)alkyl isocyanurates. Still another means to obtain the bis(hydroxybenzyl)alkyl isocyanurates is the condensation reaction of the monoalkyl isocyanurate with formaldehyde and a hindered phenol. Details of the preparation and testing of one such compound is given in the following examples.

Example 1: Bis(3,5-di-tert-butyl-4-hydroxybenzyl)hexyl isocyanurate was prepared from 100 g (0.97 mol) biuret, 66 ml nitric acid and 250 ml concentrated sulfuric acid. The cooled mixture of nitric acid and sulfuric acid were charged to the reactor containing the biuret over a 2 hr period while maintaining the temperature between about 25° and 30°C. The reaction mixture was then poured into ice and the solid produce obtained therefrom, washed several times with water and ethanol. 83.9 g of the nitrobiuret melting at 144.5°C was obtained.

Nitrobiuret (37 g, 0.25 mol) was reacted for 35 min at about 90°C with 25.25 g (0.25 mol) hexylamine in 250 ml water. The hexylbiuret (MP 126° to 127.5°C) was obtained by recrystallization from aqueous ethanol. Hexylbiuret was then condensed with ethyl carbonate to obtain hexyl isocyanurate. Sodium ethoxide was formed by reacting 2.3 g sodium metal (0.1 mol) with 100 ml of ethanol. The hexylbiuret (9.39 g, 0.05 mol) and diethyl carbonate (12.0 g, 0.1 mol) were then added to the sodium ethoxide and the reaction mixture heated to reflux for about 18 hr. The solid formed was removed by filtration and the hexyl isocyanurate obtained by the addition of 50% HCl to this filtrate. The hexyl isocyanurate, recrystallized from aqueous ethanol, had a melting point of 223° to 226°C.

Hexyl isocyanurate (10.6 g, 0.05 mol) was charged to a reactor containing about 100 ml N,N-dimethylformamide and 6.9 g potassium carbonate. This mixture was heated to about 115°C and 25.5 g (0.1 mol) 2,6-di-tert-butylbenzyl chloride dissolved in about 50 ml N,N-dimethylformamide added dropwise over a 2 hr period followed by an additional 6 hr heating at this temperature.

The reaction mixture was allowed to cool and the bis(3,5-di-tert-butyl-4-hydroxybenzyl)-hexyl isocyanurate precipitated by the addition of aqueous ethanol. The product was further recrystallized from acetone and water and had a melting point of 113° to 114.5°C. Infrared analysis and nuclear magnetic resonance spectroscopy confirmed the product to be the bis(3,5-di-tert-butyl-4-hydroxybenzyl)hexyl isocyanurate.

Example 2: The bis(3,5-di-tert-butyl-4-hydroxybenzyl)hexyl isocyanurate obtained from Example 1 was used by itself and in combination with dilauryl β-thiodipropionate, to stabilize a conventional high density polyethylene. The stabilizing additives were incorporated in the polyethylene by dissolving them in an acetone suspension of the polyethylene and then removing the acetone under vacuum with a rotary evaporator. The stabilized polyethylene was then hot milled (290° to 300°F) for 5 min, sheeted off, and placed in a warm four cavity ACS mold, shimmed to 10 mil thickness. The mold was closed and heated at 300°F for 10 min with the application of 150 tons pressure for the last 5 min.

The samples were then allowed to cool to room temperature under pressure. Oxygen absorption data was obtained for these samples by aging the samples at 140°C in pure oxygen in a modified Scott tester block. The induction periods, that is, the time required for autooxidation of the polyethylene to occur, was about 52 hr for the polyethylene samples stabilized with 0.1 part bis(3,5-di-tert-butyl-4-hydroxybenzyl)hexyl isocyanurate and about 115 hr for the sample stabilized with 0.1 part bis(3,5-di-tert-butyl-4-hydroxybenzyl)hexyl isocyanurate in combination with 0.2 part dilauryl β-thiodipropionate. A polyethylene sample which contained no stabilizer had an induction time of less than 1 hr. In addition to the stabilization of polyethylene, the isocyanurates were also stated to stabilize polypropylene, a 4-methylpentene-1/hexene-1 copolymer and EPT.

Phenylhydrazones

Many of the important applications of polyethylene such as its use in cable sheathings, depend on its good mechanical properties such as high tensile strength and abrasion resistance coupled with its resistant properties against water and water vapors. Other uses take advantage of its dielectric strength in applications such as primary insulation of metallic conductors. Such consequences of thermal oxidation in such polymers are an increase in the brittle point, impairment of tensile strength and deterioration of useful dielectric properties.

R.H. Hansen; U.S. Patent 3,809,675; May 7, 1974; assigned to Bell Telephone Laboratories, Incorporated has found that substituted phenylhydrazones have a significant antioxidant effect when added or incorporated in these polymers. The stabilizers for use herein may be selected from

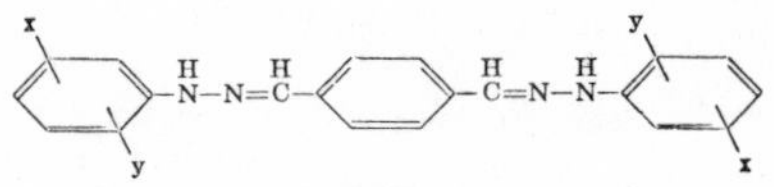

and

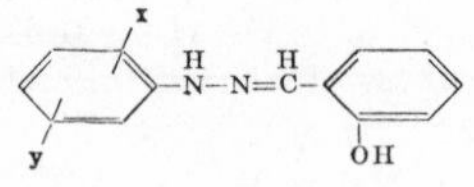

where x and y are selected from F, Cl, COOH, H and NO$_2$. These antioxidants are prepared by reacting phenylhydrazines of the formula

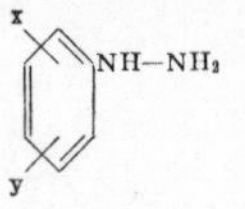

wherein x and y may be selected from among F, Cl, COOH, H and NO$_2$ with an aldehyde or dialdehyde selected from salicylaldehyde and terephthaldehyde. Reaction is effected by independently dissolving each of the reactants in an inert solvent, typically a low molecular weight aliphatic alcohol such as methanol or ethanol heated to a temperature of the order of 50°C, mixing the two solutions and refluxing the mixture for a time period ranging from 1 to 200 hr at reflux temperature.

The reaction is facilitated with an acid catalyst, for example, acetic acid. When used, the acid is employed in minimal quantities, typically a drop or two. The antioxidants are most useful between 0.002 to 10% by weight, based upon the weight of the polymer.

Example: Initially, an antioxidant was prepared by independently dissolving two mols of phenylhydrazine and one mol of terephthaldehyde in 1,000 cc of methyl alcohol heated to a temperature of approximately 50°C. Then, the two solutions were mixed and 5 drops of glacial acetic acid was added. The resultant mixture was then refluxed for 3 hr, so resulting in the preparation of bisphenylhydrazone of terephthaldehyde. Longer reflux periods enhance the yield.

The hydrocarbon polymer together with the antioxidant was prepared by mill massing on a 6" x 12" two roll mill having roll speeds of approximately 24 and 35 rpm with the rolls at a temperature of about 120°C. Various concentrations of antioxidant ranging from 0.00 (control) to 4.65% by weight, based on the weight of the polymer were incorporated into the polymer being tested. The polyethylene used in the studies was a high molecular weight, high pressure polymer obtained from commercial sources. Test samples, approximately 10 mils in thickness were obtained by molding the mill massed compositions at 125°C.

Duplicate samples of the 10 mil molded material, each weighing 0.100 g were placed in calibrated oxygen uptake burets and sealed in an atmosphere of pure oxygen. The specimens were then placed in constant temperature baths and the time required for the interaction of the polymer composition with 1 cc (or 10 cc/g) was chosen as the point at which oxidation had proceeded sufficiently to destroy useful physical and dielectric properties of the polymeric composition. Duplicate samples were prepared for each composition at a variety of temperatures both above and below the melting point of the polymer itself.

At 0.00215% by weight antioxidant, 550 hr at 90°C is required to effect oxidation in contrast with the control in which the same effect was reached after only 300 hr. At 0.01% by weight antioxidant, this effect was reached at 90°C after 1,300 hr.

ANTIOXIDANTS FOR OTHER POLYMERS

ANTIOXIDANTS FOR POLYAMIDES

Synergistic Phosphite-Diamine Mixtures for Caprolactam

Nylon 6, a nylon obtained by polycondensation of epsilon-caprolactam (aminocaproic lactam), has been stabilized by aryl phosphites and by para-phenylenediamines. The process developed by *J.H. Tazewell; U.S. Patent 3,644,280; February 22, 1972; assigned to The Firestone Tire & Rubber Company* discloses nylon 6 which contains a tri(alkylphenyl) phosphite and a para-phenylenediamine (referred to herein as PPD) which act synergistically to stabilize nylon. The tri(alkylphenyl) phosphites include those in which the alkyl group contains 8 to 12 carbons. A preferred phosphite is tri(mixed nonylphenyl) phosphite known commercially as Polygard. Other phosphites (and mixed phosphites) which may be used include the trioctylphenyl, the trinonylphenyl, the tridecylphenyl, the triundecylphenyl, and the tridodecylphenyl. They include also mixtures of phosphites containing alkyl groups of different lengths.

The PPD derivatives which may be used include N,N'-disubstituted aromatic and aliphatic derivatives. A preferred derivative is N,N'-di-beta-naphthyl PPD. Other derivatives which may be used include the other known N,N'-disubstituted PPD antioxidants (see Ambelang et al "Antioxidants and Antiozonants for General Elastomer Purposes," *Rubber Chemistry and Technology*, 36:5, page 1497, December 1963), including N,N'-diphenyl PPD, N,N'-dicyclohexyl PPD, N-cyclohexyl-N'-phenyl PPD, N,N-dihexyl PPD, N-hexyl-N'-phenyl PPD, etc. The amount of the stabilizer components used will be any stabilizing amount, such as 0.05 to 1.0 part each of the PPD derivative and the phosphite per 100 parts by weight of the nylon, 30 to 70% by weight of the one component being used with 70 to 30% of the other component.

To illustrate the process, nylon 6 (polycaprolactam) was prepared according to the following formula:

	Parts by weight
Epsilon-caprolactam	100
n-Butylamine	0.46
Acetic acid	0.26
$Na_4P_2O_7 \cdot 10H_2O$	0.0008
Water	1.4

Different samples of the reaction mixture were treated with stabilizers as shown in the table that follows. Each of the preparations was sealed and heated in a circulating air oven at 260°C for 16 hours to form a low-molecular-weight polymer. Then the condensation polymers were converted to higher molecular-weight polymer by heating to 260°C with the pressure reduced to 0.2 mm of mercury. The resultant polymers were melt spun into 18 filament yarns which were subsequently drawn 4.0/1.0 over a 310°F hot plate. The drawn yarns were aged at constant length on a metal rack in a circulating air oven at 117°C for 16 hours. The aged fiber strengths were compared with the unaged strengths, and the results are expressed as percent retained tenacity in the following table. (In the table, the parenthetical expressions stand for parts per hundred of the nylon.)

Run No.	DBNP [1] (p.p.h.)	Polygard [2] (p.p.h.)	Percent retained tenacity yarn aged 16 hours at 177° C.
1	0.1		76.3
2		0.2	20.0
3	None	None	17.0
4	0.1	0.1	95.9

[1] DBNP stands for di-N,N'-beta-naphthyl-para-phenylenediamine. (R. T. Vanderbilt Company's AGE-RITE WHITE.)
[2] Polygard is tri(mixed nonylphenyl) phosphite produced by Naugatuck Chemical Company, a division of Uniroyal.

It is seen that the di-N,N'-beta-naphthyl-para-phenylenediamine and the Polygard had a synergistic stabilizing effect, because the yarn containing the mixture lost very little tenacity.

Ternary Stabilizing Systems

H. Linhart and H. Mueller; U.S. Patent 3,787,355; January 22, 1974; assigned to Ciba-Geigy Corporation have disclosed stabilizing systems for polyamides comprising: (a) a phenolic antioxidant, (b) a derivative of phosphorus and (c) a salt of divalent manganese with inorganic or organic acids. More specifically, the system consists of: (a) a compound of the formula:

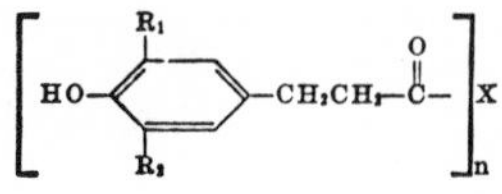

$$\left[HO \underset{R_2}{\overset{R_1}{-\!\!\!\bigcirc\!\!\!-}} CH_2CH_r \overset{O}{\overset{\|}{C}} \right]_n X$$

where R_1 is hydrogen or alkyl containing 1 to 5 carbons, R_2 is alkyl containing 1 to 5 carbons, X is one of the groups:

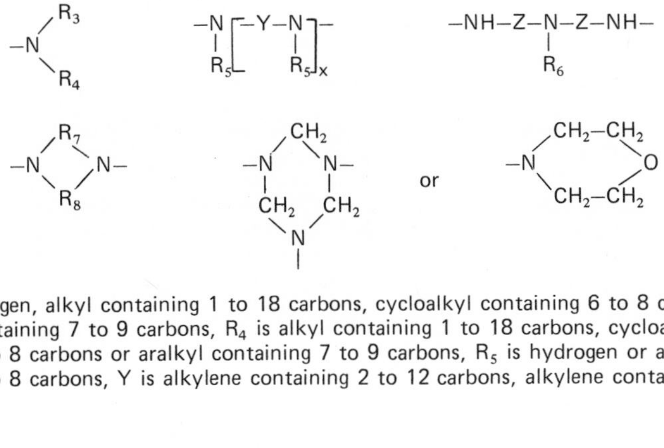

$$-N\begin{smallmatrix}R_3\\ \\R_4\end{smallmatrix} \qquad -N\left[-Y-N\right]_x \begin{smallmatrix}R_5\end{smallmatrix} \qquad -NH-Z-N-Z-NH-\\ \qquad\qquad\qquad R_6$$

$$-N\begin{smallmatrix}R_7\\ \\R_8\end{smallmatrix}N- \qquad -N\begin{smallmatrix}CH_2\\ \\CH_2 \quad CH_2\\ N\end{smallmatrix}N- \quad or \quad -N\begin{smallmatrix}CH_2-CH_2\\ \\CH_2-CH_2\end{smallmatrix}O$$

R_3 is hydrogen, alkyl containing 1 to 18 carbons, cycloalkyl containing 6 to 8 carbons or aralkyl containing 7 to 9 carbons, R_4 is alkyl containing 1 to 18 carbons, cycloalkyl containing 6 to 8 carbons or aralkyl containing 7 to 9 carbons, R_5 is hydrogen or alkyl containing 1 to 8 carbons, Y is alkylene containing 2 to 12 carbons, alkylene containing 2 to

8 carbons interrupted by cyclohexylene or phenylene or is cyclohexylene, R_6 is alkyl containing 1 to 8 carbons, the group Z—NH— or the direct bond, Z is alkylene containing 2 to 6 carbons, R_7 and R_8 are alkylene containing 1 to 4 carbons and together with both nitrogen atoms form a 6-membered ring, n = 1 to 3 and x = 1 to 3, (b) a compound of the formula:

$$(O{=})_m \overset{\overset{\textstyle R_9}{\textstyle |}}{\underset{\underset{\textstyle R_{11}}{\textstyle |}}{P}}{-}R_{10}$$

where R_9, R_{10} and R_{11} are the same or different and are alkyl containing 1 to 18 carbons, cycloalkyl containing 6 to 8 carbons, aralkyl containing 7 to 12 carbons, phenyl, alkylphenyl containing 7 to 10 carbons, hydroxy, alkoxy containing 1 to 18 carbons, cycloalkoxy containing 6 to 8 carbons, aralkoxy containing 7 to 9 carbons, phenoxy or alkylphenoxy containing 7 to 15 carbons and m represents 0 or 1, or consists of a mono- or divalent salt of a mono- or polyvalent oxyacid of phosphorus, and (c) a salt of divalent manganese with inorganic or organic acids. This mixture prevents the deleterious yellowing of polyamide fibers under thermofixing conditions and simultaneously effects good light resistance and excellent long term protection against loss of tensile properties caused by the action of heat.

Example: Long Term Protection of Nylon 6 Against Degradation by Heat — The stabilizers listed in the following table are sprinkled dry on polyamide 6 granules prepared by the conventional process in an autoclave and in which the light-protective combination of 50 ppm Mn as Mn(II) acetate and 0.025% sodium hexametaphosphate, and the delustering agent 1.87% TiO$_2$ (Anatas), have already been polymerized, and the resulting mixtures are spun directly via extruders to 20 denier monofilaments. These filaments are subsequently tempered in a forced draft oven for 24, 48, 72, 96 and 120 hours at 165°C and the relative viscosities in 1% H$_2$SO$_4$ solution are determined after the various oven aging times. The results are given in the following table.

		After Oven Aging at 165°C, hours				
Stabilizers	Untreated	24	48	72	96	120
Without stabilizer	2.40	1.45	1.39			
0.5% stabilizer 1	2.40		2.33	2.10	2.0	1.80	1.58
Comparison according to prior art; 0.5% stabilizer 2	2.40	1.92	1.60	1.45		

Stabilizer 1 is 1,6-bis[3-(3,5-di-tert-butyl-4-hydroxyphenyl)propionamido]-hexane.
Stabilizer 2 is 1,3,5-tris-(3,5-di-tert-butyl-4-hydroxy-benzyl)-2,4,6-trimethylbenzene.

ANTIOXIDANTS FOR POLYURETHANES

Hindered Hydroxybenzylanisole Antioxidants

Phenols such as 4,4'-alkylidene-bis-(6-tert-butyl-m-cresol), 2,6-di-tert-butyl-4-methylphenol or 4,4'-methylene-bis-(2,6-di-tert-butylphenol) have been tested as stabilizers but they either initially discolor polyurethane or they fail to provide protection against discoloration under the action of light or substances present in the atmosphere. The use of polyphenols such as 1,3,5-trimethyl-2,4,6-tris-(3,5-di-tert-butyl-4-hydroxy-benzyl)-benzene has also been proposed as stabilizers. Furthermore, numerous phenolic compounds are said to be suitable for stabilizing polyurethanes when used together with hydroxybenzophenones. The effect of these phenolic stabilizers, however, is not sufficient or is not wash resistant or the stabilizers themselves have a color which makes them unsuitable, e.g., for use with white elastomer threads.

R. Nast, H. Oertel and K. Ley; U.S. Patent 3,642,669; February 15, 1972; assigned to Farbenfabriken Bayer AG, Germany have developed a class of phenolic stabilizers which owing to their typical structure provide a highly effective stabilization of polyurethane in threads and foils. Moreover, these stabilizers are colorless, cause no discoloration of the polyurethane and provide substantially better, wash-resistant protection against discoloration and degradation under the action of light and/or substances present in the atmosphere. The polyurethanes are stabilized by the use of 0.05 to 10% by weight of alkoxy substituted, sterically hindered, phenols of formula

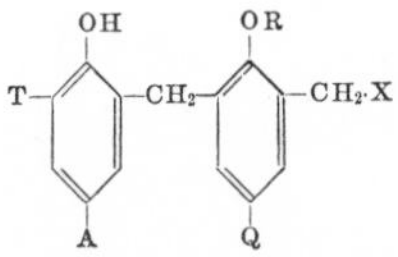

T = a tertiary alkyl group, e.g., a tert-butyl, tert-amyl, tert-octyl or tert-dodecyl radical, preferably the tert-butyl radical

A = a primary or secondary alkyl having 1 to 12 carbons, preferably methyl, isononyl or the radical T

R = a primary alkyl having 1 to 12 carbons, preferably methyl, or an aralkyl radical, preferably benzyl

Q = the group A or T, preferably methyl, isononyl, tert-butyl or tert-octyl or an OR group, preferably methoxy or benzyloxy

X = hydrogen or

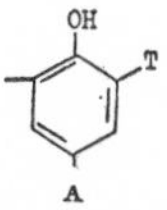

where $CH_2 \cdot X$ stands in the 6-position when Q is alkyl and in the 5-position when Q is OR.

The phenolic compounds can be prepared by reacting 2-tert-alkyl-4-alkylphenols with o-hydroxymethyl-alkoxybenzenes in the presence of catalytic quantities of strong acids, water being split off in the process. The substantial improvement which can be achieved by using the alkoxy-substituted, sterically hindered phenols is demonstrated in comparison tests using, for comparison, corresponding compounds which contain a free hydroxyl group instead of the alkoxy substituent. In the comparison tests, a phenol, namely 1,3,5-trimethyl-2,4,6-tris-(3,5-di-tert-butyl-4-hydroxybenzyl)-benzene which may be regarded as one of the most effective phenolic compounds of those previously known is also included.

It is then found, inter alia, that equivalent phenols show a strong discoloration of their own (yellow), compared with the stabilizer which contains an alkoxy group instead of the middle hydroxyl group, and they are therefore unsuitable for stabilizing colorless polyurethanes. Also the alkoxy substituted phenols show better stabilization to degradation than, for example, the pure phenolic stabilizer 1,3,5-trimethyl-2,4,6-tris-(4-hydroxy-3,5-di-tert-butyl-benzyl)-benzene.

Example 1: A solution of 200 g (1.22 mol) of 2-tert-butyl-p-cresol and 1 g of p-toluene-sulfonic acid in 500 ml of toluene is heated to boiling in a water separator. A solution of 100 g (0.55 mol) of 1-methoxy-4-methyl-2,6-di-hydroxy-methyl-benzene in 150 ml of toluene heated to 100°C is then slowly introduced dropwise in the course of 6 hours. The reaction mixture is then heated to boiling for a further 3 hours and 1.3 liters of light petrol is then added at about 80°C, the solution is cooled and after it has been left to stand for several hours the crystals which separate are removed by suction filtration. Eighty-eight grams of 4-methyl-2,6-bis-(2'-hydroxy-3'-tert-butyl-5'-methyl-benzyl)-anisole (Stabilizer A) are obtained in the form of colorless crystals. MP 188° to 190°C.

Stabilizer A

Example 2: 800 parts of a polytetramethylene ether diol (molecular weight 1,010), 17.4 parts of N,N-bis-(β-hydroxypropyl)-N-methylamine, 306.6 parts of diphenylmethane-4,4'-di-isocyanate and 284 parts of chlorobenzene are heated to 65° to 75°C for 52 minutes and then cooled at room temperature. 400 parts of this NCO prepolymer solution (1.88% NCO) are introduced in the course of 4 minutes, with rapid stirring, into a fresh suspension prepared by adding 15 parts of solid carbon dioxide to a solution of 5.93 parts of ethylene diamine in 898 parts of dimethyl-formamide, a homogeneous, viscous, slightly yellowish elastomer solution being obtained. This solution is pigmented by the addition of 4% by weight (based on the solid elastomer substance) of titanium dioxide (rutile). Portions of this elastomer solution (viscosity 423 poises) with and without stabilizer are converted into films in the usual manner and these films are cut up into threads which are then exposed to UV light (Fade-Ometer) (see table below).

In a similar reaction to that described in the above Example, 2% by weight of stabilizer A (6.52 parts) were not added subsequently to the finished elastomer solution but dissolved in dimethylformamide together with the ethylene diamine, and the elastomer solution was then prepared from the NCO prepolymer. A homogeneous, viscous, completely colorless elastomer solution which did not discolor even on exposure to air was obtained. After the solution had been cast to form films and the threads had been exposed to light, a practically identical stabilizing effect against mechanical degradation under exposure to light was measured.

	Fade-Ometer exposure									
	Before exposure to light		22 hours		44 hours		66 hours		88 hours	
Stabilizer	Tensile strength, g./denier	Elon-gation, percent	Tensile strength, g./denier	Elon-gation, percent	Tensile strength, g./denier	Elon-gation, percent	Tensile strength, g./denier	Elon-gation, percent	Tensile strength, g./denier	Elon-gation, percent
Without the addition of stabilizer.	0.60 Discoloration: almost colourless	584	<0.03 Yellow	<100	Not measurable Yellowish brown		Yellowish brown		Yellowish brown	
Plus 2% stabilizer A............	0.60 Discolouration: colourless	585	0.60 Colourless	586	0.59 Almost colourless	587	0.58 Almost colourless	580	0.18 Slightly yellowish	330

Synergistic stabilization of the polyurethanes is also obtained using a mixture of the sterically hindered anisol and a 2-(2'-hydroxyphenyl)-benzotriazole.

Mixed Phenol-Phosphite Antioxidants for Polyurethane Foam

Flexible, open-cell, polyurethane foams are prepared by reacting an aliphatic, or an aliphatic-like, organic polyisocyanate, such as dimethyl benzene ω,ω'-diisocyanate (xylylene di-isocyanate) with an active-hydrogen-containing polyol in the presence of a mixed catalyst system comprising an alkanolamine, a stannous salt of a carboxylic acid, and a stannic salt of a carboxylic acid. Discoloration of the resulting foams can be prevented by including in the reaction mixture a mixed stabilizer system disclosed by *R.J. Lamplugh and F.W. Meisel, Jr.; U.S. Patent 3,772,218; November 13, 1973; assigned to Scott Paper Company.*

This system comprises a primary antioxidant, such as a high molecular weight hindered polyphenol, a secondary antioxidant, such as a high molecular weight phosphite and an ultraviolet light absorbing compound.

Representative primary antioxidants are Irganox 1010 (a high molecular weight hindered polyphenol); Plastinox 2246 [2,2'-methylene-bis(4-methyl-6-tert-butylphenol)]; Antioxidant No. 22 (N,N'-di-sec-butyl-para-phenylenediamine); Ionox 330 [1,3,5-trimethyl-2,4,6-tris(3,5-di-tert-butyl-4-hydroxy benzyl)benzene]. It has been found that the most preferred class of primary antioxidants are the high molecular weight hindered polyphenols.

Representative secondary antioxidants are Uvi-Nox 3100, a tri(mixed mono and dinonyl phenyl)phosphite; Wytox 345 and 348, polymeric phosphites; Plastanox LTDP, dilauryl thiodipropionate. The high molecular weight phosphites are especially preferred as secondary antioxidants.

Suitable ultraviolet light absorbing compounds, also called ultraviolet absorbers, are defined and described in *Modern Plastics Encyclopedia*, 1968, pages 406-409, and are listed in variety in the chart on pages 508 and 509. Important classes of useful ultraviolet screening agents for this stabilizing system include the hydroxyphenyl benzotriazoles, such as 2-(2'-hydroxyphenyl)benzotriazoles, the 2-hydroxybenzophenones, the substituted acrylonitriles, the salicylic acid derivatives and the 2-hydroxyphenyl-triazines. It is preferred to use at least 1.0 weight percent, based on the weight of polyol in the reaction mixture, of the ultraviolet light absorbing compound and 2.0 weight percent, also based on the weight of polyol in the reaction mixture, of the combined primary and secondary antioxidants. The ratio of primary antioxidant to secondary antioxidant is preferably from about 2:1 to 5:1 with a ratio of about 2.5:1 being especially preferred.

When the mixed stabilizer system described above is incorporated into the polyurethane foam-forming reaction mixture it is preferred, to achieve a stable foam, to include a surfactant such as those which are normally employed in rigid polyether-based foam systems. These surfactants are well known in the art and include, for example, DC-193, a silicone glycol copolymer. In carrying out the process, the one-shot technique for producing foam is usually employed at room temperature. In the one-shot method all of the ingredients, that is, the polyol, the aliphatic polyisocyanate, the foaming agent, the mixed catalyst system, the surfactant and the mixed stabilizer system are simultaneously mixed with each other by any suitable means and then poured into a mold where the foaming reaction takes place.

Example: Foams were prepared from the foam formulations shown in the table below in a one-shot process carried out at room temperature. The foam formulations contained both the mixed catalyst system and the mixed stabilizer system. The results also given in the table point out the improved stability of foams containing the mixed stabilizer system. Heat stability was tested by placing the foams in an oven set at 140°C for 22 hours. Light stability was tested by placing the foams in an Atlas Weatherometer where it was exposed to radiation from an enclosed carbon arc lamp source at a temperature of 145°F for 40 hours.

	A	B	C	D	E	F	G	H
Fomrez 50	100	100	100	100	100	100	100	100.
Surfactant	1.0	1.0	1.0	1.0	1.0	1.0	1.0	1.0.1
Stannous Octoate	1.0	1.0	1.0	1.0	1.0	1.0	1.0	1.0.
T-26 stannic	1.0	1.0	1.0	1.0	1.0	1.0	1.0	1.0.
Monoethanolamine	1.0	1.0	1.0	1.0	1.0	1.0	1.0	1.0.
Antioxidant (primary)	2.5	2.5	2.5	2.5	2.5	2.5	2.5	2.5.7
Antioxidant (secondary)	1.0	1.0	1.0	1.0	1.0	1.0	1.0	1.0.1
UV absorber	3.0	3.3	3.0	3.0	3.0	3.0	3.0	3.0.1
H₂O	3.0	3.0	3.0	3.0	3.0	3.0	3.0	3.0.
Xylylene diisocyanate	43.0	43.0	43.0	43.0	43.0	43.0	43.0	43.0.
Index	105	105	105	105	105	105	105	105.
Oven aging (22 hrs. at 140° C.):								
Color change	Dark brown	Light yellow	None	None	Slight discoloration.	Slight discoloration.	Slight discoloration.	Slight discoloration.
Tensile (p.s.i.)	8.8	12.9	12.1	11.4	12.7	12.2	11.0	14.1.
Initial tensile (p.s.i.)	14.3	15.3	14.6	13.0	14.2	14.3	14.4	18.1.
Weather-Ometer (40 hr. exposure):								
Color retention	Poor	Good	Excellent	Fair	Good	Fair	Excellent	Not evaluated.
Surface tack	Melted at 20 hrs.	Negligible	None	Tacky	Negligible	Negligible	Negligible	

The key to the additives indicated in the preceding table is as follows.

Surfactants	Antioxidants (Primary)	Antioxidants (Secondary)	UV Absorbers
[1]DC-193	[1]Irganox 858	[1]Plastanox LTDP	[1]Tinuvin 328
	[2]Irganox 1010		
	[3]Irganox 1076		
	[4]Plastanox 2246		
	[5]Antioxidant No. 22		
	[6]Topanol CA		
	[7]Ionox 330		

ANTIOXIDANTS FOR POLYETHERS

Phenol-Polyvinylpyrrolidone Complex for Formaldehyde Polymers

The process disclosed by *J. Ackermann, P. Radici and F. Ferre; U.S. Patent 3,692,876; September 19, 1972; assigned to Societa Italiana Resine SDR, SpA, Italy* provides for stabilizing formaldehyde polymers by a complex of a phenolic antioxidant with polyvinylpyrrolidone. This complex is produced by dissolving a polyvinylpyrrolidone having a molecular weight of 1,100 to 90,000 and a phenolic antioxidant in a common solvent or solvent mixture, and precipitating the complex compound of the polyvinylpyrrolidone and the phenolic antioxidant by adding to the resulting solution a nonsolvent for the complex compound. The complex compound is separated from the parent liquid subsequent to precipitation so that the complex compound is substantially free of unreacted polyvinylpyrrolidone and phenolic antioxidant.

The term common solvent means solvents which fully dissolve polyvinylpyrrolidone and the phenol antioxidant. Such solvents are alcohols or alcohol-ketone mixtures with the ketone content equaling, or lower than, 60% by volume. Preferred solvents for the purpose are methanol and mixtures thereof with acetone. Any common solvent can be used which does not interfere with complex formation. Further useful solvents are dialkyl formamides (such as dimethylformamide and diethylformamide) and dialkyl acetamides (such as dimethylacetamide and diethylacetamide).

The preferred nonsolvent is water. Further nonsolvents are liquid aliphatic hydrocarbons (such as hexane and heptane) and liquid mononuclear aromatic hydrocarbons (such as benzene and toluene). Generally, addition of the nonsolvent precipitates the complex in powder form. Preparation of the solution can be carried out at room temperature or even higher temperature in order to promote dissolution of the starting compounds, whereas the complex is usually precipitated at room temperature. The dissolution temperature is normally 20° to 80°C, preferably 20° to 60°C. The precipitation temperature is normally from 20° to 60°C, preferably 20° to 40°C. In the preferred embodiment of the process, the stabilizing complex compound is precipitated in the presence of the formaldehyde polymer to thereby obtain a stabilizer-rich master batch.

Example 1: Fifteen liters of a solution in methanol containing 8.4 grams of 4,4-thio-bis-(6-tert-butyl-3-methylphenol) and 8.0 grams of polyvinylpyrrolidone (having a molecular weight of approximately 90,000) per 100 ml of solution, were fed into a thermostatically controlled vessel equipped with a stirrer. The temperature was maintained between 45° and 55°C, while 3.5 kg of powdered acetylated polyformaldehyde and then 30 liters of desalinated water were slowly added. The polyformaldehyde had a molecular weight of 35,000, and was obtained by polymerization of pure formaldehyde, in toluene and in the presence of a polymerization catalyst. The crude polymer thus obtained was then acetylated with acetic anhydride to lock the terminal groups of the macromolecules.

A fine and homogenous suspension was thus obtained, which was filtered in a centrifuge. The mother liquor after the filtration was clear, and the residue after evaporation at 110°C amounted to less than 0.02 gram per 100 ml. The batch of solid precipitate was washed thoroughly in the centrifuge with hot distilled water, scraped from the centrifuge and dried in air in a drier employing a pneumatic conveyor system. There was thus obtained 5.88 kg of a composition rich in stabilizer, in the form of a powder having a granulometry and apparent density analogous to those of the polyformaldehyde. 5 further kg of acetylated polyformaldehyde were mixed with 37 g of this composition so as to reduce the content of stabilizer to 0.7%, by weight of the polymer. The composition was extruded in the form of granules of a diameter of approximately 2 mm, in a worm-type extrusion press, at a temperature of 190° to 220°C. The following tests were performed on these granules.

(a) Thermal degradation at 220°C in a nitrogen atmosphere (K_{220}): measured by the speed of decomposition, expressed in percentage by weight of the polymer per minute during the first 30 minutes.

(b) Degradation in air at 220°C (D_{220}): measured by the loss in weight, expressed in percentage of the polymer, after 10 and 20 minutes of heating at 220°C. The color of the polymer after extrusion was also noted.

The results for Examples 1 and 2 are listed in the following table.

Example 2: Equal parts by weight of 4,4-thio-bis-(6-tert-butyl-3-methylphenol) and polyvinylpyrrolidone of a molecular weight of 90,000 were crushed and intimately mixed together, and the mixture was added to the formaldehyde polymer of Example 1 in quantities corresponding to 0.35% of each by weight of polymer. The polymer containing the stabilizer was then shaped into granules and tested as in Example 1.

Example	K_{220}	D_{220} 10 Minutes	20 Minutes	Color
1	0.07	0.4	1.0	White
2	0.12	0.8	1.5	Pink-fawn

Alkanolamines with Phosphites and Sulfides for Polyphenylene Ethers

Polyphenylene ether polymers or blends with another polymer are stabilized by *A. Katchman and R.M. Summers; U.S. Patent 3,761,541; September 25, 1973; assigned to General Electric Company* with alkanolamines, alone or with an inorganic sulfide and/or organic phosphite. A preferred composition comprises a blend of a poly(2,6-dialkyl-1,4-phenylene)ether and a polystyrene stabilized with a mixture of the alkanolamine, organic phosphite and inorganic sulfide as the combination of stabilizers. Oxides of metals such as zinc may be added to the compositions which contain inorganic sulfides to provide additional stability.

The alkanolamine stabilizer may be represented by the formula NR_3 where each R is independently hydrogen or (lower)alkanol having 1 to 4 carbons, provided that at least two Rs are alkanol. Typical alkanolamines include diethanolamine, triethanolamine, tripropanolamine, dibutanolamine and the like. In general, the alkanolamine may constitute from 0.1 to 6.0% by weight of the total formulation. The particular inorganic sulfide used in combination with the alkanolamine is not critical. Examples of suitable sulfides include the sodium, potassium, calcium, barium, zirconium, titanium, nickel, manganese, iron, cobalt, chromium, copper, zinc, cadmium, mercurous and mercuric, tin, lead, and the like. Preferred sulfides are those of zinc and cadmium. Preferably, the sulfide in the formulation comprises at least 0.1% by weight and most preferably, from 0.1 to 6.0% by weight of the total formulation.

In addition, an organic phosphite may be included in the stabilizer formulation. Phosphites include those compounds of the formula

$$RO-P\begin{matrix}OR\\ \\OR\end{matrix}$$

where R is independently selected from hydrogen and substituted and unsubstituted hydrocarbon groups containing up to 20 carbons including saturated and unsaturated, straight, branched chain and monocyclic and polycyclic groups. Suitable examples are those where R is hydrogen, straight or branched chain alkyl of 1 to 20 carbons, alkenyl of 1 to 20 carbons, (lower)-alkylphenyl, phenyl, halo alkyl of 1 to 20 carbons, and substituted phenyl where the substituents may include one or more halogen, hydroxy or (lower)alkyl groups. The permissible concentration range for the phosphite is about the same as that for the sulfide and alkanolamine, but where the three are used in combination, the lower limits of the range are preferred such as for example, between about 0.1 to 2.0% for each of the stabilizers in the combination. The following examples serve to illustrate the stabilization.

Examples 1 through 8: A blend was prepared comprising 45 parts of a poly(2,6-dimethyl-1,4-phenylene) ether (PPO polyphenylene ether, General Electric), 55 parts of a high impact polystyrene (Lustrex HT-91, Monsanto, believed to contain about 9% butadiene), 1.5 parts polyethylene, and various quantities of cadmium sulfide and diethanolamine. Test specimens were prepared by passing 25 pounds of the powder blend through a Reifenhauser S60 vented extruder to form an extruded strand which was chopped into pellets. One gram samples of these pellets were heated in a pure oxygen atmosphere at 125°C and the time necessary for uptake of 5 cubic centimeters of oxygen per gram of polymer blend (cc/g) determined. The amount of cadmium sulfide and triethanolamine used and the results obtained are set forth in the following table.

Example	Triethanolamine, phr	Cadmium Sulfide, phr	Uptake Time, hr
1	0.02	0.02	195
2	0.03	0.03	210
3	0.10	0.10	230
4	0.15	0.15	260
5	0.30	0.30	250
6	1.50	1.50	200
7	0	0.60	60
8	0.50	0	50
Control	0	0	25

From the data, it can be seen that significant improvement in resistance to oxygen uptake is realized by even small additions of triethanolamine, but combining the triethanolamine with cadmium sulfide provides substantial improvement that is greater than a merely additive effect.

Examples 9 through 14: The blending and extrusion procedures of Examples 1 through 8 are repeated with a 50/50 blend of a poly(2,6-dimethyl-1,4-phenylene) ether and a high impact polystyrene with various mixed stabilizers. The resultant pellets were molded into tensile specimens and thermal aging was carried out by placing these specimens in an air circulating oven maintained at 125°C. Samples were considered brittle when they broke without yielding. Stabilizer formulations and results are set forth in the following table.

Example	Additive, phr	Time to Embrittlement at 120°C, days
9	ZnS (0.50)	7
10	TEOA (0.50)	8
11	TEOA (0.25) ZnS (0.25)	15
12	TDP (0.25) ZnS (0.25)	14
13	TDP (0.25) TEOA (0.25) ZnS (0.25)	34
14	TDP (0.50) TEOA (0.50) ZnS (0.50)	36

TEOA – triethanolamine
TDP – tridecylphosphite

From this data, it can be seen that there is a synergism in the combination of the sulfide with the triethanolamine and there is an even greater synergism exhibited by the further combination with the phosphite.

ANTIOXIDANTS FOR POLYVINYL CHLORIDE

Mixed Liquid Stabilizers Containing Polyglycerol Esters

Multicomponent stabilizers are extensively used for the stabilization of polyvinyl chloride resins. Such stabilizer systems, sometimes referred to as stabilizer packages, are commonly used due to the inability of any one material to sufficiently protect the resins against oxidative, thermal and photochemical degradation and to impart other desirable properties to the resin.

P.H. Rhodes and R.L. Ahr; U.S. Patent 3,755,200; August 28, 1973; assigned to Emery Industries, Inc. have developed homogeneous liquid stabilizer solutions for improving the heat stability and antifogging and antistatic properties of the resin. The stabilizer solutions are comprised of a partial ester of a polyglycerol, a metal salt of a monocarboxylic fatty acid, an epoxy plasticizer and an organic phosphorous compound. They are homogeneous solutions which do not undergo phase separation when allowed to stand at ambient conditions for prolonged periods. These stabilizer compositions are obtained through the use of a specific blending technique which consists of first forming a solution of the metal salt, the epoxy compound and the organo-phosphorous compound by heating at a temperature from 125° up to 200°C to effect solution. The polyglycerol partial ester is then added to the resulting clear uniform solution and blended therewith.

Stabilizer systems prepared following this procedure are liquids which do not separate upon standing and which can be readily blended with polyvinyl chloride employing conventional process equipment. The so-prepared liquid stabilizer may also be blended with plasticizers and employed as a master-batch. Polyvinyl chloride resins compounded with these liquid stabilizers exhibit a high degree of resistivity to oxidative, thermal and photochemical degradation as well as having improved antistatic and antifogging properties. The following examples illustrate the preparation and use of these solutions. In the examples all parts and percentages are given on a weight basis unless otherwise indicated.

Example 1: A polyglycerol partial ester was prepared as follows: 1,980 grams (8.33 mol) of a polyglycerol having a hydroxyl value of about 1,280 which corresponds to about 2.3 glycerol units condensed, 1,287 grams (8.33 mol) mixed fatty acids comprised of C_8 to C_{10} normal acids and 1,155 grams (4.14 mol) oleic acid were combined in a flask. The reaction mixture was heated (235°C maximum) with stirring and allowed to react until the acid value of the mixture was substantially nil. About 30% of polyglycerol hydroxy groups were reacted. The reaction mixture was then cooled and stored for subsequent use. No catalyst was employed for this esterification reaction, however, similar esterifications were conducted employing hypophosphorous acid.

Example 2: A liquid stabilizer composition having superior antifogging and antistatic properties was prepared as follows: 280 grams zinc stearate, 200 grams epoxidized soybean oil and 520 grams tri(nonylphenyl) phosphite were heated at 150°C and the heating terminated when a clear solution was obtained. After cooling the mixture to about 60°C, 3,000 grams of the polyglycerol partial ester of Example 1 was added with stirring. The resulting clear, homogeneous liquid stabilizer was compounded with polyvinyl chloride resin to prepare a meat packaging film in accordance with the following recipe.

	Parts
Polyvinyl chloride homopolymer	100
Dioctyl adipate	18
Epoxidized soybean oil	9
Ethylene-bis-stearamide	0.25
Liquid stabilizer	2.5

The ingredients were blended and milled at 350°F for about 5 minutes. Thirty-five mil and 3 mil clear sheets were obtained. Oven heat stability tests were conducted using 1 x 1 inch squares cut from the 35 mil sheet by placing the samples on eight glass trays fitted on a rotating device in an electric oven maintained at 375°F. The heating is continued for 80 minutes with one glass slide being removed after each ten minute interval. Each slide is cooled after removal from the oven and the test specimen removed for observation and comparison. Samples stabilized with the above stabilizer withstood the entire 80-minute heating period without failure, that is, without degradation or severe discoloration and charring. After 80 minutes the samples were clear and had an amber color.

Liquid stabilizer compositions are also provided by *P.H. Rhodes and R.L. Ahr; U.S. Patent 3,759,856; September 18, 1973; assigned to Emery Industries, Inc.* which are obtained by mixing a Group II metal halide with a polyglycerol partial ester. This discovery is particularly surprising when it is considered that Group II metal halides have heretofore generally been thought to be detrimental to vinyl halide resins. The liquid stabilizers are solutions, achieved by first dissolving the metal halide in a small amount of water and then mixing with the partial ester, which do not undergo phase separation when allowed to stand at ambient conditions for prolonged periods. Preferred compositions consist of zinc chloride or zinc chloride in combination with one or more other metal chlorides with a polyglycerol partial ester derived from a polyglycerol containing 2 to 10 condensed glycerol units and an aliphatic or aromatic monocarboxylic acid containing 6 to 24 carbons.

The polyglycerol partial esters will have no more than 75%, and preferably less than 50%, of the hydroxyl groups reacted to the ester. The metal halide to polyglycerol partial ester ratio is such that the metal content in the liquid stabilizer is between 0.1 and 10% by weight. The stabilizers are used in amounts so that between about 0.01 and 2% of the metal is present in the compounded resin which is preferably a vinyl chloride homopolymer or copolymer.

In another embodiment of this process an organophosphorous compound may be included in the liquid stabilizer in an amount up to about 25% by weight. The following examples illustrate the preparation of the polyglycerol ester and uses of the combined liquid stabilizer in polyvinyl chloride. In the examples all parts and percentages are given on a weight basis unless otherwise indicated.

Example 1: A polyglycerol partial ester was prepared as follows: 1,920 grams of a polyglycerol having a hydroxyl value of about 1,280 (an average of 2.3 condensed glycerol units), and 2,496 grams mixed C_{8-10} normal fatty acids were combined in a flask. The reaction mixture was heated at a maximum temperature of 240°C with continuous stirring in the presence of 8 grams of a 30% solution of hypophosphorous acid. The resulting ester contained about 55% unreacted hydroxyl groups.

Example 2: A liquid stabilizer was prepared by dissolving 2.75 parts anhydrous zinc chloride in 2.75 parts water. When the zinc chloride had dissolved and the solution cooled to room temperature 94.5 parts of the polyglycerol partial ester of Example 1 was added with stirring. The resulting clear light amber liquid was used to stabilize polyvinyl chloride resin. The formulation used to obtain a semirigid composition was as follows.

	Parts
Polyvinyl chloride homopolymer	100.0
Impact modifier (Blendex 401)	17.0
Epoxidized soybean oil (6.8 – 7.0 oxirane value)	15.0
Stearic acid	0.5
Liquid stabilizer	2.0

The ingredients were blended and milled at 350°F for about 5 minutes. Water-white films suitable for vacuum forming and having excellent heat stability and antifogging and antistatic properties were obtained. To demonstrate the heat stability of the stabilized resins, 1" x 1" squares were cut from 35 mil sheet and the samples placed in eight glass trays which were fitted in a rotating device in an electric oven maintained at 375°F. The heating was conducted for 80 minutes and a single sample removed at ten-minute intervals. After cooling the test specimens were observed for discoloration and other signs of polymer degradation. Samples stabilized with the above liquid stabilizer withstood the entire 80-minute heating without failure, that is, without degradation and severe discoloration and charring. After 80 minutes the samples were clear with only slight coloration (light amber).

Synergistic Stabilizers Containing Phenolic Antioxidant

R.D. Dworkin and C.H. Stapfer; U.S. Patent 3,649,577; March 14, 1972; assigned to Carlisle Chemical Works, Inc. have developed synergistic stabilizers containing low cost metal soaps for the stabilization of halogenated resins against thermal degradation. It was found that various polyvinyl chloride formulations could be effectively stabilized against heat degradation by incorporating a mixture of magnesium maleate and a zinc carboxylate and, optionally, a phenolic antioxidant to the resin blend. The addition of small amounts of a zinc soap to magnesium maleate increases the long term stability of a resin formulation as well as improves its early color. This discovery was unexpected, since most magnesium salts have very little if any stabilizing activity when used by themselves.

The addition of zinc salts of carboxylic acids such as stearic or 2-ethylhexoic acids exhibits a synergistic influence on the efficacy of the magnesium salt thus improving the long term stability of the resin blend by nearly 100%. The early color is also significantly improved by these synergistic stabilizers. The resins stabilized with these synergistic combinations may also contain conventional lubricants, pigments, plasticizers, solvents and the like. These materials, like the resins, are preferably those sanctioned for food packaging use.

Example: Formulations were prepared containing 100 parts of VC-80, a suspension polyvinyl chloride resin (Borden), 10 parts of dioctyl phthalate, 5 parts of an epoxidized soybean oil, and 0.25 part of stearic acid. These were respectively stabilized with 1.5 parts of magnesium maleate alone, the same amount of a mixture of magnesium maleate with 2.5% of zinc stearate, the same amount of a mixture of magnesium maleate with zinc octoate, the same amount of each zinc carboxylate-magnesium maleate mixture containing 5% of para nonyl phenol and the same amount of each zinc carboxylate-magnesium maleate mixture containing 2,6-di-tert-butyl-para-cresol.

The very slow color development of the formulations containing the magnesium maleate-zinc carboxylate or magnesium maleate-zinc carboxylate-phenol systems as compared with the formulation containing magnesium maleate as sole stabilizer is shown by the results in the following table.

Resin formulation containing—	Time in minutes of exposure at 370° F. leading to—		
	First discoloration	Medium discoloration	Strong discoloration
1.5 parts of—			
Magnesium maleate		10	20
Mg mal.+Zn stearate	20		40
Mg mal.+Zn octoate	20		40
Mg mal.+Zn stear.+BHT	20	40	50
Mg mal.+Zn stear.+non. ph.	20	40	50
Mg mal.+Zn oct.+BHT	30		40
Mg mal.+Zn oct.+non. ph	20	40	50

The formulations were processed on a two roll mill at 320°F for 5 minutes, and exposed for one hour at 370°F in an air circulation oven. At 10 minute intervals a sample of each formulation was removed from the oven and compared for relative discoloration with the formulation containing no stabilizer.

ANTIOXIDANTS FOR FOODS

With the current restrictions placed on food additives, the emphasis in recent patents is on natural products for use as antioxidants in foods. Throughout this section, references are made to the following known food antioxidants by their codes or abbreviations: BHA, butylated hydroxanisole; BHT, butylated hydroxytoluene; NDGA, nordihydroguaiaretic acid; PG, propyl gallate.

SYNERGISTIC TOCOPHEROL MIXTURES FOR LIPIDS

Colamine and Ascorbic Acid Esters

The most frequently employed antioxidants for fats and vitamin A are tocopherols such as α- and γ-tocopherol and related compounds such as α-tocopheramine, N-methyl-γ-tocopheramine, BHA, BHT, NDGA, gallates, especially those esters of gallic acid with alcohols having at least 3 carbons, for example, propyl gallate, octyl gallate, decyl gallate, dodecyl gallate and 6-ethoxy-2,2,4-trimethyl-1,2-dihydroquinoline, as well as mixtures thereof.

Improved tocopherol antioxidant mixtures have been developed by *H. Klaui and W. Schlegel; U.S. Patent 3,637,772; January 25, 1972; assigned to Hoffmann-La Roche Inc.* In its broadest aspect, these mixtures are antioxidation compositions containing an antioxidant, colamine and/or a higher fatty acid salt thereof and a higher fatty acid ester of ascorbic acid.

It has been found that a particularly strong synergistic action is achieved with tocopherols, which in view of the physiological acceptability of these materials is of extraordinary importance. In this respect, α- and γ-tocopherol are advantageously utilized. Thus, the preferred composition contains as the antioxidant either α- or γ-tocopherol.

Colamine can be used as the base or as a salt with a higher fatty acid having 10 to 20 carbons. The palmitate and the stearate are the preferred salts. The ascorbic acid esters used are esters of higher fatty acids having from 10 to 20 carbons, preferably palmitic or stearic acid.

The amount of ingredients in the antioxidation compositions are suitable within broad ranges. Thus, for every part by weight of antioxidant, the amount of colamine or colamine salt can be from 0.1 to 50 parts by weight with 1 to 10 parts by weight preferred and the amount of ascorbic acid ester can be from 0.5 to 100 parts by weight with 1 to 10 parts by weight preferred. The amount of antioxidation composition used depends on the requirements of the substrate to be stabilized. Amounts between 0.01 and 0.1% by weight are generally sufficient with oils and fats, and amounts between 0.5 and 30% by weight are sufficient in the case of vitamin A preparations.

Example 1: Two grams of ascorbyl palmitate, 3 grams of sodium ascorbate, 0.5 gram of α-tocopherol, 0.6 gram of colamine and 1 gram of dextrin are dispersed in 20 milliliters of water at 50°C. The emulsion obtained is blended into 10 kilograms of sausage meat for hard sausages. The sausages manufactured therefrom have stability equivalent to those whose filling contains double the amount of ascorbyl palmitate and no colamine or α-to copherol.

Example 2: 1.5 grams of vitamin A palmitate, 1.5 grams of sunflower oil, 50 milligrams of α-tocopherol, 250 milligrams of ascorbyl palmitate, 250 milligrams of colamine palmitate, 200 milligrams of polyoxyethylene (2) oleyl ether (HLB value 4.9) and 0.3 milligram of copper oleate are heated to 60°C and homogeneously mixed. This mixture is stored in air at 45°C and the vitamin A retention is measured and compared to compositions without colamine and compositions without ascorbyl palmitate. After a storage time of 600 hours, the vitamin A retention in the composition prepared according to this example is 96%. In the composition without colamine, the vitamin A retention is 0% and in compositions without ascorbyl palmitate the vitamin A retention is about 10%.

Example 3: One kilogram of safflower oil with a natural content of tocopherols of about 400 milligrams per kilogram (about 320 milligrams thereof α-tocopherol) is treated with 100 milligrams of α-tocopherylamine, 200 milligrams of ascorbyl laurate and 20 milligrams of colamine palmitate. The stabilized oil is stored open in daylight at room temperature. The time lapse until the attainment of a peroxide number of 10 is 3.6 times longer than that for an oil without the addition of tocopherylamine, ascorbyl laurate and colamine palmitate, while without addition of ascorbyl laurate this protection factor is 3.3 and without colamine palmitate it is 3.1.

Unsaponifiable Component of Rice Oil

To prevent oxidation of lipid, for example, in instant fried vermicelli, it has been proposed to use an antioxidant made from BHA or BHT. Attempts have been made to find some natural substance to serve as antioxidant in place of a chemical antioxidant. In particular, it would be desirable to select a naturally occurring substance which eliminates the drawbacks of the above antioxidants. However, this has proved difficult in the light of the efficiency for antioxidation of BHA and BHT as well as the economical considerations involved.

S. Maruyama and T. Wakayama; U.S. Patent 3,752,832; August 14, 1973; assigned to Kongo Yakuhin KK, Japan have found that unsaponifiable matter of rice oil and tocopherol if used together have a remarkable effect in imparting lipids with heat resisting property in addition to antioxidation equal to BHA and BHT under the effect of synergism. Their use is also exceedingly economical. Furthermore, the effect of antioxidation for animal oil and fat such as lard and the like as well as vegetable oil and fat is increased by additionally using a synergist.

The quantities of unsaponifiable matter of rice oil and tocopherol may vary within wide limits, but it is desirable that the former be added in the range of 0.01 to 2% calculated on the amount of lipid while for the latter a range of 0.01 to 15% is advantageous. The ratio between the unsaponifiable matter of rice oil and the tocopherol is preferably in the range of 1:0.1 to 10:0.1.

As synergists may be used citric acid, ascorbic acid and their salts or esters, isoascorbic acid, phosphoric acid, condensed phosphate, cephalin and tartaric acid. Among them citric acid is most effective for vegetable lipid (such as cooking oil or margarine) where it forms a stable chelate compound with calcium, iron and nickel causing these trace metals to become inactive. Ascorbic acid and salts thereof, esters (vitamin C palmitate and stearate) and physiologically inactive isoascorbic acid (erythorbic acid, 2-ascorbic acid) are effective as the foregoing and are excellent synergists in phenolic antioxidants. Vitamin C is good for lactic liquid, powdery cereals and fatty fishes. Besides the foregoing as good synergist, phosphoric acid and condensed phosphate are good for maintaining the hue and color of edibles. Moreover, the effects of cephalin and tartaric acid of phosphatide containing N which are found in brain cells, nervous tissues and the yoke of an egg are considered suitable. In recent years, a very good effect of salts of cytracon (methyl maleic acid and phitinic acid, salt of inomitol, hexaphosphoric, Ca-Mg) was found.

Antioxidants made from unsaponifiable matter of rice oil, tocopherol and synergist exert high antioxidation power against lipid not only in heat treatment, but also in low temperature treatment (refrigeration) thereby. They have thus proved to be useful as stabilizers for refrigerated edibles.

Example: The test sample to be used is instant fried vermicelli, genuine lard (standard grade defined by JAS). The antioxidant to be applied is a mixture of unsaponifiable matter of rice oil and tocopherol, additive quantity of each of which is 0.2% and 0.05%. (Mixture of BHA and BHT at the rate of 400 ppm, 1:1 of additive quantity). Peroxide value (POV), functional test (luster of color, scent and condition), and the content of unsaponifiable matter of rice and oil and tocopherol are the categories of the test.

Test Conditions — The two kinds of instant fried vermicelli which served as samples are separately placed in lard baths. One of the lard baths contains the antioxidant while the other lard bath is devoid of antioxidant. After the immersion in the baths, the samples are fried well in the respective lard bath for 3 minutes at a temperature of 145 ± 3°C. The peroxide value measurement test and the odor-color-taste test are made immediately after the frying of the samples and under constant temperature and humidity conditions. The samples are then inspected for POV and are appraised for function. Test for variation of lapsed time is carried out under the following three different conditions with the constant temperature at 40°C, constant humidity (RH 60%) resulting in the data listed in the following table.

Sample	Reserving term of days	Oil solution—Lard solution					
		0 hour		5 hours		24 hours	
		POV	Function	POV	Function	POV	Function
Comparison	0	5.00	Good	8.11	Good	10.2	Good.
	7	10.9	do	31.2	Not so good	52.0	No good.
	14	55.0	No good	89.1	No good	138.0	Do.
	21	153.0	do	437.0	do	505.0	Do.
Unsaponifiable matter of rice oil and tocopherol.	0	4.50	Good	7.34	Good	8.96	Good.
	7	5.50	do	11.8	do	13.0	Do.
	14	6.20	do	14.0	do	16.3	Do.
	21	7.80	do	20.6	do	25.7	Do.
(BHA) and (BHT)	0	3.74	do	7.43	do	8.00	Do.
	7	3.90	do	13.0	do	15.1	Do.
	14	4.23	do	15.4	do	17.9	Do.
	21	4.60	do	23.7	do	24.3	Do.

REMARKS.—"Not so good" set forth in function column of the above table means inferiority of scent, "no good" means strong bad smell caused by rancidity.

ANTIOXIDANTS FROM RED CEDAR

The results of investigations relating to the extraction of chemicals such as plicatic acid and the polyphenols from western red cedar wood, the identification of these chemical constituents, the yields obtained and the methods used for the separation of the extract into its various components have been discussed in two articles entitled "The Polyphenols of Western Red Cedar" by Gardner, Barton and MacLean, *Can. J. Chem,* volume 37, pages 1703 to 1709, (1959), and "The Chemistry and Utilization of Western Red Cedar" by Dr. J.A.F. Gardner, *Department of Forestry Publication No. 1023,* 1963, Department of Forestry, Canada. These materials have shown value as natural antioxidants for food products.

Cedar Polyphenols—Thiodipropionic Acid Mixtures

The major portion of the cedar polyphenols is believed to be open chain substituted 2,3-dibenzyl butyrolactones having the following structural formula:

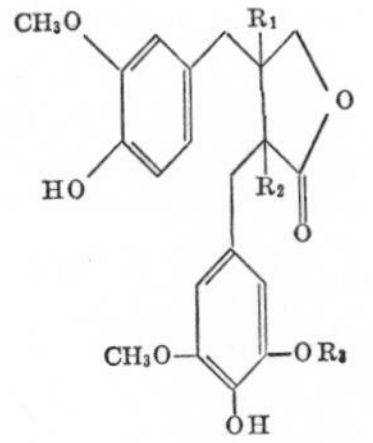

where R_1 is either H or OH, R_2 is either H or OH, and R_3 is either H or CH_3.

A. Karchmar; U.S. Patents 3,784,480; January 8, 1974; 3,628,971; December 21, 1971; both assigned to International Telephone and Telegraph Corporation has found that mixtures of cedar polyphenols and thiodipropionic acid where the amount of polyphenols in the mixtures is at least substantially equal to the amount of thiodipropionic acid therein, are synergistically more effective antioxidants for edible oils and fats than equivalent amounts of either component taken separately or in combination with other known antioxidants. It is preferred that the ratio of polyphenols to thiodipropionic acid used in antioxidant mixtures should be in a range of from 1:1 to 2:1.

Example: For purposes of study, the samples of fats and oils selected were free of antioxidants; commercial lard and oils of the same type containing antioxidants were used as subcontrols. BHT and BHA combined, cedar polyphenols and methionine combined, cedar polyphenols and 1-proline combined, methionine alone and 1-proline alone were introduced into antioxidant-free fat and oil samples for a straight comparison with polyphenol-thiodipropionic acid antioxidant mixtures.

A total of 40 samples of lard and oils was weighed into 150 milliliter beakers. A total of 40 samples of the various antioxidants was weighed, all in the same concentration of 0.015% based on the weight of lard or oil. Wherever a combination of two antioxidants was used (BHT + BHA, cedar polyphenols + methionine, and cedar polyphenols + 1-proline) or an antioxidant and a synergist (cedar polyphenols + thiodipropionic acid), respectively, the total mixture was weighed to represent 150 parts per million.

The various antioxidant samples were weighed into microbeakers, dissolved in a small amount of absolute ethanol and transferred quantitatively into the oil and lard. The latter were then slightly heated to evaporate the ethanol and placed in an air-aerated oven at 58°C (± 2°C). All samples in beakers were mixed with glass rods twice a day to permit an even exposure of oils and fats to the oven temperature.

The following table represents the effect of the various antioxidant additives in a sample of fresh lard as measured by its peroxide value (a measure of its oxidation) after a given period of time. It will be seen that the cedar polyphenols and thiodipropionic acid antioxidant additive was the most effective antioxidant tested.

Sample	Antioxidant additive	Concentration of antioxidants (p.p.m.)	Time (hrs.)	Peroxide test (m.e./ 1,000 gr.)
Lard [1]	Control	0	200	105.0
	Cedar polyphenols	150	500	100.0
	Thiodipropionic acid	150	300	102.5
	Methionine	150	200	82.5
	1-proline	150	200	95.0

(continued)

Sample	Antioxidant additive	Concentration of antioxidants (p.p.m.)	Time (hrs.)	Peroxide test (m.e./ 1,000 gr.)
Lard [1]	Cedar polyphenols ...	100		
	plus		500	92.5
	Methionine	50		
	Cedar polyphenols	100		
	plus		500	92.5
	1-proline	50		
	BHT	75		
	plus		500	82.5
	BHA	75		
	Cedar polyphenols	100		
	plus		500	50.0
	Thiodipropionic acid	50		

[1] Fresh deodorized initial peroxide value=0.5 m.e. per 1,000 gr.

Data on the stabilization of safflower oil were also included in both patents.

Plicatic Acid—Thiodipropionic Acid Mixtures

A. Karchmar and K.L. McDonald; U.S. Patent 3,573,936; April 6, 1971; assigned to Rayonier Incorporated have also found that a mixture of plicatic acid and thiodipropionic acid exhibits a synergistic antioxidant effect when added to animal fats and vegetable oils and foodstuffs containing these materials. The plicatic acid-thiodipropionic acid additive, which comprises substantially equal amounts of each component, greatly increases the storage life of fats and oils when added in amounts approximating 100 parts per million.

Plicatic acid has the following structure as shown by its chemical degradation products and x-ray crystallography in investigations by Gardner, Barton and MacLean, *Can. J. Chem.* 37, pages 1703 to 1709, (1959); Gardner, MacDonald and MacLean, *Can. J. Chem.* 38, pages 2387 to 2394, (1960) and Gardner, Swan, Sutherland and MacLean, *Can. J. Chem.* 44, pages 52 to 58, (1966).

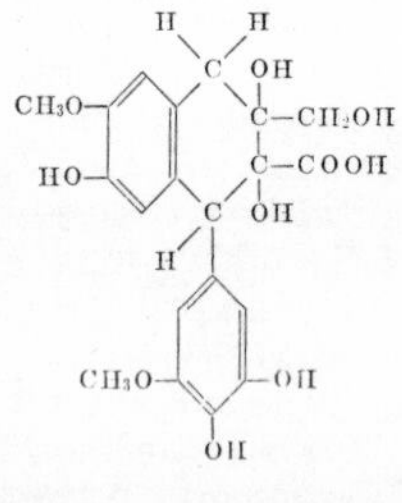

For purposes of the study, the samples of fats and oils selected were free of antioxidants; commercial lard and oils of the same type containing antioxidants were used as subcontrols. BHT and BHA combined with NDGA alone were introduced in antioxidant-free fat and oil for a straight comparison with plicatic acid.

A total of 54 samples of lard and oils was weighed into 150 milliliter beakers. A total of 54 samples of the various antioxidants was weighed, all in the same concentration of 0.01% based on the weight of lard or oil. Wherever a combination of two antioxidants was used (BHT + BHA) or an antioxidant and a synergist (plicatic acid + TDPA), respectively, each compound was weighed to represent 50 ppm or a total of 100. The antioxidants were weighed into microbeakers, dissolved in a small quantity of absolute ethanol, and transferred quantitatively into the lard and oils. The latter were then slightly heated to evaporate the ethanol and placed in an air-aerated oven at 57°C (± 2°C). All samples in beakers were mixed with glass rods twice a day to permit an even exposure of oils and fats to the oven temperature.

The table shown on the following page represents the effect of various antioxidant additives in a sample of fresh lard as measured by its peroxide value (a measure of its oxidation) at 450 hours. It will be seen that the plicatic acid plus TDPA antioxidant additive was the most effective antioxidant tested. Generally, the plicatic acid is used in amounts of from 50 to 150 ppm. More or less plicatic acid, however, can be used if desired. Concentrations of plicatic acid below 20 ppm are relatively ineffective, however, while it is soluble in oils to a concentration of the order of 150 ppm. Preferably, the ratio of TDPA to plicatic acid will vary from about 1:10 to 1:0.5. The sample of fresh, deodorized lard had an initial peroxide value of 0.5 milliequivalent per 1,000 grams.

Compound	Time (hours)	Peroxide Test meq per 1,000 grams
Plicatic acid, pure	450	32.5
Plicatic acid, crude	450	40.5
BHT + BHA	450	47.5
NDGA	450	37.5
Plicatic acid + TDPA	450	17.5
Commercial lard containing BHT + BHA + PG	450	25.0

The stabilization of safflower oil is also illustrated in the original patent.

Plicatic Acid Esters

Alkyl and aryl esters of plicatic acid and the use of these esters as antioxidants for fats and oils are disclosed by *J. Howard and T.D. McIntosh; U.S. Patent 3,644,481; February 22, 1972; assigned to ITT Rayonier Incorporated and U.S. Patent 3,754,937; August 28, 1973.*

The alkyl and aralkyl plicatates have been prepared by one or more of the following methods: (1) the direct esterification of pure plicatic acid tetrahydrate with the appropriate alkyl alcohol in the presence of an acid catalyst, (2) the direct esterification of crude red cedar extracts with methyl alcohol in the presence of an acid catalyst, (3) the replacement of the methyl group in methyl plicatate with a higher alkyl group by heating with a higher alcohol in the presence of an acid catalyst, (4) the acid catalyzed alcoholysis of plicatin (the lactone of plicatic acid) with an appropriate alkyl alcohol, and (5) the reaction of potassium plicatate with an appropriate alkyl or aralkyl halide. A large number of plicatic acid esters have been prepared by the foregoing methods and the antioxidant properties of these esters have been confirmed.

Example 1: Crystalline plicatic acid tetrahydrate (4.94 grams, 10 mmol) was dissolved in 25 ml of methanol containing 2.0 ml of concentrated sulfuric acid. The mixture was then seeded and set aside at room temperature in a stoppered flask for 4 days. During this time the white crystals of methyl plicatate which had deposited were removed by filtration, washed free of sulfuric acid, dried under high vacuum at 100°C and found to weigh 3.7 grams (85% yield). The melting point was 227° to 230°C with some decomposition (Leitz hot stage apparatus).

Example 2: A solution of 4 grams of plicatin (the lactone of plicatic acid, 10 mmol) in 15 ml of methanol containing 0.2 ml of concentrated sulfuric acid was gently refluxed with stirring. Within 10 minutes crystalline methyl plicatate began to separate from the reaction mixture. After 4 hours the reaction mixture was cooled and the product separated and washed with a little methanol. After drying, 3.5 grams of pure white material melting at 227° to 230°C were obtained (80% yield). This material was identical to methyl plicatate prepared as in Example 1.

Example 3: The plicatic acid esters were tested to determine the antioxidant properties or activity of these compounds. The antioxidant activity was evaluated by the standard AOCS method in which the relative worth of a particular compound is determined by the number of hours it takes for a sample of a given fat or oil containing 0.01% by weight of the compound to develop a peroxide value of 100 milliequivalents per 1,000 grams of oil or fat. This value of 100 is referred to as the standard of rancidity. The table shown below sets forth the relative effectiveness of the esters as compared with plicatin, plicatic acid and the pure substrate as antioxidants for lard based on the aforementioned standards of rancidity for these substrates.

Compound	Time in Hours to Standard Rancidity Value (100)
n-Propyl plicatate	37.5
Iso-propyl plicatate	37
Plicatin	36
n-Butyl plicatate	36
Plicatic acid	34.5
Ethyl plicatate	33
Methyl plicatate	32.5
Benzyl plicatate	31
n-Hexyl plicatate	30.5
Dodecyl plicatate	30.5
Octadecyl plicatate	29.5
Control (pure lard)	9

Data were also shown for the stabilization of safflower oil in the complete patents.

MISCELLANEOUS FOOD STABILIZERS

Isoascorbic Acid Phosphates

The use of ascorbic and isoascorbic acids and their salts as antioxidants in the processing of food and beverages is widely known. Notwithstanding the antioxidative characteristics of these agents, experience has also shown that isoascorbic and ascorbic acids possess inherent properties that detract from their usefulness. For example, although in the dry form both ascorbic and isoascorbic acid and their salts are stable for long periods when stored under cool, dry conditions, discoloration may occur during prolonged storage and this decomposition is accelerated by the presence of moisture or elevated temperatures and exposure to air. Likewise, solutions of these acids will rapidly undergo oxidation if exposed to air, alkaline conditions or high temperatures, even for relatively short periods.

The instability of both isoascorbic and ascorbic acids is known to be due to the high sensitivity of the enolic hydroxyl groups of the lactone ring to oxidative influences. To prevent this oxidation, one or both of the enolic hydroxyl groups may be blocked, for example, by formulation of an ester or ether. Unfortunately the esterification or etherification of these hydroxyl groups often renders isoascorbic or ascorbic acid unsatisfactory or useless as an antioxidant for different reasons, namely, the resistance to in vitro or in vivo cleavage of the ether or ester group. Thus, it is desirable to protect the enolic hydroxyls on the lactone ring by means of a group which is stable to air or other oxidation influences, yet is slowly hydrolyzed under in vitro or in vivo conditions by enzymatic or other controlled mechanisms.

D.F. Hinkley; U.S. Patents 3,749,680; July 31, 1973; and 3,718,482; February 27, 1973; both assigned to Merck & Co., Inc. has found that the phosphate esters of isoascorbic acid meets these desired criteria of stability and availability. The compounds of the present process are, namely, isoascorbic acid-2-phosphate, isoascorbic acid-3-phosphate, isoascorbic acid-2,3-diphosphate, and isoascorbic acid-2,3-cyclic phosphate, and the mono, di or tri alkali and alkaline earth metal salts thereof.

These compounds of the present process function as antioxidants via the slow liberation of isoascorbic acid by medium hydrolysis or enzymatic cleavage. By this ability to slowly hydrolyze to isoascorbic acid, these compounds offer many advantages over the free ascorbic and isoascorbic acids when used as antioxidants in food and beverage processing, since for the most part, they are stable for longer periods towards oxidative influences that ordinarily lead to the premature decomposition of isoascorbic acid.

Example 1: Step 1, The Phosphorylation of 5,6-O-Isopropylidene Isoascorbic Acid to Form the Phosphate Esters — 195 grams (0.9030 mol) of 5,6-isopropylidene isoascorbic acid is dissolved in 6,700 ml of dry acetone at 40°C under nitrogen and the solution is subsequently cooled to –5°C. To this solution is then added, via a dropping funnel over a 45 minute period, a freshly prepared solution containing 97.5 ml (1.005 mols) of phosphorus oxychloride and 273 ml (3.46 mols) of pyridine which has been cooled to 10° to 15°C. The batch is then aged for another 45 minutes during which time the temperature is maintained at –5° to 2°C. To the aged batch is then added 341 grams (4.06 mols) of sodium bicarbonate followed by a careful addition of 560 ml of water. The resulting slurry is then aged for 1 hour, filtered, and the resulting salt cake washed twice with 600 milliliters of acetone.

The combined filtrates contain a mixture primarily of the 2- and 3-enol phosphate esters of of 5,6-O-isopropylidene isoascorbic acid and the 2,3-diphosphate and 2,3-cyclic phosphate esters of 5,6-O-isopropylidene isoascorbic acid in lesser amounts. The combined filtrates are then concentrated on a bath under vacuum by a heavy oily syrup containing a mixture of the 2- and 3-enol phosphate esters of 5,6-O-isopropylidene isoascorbic acid and the 2,3-diphosphate and 2,3-cyclic phosphate esters of isoascorbic acid.

Step 2, The Cleavage of 5,6-O-Isopropylidene Protecting Group — The mixture containing the phosphate esters of 5,6-isopropylidene ascorbic acid is dissolved rapidly in 1,200 ml of 0.1 N hydrochloric acid. The batch is then aged at room temperature for one-half hour after which it is diluted with 4,160 ml of methanol (precooled in an acetone wet ice bath) and the pH slowly adjusted to 5.5 with about 825 ml of 50% aqueous sodium hydroxide, while the temperature is maintained at about 10° to 15°C. The mixture is then aged for 1 hour, filtered, and the precipitate containing sodium chloride is washed with 700 ml of methanol. The filtrate and washings contain the crude phosphate esters of isoascorbic acid, traces of free isoascorbic acid and inorganic phosphate salts.

Step 3, The Isolation of Crude Isoascorbic Acid Phosphates — The pH of the filtrate obtained in the step above is slowly adjusted from 5.5 to 6.5 to 7.0 with 50% sodium hydroxide solution, and the pH is slowly raised to 10.0 using 50% sodium hydroxide. The resulting slurry is then aged for 12 to 20 hours at room temperature, after which it is filtered (filtrate contains traces of isoascorbic acid in the form of its sodium salt) and the solid obtained thereby washed twice with 500 ml of methanol followed by 500 ml of ether and sucked dry on the funnel under nitrogen, the precipitate obtained contains a mixture of crude 2- and 3-enol phosphate ester of isoascorbic acid trisodium salt, 2,3-diphosphate isoascorbic acid tetrasodium salt and 2,3-cyclic phosphate isoascorbic acid monosodium salt.

Step 4, The Separation of Phosphate Esters of Isoascorbic Acid — The mixture obtained in Step 3 is placed on a 1¼ inch by 20 inch silica gel column prepared in the manner described by B. Love and M. Goodman, *Chem. and Ind.*, (December 2, 1967), "Dry Column Chromatography", and eluted with a solvent comprising isopropanol:water:acetic acid:ammonium hydroxide (65:30:30:30).

The eluate is collected in 20 ml fractions whose composition is evaluated via their layer chromatography on silica gel using a similar solvent system. The fractions containing each isomer are combined and evaporated to small volume and diluted with 50% sodium hydroxide to pH 10. The solutions are then mixed with 5 volumes of methanol and allowed to stand overnight. The resulting precipitates of sodium salts are filtered and washed with a little aqueous methanol to give, after drying, the several isomeric phosphates, respectively.

Example 2: Stabilization of Beer — The beer is fermented in the usual manner. At the end of the fermentation period, there is added one-half pound of a mixture containing 10% sodium isoascorbate and 90% of trisodium isoascorbic acid-3-phosphate per 100 barrels of beer. Prior to final filtration, there is added three-quarters of a pound of a mixture containing 90% sodium isoascorbate and 10% trisodium isoascorbic acid-3-phosphate per 100 barrels of beer. The beer is bottled or canned immediately in the usual manner.

Examples are also included in the complete patent on the stabilization of oil, mushrooms, frozen clams, liver sausage and canned peaches with these phosphate esters.

Isoprenoid Substituted Quinones and Hydroquinones

Synthetic methods have been disclosed by *U. Gloor, R. Ruegg and U. Schwieter; U.S. Patents 3,517,070; June 23, 1970; 3,118,914; January 21, 1964; and 3,670,031; June 13, 1972; all assigned to Hoffmann-La Roche Inc.* for the preparation of isoprene-hydroquinone condensates. The process comprises reacting 2,3-dimethoxy-5-methyl-1,4-benzohydroquinone or its 4-monoacyl derivative in the presence of an acidic condensing agent with a compound represented by the formula:

(1)
$$CH_2=CH-\underset{\underset{C}{|}}{\overset{\overset{X}{|}}{C}}-\left[CH_2-CH_2-CH-\overset{\cdots}{C}-\right]_n CH_3$$
$$\qquad\qquad\qquad\qquad\qquad CH_3$$

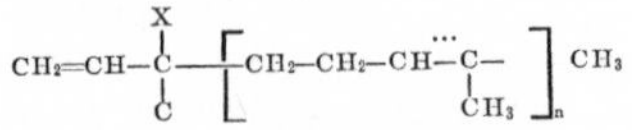

where the double bond shown by the dotted line can optionally be fully hydrogenated, n represents a number from 0 to 9 inclusive, and X is halogen, hydroxy, or acyloxy, or with an allyl-rearrangement product thereof. An optional further step comprises saponifying the condensation product obtained. Still a further optional step comprises oxidizing the condensation product (or the saponification product) to the correspondingly substituted 1,4-benzoquinone. Still a further optional step comprises cyclizing the condensation product, before or after saponification, to the correspondingly substituted chroman derivative. The products are represented by the following formulas:

(2)

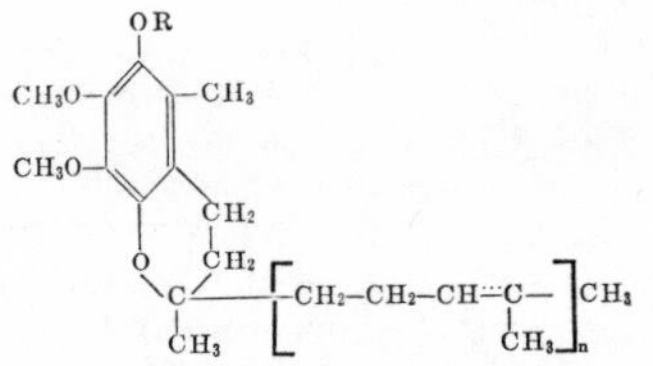

where R is hydrogen, lower alkanoyl or benzoyl, n represents a number from 0 to 9 inclusive, and the double bond shown by the dotted line can optionally be fully hydrogenated,

(3)

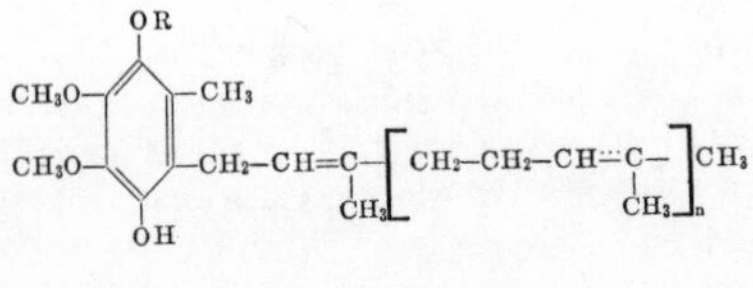

where R, n and double bond are the same as in Formula 2, or

(4)

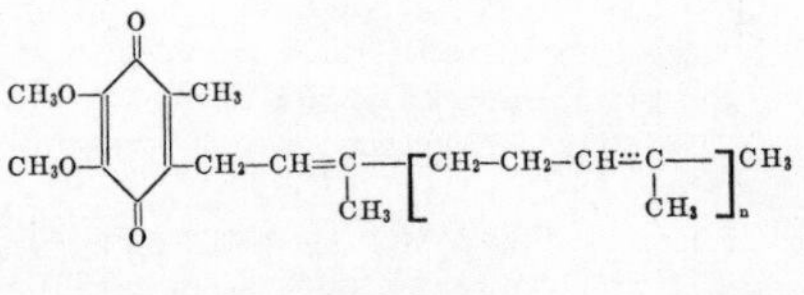

where n represents an integer from 1 to 5 inclusive and the double bond shown by the dotted line can optionally be fully hydrogenated.

The compounds of Formulas 2, 3 and 4 are fundamental components of biological oxidation systems. The benzoquinone and benzohydroquinone portions are essential as they cannot be synthesized by higher organisms but must be supplied from outside these organisms as vitamins. These substituted benzohydroquinones and substituted chromanols are useful as antioxidants for foodstuffs, feedstuffs, and vitamin preparations. The reaction of the 2,3-dimethoxy-5-methyl-1,4-benzohydroquinone or 4-monoacyl derivative with the compound of Formula 1 or allyl rearrangement product thereof is effected in the presence of an acidic condensing agent under either mild or energetic reaction conditions.

Upon employment of mild reaction conditions, the hydrogen atom in the nuclear 6-position of the 1,4-benzohydroquinone derivative is substituted by the aliphatic rest of the compound of Formula 1 used for the condensation. This reaction is preferably effected in the presence of an inert solvent, e.g., diethyl ether, diisopropyl ether or dioxane, at room temperature, or at the reflux temperature of diethyl ether. To avoid side reactions, heating the reaction above 40°C should be avoided. As the acidic condensing agent, zinc chloride with an addition of glacial acetic acid is especially suitable. In a preferred mode of execution, an alcohol of Formula 1 is employed, and zinc chloride is employed as the condensing agent in absolute ether with addition of a little glacial acetic acid, at a temperature below 40°C.

In the case where the starting material is the acyl derivative, the hydroxy group in the 4-position of the condensation product can be liberated by saponification. Saponification is suitably effected by means of alkaline solutions, e.g., by means of methanolic potassium hydroxide solution, advantageously in an inert gas atmosphere, e.g., under nitrogen.

The condensation products obtained are yellow to orange, 6-substituted-2,3-dimethoxy-5-methyl-1,4-benzohydroquinones, which can suitably be purified by chromatography. They can either be oxidized to the corresponding quinones or cyclized to the correspondingly substituted chroman derivatives.

To oxidize the substituted 1,4-benzohydroquinones obtained, known methods are employed, e.g., by shaking the substituted 1,4-benzohydroquinone in ethereal solution with silver oxide at room temperature. The crude products can be purified by known methods, suitably by chromatography. They are yellow compounds and exhibit typical maxima in the ultraviolet absorption spectrum.

If the 6-substituted-2,3-dimethoxy-5-methyl-1,4-benzohydroquinones are to be cyclized to the substituted chroman compounds, they are treated with an acidic cyclizing agent under energetic reaction conditions. It is appropriate to effect the reaction in an inert solvent, e.g., in petroleum ether, at a temperature above 40°C, e.g., at the reflux temperature of the reaction mixture. In the case where the substituent in the 6-position of the hydroquinone is unsaturated, the reaction conditions must be so selected that the unsaturated substituent is not attacked during the reaction. The use of boron trifluoride etherate in petroleum ether solution has been found to be especially suitable.

In the event that the substituent in the 6-position of the hydroquinone is (aside from the β,γ-double bond) saturated, other acidic agents can also be employed, e.g., zinc chloride in the presence of hydrochloric acid. By the cyclization reaction, a chroman ring is formed, wherein the oxygen-containing 6-membered ring is formed from the 1- and 6-carbon atoms of the hydroquinone, the oxygen atom attached to the 1-carbon atom and also the first three carbon atoms of the side chain introduced by the reagent of Formula 1. The products obtained are yellow compounds which can suitably be purified by chromatography or distillation.

These cyclized products can also be obtained directly, by applying the reaction conditions described in the preceding paragraph to 2,3-dimethoxy-5-methyl-1,4-benzohydroquinone or, respectively, a 4-monoacyl derivative thereof and a compound of Formula 1 or, respectively, an allyl rearrangement product thereof.

Example 1: Five grams of 2,3-dimethoxy-5-methyl-1,4-benzohydroquinone are shaken overnight in a nitrogen atmosphere with 2.7 grams of anhydrous zinc chloride, 12 grams of phytol, 150 ml of absolute ether and 0.3 ml of glacial acetic acid and then the mixture is refluxed for 1½ hours. The solvent is evaporated at room temperature under a water pump vacuum, the residue is dissolved in a mixture of 500 ml of petroleum ether (boiling range, 40° to 45°C) and 250 ml of 75% methanol and the petroleum ether solution is washed 3 times with 250 ml portions of 75% methanol.

The methanol solutions are extracted one after the other in a second separatory funnel with 250 ml of petroleum ether. By dilution of the methanol solutions with water and extraction with ether some starting material can be recovered. The petroleum ether solutions are combined, washed with water, dried with sodium sulfate and the solvent is evaporated. The crude product is dissolved in petroleum ether and chromatographed on a column of 300 grams of aluminum oxide (Brockmann activity I, deactivated with 4% of water). By elution with 3 liters of petroleum ether there is obtained 3 grams of a yellow oil and then by elution with 1 liter of ether there is obtained 9.5 grams of red 2,3-dimethoxy-5-methyl-6-phytyl-1,4-benzohydroquinone.

Example 2: 9.5 grams of 2,3-dimethoxy-5-methyl-6-phytyl-1,4-benzohydroquinone is dissolved in 200 ml of ether and shaken for 2 hours at room temperature with 20 grams of silver oxide. Then the solution is filtered and the solvent is evaporated. The crude product is chromatographed on a column of 250 grams of aluminum oxide (Brockmann activity I, deactivated with 7% of water) and then 2,3-dimethoxy-5-methyl-6-phytyl-1,4-benzoquinone is eluted with petroleum ether. There is thus obtained 2,3-dimethoxy-5-methyl-6-phytyl-1,4-benzoquinone as a yellow product.

Example 3: Three grams of 2,3-dimethoxy-5-methyl-1,4-benzohydroquinone in a mixture of 20 ml of absolute benzene and 10 ml of absolute ether is refluxed, while stirring, with 1 gram of zinc chloride, while passing through hydrogen chloride gas. A solution of 5 grams of isophytol in 10 ml of benzene is added dropwise over a period of 30 minutes, and the mixture is refluxed for an additional 3 hours.

Then the mixture is allowed to cool, diluted with 100 ml of petroleum ether (boiling range 40° to 50°C) and washed in turn with water, 80% methanol, and then again with water. It is dried with sodium sulfate and the solvent is evaporated. There is obtained 8.1 grams of a brown oil of 2-(4,8,12-trimethyltridecan-1-yl)-2,5-dimethyl-7,8-dimethoxy-6-chromanol. The crude product can be purified by adsorption on aluminum oxide (activity IV, Brockmann).

Solid Antioxidants for Milk Substitutes

The antioxidant preferably used in the food industry is 5-ethoxy-2,2,4-trimethyl-1,2-dihydroquinoline. Antioxidants of this type are normally added to the feed composition in liquid form in amounts below 0.5% by weight of the total composition. A homogeneous mixture between the liquid additive and the solid components of the feed composition in these cases can be attained only with difficulty where the liquid is used in very small amounts.

K.-H. Muller; U.S. Patent 3,644,215; February 22, 1972; assigned to Deutsche Gold-und Silber-Scheideanstalt vormals Roessler, Germany has found that the above antioxidants can be converted to a finely dispersed 70% powdery concentrate by addition of silica. This concentrate can be mixed with the other food composition additives in a completely homogeneous manner within a very short period of time if the liquid additive is incorporated into a finely divided synthetic silica, which has been preplaced into a mixer, by spraying or pouring into the mixer and using a continuous mixing operation.

The amount of the carrier preferably is between 10 and 50% by weight relative to the total weight of the antioxidant-silica mixture. The quality of the silicon dioxide used as the carrier is of substantial significance. It should be a powder where the primary particle size is below 500 mμ and preferably is between 3 and 40 mμ. The surface of the material should be between 50 and 500 square meters per gram and preferably should be between 50 and 300 square meters per gram and most preferably between 150 and 250 square meters per gram (measured by the BET method).

Particularly suitable is a precipitation-formed, spray dried, highly dispersed silica of super-fine particle size which has a BET surface between 50 and 300 square meters per gram and a mean particle size between 10 and 150μ. The significant features of this type of product are a high absorption property for liquids of all kinds, a good compatibility with almost all kinds of materials, physiological acceptability and good mixing properties with dry materials.

The silica may, however, also be finely divided, pyrogenically obtained silica having a mean particle size below 500 mμ and preferably between 3 and 40 mμ and a specific BET surface between 50 and 300 square meters per gram, preferably between 150 and 250 square meters per gram.

Example: Thirty kilograms of a precipitated and spray dried silica was placed in a paddle mixer (a so-called Loedige mixer). The 70 kilograms of the liquid antioxidant referred to above was then added by spraying and continued mixing. After completion of the addition, stirring was continued for 3 minutes.

There was thus obtained a powder containing 70% of antioxidant which had excellent flow properties and could be packed in bags. Instead of the paddle mixer, there also could have been used a so-called Nauta mixer, which consists of a cone-shaped receptacle provided with a rotating mixing screw as its interior wall. Also, a fluidizing bed mixer could be used.

Oil-Soluble Spice Extract

A process for extracting an antioxidant principle from spices has been developed by *D.L. Berner, G.A. Jacobson and C.D. Trombold; U.S. Patent 3,732,111; May 8, 1973; assigned to Campbell Soup Company.*

In accordance with this process, the antioxidant principle is obtained by extracting the spice with an edible animal or vegetable oil at a temperature sufficient to extract the oil-soluble volatile and nonvolatile components from the spice, separating the oil extract containing the oil-soluble volatile and nonvolatile spice components from the spent spice solids, deodorizing the oil extract by heating under vacuum while simultaneously sparging with steam, the quantity of heat, vacuum and steam being sufficient to drive off the volatile spice components and recovering the nonvolatile, oil-soluble, deodorized spice antioxidant principle.

The present process is adaptable for extracting the antioxidant principle from any spice, however, it is particularly useful in extracting the antioxidant principle from those spices noted for their antioxidant activity. Members of the Labiatae family such as sage, rosemary, basil, peppermint, spearmint, and blends of these spices may be used to provide the desired spice antioxidant principle. The antioxidant principle extracted from these spices has been found to exhibit greater antioxidant activity in comparison with an equivalent amount of the dry spice.

While whole spice may be used in the process, it is preferred that the spice or mixture of spices should be coarsely ground to aid extraction of the antioxidant principle. The oil selected for extraction of the antioxidant may be a liquid vegetable oil such as cottonseed oil or peanut oil or it may be a solid animal oil such as beef or mutton tallow. Hydrogenated or saturated oils may also be utilized. The preferred oils are cottonseed oil and peanut oil.

It has been found that the oil-soluble spice components are extracted most efficiently when the oil is heated to 80° to 180°C, preferably 120° to 125°C during the extraction step. In practice, it is preferred to heat the vegetable oil prior to the addition of the ground spice. The extraction takes place in from one-half to three hours, preferably two hours, with continuous agitation of the oil-spice mixture, however, the agitation should not cause aeration of the oil.

Following the oil extraction, the extract containing the volatile and nonvolatile spice components is separated from the spent spice solids. One convenient means involves centrifuging the mixture followed by isolation of the oil phase from the spent spice solids. Any fine spice particles found in the isolated oil which were not removed by the centrifugal separation may be easily removed from the oil by filtration.

While not a necessary feature of this process, if the oil extract has a color which would be undesirable in use, the oil extract can be decolorized by passing it through a bed of any well-known decolorizer or by forming a slurry of the oil and solid decolorizer and separating the oil from the decolorizer.

After separating the oil extract from the spent spice solids, the oil extract is deodorized to recover the desired spice antioxidant principle. The goal of the deodorization step is to remove the more volatile spice components from the less volatile spice components of the oil extract. Deodorization involves three interrelated parameters, temperature, vacuum and steam sparging. By the proper combination of these three factors, the more volatile spice components, including any unwanted flavor and aroma characteristics extracted by the oil, are removed from the oil extract producing a deodorized, bland oil extract.

The oil extract of the spice antioxidant principle can be added to food products in a wide range of amounts to provide antioxidant activity. For example, about ½% by weight of the spice antioxidant principle provides antioxidant activity in candy, while about 1½% and 5% by weight of the spice antioxidant principle based on the weight of the raw materials is required to provide antioxidant activity in sausage and chicken batter, respectively.

Example: Two hundred and twenty-five grams of cottonseed oil is heated in an open container to about 125°C. Forty-five grams of sage (20 to 60 mesh) is added to the oil and the mixture is continuously agitated without significant aeration of the oil for three hours while maintaining the mixture at 125°C.

The mixture is transferred to a centrifuge, and the oil extract phase is separated from the spent spice solids. The oil extract is filtered to remove fine spice particles, transferred to a closed deodorized vessel and heated to 175°C with steam sparging for one-half hour under 2 to 4 mm mercury. One hundred eighty grams of oil having a bland taste and little or no aroma is recovered.

Varying amounts of the spice antioxidant principle are added to pork fat and evaluated for antioxidant activity. Comparisons are made with a control sample containing no antioxidant principle and with pork fat containing synthetic antioxidants. The results are set forth in the table on the following page.

Active Oxygen Method (AOM) Evaluation of Antioxidants

Percent antioxidant principle in pork fat	AOM time,[1] min.	Antioxidant index [2]
Control (no antioxidant)	20	1.0
1.25% extract	480	24.0
2.50% extract	1,050	32.5
3.75% extract	1,290	64.5
5.00% extract	1,110	55.5
7.50% extract	1,620	81.0
0.05% mixture [3]	1,725	86.3
0.02% BHA (butylated hydroxyanisole)	570	28.4
0.02% PG (propyl gallate)	940	47.0

[1] Time to reach a peroxide value (PV) of 20 at 110° C. and 2.33 cc. air per sec.

[2] Antioxidant index = $\dfrac{\text{Sample time required to reach PV 20}}{\text{Control time required to reach PV 20}}$

[3] The mixture consisted of 20% BHA, 6% propyl gallate, 4% citric acid, and 70% propylene glycol.

Green Coffee Bean Extract

G. Lehmann, O. Neunhoeffer, W. Roselius and O. Vitzhum; U.S. Patent 3,663,581; May 16, 1972; assigned to Hag AG, Germany have found that substances that are susceptible to autoxidation can be protected against impairment resulting from such oxidation by the addition of an antioxidative extract of green coffee beans.

This extract is advantageously obtained by:

(a) dissolving in hot water the caffeine extract obtained in a known manner from green coffee beans,

(b) cooling the hot aqueous phase whereby coffee wax is separated on the surface and the caffeine is deposited as a sediment,

(c) removing the caffeine, making the aqueous solution containing the coffee wax strongly alkaline and separating the aqueous alkaline phase,

(d) extracting the separated aqueous alkaline phase with an aliphatic halohydro-carbon and separating the aqueous alkaline phase from the organic phase,

(e) acidifying this aqueous alkaline phase with a mineral acid,

(f) extracting the acid aqueous solution with a water-immiscible solvent, drying the solvent phase and drawing off the solvent.

The residue remaining after the solvent is drawn off is a brown substance of oily consistency having an exceedingly pronounced antioxidative action.

In the past it was commonly believed that the antioxidative properties (substances) of coffee developed only upon roasting (see *Journal Sci. Ind. Res. India*, 17c, page 147, 1958, right column, item 5 of the abstract). It was, therefore, very surprising to find that it is possible to obtain from green coffee beans a highly antioxidative active principle.

The green coffee beans used as starting material (which may or may not be comminuted) are extracted in a known manner, for example, in accordance with German Patents 198,279 and 538,439 and British Patent 625,365, with a caffeine extraction solvent (aliphatic halo-hydrocarbons such as $CHCl_3$, CH_2Cl_2, CCl_4, dichloroethylene, trichloroethylene, benzene, ethyl acetate, under certain conditions, also ether, etc. The extract is treated for the removal of the solvent and then dissolved in hot water. Beneficial effects are obtained, if the extract at first is not completely thickened by evaporation and if the residual caffeine extraction solvent is removed by a jet of steam. The steam that condenses at the surface of the extract serves at the same time to make up the caffeine extraction residue. At this point, the hot aqueous phase is allowed to cool to about room temperature whereby coffee wax is separated on the surface and the caffeine is deposited as a sediment.

A preferred way of carrying out the process is as follows. After dissolving the caffeine extraction residue obtained from the green coffee beans with hot water, and after cooling the hot aqueous phase, the resulting three-phase mixture (precipitated caffeine, aqueous phase, coffee wax) is separated. The aqueous phase is made strongly alkaline, so as to arrive at a preferred pH value in the range from 12 to 14, the optimum value being 13. The coffee wax layer is also made alkaline with strong aqueous lye, preferably NaOH or KOH, having a pH value in the range from 12 to 14, preferably 13, is extracted, and the two aqueous alkaline phases are treated separately in the manner described for the joint treatment thereof (extraction with aliphatic halohydrocarbons, etc.) whereupon the two end products, after the removal of the solvent, are united.

Example 1: Fifty liters of the aqueous phase obtained as a result of the caffeine extraction as described above, and after removal of the caffeine precipitated in the course of cooling, is made alkaline with 1 liter of 5 N NaOH. Residual caffeine is removed by consecutive agitations carried out with 25 liters, 20 liters, 15 liters, 15 liters, 10 liters, 10 liters of chloroform. The aqueous alkaline phase is acidified with 3.5 liters 5 N HCl and the acid solution is agitated by shaking with 35 liters, 25 liters, 15 liters, 15 liters of ether. The combined ether extracts are dried over sodium sulfate and the ether is distilled off. This leaves behind 140 grams of a brown oil having high antioxidative activity.

Example 2: To a roasted coffee extract containing 18% by weight of solid matter, there is added 0.1% by weight, based upon the total coffee extract, of the oil obtained in accordance with Example 1. The extract is then concentrated in a vacuum to a solids content of 30%, whereby the volatile aromatic substances are recovered separately by condensation into a cooling device. These are combined with the same amount by weight of the antioxidant that was used for the coffee extract and this mixture is applied as a spray onto the dry powder of the roasted coffee extract. There is obtained a highly aromatic stable product.

Example 3: Linseed oil to be used for dietary purposes is mixed with 0.1% by weight of the oil obtained as by Example 1. The resulting product is stable even in containers that were opened.

PRODUCT STABILIZATION INDEX

This index is designed to help the user find antioxidants for a specific substrate. The following patents are indexed according to the materials stabilized by the antioxidant disclosed by examples in the patents. This list does not include all patents covered in the book. For example, in the section on the stabilization of polyolefins, patent numbers are included in this index only if there are also examples in the original patent describing the stabilization of materials other than polyolefins. This also holds true for the sections on petroleum products, synthetic lubricants, elastomers, other polymers and foods.

The index is organized by patent number. The substrates to be stabilized are coded by the numbering system below. The asterisk following a coded number in the index indicates that the example describing this substrate is included in the book. The original document must be consulted for examples of other substrates.

Polyolefins

Polyethylene - **1**
Polypropylene - **2**
Polyisobutylene - **3**
Other Olefin Polymers
   and Copolymers - **4**

Addition Polymers

Polystyrene - **11**
High Impact Polystyrene - **12**
ABS Polymer - **13**
Polyvinyl Chloride - **14**
Vinyl Acetate Polymers - **15**
Acrylate Polymers - **16**
Fluorocarbon Polymers - **17**
Acrylonitrile Polymers - **18**

Condensation Polymers

Nylon 6 - **20**
Nylon 66 - **21**
Polyesters - **22**
Polyurethanes - **23**
Polycarbonates - **24**
Polyethers - **25**

Elastomers

Natural Rubber - **30**
SBR - **31**
NBR - **32**
EPT - **33**
Butyl Rubber - **34**
Polyisoprene - **35**
Polybutadiene - **36**
Neoprene - **37**

Petroleum (Synthetic) Products

Gasoline - **70**
Diesel Fuel - **71**
Antiknock Fluid - **72**
Petroleum Oil, Lubes and
   Greases - **73**
Synthetic Polyester Lubricants - **74**
Functional Fluids - **75**
Phosphates - **77**
Silicones - **78**
Fuel Oil - **79**

Foods and Vitamins

Lard - **80**

Foods and Vitamins (continued)

    Oils - **81**

    Vitamins - **82**

Chemicals

    Cyclohexene - **90**

    Toluene - **91**

    Aldehydes - **92**

    Other Unsaturates - **93**

CROSS REFERENCE LIST

U.S. Patents   **Code Number**

3,285,855 - 1,2*, 11, 12, 14, 20, 23, 70, 73, 74, 80, 90, 92

3,442,806 - 1, 2, 11, 14, 15, 16, 17, 22, 30, 31, 32, 78

3,445,391 - 73

3,446,808 - 1, 2, 11

3,452,056 - 30*

3,465,029 - 30, 31, 32, 70, 73, 74, 75

3,476,699 - 14

3,476,814 - 30, 31, 32, 33, 34, 70, 71, 72, 73, 74, 80, 81

3,480,698 - 1, 2*, 11, 13, 73, 79

3,481,978 - 2, 31, 73

3,483,260 - 1, 2, 13, 70, 71, 73, 74, 80, 81

3,488,368 - 1, 2*, 13, 14, 20, 23, 70, 73, 74, 80, 92

3,491,137 - 30, 31, 32, 33, 70, 71, 72, 73, 74

3,505,225 - 1*, 2, 13, 25, 33

3,522,315 - 1, 2*, 13, 30, 31, 32, 70, 71, 72, 73, 74, 80, 81

3,530,069 - 1, 2, 11, 14, 15, 16, 17, 22, 30, 31, 32, 78

3,531,483 - 1, 2*, 4, 13, 14, 18, 23, 25, 30, 31, 33, 35

3,533,992 - 30*

3,536,706 - 74*

3,542,679 - 74

3,567,682 - 1, 2*, 13, 30, 31, 32, 70, 71, 72, 73, 74, 80, 81

3,567,724 - 1, 2*, 11, 13, 14, 20, 22, 25, 30, 33, 36, 31, 73, 74, 90

3,579,561 - 1, 2, 3, 70, 73, 74, 80, 81

3,584,047 - 2*, 12, 21, 25, 70, 73, 80

3,590,083 - 1, 2*, 12, 21, 30, 73

3,598,855 - 2*, 31, 70, 74, 79

3,600,411 - 22, 23, 24

3,629,190 - 2, 31, 70

3,632,631 - 2*

3,637,585 - 30, 31, 32, 70, 73, 74, 75

3,637,586 - 30, 31, 32, 33, 34, 70, 71, 72, 73, 74, 80, 81

3,637,587 - 1, 2*, 11, 13, 73, 79

3,639,336 - 1, 2*, 11, 13, 14, 20, 22, 25, 30, 31, 33, 36, 73, 74, 90

3,641,218 - 2*, 14*, 31*

3,642,629 - 74*

3,642,691 - 1, 2, 13, 70, 71, 73, 74, 80, 81

3,644,217 - 2*, 11, 13, 20, 22, 25

3,644,278 - 2*, 13, 73, 80, 90

3,644,281 - 1, 2, 3, 70, 73, 74, 80, 81

3,644,540 - 92, 93*

3,647,749 - 30, 31, 32, 33, 70, 71, 72, 73, 74

3,649,690 - 2*, 25, 33, 74

3,651,093 - 73*

3,652,561 - 1, 2*, 12, 13, 70, 73, 74, 80, 81

3,655,559 - 2, 31

3,655,560 - 74

3,655,832 - 14

3,658,702 - 73

3,660,289 - 74

U.S. Patents   Code Number

3,660,352 - 2*, 13
3,660,438 - 2*, 12, 21, 25, 30
3,665,031 - 18, 20*, 21, 23
3,666,716 - 1*, 2, 13, 25, 33
3,666,837 - 2*, 14, 30, 33
3,668,237 - 74
3,673,186 - 2*, 79
3,676,449 - 2*, 81
3,676,494 - 1, 2*
3,676,530 - 1, 2*
3,676,531 - 2*, 12, 21, 25, 70, 73, 74
3,677,945 - 73
3,677,965 - 2*, 12, 21, 25, 70, 73, 80
3,678,047 - 1, 2*, 11, 13, 14, 16, 20, 23, 25, 30, 33, 35, 37, 75
3,679,744 - 2*, 12, 30
3,681,435 - 92
3,682,980 - 73
3,683,033 - 2*
3,683,054 - 30, 31, 32, 70, 73, 74, 75
3,686,312 - 35*
3,686,313 - 33*
3,686,367 - 2*
3,687,892 - 1, 2*, 12, 21, 30, 73
3,689,513 - 30*
3,692,679 - 1, 2, 11, 14, 15, 16, 17, 22, 30, 31, 32, 78
3,692,680 - 2*, 31, 70, 74, 79
3,692,691 - 73, 31
3,692,879 - 2*, 14, 30, 33
3,694,357 - 73, 74
3,694,374 - 11, 14
3,694,375 - 2*, 12, 30
3,694,440 - 2*, 12, 21
3,696,851 - 74
3,699,152 - 2, 15, 30, 31
3,700,666 - 1, 2*
3,704,326 - 2*
3,706,740 - 1, 2*, 12, 13, 20, 21, 25, 31, 73, 74, 90
3,706,798 - 2*
3,706,802 - 31*
3,707,488 - 22, 23, 24
3,709,884 - 1, 2*, 12, 21, 25, 31, 73, 74, 90
3,714,300 - 2*, 12, 21, 22, 23, 25, 35, 70, 73, 74
3,716,603 - 1, 2*, 30, 31, 32, 33, 70, 71, 72, 73, 74, 80, 81
3,721,704 - 2*, 12, 13, 73, 90
3,723,316 - 80, 91
3,723,427 - 2*
3,723,428 - 2*
3,729,471 - 1, 2*
3,734,884 - 2*
3,734,926 - 1, 2*, 21, 31
3,741,909 - 13, 74
3,742,096 - 2*, 21, 73
3,745,148 - 1, 2, 70, 71, 73, 74, 78, 80, 81
3,746,654 - 36*
3,746,721 - 1, 2*, 21, 31
3,751,472 - 1, 2, 13, 25, 33*, 74
3,754,031 - 2*, 12, 30
3,755,171 - 73

U.S. Patents   Code Number

3,755,250 - 30, 31, 32, 70, 73, 74, 75
3,755,549 - 1, 2*, 12, 31, 73, 74, 90
3,763,093 - 1, 2*, 11, 13, 14, 16, 20, 23, 25, 30, 33, 35, 37, 75
3,763,094 - 2*, 12, 21, 25
3,763,287 - 2*, 70, 73
3,764,534 - 74
3,769,372 - 1, 2*, 12, 21, 25, 31, 73, 74, 90
3,773,722 - 2*, 12, 21, 25, 30, 90
3,773,830 - 2*
3,775,411 - 2*
3,778,464 - 2*, 13, 73, 80, 90
3,779,945 - 2*, 33
3,780,103 - 2*, 90
3,781,361 - 2*, 25, 33, 74
3,787,416 - 2*, 79
3,790,597 - 1, 2*, 12, 13, 21, 31, 73, 90
3,795,700 - 13*
3,796,685 - 2*, 35
3,809,719 - 74
3,810,929 - 2*

COMPANY INDEX

The company names listed below are given exactly as they appear in the patents, despite name changes, mergers and acquisitions which have, at times, resulted in the revision of a company name.

INVENTOR INDEX

U.S. PATENT NUMBER INDEX

NOTICE

Nothing contained in this Review shall be construed to constitute a permission or recommendation to practice any invention covered by any patent without a license from the patent owners. Further, neither the author nor the publisher assumes any liability with respect to the use of, or for damages resulting from the use of, any information, apparatus, method or process described in this Review.

FOOD ADDITIVES
TO EXTEND SHELF LIFE 1974

by Nicholas D. Pintauro

Food Technology Review No. 17

Aside from freezing, canning and sophisticated methods of packaging, food is preserved by dehydration, salting, sugaring, smoking, curing, and certain types of fermentation.

A newer effective approach toward prevention of spoilage is by the use of chemical additives other than sugar, salt, vinegar, and spices.

Food additives, as defined by the National Academy of Sciences are those relatively nontoxic chemicals that may be incorporated into foodstuffs during the growing, processing, or storing periods. Every chemical added must serve one or more of these general purposes: Improve or maintain nutritional value, enhance quality, increase consumer acceptability, and facilitate preparation. In modern applications food additives are combined with established, classical methods of food preservation to maximize stability for extended shelf life. There is a great demand for additives to prevent or retard food deterioration. These additives include antioxidants, antibacterial agents, mold inhibitors, color stabilizers, anticaking agents, antibrowning agents, cloud stabilizers, metal scavengers, enzyme inhibitors.

This book describes over 140 processes involving the newest technology available in the U.S. patent literature using food additives. A partial and condensed table of contents follows here. Chapter headings are given, followed by examples of important subtitles.

ISBN 0-8155-0548-0

402 pages

FUEL ADDITIVES 1974

by M. William Ranney

Chemical Technology Review No. 26

The search for improved fuel additives has taken on new and significant dimensions with the pending world-wide fuel shortage. The mid-seventies are expected to be a time of increasingly short fuel supplies which could drastically curtail our production capability, our personal travel patterns, and in the long run, our gross national product and our very way of life, while at the same time reversing the ecological progress made to date.

Successful research for more effective additives, which really increase mileage or BTU output of the fuels in question, will provide many new business opportunities in the next few years. Fuel additives manufacture and sales can be expected to show well above normal growth over the next decade.

This book describes almost 200 processes, including many fuel additive formulations which appeared in the U.S. patent literature during just the past three years. A partial and condensed table of contents follows. Numbers in ( ) indicate the number of processes per topic. Chapter headings are given, followed by examples of important subtitles.

ISBN 0-8155-0525-6

FIRE RESISTANT

AND

FLAME RETARDANT POLYMERS 1974

by Maurice William Ranney

Chemical Technology Review No. 35

The U.S. market for these materials is a hundred million dollar annual business and is expected to double within the next three years. This includes reactive intermediates and non-reactive additives which impart fire retardance to plastics, foams, textile fibers and paints.

Such flame retardant additives and reactive intermediates are now available for most polymer systems. While many proven formulations rely on additives containing halogen, such as chlorinated wax and tris-(dibromopropyl) phosphate, commonly in combination with antimony oxide, much recent technology has been directed toward building flame retardance into the polymer nucleus, using reactive intermediates.

Self-extinguishing polyesters, employing halogenated dicarboxylic acids or anhydrides, and polyurethanes based on phosphorus-containing polyols are now finding increased use by the industry.

This book provides an in-depth look at over 250 processes. Directions are adequate enough to make manufacturing decisions by an industry which is faced with great responsibilities and opportunities as increasing public and governmental attention is focused on the need for improved flame retardant products.

A partial and condensed table of contents follows. Numbers in ( ) indicate the number of processes per topic.

ISBN 0-8155-0541-8

395 pages.